Monica

Kinesiology for Manual Therapies

Nancy W. Dail, BA, LMT, NCTMB
Downeast School of Massage
Waldoboro, Maine

Timothy A. Agnew, BA, LMT, ACSM, NCTMB
Timothy Agnew Therapy
Sarasota, Florida

R. T. Floyd, EdD, ATC, CSCS
University of West Alabama
Livingston, Alabama

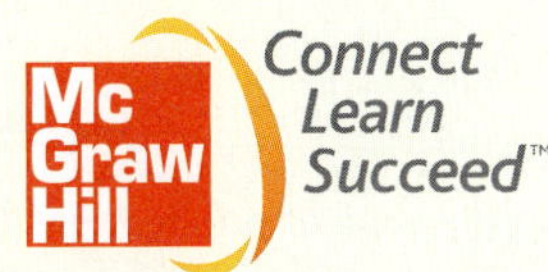

The McGraw-Hill Companies

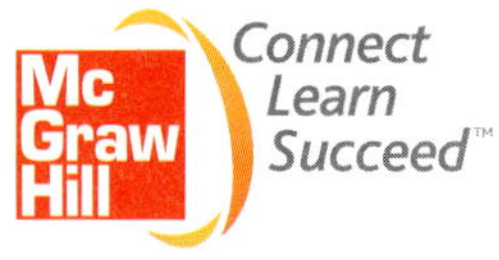

KINESIOLOGY FOR MANUAL THERAPIES
Published by McGraw-Hill, a business unit of The McGraw-Hill Companies, Inc., 1221 Avenue of the Americas, New York, NY, 10020.

This book is printed on acid-free paper.

2 3 4 5 6 7 8 9 0 DOW/DOW 1 0 9 8 7 6 5

ISBN 978-0-07-340207-9
MHID 0-07-340207-9

Vice president/Editor in chief: *Elizabeth Haefele*
Vice president/Director of marketing: *John E. Biernat*
Publisher: *Kenneth S. Kasee Jr.*
Senior sponsoring editor: *Debbie Fitzgerald*
Director of development, Allied Health: *Patricia Hesse*
Developmental editor: *Connie Kuhl*
Marketing manager: *Mary Haran*
Lead media producer: *Damian Moshak*
Media producer: *Marc Mattson*
Director, Editing/Design/Production: *Jess Ann Kosic*
Project manager: *Marlena Pechan*
Senior production supervisor: *Janean A. Utley*
Senior designer: *Srdjan Savanovic*
Lead photo research coordinator: *Carrie K. Burger*
Media project manager: *Cathy L. Tepper*
Outside development house: *Andrea Edwards*
Cover design: *Kay D. Lieberherr*
Interior design: *Kay D. Lieberherr*
Typeface: *10/12 New Aster*
Compositor: *MPS Limited, A Macmillan Company*
Printer: *R. R. Donnelley*
Cover credit: Illustration: © 3D4Medical.com, Getty. Photos: © The McGraw-Hill Companies, Inc./Leigh Kelly Monroe, photographer
Credits: The credits section for this book begins on page 516 and is considered an extension of the copyright page.

Library of Congress Cataloging-in-Publication Data

Dail, Nancy W.
Kinesiology for manual therapies / Nancy W. Dail, Timothy A. Agnew, R.T. Floyd.
p. ; cm.
Includes bibliographical references and index.
ISBN-13: 978-0-07-340207-9 (alk. paper)
ISBN-10: 0-07-340207-9 (alk. paper)
1. Kinesiology. 2. Manipulation (Therapeutics) I. Agnew, Timothy A. II. Floyd, R. T. III. Title.
[DNLM: 1. Kinesiology, Applied—methods. 2. Musculoskeletal Manipulations—methods. 3. Movement—physiology. 4. Muscles—physiology. WB 890 D133k 2011]
QP303.D35 2011
612.7'6—dc22

2009036330

www.mhhe.com

Dedication

To my mother, Mildred Waltz Newcomb, 1907–1974, who pioneered the path of women aviators and believed in the independence of women. Her philosophy, "You can do what you want to do in life; you just have to choose a path and do it," underlined all that she did. Fear and doubt were not in her vocabulary. She helped me find the tools to accomplish my goals in life and to believe in myself; it is the ultimate gift.

Nancy Dail

To my mother, Nancy Wren Cheatham, who taught me to swim in the ocean of words.

Timothy Agnew

To my students and professional colleagues, who taught me to think on a different level.

R. T. Floyd

About the Authors

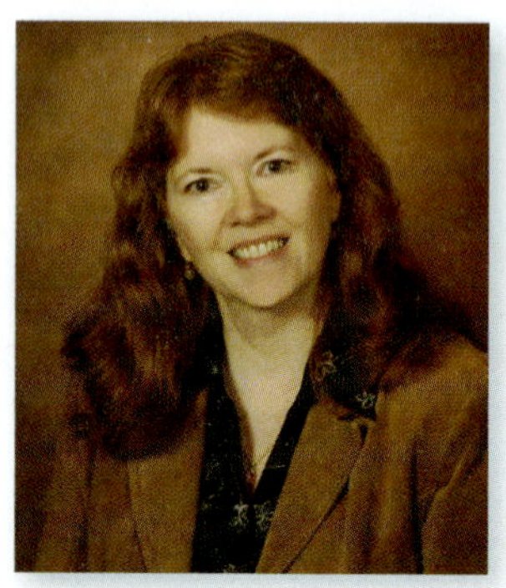

Nancy Dail, BA, LMT, NCTMB, is a co-author, with Timothy Agnew and R. T. Floyd, of McGraw-Hill's *Kinesiology for Manual Therapies.* She began her professional massage therapy career in 1974 in New Mexico, combining her education in acupuncture, aikido, and Western massage. After returning to Maine, Nancy built her massage therapy practice, became an EMT, served with the local ambulance service, and worked with two chiropractors in the midcoast region. In 1980, she founded and developed the comprehensive COMTA accredited program at the Downeast School of Massage in Waldoboro. A leader in her field, she helped create the AMTA National Sports Massage Team, the Commission on Massage Therapy Accreditation, and the AMTA Council of Schools. She has served on the AMTA National Board, has participated on numerous committees, and was the charter president of the Maine AMTA chapter. As a sports massage therapist, she volunteered her services at the 1996 Atlantic Olympic Games in the Olympic Village Sports Medicine Clinic, numerous Boston marathons, and local Maine events. An international representative for massage, Nancy has presented workshops at the University of Belgorod in Belgorod, Russia, in the fall of 1997; at the Complementary Medicine Symposia for Harvard Medical in Boston, annually for nine years; at many New England AMTA conferences; for Colby College; and at many more educational venues. She has been a consultant for several Maine hospitals on integrating massage clinically and has assisted the credentialing of massage therapists in many institutions. At home in Waldoboro, she reviews and has written books and articles for the industry, including her college thesis "Tension Headaches," and she edits the Downeast School of Massage *In Touch* newsletter. In July 2008 she directed and produced, with her daughter Emily Waltz, *A Gift of Touch,* a DVD on foundational massage, and the accompanying *Manual for A Gift of Touch.* The DVD is used as a teaching tool at the Downeast School of Massage and is internationally sold through the DSM Bookstore. Her BA degree in health, arts, and science from Goddard College helps her balance her DSM administrative duties as director with her teaching of dimensional massage, advanced skills, kinesiology, and other related subjects. Nancy is licensed in massage therapy in the state of Maine and has been nationally certified in therapeutic massage and bodywork since 1993. She is certified in orthopedic massage and has taken countless workshops in continuing education at Downeast and internationally over the years. Her education, background, and experience are the foundation of her contributions and her success as a therapist, writer, and teacher in the field of massage therapy. Nancy can be reached through the Downeast School of Massage in Waldoboro and through the school's Web site at www.downeastschoolofmassage.net.

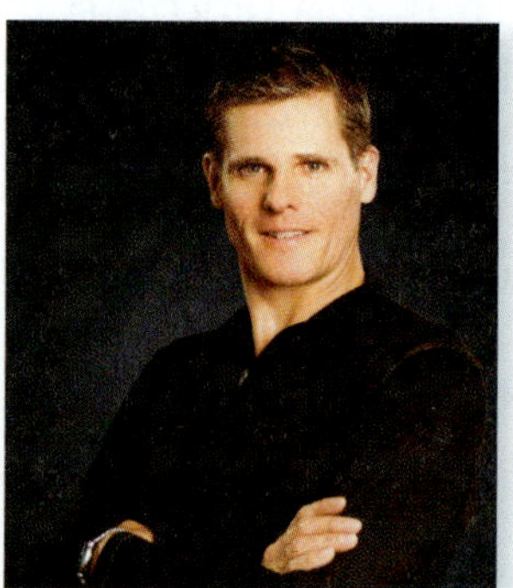

Timothy Agnew, BA, NCTMB began his study of human anatomy in 1982 at the Ringling College of Art and Design in Sarasota, Florida. In drawing the human figure, he realized he could apply his new knowledge to help his occasional competitive running injuries. After working in the art field in various capacities, he returned to school and earned a degree in English literature while working as a certified personal trainer. Seeing a need for a more hands-on approach to wellness, Timothy shifted his studies to physical therapy, and applied to different programs in the hope of once again returning to school. When a client introduced him to renowned kinesiologist Aaron L. Mattes, he became fascinated with kinesiology and its more specific focus on human movement. After serving an internship with him, Aaron convinced Timothy to pursue kinesiology as a course of study. He completed the ATC (Athletic Trainer Certified) course requirements under the guidance of Dr. Carl Cramer at

Barry University in Miami, and finished the program at the University of South Florida. Upon completing his college track, he became a nationally certified massage therapist. He continued his studies in orthopedic rehabilitation, including symposiums with the Cleveland Clinic of Sports Health, focusing on upper- and lower-extremity dysfunctions. Having begun training in the Japanese martial art aikido in 1991, he applied the philosophy of aikido to his kinesiology knowledge and opened a private practice concentrating in rehabilitation. At his clinic in Sarasota, he specializes in improving the quality of life for his patients, which include Olympic athletes, renowned artists and dancers, as well as stroke, MS, and Parkinson's patients. Timothy has been an educator in the health field for over 15 years, presenting his modality *Clinical Flexibility and Therapeutic Exercise (CFTE)* seminars to international and regional conferences, students, and the general public. He is a member of the American College of Sports Medicine (ACSM) and served as a continuing education provider for the American Council on Exercise (ACE) and currently the National Certification Board for Therapeutic Massage and Bodywork (NCBTMB). In 1998, Timothy formed Intent Multimedia, an educational media company that produced the DVDs *CFTE: Assisted Clinical Flexibility* and *Dynamic Flexibility: A Safe and Effective Self-Stretching Program,* as well as *The Dynamic Flexibility Manual: A Safe and Effective Self-Stretching Program.* Timothy continues to play an active role in the production of his media, including human anatomy animations used in his videos. He also wrote, directed, and edited his most recent DVD, designed for the general public. His current project is a brand-new edition of *The Dynamic Flexibility Manual* that is to be used with the *Dynamic Flexibility* DVD. An avid reader and writer, Timothy's short stories have appeared in *The Roanoke Review, Skylark (Purdue University Calumet),* and the anthology *A Cup of Comfort,* and he has won regional awards for his fiction. He continues to teach and train in aikido, a true study of human movement. He lives with his family in Sarasota and can be reached at www.stretchme.com.

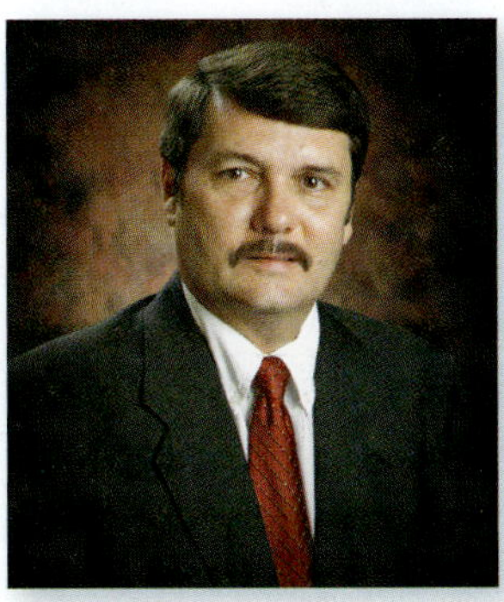

R. T. Floyd, EdD, ATC, CSCS, is in his 35th year of providing athletic training services for the University of West Alabama (UWA). Currently, he serves as the director of athletic training and sports medicine for the UWA Athletic Training and Sports Medicine Center, the program director for UWA's CAATE accredited curriculum, and a professor in the Department of Physical Education and Athletic Training, which he chairs. He has taught numerous courses in physical education and athletic training, including kinesiology at both the undergraduate and graduate levels since 1980.

Floyd has maintained an active career throughout his working life. He was recently reelected to serve on the National Athletic Trainers' Association (NATA) Board of Directors as the representative for District IX, the Southeast Athletic Trainers' Association (SEATA). He served two years as the NATA District IX chair on the NATA Research and Education Foundation Board before being elected to his current position as the Member Development chair on the board. Previously, he served as the District IX representative to the NATA Educational Multimedia Committee from 1988 to 2002. He has served as the Convention Site Selection chair for District IX from 1986 to 2004 and has directed the annual SEATA Competencies in Athletic Training student workshop since 1997. He has also served as a NATA BOC examiner for well over a decade and has served as a Joint Review Committee on Educational Programs in Athletic Training site visitor several times. He has given over 100 professional presentations at the local, state, regional, and national levels and has also had several articles and videos published related to the practical aspects of athletic training. He began authoring *Manual of Structural Kinesiology* in 1992, which is now in its 17th edition.

Floyd is a certified member of the National Athletic Trainers' Association, a certified strength and conditioning specialist, and a certified personal trainer in the National Strength and Conditioning Association. He is also a certified athletic equipment manager in the Athletic Equipment Managers' Association and a member of the American College of Sports Medicine, the American Orthopaedic Society for Sports Medicine, the American Osteopathic Academy of Sports Medicine, the American Sports Medicine Fellowship Society, and the American Alliance for Health, Physical Education, Recreation and Dance. Additionally, he is licensed in Alabama as an athletic trainer and an emergency medical technician. Floyd was presented the NATA Athletic Trainer Service Award in 1996, the NATA Most Distinguished Athletic Trainer Award in 2003, and the NATA Sayers "Bud" Miller Distinguished Educator Award in 2007. He received the SEATA District IX Award for Outstanding Contribution to the Field of Athletic Training in 1990 and the Award of Merit in 2001 before being inducted into the organization's Hall of Fame in 2008. He was named to *Who's Who Among America's Teachers* in 1996, 2000, 2004, and 2005. In 2001, he was inducted into the Honor Society of Phi Kappa Phi and the University of West Alabama Athletic Hall of Fame. He was inducted into the Alabama Athletic Trainers Association Hall of Fame in May 2004.

Brief Contents

Contents

Foreword

Musculoskeletal disorders are one of the most pervasive health care challenges we currently face. The frequency of these disorders highlights the need for a greater focus on them as a primary health care challenge. Health and impairment of the musculoskeletal system is addressed by numerous professions and is truly an interdisciplinary exploration. Learning the essentials of anatomy and kinesiology can be a daunting task for any student of the health sciences. Unfortunately, in many educational environments this study often degrades into a process of content memorization in which the greater purpose of applying clinical knowledge is lost.

Using R. T. Floyd's *Structural Kinesiology* as a foundation, Dail and Agnew have taken a fresh approach and made a concerted effort to bring this interesting study to life. Human movement is fascinating, and they do its study justice in this text. They have presented complex and valuable information about human movement with an ease of readability and a visual approach that is truly engaging.

From the first glance, what catches your eye is the abundant use of high-quality color illustrations, photographs, and diagrams. In kinesiology the study of movement is the primary focus. Movement is difficult to convey in a book, but these visual aids go a long way to achieving that goal and make the book a valuable resource for the student and professional clinician.

The complexities of human movement are quite intricate, so it is challenging to determine how much detail to include. This text strikes a great balance, as there is a rich depth to the content but it is not overwhelming. The technical content is equally balanced by the clinical applications of massage, stretching, and soft-tissue manipulation that help the reader see exactly how these concepts are put into action.

This book is unique among other kinesiology texts because of its inclusion of massage therapy techniques for muscles that have been presented in each regional body section. Presentation of treatment methods for these tissues makes the book a valuable classroom and clinical reference for both student and practitioner alike. Throughout the section on treatment approaches, real-life clinical pearls are shared, which reinforce the concepts of structure and function and make those concepts directly applicable to clinical practice. A wide variety of study questions are included at the end of each chapter and can be used by instructors or professionals in practice who want to solidify their understanding of the material.

Tackling a topic as expansive as human movement is a challenge for any author. Knowing authors Dail and Agnew, and being familiar with their work for many years, I recognize that they have put forth a tremendous effort in producing a great contribution to our professional literature. Dail, Agnew, and Floyd provided an educational mechanism to open new horizons in studying kinesiology with *Kinesiology for Manual Therapies*. It is destined to remain a classic of study for a wide spectrum of professionals who work with the musculoskeletal system.

Whitney Lowe
Fritz Creek, AK

Foreword

Kinesiology for Manual Therapies by Dail, Agnew, and Floyd is a well-illustrated, user-friendly text that will be especially helpful to soft-tissue investigation and treatment of muscles that affect movement, elicit pain, and establish sound posture and precise locomotion. Doctors, nurses, athletic trainers, teachers, and physical and massage therapists will benefit from this uniquc approach to understanding and improving movement. With the inclusion of my lifework in Active Isolated Stretching (AIS), and the book's focus on the importance of a safe method of the clinical stretching of patients, this book breaks new ground in the field of manual therapies. When Timothy Agnew began his training with me many years ago, and then continued his college studies, I knew he was an exceptional student. While I taught him the principles of AIS, Timothy chose to continue his studies in human movement and physiology and applied the knowledge to his own clinical practice. He is now well known as one of the leading AIS teachers and practitioners.

We now view human motion as the consequence of the interaction between muscles and the external forces acting on the anatomical system. It must be remembered that the analysis of motion is not an end in itself but a means to the learning of new movement patterns and the improvement of previously learned patterns. Kinesiologists were introduced to the anatomical and physiological works by numerous research studies and textbooks that influenced kinesiology as we know it today. New textbooks that offer this valuable information are necessary for the advancement of the field. The ever-changing health care profession will benefit from the concentrated information in *Kinesiology for Manual Therapies*.

I began developing "Active Isolated Stretching: The Mattes Method" in 1970 while teaching at the University of Illinois, at Urbana-Champaign. After finding traditional static stretching with long holds ineffective, and observing that this stretch method frequently caused injury, I began to examine short-stretch holds. Teaching and supervising students and working with prescribed patients, I began clinically experimenting with short-duration stretches of 2 seconds while using electromyography. I also examined the stretching relationship between agonist and antagonist muscles. From studying the prime mover muscles, it became apparent that short-duration stretching, as well as engaging the opposite-side muscles in contraction, allowed a more rapid progression in muscle length. Also, there was minimal tenderness in the lengthened muscles, even when injuries were present in the muscles stretched.

Since 1979, emphasis on tissue elasticity of all the joints has resulted in muscle and fascial specificity, creating exciting results within sports medicine, including muscle diseases and spinal cord problems. This specificity and focus on tissue elasticity is now included in programs of all phases of training and is a dynamic modality in rehabilitation.

The use of clinical flexibility in this text, as well as specific strengthening, is a profound addition to the advancement of the field of manual therapies. It encourages the mind-set of a specific, proactive approach for soft-tissue injuries in a myriad of practices.

Aaron L. Mattes, MS, RKT, LMT
Developer, Active Isolated Stretching (AIS):
The Mattes Method

Preface

In the ever-expanding fields of allied health occupations, knowledge of the human body is tantamount. Indeed, professions in manual therapies are founded on the principles of science and the study of anatomy, physiology, and kinesiology. In the educator's quest for greater understanding of human anatomy, clinical tools such as cadaver studies help provide research for textbooks, in the hope that new comprehensible learning will take place from those texts. It is important that the student and professional have books, charts, and maps to guide them to learn the breadth and depth of the skeletal, articular, muscular, and nervous systems. Without them we would be unable to begin our explorations and develop our treatment goals.

This book has been written to assist and guide the student and the professional in their journey of anatomical study and manual therapy practice and to be a resource for continuing education. Its contents provide the information that will assist you in making science a foundation for therapeutic practices and encourage the development of your creative art for therapy. Science is the foundation of our art in manual therapy, and this text represents this philosophy on every page.

Structural Kinesiology was written over 60 years ago, and since then it has become a standard for teaching kinesiology to multiple students and occupations. R. T. Floyd used that book in his undergraduate work and later in his teachings. Like R. T., at the Downeast School of Massage (DSM), we used *Structural Kinesiology* as a text for years. We developed a handbook that was a useful tool for the student as an accompanying product. It was an outline, workbook, study tool, and technique detail all in one. It seemed logical to approach McGraw-Hill about writing an accompanying workbook. From workbook to actual text, the project grew to include DSM's dimensional massage therapy philosophy and accompanying techniques, but this project needed to add the aspect of kinesiology and physiology. With the addition of clinical flexibility and therapeutic exercise techniques, the capable McGraw-Hill staff has taken us on a whirlwind ride through textbook publication. The reviewers agreed there is a demand, indeed a niche, for this text within the science and manual therapy world.

We approached this book from a wide perspective of needs in multiple manual therapies, massage therapy and bodywork, athletic training, physical therapy, occupational therapy, and physical fitness. This book helps bridge the gap between basic anatomy and physiology courses and continuing education after graduation. Therapists will be able to use this text as a reference for their clients, for national exams, and for workshops with high science content. Kinesiology has not always been a part of every basic massage therapy program. Other professionals of manual therapies may not have had the appropriate textbooks to explore how massage therapy may enhance their practice. The information provided in this text will serve the expansion of education to the field of massage therapy as well as to additional manual therapies.

Our rationale with this text is to provide an advanced look at kinesiology and functional anatomy. Included are learning-intensive guides that will help students develop palpation skills, support their knowledge base of anatomy, and build a toolbox of techniques that provide a mechanism for specializing treatments. This text is a collective effort to explore the curriculum of kinesiology along with massage techniques, therapeutic exercises, and flexibility for multiple manual therapies.

This book is divided into chapters that provide a close anatomical look at each major joint of the body. Some chapters explore the skeletal structure and all the involved articulations, muscular attachments, functions, and nerve innervations. There are Clinical Notes featuring real-life examples about each muscle and its postural impact. Massage techniques, known as *dimensional massage,* are introduced to assist palpation skills, explore the structure, and develop a philosophical approach for treatment. Other chapters introduce students to specific, concentrated stretching and strengthening exercises as a modality, all of which follow the body's natural kinesthetic movements. Learning these techniques, known as *clinical flexibility and therapeutic exercise,* will help students understand anatomy from a *functional* standpoint—that is, how the muscles move the body in gravity—a focus that is often lacking in many curricula.

Dimensional Massage

The body is all connected; it has depth, width, and length. The joints in the body provide a network of anatomical structures designed for constant use. To properly relax and unwind soft tissue, the massage therapist must manipulate as many of these structures as possible. Each joint is a collection of muscles that work in groups and in paired opposition. By systematically working on specific muscles that share contraction and opposite action, dimensional massage helps to create balance in the joint structures. Dimensional massage encompasses an approach to technique and structure as well as to the sequence of the specific techniques for a particular soft-tissue problem. The techniques are a collection of soft-tissue manipulations that are designed to be efficient and sequentially specific to unwind the most resistant hypertonicities. Dimensional massage should provide the least amount of discomfort to the client in the therapeutic process, and if performed correctly, the techniques should be easy on the therapist's hands and body. Many dimensional massage techniques first utilize passive shortening of the length of the muscle to efficiently soften fibers. Other dimensional massage manipulations require rhythmically moving a joint at the same time as unwinding specific muscles or alternating clockwise and counterclockwise movements to joints or muscles. These "distractions" provide a mechanism for the client to give up "holding" patterns and for the soft-tissue fibers to release built-up tension. All techniques should be sequenced according to the individual structure of the client. Therapists need to build a large "tool belt" of many techniques to adapt to the wide variety of structures and repetitive actions that plague humanity. Dimensional massage provides a philosophical approach, sequence, and methodology of techniques for the massage therapist to utilize in a therapeutic practice.

Clinical Flexibility and Therapeutic Exercise

Clinical flexibility and therapeutic exercise (CFTE) is a modality that utilizes the body's natural movements to help restore muscle and movement function. While it involves assessment, muscle testing, and other clinical protocols, in its simplest form it is a method of stretching and strengthening the body in a clinical setting. One part of its components is the Active Isolated Stretching method, in which every joint is isolated and moved into a position for muscles to be lengthened. Because this method is active and the patient is always performing the movements, circulation is increased and muscles are strengthened. Much like massage therapy, increasing circulation is a goal in healing injuries. Yet this modality also induces muscle reeducation and strengthening of muscles because of its active element, a beneficial component to patients of stroke. The dynamic element of this modality of manual therapy is its use of specific movement. CFTE utilizes every direction a muscle can move a joint: flexion, extension, rotation, and so on, and restores range of motion very quickly. The strengthening component offers specific isolation of muscles to better challenge them for strengthening, and it focuses on restoring imbalances within the body. From a learning standpoint for students, CFTE offers a different approach to learning muscle attachments and actions because it is the study of functional anatomy, kinesiology in its truest form.

Organization and Structure

This book has been designed for the student's optimal learning experience and is divided into four parts. Part One includes the first three chapters, which are in part a review for the reader and an introduction to the theory and principles of movement and kinesiology. Part Two takes the student through the upper extremities, starting with the shoulder girdle and following with the shoulder joint, elbow and radioulnar joints, and hand and wrist joints. After each joint and muscle chapter, there is a technique chapter specific to the area of the body just studied. The last chapter in Part Two concentrates on the concepts of muscular analysis and clinical flexibility of the upper extremities. Part Three isolates the trunk, spine, and head movements, joints, and muscles. It concludes with a special chapter on the structural perspectives of the head and neck, tension headaches, and techniques specific for this region. Part Four explores the structure of the lower extremities, starting with the hip and pelvic girdle and moving to the knee joint and the ankle and foot. Again, each chapter is followed by a technique chapter specific for the region. A muscular analysis of the lower extremities and clinical flexibility ends Part Four.

Features of the Book

All chapters are carefully designed with student learning in mind. Color photos and illustrations give depth and dimension to the visual education of the reader. Any book is more interesting in color, but in an anatomy text color raises learning to a higher level. Color helps students remember the art, and in a structural text that is a necessity.

Each chapter opens with special features designed to enhance learning:

- *Learning Outcomes* at the beginning of each chapter show important points for a quick understanding of the chapter's contents.

- The *Key Terms* list presents important words that are bolded and defined in the text. All the key terms are also defined in the Glossary at the end of the book.
- The *Introduction* assists the student to ease into the body of the chapter.

The chapters feature specific types of boxes that enhance the information in the text and capture the interest of the reader:

- *Clinical Notes* boxes are presented throughout the text to further student learning and interest in the content. The clinical notes link the structure being discussed to pathologies, postural issues, and anatomical facts by presenting information that is useful in practice. Each muscle has a Clinical Notes box as part of its description.
- *Muscle Specific* boxes include very useful information on the actual location of the muscles. This helps the student to have a visual snapshot of the locations of the agonist and antagonist muscles of each joint, matched with their actions.
- *Flexibility & Strength* boxes include all the movements of the described joint in detail. Some boxes feature accompanying pictures that provide a clear visual of the emphasized movements.
- *OIAI Muscle Chart* boxes present a brief description and color illustration of every muscle discussed in the text. The boxes are easy to see and refer to. Each box includes the origin, insertion, action, and innervation of the described muscle. A complete table of the muscles is also included to provide information on all the agonists and antagonists of the particular joint.
- *Treatment Protocol* boxes enable the student to prepare for the utilization of the techniques explained in the chapter.
- *A Technique* box gives definitions of hands-on applications in the text. Deep-tissue definitions are concise and easy to read, and tips are given on surface applications.

The muscle and joint chapters are organized by location of specific structures. Within chapters, the muscles are presented according to location and in groups based on action for better student learning. For example, all the flexors of the forearm that have action on the hand and wrist joints are grouped together, listed superficially to deep. This way, the student can unwrap the forearm layer by layer and learn the muscles according to location and action, an approach that helps with memorization skills. The discussion of each muscle includes an OIAI box, which provides an overview of key facts. In addition to the box there is a section on palpation of the muscle, designed to enhance kinesthetic learning; a Clinical Notes box; and sections on muscle specifics, clinical flexibility, and strengthening relevant to the muscle. The Muscle Specifics section is filled with a variety of details and interesting facts pertinent to the movement, structure, and posture of the muscles. To assist the student in learning functional anatomy, the Flexibility & Strength boxes outline detailed joint and muscle movements in most of the muscle chapters. Learning is reinforced from a kinesthetic perspective by a specific focus on exercises to demonstrate muscle action. Clinical flexibility is further explored in special chapters on the upper and lower extremities.

The technique chapters contain postural information and discussions on pathology, treatment protocol, body mechanics, and technique definitions and sequences to support the dimensional massage applications. Each technique chapter has a section before the hands-on applications that discusses an appropriate protocol and sequence for the area of the body emphasized in the text. It includes tips on appropriate protocol, palpation skills, warm-up techniques, determination of pressure, passive shortening of tissues, the use of critical thinking, and more.

Hands-on applications are included in every technique chapter. The technique chapters follow each major anatomy chapter to expand the knowledge base, palpation skills, and practical skills of the student. All the photos for the techniques are in color.

Body mechanics are the basis for safely applying techniques in practice. Good body mechanics utilize ergonomically safe methods and practices of executing techniques to prevent injury, support self-care, provide balanced energy, and promote a long career in therapeutic practices. Appropriate body mechanics are emphasized throughout the text in the technique applications.

At the end of every chapter are Chapter Summary, Chapter Review, and Explore & Practice sections:

- Each *Chapter Summary* provides a concise review for the student. The summary repeats the main headings from the chapter and outlines the information in an organized manner. The summaries are easy to read and refer to.
- *Chapter Review* questions reinforce the concepts that the students have learned in the chapter. They include true or false, short answer, and multiple-choice questions. Answering the review questions is a helpful way for students to prepare for tests and exams.
- Each *Explore & Practice* section offers demonstrable and practical activities for student participation. The activities enable students to develop their palpation skills, practice techniques, and use critical-thinking skills to answer challenging

questions. They promote a kinesthetic learning style that is all-important in manual therapy education. Some Explore & Practice sections feature fill-in charts that draw on students' overall knowledge of the muscle concepts discussed in the chapter.

The book includes two appendixes. Appendix A lists numerous resources for additional reading. As a special addition, Appendix B presents a medical history questionnaire specific to head, neck, and shoulder pain that is useful for headache and migraine clients.

Worksheets at the end of the book enable students to become creative in a kinesthetic manner. On some worksheets, students locate and draw muscles on the applicable skeletal bones. Other worksheets enhance understanding of the movements of the joints. Worksheets are yet another way to utilize different learning styles.

A hardbound spiral cover allows the book to lie flat for easy reference while the student is studying or doing practical applications.

Packaged with the book are Muscle Cards that are designed after the detailed OIAI charts. Muscle Cards provide the students with a convenient tool that displays the origin, insertion, action, and innervation of each muscle studied in the text.

The Online Learning Center provides links to supplemental educational materials.

Online Learning Center (OLC), www.mhhe.com/dailkinesiology

The OLC consists of the Instructor's Manual, PowerPoint presentations, an image bank of all illustrations, and EZ Test for the instructor. McGraw-Hill's EZ Test is a flexible and easy-to-use electronic testing program. The program allows instructors to create tests from book-specific items. It provides a wide range of question types, and instructors can add their own questions as well. Multiple versions of the test can be created, and any test can be exported for use with course-management systems such as WebCT, BlackBoard, or PageOut. EZ Test Online is a new service that gives instructors a place online where they can easily administer EZ Test–created exams and quizzes. The program is available for both PC and Macintosh operating systems.

The OLC also has a student section that consists of PowerPoint presentations, flashcards, and quizzes.

In Conclusion

Although we are targeting the massage therapy field, our expectation is that many health professional occupations will benefit from the content of this text. We expect that athletic trainers, physical therapists, kinesiologists, health club instructors, strength and conditioning specialists, personal trainers, physicians, and occupational therapists will be able to utilize the philosophy of our approach to exercise and flexibility. We strived to provide a real-world approach that clinicians might see in their practices. We hope that this book will serve the advancement of massage therapy and bodywork, as well as the supportive education of other health occupations.

Remember, science is the foundation of your art in manual therapies. It is this factual information that gives us the ability to perform our therapy on and with the human body. Knowledge only becomes more profound as you seek it again and again.

Acknowledgments

Author Acknowledgments

Nancy Dail: Great therapy does not come from isolation; it is encouraged and developed over time by teachers, mentors, peers, and multiple clients. From the beginning of my career with Jay Victor Scherer and Sensai Nakazono to now, there have been many influences that have affected and developed the philosophy of dimensional massage therapy. Benny Vaughn was the first person to give a name to elliptical movement, and I took his instructions on compressive effleurage to heart. He inspired me with his knowledge of science and dedication to manual therapies. He is still one of my heroes. I would like to thank Bob King for his encouragement and support, his myofascial techniques, and his legendary workshops. My appreciation goes to my Russian connection, author and teacher Vladimir Savchenko. Special thanks and appreciation go to Whitney Lowe, author, scientist, and presenter, for being a part of this effort to help educate the industry. My gratitude goes to Ruth Werner for her support, advice, and great pathology text. I would also like to acknowledge the great work of Dr. Janet Travell for trigger points, myofascial pain, and dysfunction. Her research has given us all a foundation to grow from.

I would like to thank Connie Kuhl, Andrea Edwards, Marlena Pechan, and the staff from McGraw-Hill; George Stamathis and Steve Capellini, who gently pushed me in the right direction; and the reviewers for their hard work and great suggestions.

Special thanks to my family and fan club, Bill, Emily, Amber, and William; to my brother Frederick Newcomb, for his expertise with aikido; and to my friends and advisers, Kate Waltz-Hixon, Sue Faust, Nancy Terrell Hall, Jen Merritt, Elliot Greene, Ray Moriyasu, Grace Chan, Margaret Avery-Moon, Ruth Marion, and Sally Niemand. Gratitude and thanks go to all my students, graduates, staff, especially to Suzanne Ash, and to the faculty of the Downeast School of Massage. I would like to acknowledge Leigh Kelly-Monroe from Image Catcher for great photography and Chad Murillo, Teneisha Lattibeaudiere, William Dail, and Emily Waltz for expert modeling.

My very special thanks and gratitude go to my writing partners Tim Agnew, and to R. T. Floyd for his patience and support, and to Clem Thompson for the development of his original work. Thank you all!

Timothy Agnew: Over the course of two years, this book has finally birthed, yet it would have been impossible without help and support. I am forever indebted to my friend, brilliant educator, and co-writer Nancy Dail. Without you, I would not be part of this book. Thank you for believing in me and allowing me to watch your children grow up on Moose Meadow Pond. I am in gratitude to the great kinesiologist Aaron L. Mattes, my friend and mentor; you gave me the spark that ignited my quest in kinesiology. I also thank you for your generous counsel and for lending me books from your extensive library. Thank you to Whitney Lowe, who gave us feedback on early drafts. This book would not have made it to the printer without our editor Connie Kuhl, Andrea Edwards, Marlena Pechan, and the great staff from McGraw-Hill. A special thanks to R. T. Floyd for his original text; I am humbled. I am grateful to model Cindi Carroll and photographer Barbara Banks for the beautiful pictures. A thanks to my Monday night aikido students, who threw me around every week just when I needed it. Thanks to my friends, colleagues, and patients; without all of you I would have had no motivation to complete this text. I am most grateful to my wife, Suzanne, who put up with the hours of isolation, and my son, Liam, who let me build Legos with him another day.

Reviewer Acknowledgments

Laura A. Abbott, MS, LMT
Georgia State University

Denise Abrams PT, DPT, MA
Broome Community College

Michelle J. Alley, MS, AP, LMT
High-Tech Institute

Patricia C. Berak, NCTMB, BHSA, MBA
Baker College

Kathy Bertolini, LMT
The Salter School

Paul Bolton, DC, BS
National Holistic Institute

Susan L. Bova
Penn Commercial, Inc.

Rebecca Buell, BS
McIntosh College

Iris Burman
Educating Hands School of Massage

Michelle Burns, BSN, BS Alt. Med, LMT, MTI
Advanced Holistic Healing Arts

Nathan Butryn
Boulder College of Massage Therapy

Gregory J. Brink, BS
University of Pittsburgh at Titusville

Jean Capretti, BFA
Career Training Academy

KC Chambers, NCTMB, NMT
Atlanta School of Massage

Carl Christie, NMT, LMT
Gwinnett College, Rising Spirit School of Massage

Suzanne Costa, BA
Baltimore School of Massage

Nathan Cuddihy-Garner, BA, CMT
Boulder College of Massage Therapy

Sheryl Daniel
Bear Mountain School of Massage

Deanne DeBerry, LMT
American Career College

Jennifer M. DiBlasio, AST, ACMT
Career Training Academy, Inc.

Marc Ellis, NMT, D.C., DACNB
Gwinnett College

Nate Ewert, AOS
Heritage College

Catherine A. Follis, D.C., CCSP, CIMI
Everest College

Cindi Gill
Body Business School of Massage Therapy

Sam Gill
Body Business School of Massage Therapy

Rebecca Giuliante, MS, RN, LMT
Our Lady of the Lake College

Ginny Hoeschen, LMT
Apollo College

Susan Hughes
Southeastern Community College

Lisa Jakober
National Massage Therapy Institute

Mary E. Larsen, CMT, AHI, RMA
C.E.R.A.H. of Idaho

Gerald Larson
National American University

Jennifer Opfer, AST
Pittsburgh Technical Institute

Cindy Pavel, MPA, CMT
Davenport University

Jeffery Penton, LMT
Capps College

Lee Phillips, BS, CMT
Lincoln Educational

Gilbert C. Rivera
Apollo College

Charlene Hebert Russell, BS, LMT
Virginia College

Brian Sacks, MS, BS
Southwest Institute of Healing Arts

Richard Sager, BA, LMT
Community College of Vermont

Dorothy Sala
Branford Hall

Laura Santen, BA
Allied College

Rosemary Schliep, BS, AS
Minnesota State SE Technical

Sandy Scott, RMTI-I
Allied College

Jacqueline Shakar, PT, MS, AT, CMT
Mount Wachusett Community College

Cheryl Siniakin, PhD, LMTI, NCTMB
Community College of Allegheny County

Michael P. Sliman, D.C.
Capps College

Nancy Smeeth
Connecticut Center for Massage Therapy

Jaclyn Taylor, LMT
Penn Commercial Business/Technical School

Nancy A. Tegan
National American University

Greg Turpin, LMT
Southeastern School of Neuromuscular Massage Therapy

Sandra V. Valdebenito, BA
High-Tech Institute
Marilyn S. Veselack, DA, RMT
Institute of Therapeutic Massage of Western Colorado
William Vogel
Western School of Health and Business
Brad Welker, BS, D.C.
Central Oregon Community College
Steve Wiley, LMT, MTI, CEP
American Institute of Allied Health
Kim D. Woodcock, NCBTMB
McCann School of Business and Technology

A Visual Guide to *Kinesiology for Manual Therapies*

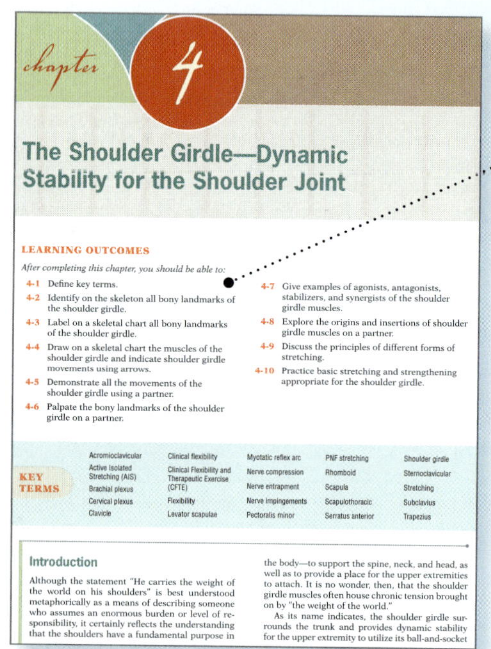

chapter 4

The Shoulder Girdle—Dynamic Stability for the Shoulder Joint

LEARNING OUTCOMES

After completing this chapter, you should be able to:

- 4-1 Define key terms.
- 4-2 Identify on the skeleton all bony landmarks of the shoulder girdle.
- 4-3 Label on a skeletal chart all bony landmarks of the shoulder girdle.
- 4-4 Draw on a skeletal chart the muscles of the shoulder girdle and indicate shoulder girdle movements using arrows.
- 4-5 Demonstrate all the movements of the shoulder girdle using a partner.
- 4-6 Palpate the bony landmarks of the shoulder girdle on a partner.
- 4-7 Give examples of agonists, antagonists, stabilizers, and synergists of the shoulder girdle muscles.
- 4-8 Explore the origins and insertions of shoulder girdle muscles on a partner.
- 4-9 Discuss the principles of different forms of stretching.
- 4-10 Practice basic stretching and strengthening appropriate for the shoulder girdle.

KEY TERMS

Acromioclavicular
Active Isolated Stretching (AIS)
Brachial plexus
Cervical plexus
Clavicle
Clinical flexibility
Clinical Flexibility and Therapeutic Exercise (CFTE)
Flexibility
Levator scapulae
Myotatic reflex arc
Nerve compression
Nerve entrapment
Nerve impingements
Pectoralis minor
PNF stretching
Rhomboid
Scapula
Scapulothoracic
Serratus anterior
Shoulder girdle
Sternoclavicular
Stretching
Subclavius
Trapezius

Introduction

Although the statement "He carries the weight of the world on his shoulders" is best understood metaphorically as a means of describing someone who assumes an enormous burden or level of responsibility, it certainly reflects the understanding that the shoulders have a fundamental purpose in the body—to support the spine, neck, and head, as well as to provide a place for the upper extremities to attach. It is no wonder, then, that the shoulder girdle muscles often house chronic tension brought on by "the weight of the world."

As its name indicates, the shoulder girdle surrounds the trunk and provides dynamic stability for the upper extremity to utilize its ball-and-socket

Every chapter opens with Learning Outcomes, Key Terms, and an Introduction that prepare the students for the learning experience.

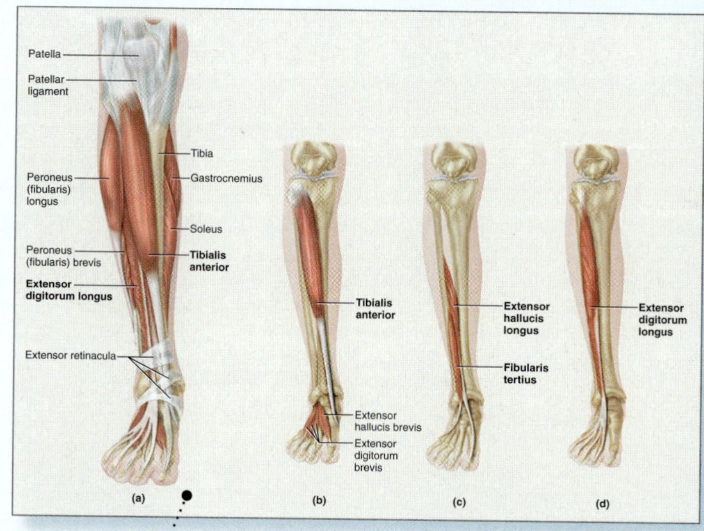

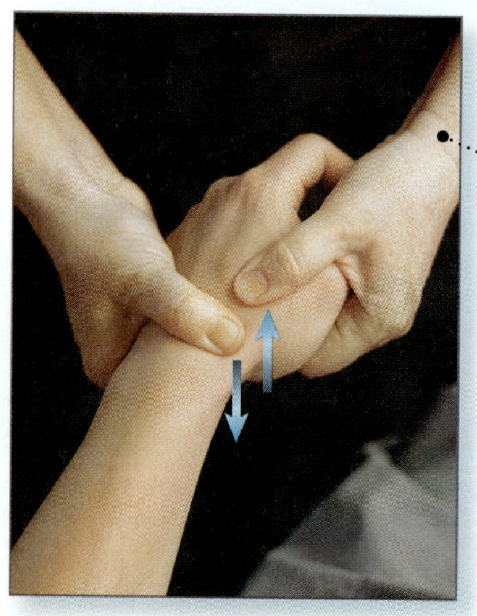

Color photos and illustrations give depth and dimension to the visual learning experience.

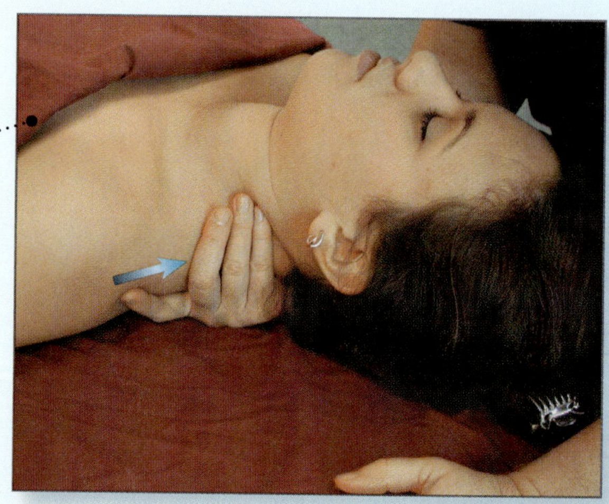

The anatomy chapters have unique features.

Flexibility & Strength boxes assist students in learning functional anatomy by presenting detailed joint and muscle movement information.

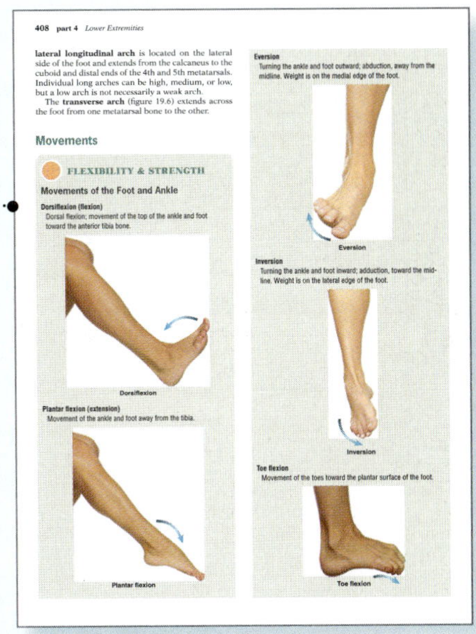

408 part 4 *Lower Extremities*

lateral longitudinal arch is located on the lateral side of the foot and extends from the calcaneus to the cuboid and distal ends of the 4th and 5th metatarsals. Individual long arches can be high, medium, or low, but a low arch is not necessarily a weak arch.

The **transverse arch** (figure 19.6) extends across the foot from one metatarsal bone to the other.

Movements

FLEXIBILITY & STRENGTH

Movements of the Foot and Ankle

Dorsiflexion (flexion)
Dorsal flexion; movement of the top of the ankle and foot toward the anterior tibia bone.

Dorsiflexion

Plantar flexion (extension)
Movement of the ankle and foot away from the tibia.

Plantar flexion

Eversion
Turning the ankle and foot outward; abduction, away from the midline. Weight is on the medial edge of the foot.

Eversion

Inversion
Turning the ankle and foot inward; adduction, toward the midline. Weight is on the lateral edge of the foot.

Inversion

Toe flexion
Movement of the toes toward the plantar surface of the foot.

Toe flexion

"The Clinical Flexibility and Strengthening Exercises are a fantastic way to allow the students to learn a therapeutic approach to massage therapy." **Laurie Santen, BA, Allied College**

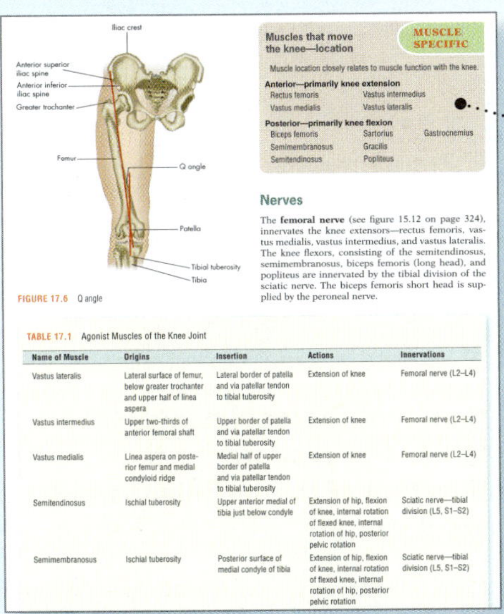

FIGURE 17.6 Q angle

Muscles that move the knee—location MUSCLE SPECIFIC

Muscle location closely relates to muscle function with the knee.

Anterior—primarily knee extension
Rectus femoris, Vastus intermedius, Vastus medialis, Vastus lateralis

Posterior—primarily knee flexion
Biceps femoris, Sartorius, Gastrocnemius, Semimembranosus, Gracilis, Semitendinosus, Popliteus

Nerves

The **femoral nerve** (see figure 15.12 on page 324), innervates the knee extensors—rectus femoris, vastus medialis, vastus intermedius, and vastus lateralis. The knee flexors, consisting of the semitendinosus, semimembranosus, biceps femoris (long head), and popliteus are innervated by the tibial division of the sciatic nerve. The biceps femoris short head is supplied by the peroneal nerve.

TABLE 17.1 Agonist Muscles of the Knee Joint

Name of Muscle	Origins	Insertion	Actions	Innervations
Vastus lateralis	Lateral surface of femur, below greater trochanter and upper half of linea aspera	Lateral border of patella and via patellar tendon to tibial tuberosity	Extension of knee	Femoral nerve (L2–L4)
Vastus intermedius	Upper two-thirds of anterior femoral shaft	Upper border of patella and via patellar tendon to tibial tuberosity	Extension of knee	Femoral nerve (L2–L4)
Vastus medialis	Linea aspera on posterior femur and medial condyloid ridge	Medial half of upper border of patella and via patellar tendon to tibial tuberosity	Extension of knee	Femoral nerve (L2–L4)
Semitendinosus	Ischial tuberosity	Upper anterior medial of tibia just below condyle	Extension of hip, flexion of knee, internal rotation of flexed knee, internal rotation of hip, posterior pelvic rotation	Sciatic nerve—tibial division (L5, S1–S2)
Semimembranosus	Ischial tuberosity	Posterior surface of medial condyle of tibia	Extension of hip, flexion of knee, internal rotation of flexed knee, internal rotation of hip, posterior pelvic rotation	Sciatic nerve—tibial division (L5, S1–S2)

Muscle Specific boxes help students to have a visual snapshot of the locations of the agonist and antagonist muscles of each joint, matched with their actions.

The OIAI boxes provide students with an easy-to-read description of every muscle in the text.

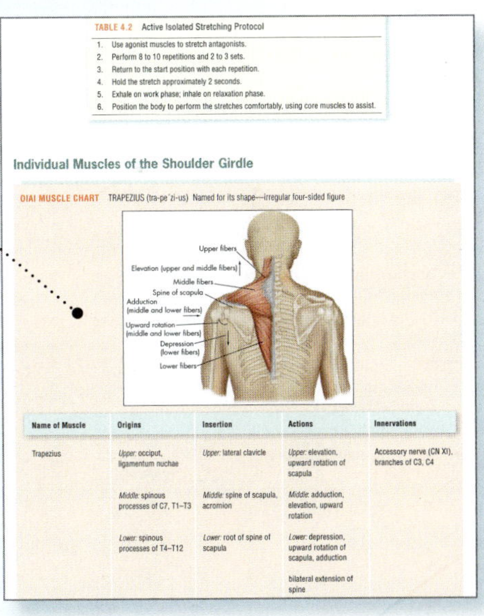

TABLE 4.2 Active Isolated Stretching Protocol

1. Use agonist muscles to stretch antagonists.
2. Perform 8 to 10 repetitions and 2 to 3 sets.
3. Return to the start position with each repetition.
4. Hold the stretch approximately 2 seconds.
5. Exhale on work phase; inhale on relaxation phase.
6. Position the body to perform the stretches comfortably, using core muscles to assist.

Individual Muscles of the Shoulder Girdle

OIAI MUSCLE CHART TRAPEZIUS (tra-pe´zi-us) Named for its shape—irregular four-sided figure

Name of Muscle	Origins	Insertion	Actions	Innervations
Trapezius	*Upper:* occiput, ligamentum nuchae	*Upper:* lateral clavicle	*Upper:* elevation, upward rotation of scapula	Accessory nerve (CN XI), branches of C3, C4
	Middle: spinous processes of C7, T1–T3	*Middle:* spine of scapula, acromion	*Middle:* adduction, elevation, upward rotation	
	Lower: spinous processes of T4–T12	*Lower:* root of spine of scapula	*Lower:* depression, upward rotation of scapula, adduction	
			bilateral extension of spine	

"The OIAI Charts are a huge plus because they put a lot of information in a nice, organized, convenient chart." **Rebecca Giuliante, MS, RN, LMT, Our Lady of the Lake College**

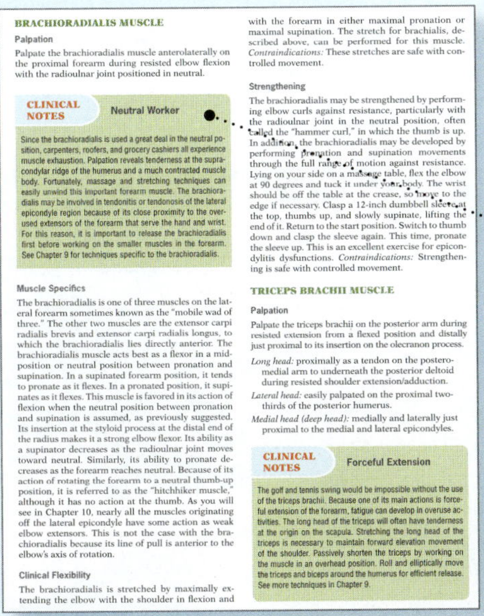

BRACHIORADIALIS MUSCLE

Palpation

Palpate the brachioradialis muscle anterolaterally on the proximal forearm during resisted elbow flexion with the radioulnar joint positioned in neutral.

CLINICAL NOTES — Neutral Worker

Since the brachioradialis is used a great deal in the neutral position, carpenters, roofers, and grocery cashiers all experience muscle exhaustion. Palpation reveals tenderness at the supracondylar ridge of the humerus and a much contracted muscle body. Fortunately, massage and stretching techniques can easily unwind this important forearm muscle. The brachioradialis may be involved in tendonitis or tendonosis of the lateral epicondyle region because of its close proximity to the overused extensors of the forearm that serve the hand and wrist. For this reason, it is important to release the brachioradialis first before working on the smaller muscles in the forearm. See Chapter 9 for techniques specific to the brachioradialis.

Muscle Specifics

The brachioradialis is one of three muscles on the lateral forearm sometimes known as the "mobile wad of three." The other two muscles are the extensor carpi radialis brevis and extensor carpi radialis longus, to which the brachioradialis lies directly anterior. The brachioradialis muscle acts best as a flexor in a midposition or neutral position between pronation and supination. In a supinated forearm position, it tends to pronate as it flexes. In a pronated position, it supinates as it flexes. This muscle is favored in its action of flexion when the neutral position between pronation and supination is assumed, as previously suggested. Its insertion at the styloid process at the distal end of the radius makes it a strong elbow flexor. Its ability as a supinator decreases as the radioulnar joint moves toward neutral. Similarly, its ability to pronate decreases as the forearm reaches neutral. Because of its action of rotating the forearm to a neutral thumb-up position, it is referred to as the "hitchhiker muscle," although it has no action at the thumb. As you will see in Chapter 10, nearly all the muscles originating off the lateral epicondyle have some action as weak elbow extensors. This is not the case with the brachioradialis because its line of pull is anterior to the elbow's axis of rotation.

Clinical Flexibility

The brachioradialis is stretched by maximally extending the elbow with the shoulder in flexion and with the forearm in either maximal pronation or maximal supination. The stretch for brachialis, described above, can be performed for this muscle. *Contraindications:* These stretches are safe with controlled movement.

Strengthening

The brachioradialis may be strengthened by performing elbow curls against resistance, particularly with the radioulnar joint in the neutral position, often called the "hammer curl," in which the thumb is up. In addition, the brachioradialis may be developed by performing pronation and supination movements through the full range of motion against resistance. Lying on your side on a massage table, flex the elbow at 90 degrees and tuck it under your body. The wrist should be off the table at the crease, so move to the edge if necessary. Clasp a 12-inch dumbbell sleeve at the top, thumbs up, and slowly supinate, lifting the end of it. Return to the start position. Switch to thumb down and clasp the sleeve again. This time, pronate the sleeve up. This is an excellent exercise for epicondylitis dysfunctions. *Contraindications:* Strengthening is safe with controlled movement.

TRICEPS BRACHII MUSCLE

Palpation

Palpate the triceps brachii on the posterior arm during resisted extension from a flexed position and distally just proximal to its insertion on the olecranon process.

Long head: proximally as a tendon on the posteromedial arm to underneath the posterior deltoid during resisted shoulder extension/adduction.

Lateral head: easily palpated on the proximal two-thirds of the posterior humerus.

Medial head (deep head): medially and laterally just proximal to the medial and lateral epicondyles.

CLINICAL NOTES — Forceful Extension

The golf and tennis swing would be impossible without the use of the triceps brachii. Because one of its main actions is forceful extension of the forearm, fatigue can develop in overuse activities. The long head of the triceps will often have tenderness at the origin on the scapula. Stretching the long head of the triceps is necessary to maintain forward elevation movement of the shoulder. Passively shorten the triceps by working on the muscle in an overhead position. Roll and elliptically move the triceps and biceps around the humerus for efficient release. See more techniques in Chapter 9.

Clinical Notes enhance student learning and interest by linking the structure to pathologies, postural issues, and anatomical facts and depicting information useful in practice.

"The Clinical Notes sections take the information and make it applicable to the client's health. Most students need to see the 'big picture,' meaning they need to see how this information applies to their work." **Jennifer Opfer, AST, Pittsburgh Technical Institute**

The technique chapters have special features.

102 part 2 *Upper Extremities*

client's need. Using deep-tissue techniques means that the practitioner is not randomly using a sequence but is, instead, critically thinking about a specific result. Compressive effleurage is an example of a valuable deep-tissue technique. Deep-tissue techniques do not have to be complicated; they are simply additional techniques that could be part of every practitioner's tool belt. Because each client is unique and has his own set of injuries, chronic and/or repetitive conditions, and specific structure, the same set of techniques is not likely to work on everyone. Practitioners need to practice with a wide variety of techniques and modalities in order to serve the tremendous variations they will inevitably find in their clients. The success of a practitioner's session depends on the critical use of her therapeutic skills.

Before beginning with the sequence itself, students are encouraged to read the following definitions, as well as "Sequence" later in the chapter, for more information on how to use the techniques in an orderly, intelligent fashion.

Dimensional massage therapy is a philosophical approach to therapy that is based on science, structure, and soft-tissue functions and that uses a variety of techniques for the client's benefit.

DEEP-TISSUE TECHNIQUES

Jostling rattles the fibers back and forth and is a form of vibration. Grasp the muscle loosely closest to the origin, apply a slight traction, and shake toward the insertion. For a better grasp of the tissues, do not use lubrication.

Compression efficiently speeds circulation to the area when executed correctly. This stroke can be combined with petrissage to make a dual-hand distraction technique. Press the muscle and soft tissue straight down against the bone, flattening and spreading tissues repeatedly with the palm and heel of the hand. Make sure that the surface is not slippery when applying compression.

Stripping is a deep-tissue technique that lengthens fibers and empties or pushes fluids. Place your thumb or forefinger of one or both hands at the distal end of the muscle and then slowly and deeply glide along the length of the muscle toward the origin. Use a minimal amount of lubrication. This technique should be used intelligently in the order of a sequence.

Deep transverse friction, or **cross-fiber friction,** is useful at tendinous attachments for releasing spasms and reducing adhesions; it can often be substituted with digital circular friction. Apply the technique against the fibers at a right angle with the fingers or thumb, using enough pressure to separate and flatten the fibers. Be careful, as the technique may be painful. Adjust pressure, and use the technique appropriately in the order of a sequence. (*Note to students:* This technique should be practiced only under the supervision of an instructor.)

Myofascial stretches are a series of techniques designed to stretch and warm up the tissues. The fascia is literally pulled off the structures in a rhythmic pace. As the fascia warms, it becomes more pliable, stretchy, and less "stuck" to the underlying soft tissue. Myofascial stretches are usually performed with little to no lubrication.

Elliptical movement is an alternating clockwise and counterclockwise distraction movement sometimes executed on joints such as the shoulder girdle and done most often while the therapist is engaged with muscles. The two alternating directions release any tension the client may be holding onto; this is because the client cannot focus on the direction of the movement and hold the tension at the same time. For a better grip, try to use this technique before applying lubrication.

Trigger points are irritated or hyperactive areas, often located in hypertonic tissue, that are either *active* (refer pain to a specific area) or *latent* (have a positive reaction to pain in the area of the trigger point). Sometimes trigger points form palpable nodules, but most often the therapist must rely on client feedback. *Satellite* trigger points are often located in functional units of synergistic muscles. **Ischemic compression,** or **trigger point release,** applies digital pressure, whereas a *pincer palpation* places the tissue between the thumb and the forefinger. The purpose of the digital pressure is to try to interrupt the pain pattern by robbing the tissue of oxygen for a short period of time. (*Note:* This book does not offer an exhaustive study on trigger points. Students seeking complete information about trigger points and treatment options for them should refer to books devoted to that topic. See Appendix A for suggested texts.)

Parallel thumbs is a deep-tissue technique executed by alternately applying pressure with the thumbs in a rolling-over motion. The thumbs face and are parallel to each other; they should be at a right angle to the muscle fibers.

Sequence

Sequence is a specific series of techniques chosen to accomplish a particular goal in a session. It is determined by the client's medical history, the structure, and the area of the body needing the work. Evaluation of pressure and technique may be determined by the stage of the condition: acute, subacute, or chronic. Therapists

Technique sections give students definitions of hands-on applications.

A Few Words about Body Mechanics

How many treatments does a massage therapist complete in a day, week, month, or year? It would be easy to add them up, but the equation of repetitive action times the amount of clients sometimes equals injury instead of a successful practice. Fortunately, good **body mechanics** that utilize ergonomically safe methods and practices to execute techniques can prevent injury, support self-care, provide balanced energy, and promote a long career in the massage therapy industry.

Practicing *aikido*, a special form of martial arts, teaches balance, the location of one's center of energy, and effortless movement. Applied to massage therapy, aikido teaches the therapist how to utilize the body's momentum for strength by applying an Eastern philosophy to a Western style of bodywork so that, ultimately, the massage therapist sinks into the soft tissue rather than pressing into it. Achieving and practicing good body mechanics is actually quite easy. Lower the massage table to enable your fingertips to just brush the top of the table when you are standing by its side. Remember that adding a person to the table means you will actually be working higher. The larger the person, the lower the table has to be set. If a client requires a side-lying position, the table should be adjusted to an appropriate lower level.

Aikido teaches that when the body moves, it should be relaxed, and that strength is not in how much force one uses but is in how the body's momentum is utilized. It is a silent strength that comes from balance and movement from the center of one's energy. The "center" of energy in the abdominal area is a Japanese concept referred to as the *hara*. Shiatsu (the Japanese rendition of acupressure), aikido, and other modalities and martial arts utilize this philosophy. The energy itself is called *chi* (Chinese) or *ki* (Japanese). How a person directs her ki forms the basis of her body mechanics.

Here are some general principles of good body mechanics:

- Always keep your back as straight as possible. As soon as you find yourself bending at the waist, your body mechanics have been compromised.
- Always move with your technique, using the momentum of movement to assist in the action. Your ki will follow your momentum as long as you are in balance. For effleurage of the extremities, for example, keep your back straight and lunge with your lower extremities, using mostly the quadriceps for strength. Relax your hands, and use your body weight over your hands to sink into the soft tissues as your momentum carries you forward.
- Always maintain balance so that you do not fall over if you need to step back for a moment.
- When you are standing straight, bend your knees so that movement is easier and springier.
- Stay over your hands as much as possible. As soon as your hands are reaching out in front of your body (a position known as the "Superman complex"), you have lost the center of balance and have no body strength to support the technique.
- Relax your thumbs, hands, and arms between techniques. Bodyworkers tend to hurt themselves with the repetitive holding of tension in their hands and arms. Do not hold your fingers or thumbs in extension while you are executing techniques.
- Always place your feet in the direction you are headed so that your body can move in that direction efficiently and easily.
- Try not to press into soft-tissue structures. Lean or sink into the tissues with your body weight. Ki extends from the center of your body, allowing you to move into the tissues. You will be surprised at how much deeper the tissues will allow you to go when you do not force your way into their fibers. It is a myth that one must be Hercules to do bodywork! Too much pressure applied incorrectly will cause discomfort and invoke immediate instinctive tension in the client's tissues. If you do not have passive tissues to work with, it is very difficult to get an effective result.
- Never sacrifice yourself to a technique or to the client's structure.
- Breathe. Students often forget the importance of breathing. Breathing is rhythmic; it silently teaches grace, promotes relaxation, and makes centering easier.
- Center yourself often. Remember that the person on the table has engaged your services. Thus, you need to be "present" for that person.

If you have no experience with any martial arts, *tai chi* will add to your practice by helping you to understand energy, discipline, balance, and movement. Tai chi is meditation, grace, and dance. It is good for the soul. In *Care of the Soul*, Thomas Moore says, "Care of the soul requires craft—skill, attention, and art. To live with a high degree of artfulness means to attend to the small things that keep the soul engaged in whatever we are doing." Massage therapy is the art of touching other human beings; thus, therapists are engaged in a relationship of response. It is the therapists' ethical duty to prepare themselves well and practice self-care. Paying such attention to your craft will feed your soul.

Good body mechanics are the basis of your success with any type of bodywork. Having someone videotape you working will help you determine whether your body mechanics are still in good form. Are your shoulders elevated while you work? Are you bending over at the waist? More to the point, does your back hurt? Do your forearms or hands hurt anywhere? If the answer is yes to any of these questions, you need to revisit your body mechanics and take a critical look at how you are executing your techniques. Becoming a "wounded healer" makes it very difficult, if not impossible, to continue in your chosen profession.

If you are already injured, seek a diagnosis and appropriate care.

Body Mechanics box emphasizes to students the basis of safely applying techniques in practice.

Treatment Protocol boxes enable students to prepare for the utilization of the techniques with useful tips.

TREATMENT PROTOCOL

- Take the client's medical history, interview the client, and record SOAP notes.
- Observe postural assessment, gait, and the range of motion of joints.
- Perform palpation.
- Passively shorten muscles and/or position shoulders and scapula whenever possible.
- Work superficial to deep.
- Release hypertonic muscles.
- Use dual-hand distraction methods when possible.
- Work individual muscles, their attachments, synergists, stabilizers, and antagonists; study the functional unit.
- Do not overwork areas.
- Do trigger point work last on passively shortened muscles.
- Stretch tissue and joints as appropriate.
- Discuss additional massage sessions and suggested self-help measures.
- Refer to other health professionals when necessary.

"The step-by-step instructions in the Treatment Protocol boxes show what to palpate and how it is important to the students so they can quickly be effective in treating a muscle." **Sandra V. Valdebenito, BA, High-Tech Institute**

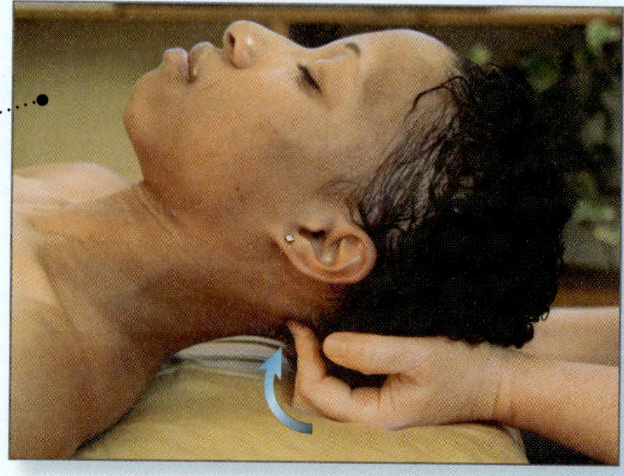

Hands-on applications expand the knowledge base, palpation skills, and practical skills of students.

Every chapter ends with special features to enhance the learning experience.

Chapter Summaries provide a concise review for the students in an organized, bulleted list.

CHAPTER summary

Introduction
✔ The mobile shoulder joint enables multiple movements, but it can sustain many injuries due to its lack of stability.

Bones
✔ The three bones that make up the shoulder joint are the clavicle, scapula, and humerus. Bony landmarks provide muscular attachment to make movement possible.

Joint
✔ The glenohumeral joint is a multiaxial, enarthrodial ball-and-socket joint.

Movements
✔ The glenohumeral joint enjoys complete range as a ball-and-socket joint. Shoulder joint actions include flexion, extension, abduction, adduction, and medial and lateral rotation. Other movements of this diarthrodial joint include horizontal adduction and abduction and diagonal plane movements.

Muscles
✔ The pectoralis major and coracobrachialis are located anteriorly, whereas the deltoid is located laterally. The rotator cuff includes supraspinatus, infraspinatus, teres minor, and subscapularis. Supraspinatus is located superior to the spine of the scapula, and infraspinatus is located posteriorly below the spine of the scapula. Teres minor is located laterally and posteriorly on the scapula, whereas the subscapularis has an anterior location on the scapula. Teres major is located inferiorly on the posterior scapula; latissimus dorsi is located posteriorly on the trunk.

Nerves
✔ The nerves for the shoulder joint muscles stem primarily from the brachial plexus.

Individual Muscles of the Shoulder Joint
✔ *Deltoid* is a superficial lateral muscle that is divided into three sections: anterior, middle, and posterior. The deltoid originates on the clavicle and scapula and inserts on the humerus. It is a major abductor of the humerus and is its own agonist and antagonist, as the anterior deltoid and posterior deltoid perform opposite actions. The anterior deltoid performs flexion, medial rotation, and horizontal adduction, whereas the posterior deltoid performs extension, lateral rotation, and horizontal abduction. The middle deltoid has very strong abduction to 90 degrees.
✔ *Rotator cuff* is composed of the supraspinatus, infraspinatus, teres minor, and subscapularis (SITS). These stabilize the head of the humerus. The supraspinatus originates on the supraspinous fossa, and its insertion lines up next to the infraspinatus and teres minor on the greater tubercle of the humerus. Infraspinatus originates on the infraspinous fossa; the teres minor attaches to the superior axillary border of the scapula. Supraspinatus performs weak abduction; infraspinatus and teres minor perform extension, lateral rotation, and horizontal abduction. Subscapularis originates on the subscapular fossa and inserts on the lesser tubercle. It adducts, extends, and medially rotates the humerus.
✔ *Latissimus dorsi* means "broad flat back." It spans superficially over most of the posterior trunk and inserts on the bicipital groove of the humerus. Its functions are adduction and extension, medial rotation, and horizontal abduction of the humerus. It is easily injured when used to pick up too much weight in an unbalanced position.
✔ *Teres major* is a posterior muscle that originates on the inferior angle of the scapula and inserts on the bicipital groove of the humerus. It forms the back aspect of the axilla region with the latissimus dorsi. It is a strong extensor and adductor and medially rotates the humerus.
✔ *Pectoralis major* has attachments on the clavicle, sternum, and costal ribs of the anterior trunk. Because of its fanlike structure coming from different directions on the trunk, it performs all shoulder joint movements with the exception of lateral rotation and horizontal abduction.
✔ *Coracobrachialis* is named for its attachments on the coracoid process of the scapula and the humerus. It flexes and horizontally adducts the humerus.

"The summaries are very good and clearly reflect what was learned in the chapters. It is the best summary format I have seen in a while." **Dorothy Sala, LMT, Branford Hall**

Chapter Review questions reinforce the concepts that students have learned in the chapter.

CHAPTER review

Worksheet Exercises
As an aid to learning, for in-class or out-of-class assignments, or for testing, tear-out worksheets are found at the end of the text, on pages 531–534.

True or False
Write true or false after each statement.
1. The pronator teres can entrap the radial nerve.
2. There are 10 carpal bones in the hand.
3. The radial nerve goes through the carpal tunnel.
4. The wrist is a condyloid joint that performs flexion, extension, abduction, and adduction.
5. The palmaris longus is a superficial muscle and performs weak flexion of the wrist.
6. The capitate can sometimes depress the carpal tunnel.
7. The flexor digitorum profundus controls flexion at the distal end of the four phalanxes.

222 part 2 *Upper Extremities*

8. The tendons of extensor pollicis longus and brevis and the abductor pollicis longus form a depression in the hand called the anatomical snuffbox.
9. The thumb extensors assist in wrist adduction.
10. The extensor digiti minimi assists in extension of the wrist as well as of the little finger.
11. Flexor carpi ulnaris does not go through the carpal tunnel.
12. Flexors and extensors of the wrist work together to cause wrist abduction and adduction.

Short Answers
Write your answers on the lines provided.
1. Discuss why the thumb is the most important part of the hand.
2. What muscles work together to complete ulnar flexion of the wrist?
3. Name a common origin of many flexors of the hand and wrist.
4. What extensor muscles work together to complete radial flexion of the wrist?
5. Name the common origin of many extensors of the hand and wrist.
6. What muscle of the forearm could be used for tendon repair?
7. Name three nerves that primarily innervate the muscles that have action on the hand and wrist.
8. Name the nerve that goes through the carpal tunnel.
9. What special function does the saddle joint allow the thumb to perform?
10. How many bones are in the hand and wrist, including the ulna and radius? Name them, and give the number of each in the cases of multiple similar bones.
11. Name the two muscles that are the *strongest* flexors of the wrist.

Multiple Choice
Circle the correct answers.
1. The distal interphalangeal joints are which classification of joint?
   a condyloid
   b. ginglymus
   c. saddle
   d. pivot

EXPLORE & practice

1. Locate the following parts of the spine on a human skeleton and on a partner:
   a. Cervical vertebrae
   b. Thoracic vertebrae
   c. Lumbar vertebrae
   d. Spinous processes
   e. Transverse processes
   f. Sacrum
   g. Manubrium
   h. Xiphoid process
   i. Sternum
   j. Rib cage (various ribs)
2. Palpate the following muscles on a partner:
   a. Rectus abdominis
   b. External oblique abdominal
   c. Internal oblique abdominal
   d. Erector spinae
   e. Sternocleidomastoid
3. Contrast crunches, bent-knee sit-ups, and straight-leg sit-ups. Which muscles are you feeling more in which exercise? Explain.
4. Have a partner stand and assume a position exhibiting good posture. What motions in each region of the spine does gravity attempt to produce? Which muscles are responsible for counteracting these motions against the pull of gravity?
5. Compare and contrast the spinal curves of a partner sitting erect with those of one sitting slouched in a chair. Which muscles are responsible for maintaining good sitting posture?
6. Which exercise is better for the development of the abdominal muscles—leg lifts or sit-ups? Analyze each one in regard to the activity of the abdominal muscles. Defend your answer.
7. Why is good abdominal muscular development so important? Why is this area so frequently neglected?
8. Why are weak abdominal muscles frequently blamed for lower-back pain?
9. Prepare an oral or a written report on abdominal or back injuries found in the literature.

Explore & Practice sections provide demonstrable and practical activities for student participation.

EXPLORE & practice

1. Locate the bony landmarks of the cervical vertebrae on a partner.
2. Locate on a partner the origins and insertions of the muscles discussed in this chapter and in Chapter 13.
3. Demonstrate how to passively shorten the flexors and extensors of the head and neck on a partner.
4. Demonstrate passive range of motion of the head and neck with a partner.
5. Demonstrate active range of motion of the head and neck with a partner.
6. List which muscles are agonists and synergists for flexion of the head and neck.
7. List which muscles are agonists and synergists for extension of the head and neck.
8. Describe how you would work on a client who has a tension headache.
9. Practice dimensional techniques individually and in a sequence on a partner.
10. Explain the precautions you would take if a client presents with a headache.

"The Explore & Practice questions are wonderful. They take the student beyond the book and into the daily hands-on information that they need to really comprehend what massage therapy is all about."
Nate Ewert, AOS, Heritage College

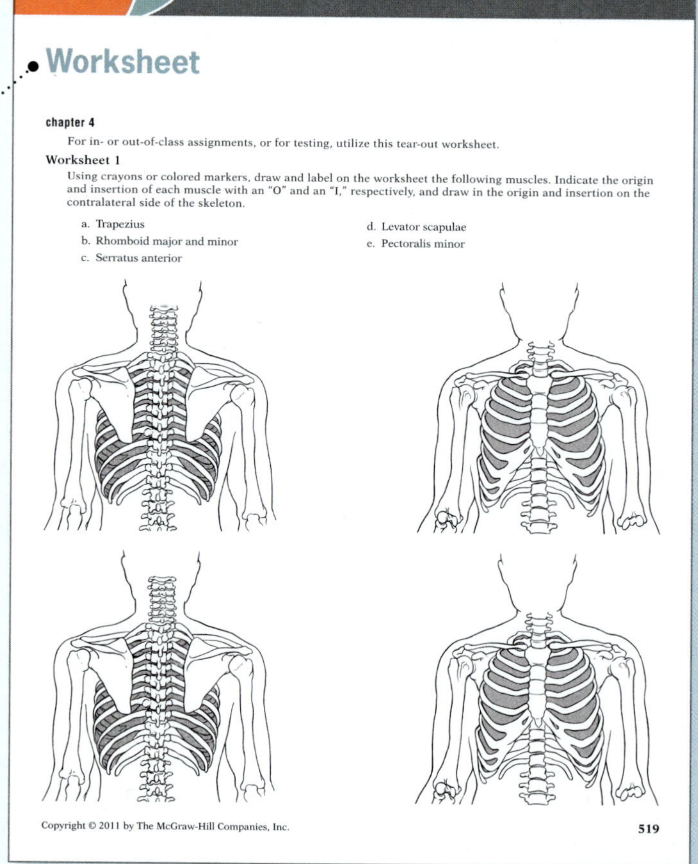
Worksheet

chapter 4

For in- or out-of-class assignments, or for testing, utilize this tear-out worksheet.

Worksheet 1

Using crayons or colored markers, draw and label on the worksheet the following muscles. Indicate the origin and insertion of each muscle with an "O" and an "I," respectively, and draw in the origin and insertion on the contralateral side of the skeleton.

a. Trapezius
b. Rhomboid major and minor
c. Serratus anterior
d. Levator scapulae
e. Pectoralis minor

519

Worksheets enhance students' understanding of the material by utilizing different learning styles.

Name of Muscle	Origins	Insertion	Actions	Innervations
TRAPEZIUS	*Upper:* occiput, ligamentum nuchae *Middle:* spinous processes of C7, T1–T3 *Lower:* spinous processes of T4–T12	*Upper:* lateral clavicle *Middle:* spine of scapula, acromion *Lower:* root of spine of scapula	*Upper:* elevation, upward rotation of scapula *Middle:* adduction, elevation, upward rotation *Lower:* depression, upward rotation of scapula, adduction bilateral extension of spine	Accessory nerve (CN XI), branches of C3, C4

Shoulder Girdle Joint
TRAPEZIUS
3

Muscle Cards that are packaged with the book provide the students with a convenient tool that displays the origin, insertion, action, and innervation of each muscle studied in the text.

"The text has all the necessary topics needed for a well-rounded, comprehensive kinesiology text." **Brian Sacks, MS, BS, Southwest Institute of Healing Arts**

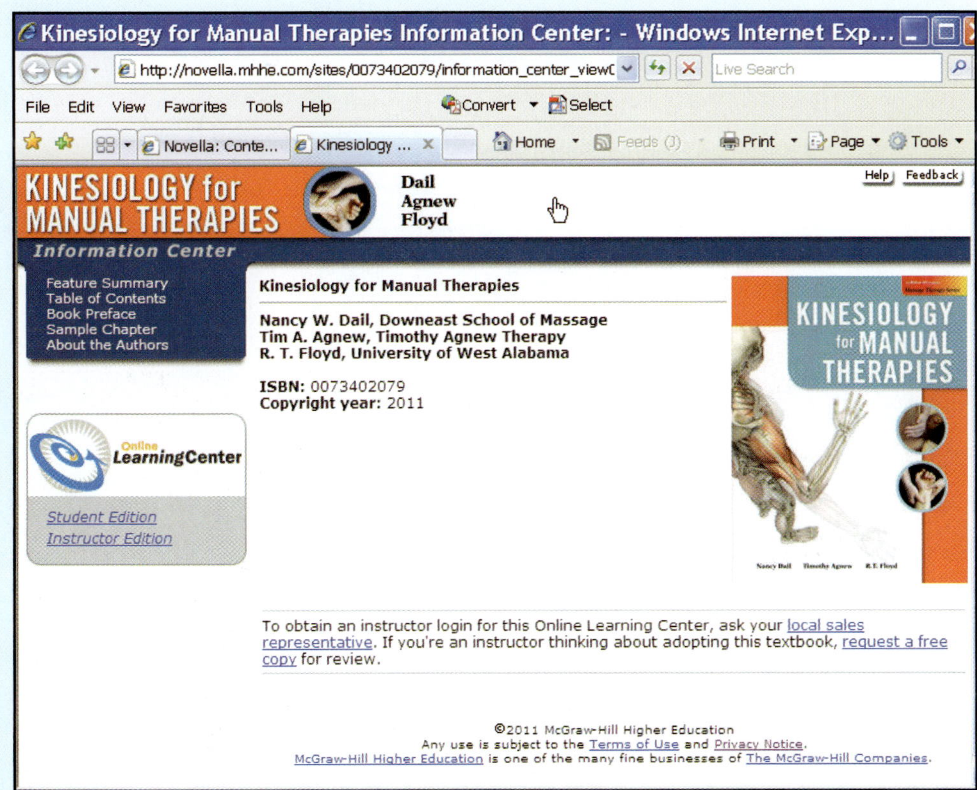

Online Learning Center, www.mhhe.com/dailkinesiology.com, offers additional learning and teaching tools.

part I

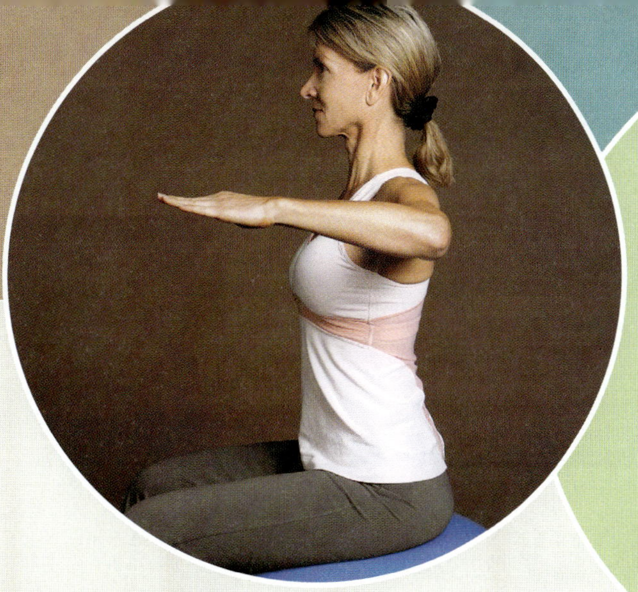

INTRODUCTION TO STRUCTURAL KINESIOLOGY

chapter 1

Foundations of Structural Kinesiology

LEARNING OUTCOMES

After completing this chapter, you should be able to:

1-1 Define *structural kinesiology* and *functional anatomy*.

1-2 Review the terminology used to describe body-part locations, reference positions, and anatomical directions.

1-3 Recognize the planes of motion and their respective axes of rotation in relation to human movement.

1-4 Identify the various types of bones and joints in the human body and their characteristics.

1-5 Describe and demonstrate the joint movements.

KEY TERMS

Abduction
Adduction
Amphiarthrodial joints
Anatomical position
Arthrodial joint
Arthroses
Articulation
Axis of rotation
Cardinal planes
Circumduction
Condyloid joint
Contralateral
Depression
Diagonal plane
Diarthrodial joints
Dorsiflexion
Elevation
Enarthrodial joint
Eversion
Extension
External rotation
Flexion
Frontal plane
Functional anatomy
Ginglymus joint
Gomphoses
Goniometer
Horizontal abduction
Horizontal adduction
Internal rotation
Inversion
Ipsilateral
Joint capsule
Kinesiology
Lateral flexion
Planes of motion
Plantar flexion
Pronation
Protraction
Range of motion
Retraction
Rotation
Rotation downward
Rotation upward
Sagittal plane
Sellar joint
Skeletal system
Structural kinesiology
Supination
Sutures
Symphysis
Synarthrodial joints
Synchondrosis
Syndesmoses
Transverse plane
Trochoid joint

Introduction

The study of human movement is an endless and challenging task. To study **kinesiology,** or the science of muscle movement, the student must have a thorough knowledge of the hundreds of muscles and bones yet also understand the physical laws that act on the body. This can be both a fascinating and daunting journey. This chapter introduces the student to the basic foundations of structural kinesiology, including planes of motion, axes of rotation, joint types, and possible movements. It also prepares the student for the subsequent chapters in this book, which support other concepts related to the study of kinesiology, in the hope that they can all be fully understood.

There are more than 600 muscles and 206 bones in the human body; each muscle has a specific responsibility to act on or move a bone. **Structural kinesiology** is the study of muscles, bones, and joints as they are involved in the science of movement. Bones vary in size and shape, and this affects the type of movement that occurs between them at the joints. The types of joints vary in both structure and function. Muscles also vary greatly in size, shape, and structure from one part of the body to another.

This text considers many of the largest and most important muscles, called *primary movers*. Since many muscles control joint movement, the text also examines some of the smaller intrinsic muscles. The six deep external hip rotators, for example, are often overlooked in a clinical setting, yet understanding their effects on joint movement and pathology in the hip is imperative in the study of structural kinesiology.

If it is within one's scope of practice, athletic trainers, physical therapists, massage therapists, personal trainers, and those in other related health fields should teach others how to strengthen, improve, and maintain muscles, bones, and joints. But first, clinicians must have an adequate knowledge and understanding of all muscle groups and their functions. This knowledge forms the basis not only of the *Clinical Flexibility and Therapeutic* exercises included in this text, which are designed to help one learn how to stretch, strengthen, and maintain the muscles, but also of *Dimensional Massage*, a modality covered in Parts Two through Four of the text. In most cases, exercises that involve the larger primary movers also involve the smaller muscles. This text discusses the important roles of some of these smaller, underdeveloped muscles, especially in examining particular movements and treating dysfunction.

Kinesiology students frequently become so engrossed in learning individual muscles that they lose sight of the total muscular system. Often, this is not the student's fault, as many curricula stress "memorizing" attachments to muscles, with little focus on the functional actions of the muscles. It is easy to forget that muscles work in groups and in paired opposition to achieve dynamic movement, whether walking, sprinting, or lifting a child. Although it is important to learn the minute details of muscle attachments, it is also critical to be able to apply the function of muscles to real-life situations. This is one of the benefits of this text: Real-life examples are discussed in the clinical notes and elsewhere throughout the text. Once the student understands the functional actions of muscles, or the **functional anatomy**, learning anatomy becomes easier. Functional anatomy allows the student to gain a new appreciation for how the human body moves.

Reference Positions

To better understand the musculoskeletal system, planes of motion, joint classification, and joint movement terminology, it is crucial that kinesiology students begin with a reference point. There are two reference positions that may be used as a basis for describing joint movements. The **anatomical position** is the most widely used and most accurate for all aspects of the body. Figure 1.1 demonstrates this reference position, with the subject standing in an upright posture, facing straight ahead, feet parallel and close, and palms facing forward. Some kinesiologists prefer to use the *fundamental* or *functional* position, which is similar to the anatomical position except that the body is in a more relaxed posture, with the palms facing the body. Since most humans walk and move with the palms facing the body, using this position offers a real-life approach to analyzing movements. The *midline* of the body is an imaginary line that divides the body into left and right sides; this term is used throughout the text.

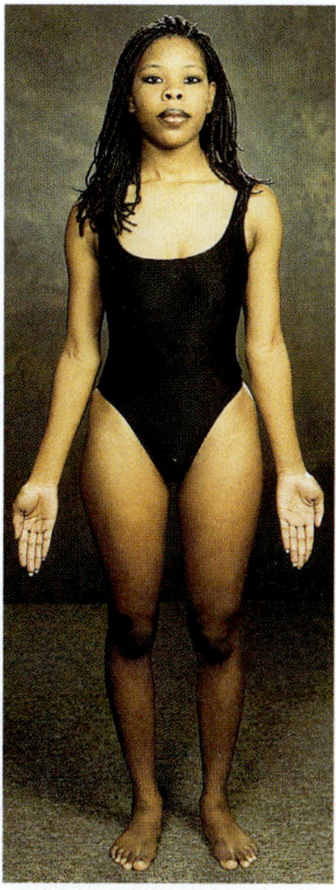

FIGURE 1.1 Anatomical position

Anatomical Directional Terminology

In order to study the human body, students must understand the directional terminology applied to it. Because students often get confused by the multiple terms used to describe areas of the body, it is important and necessary to start with the basics.

The term *medial* describes the body, or an object moving toward or located near the midline, or medial plane (see below) of the body. For example, the adductors are on the *medial* side of the femur. The opposite of medial is *lateral,* or movement or position *away* from the midline: The tensor fascia latae is located on the *anterior* and *lateral* femur, for example.

Proximal and *distal* describe positions relative to a reference point; they generally apply to the arms, hands, and feet. For example, the *proximal (closer)* attachment of the hamstring group is the ischial tuberosity; the *distal (distant)* attachments are the tibia and fibula. Also important are the terms *superior* and *inferior*. *Superior* refers to the location above a particular landmark or reference point; for example, the *superior* aspect of the foot is the top, or dorsal side. *Inferior* means lower and refers to any structure or movement lower than the landmark; for example, the medial epicondyle of the femur is located on the *inferior* end of the femur.

Anterior and *posterior* refer to the direction that a body part moves in relation to front and back, respectively. For example, the quadriceps are on the *anterior* thigh, and the hamstrings are on the *posterior* thigh.

The term **ipsilateral** describes a movement, position, or landmark location that is on the same side as a reference point. As the elbow flexes, the biceps contracts; thus this muscular activity is on the *ipsilateral* humerus. Movement, position, or landmark locations on the opposite side are described as **contralateral.** As the elbow flexes, the triceps actively lengthens on the *contralateral* humerus.

To further understand terms used in direction, see table 1.1.

Body Regions

The body can be divided into axial and appendicular regions. Each of these regions may be further divided into different regions such as the cephalic, cervical, trunk, upper limbs, and lower limbs. Within each of these regions are many more subregions. See figure 1.2 for a breakdown of these regions and their common names.

Planes of Motion

For the clinician to analyze human movement, it is necessary to understand the **planes of motion** (see figure 1.3). A plane of motion may be defined as an imaginary two-dimensional surface through which a limb or body segment moves.

There are three specific planes, or **cardinal planes**, of motion into which the various joint movements can be classified. They are the *sagittal, frontal,* and *transverse planes,* and each divides a segment of the body into halves.

TABLE 1.1 Directional Terms in Human Anatomy

Term	Meaning	Example of Usage
Ventral	Toward the front* or belly	The aorta is ventral to the vertebral column.
Dorsal	Toward the back or spine	The vertebral column is dorsal to the aorta.
Anterior	Toward the ventral side*	The sternum is anterior to the heart.
Posterior	Toward the dorsal side*	The esophagus is posterior to the trachea.
Superior	Above	The heart is superior to the diaphragm.
Inferior	Below	The liver is inferior to the diaphragm.
Medial	Toward the median plane	The heart is medial to the lungs.
Lateral	Away from the median plane	The eyes are lateral to the nose.
Proximal	Closer to the point of attachment or origin	The elbow is proximal to the wrist.
Distal	Farther from the point of attachment or origin	The fingernails are at the distal ends of the fingers.
Superficial	Closer to the body surface	The skin is superficial to the muscles.
Deep	Farther from the body surface	The bones are deep to the muscles.

*In humans only; definition differs for other animals.

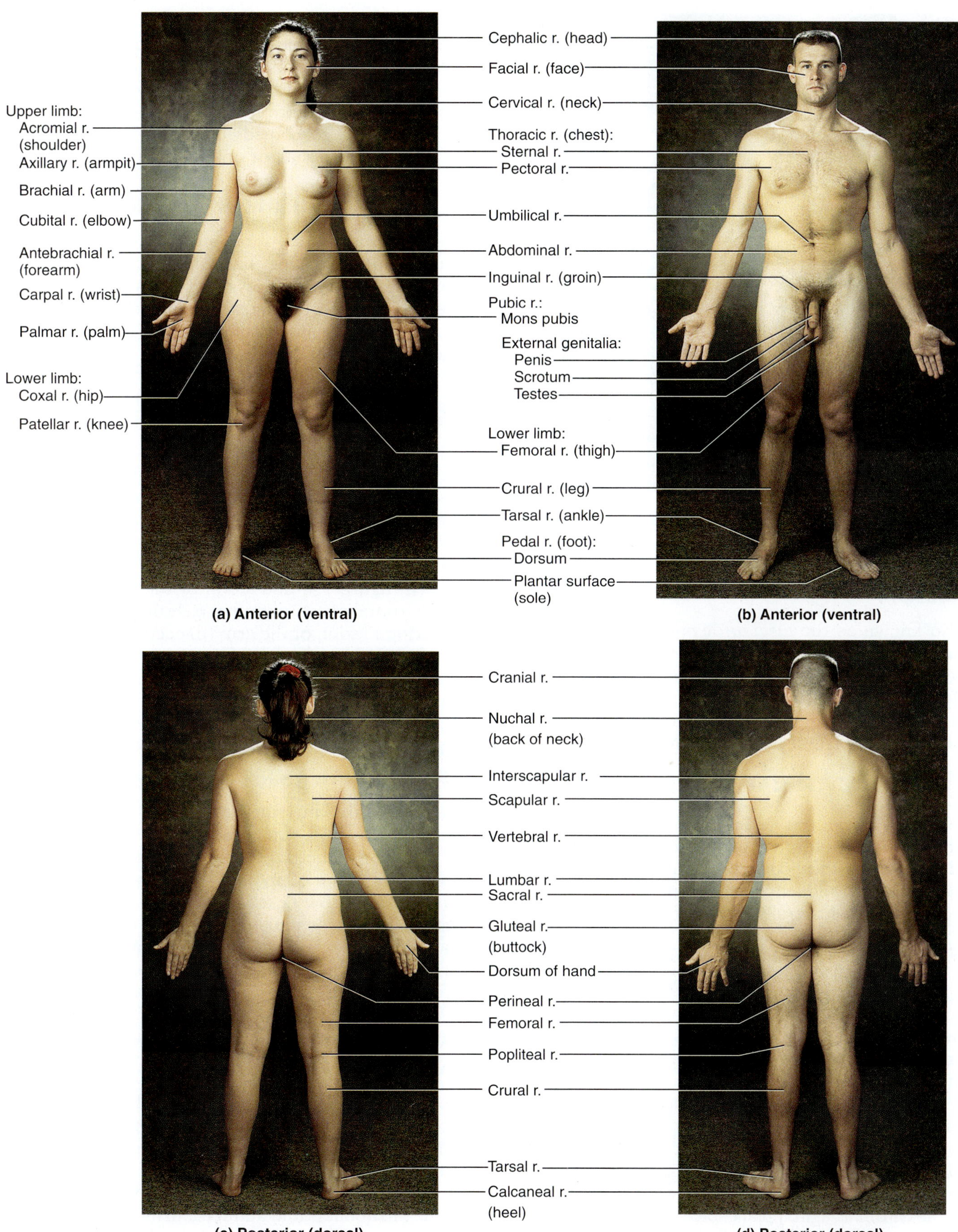

FIGURE 1.2 The adult female and male bodies

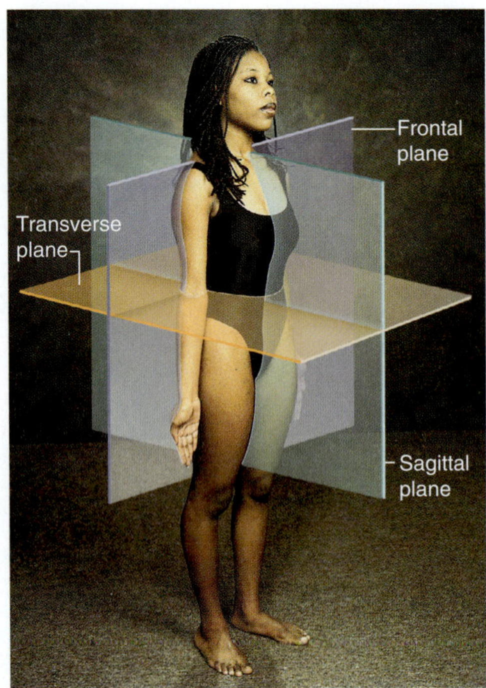

FIGURE 1.3 Anatomical planes of reference

SAGITTAL OR ANTEROPOSTERIOR PLANE

Also known as the *median* or *midsagittal plane,* the **sagittal plane** is the anteroposterior (AP) plane that divides the body into right and left symmetrical halves. Generally, flexion and extension movements, such as biceps curls, knee extensions, sit-ups, and ankle dorsiflexion and plantar flexion, occur in this plane.

FRONTAL, LATERAL, OR CORONAL PLANE

Also known as the *lateral* or *coronal plane,* the **frontal plane** divides the body into front and back halves. Abduction and adduction movements, such as jumping jacks and spinal lateral flexion, occur in this plane.

TRANSVERSE OR HORIZONTAL PLANE

The **transverse plane**, or *horizontal plane,* divides the body horizontally into superior and inferior halves. Generally, rotational movements, such as forearm pronation, supination, and spinal rotation, occur in this plane.

Additionally, there are an infinite number of planes within each half of the body that run parallel to the cardinal planes. This is best understood through the following examples of movements in the sagittal plane: Sit-ups involve the spine and, as a result, are performed in the cardinal sagittal plane; biceps curls also occur in the sagittal plane, even though the action does not technically pass through the center mass of the body.

Although each specific joint movement can be classified as being in one of the three planes of motion, body movements are not usually contained in one specific plane. Rather, they occur as a combination of motions from more than one plane. These movements from the combined planes may be described as occurring in diagonal, or oblique, planes of motion.

DIAGONAL OR OBLIQUE PLANE

The **diagonal plane**, or *oblique plane,* is a combination of more than one plane. In reality, most movements in sports activities fall somewhere less than parallel or perpendicular to the previously described planes and occur in a diagonal plane. A golf swing is a good example of this concept.

Axes of Rotation

As movement occurs in a given plane, the joint moves or turns around an **axis of rotation** that has a 90-degree relationship to that plane. The axes are named in relation to their orientations to planes of motion. It is helpful to visualize a steel pole as the axis and see the action of the joint rotating around this pole. In figure 1.4, abduction of the arm (a) occurs in the frontal plane, with the axis running anterior to posterior. Flexion of the arm (b) occurs in the sagittal plane, with the axis running lateral to the midline. Internal rotation of the arm (c) occurs in the transverse plane, with the axis running superior to inferior.

FRONTAL, LATERAL, OR CORONAL AXIS

If the sagittal plane runs from anterior to posterior, then its axis must run from side to side. Since this axis has the same directional orientation as that of the frontal plane of motion, its name is the *frontal axis.* As the elbow flexes and extends in the sagittal plane when performing a biceps curl, the forearm actually rotates around a frontal axis that runs laterally through the elbow joint. The frontal axis may also be referred to as the *bilateral axis* or *coronal axis.*

SAGITTAL OR ANTEROPOSTERIOR AXIS

Movement occurring in the frontal plane rotates around the *sagittal,* or *anteroposterior, axis.* This sagittal axis has the same directional orientation as that of the sagittal plane of motion and runs from front to back at a right angle to the frontal plane of motion. As the hip abducts and adducts during jumping jacks, the femur rotates around an axis that runs front to back through the hip joint.

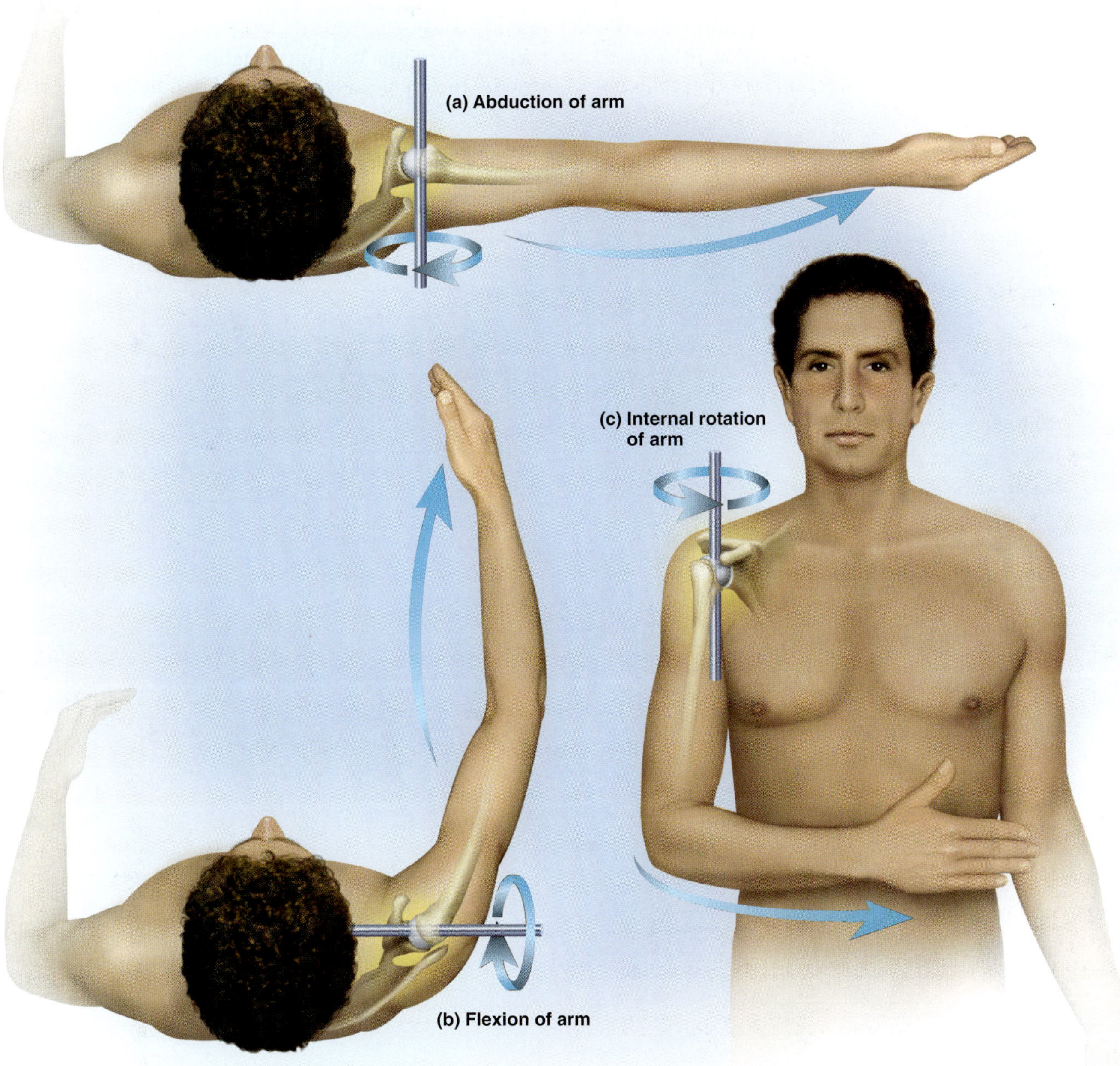

FIGURE 1.4 Axes of joint rotation

VERTICAL OR LONGITUDINAL AXIS

The *vertical axis,* also known as the *longitudinal* or *long axis,* runs straight down through the top of the head and is at a right angle to the transverse plane of motion. As the head rotates or turns from left to right, the skull and cervical vertebrae rotate around an axis that runs down through the spinal column.

DIAGONAL OR OBLIQUE AXIS

The *diagonal axis,* also known as the *oblique axis,* runs at a right angle to the diagonal plane. As the glenohumeral joint moves from diagonal abduction to diagonal adduction in overhand throwing, its axis runs perpendicular to the plane through the humeral head.

Skeletal System

The skeletal system of a typical adult is made up of approximately 206 bones; however, there are about 270 bones present at birth, with more bones forming during growth spurts, before fusing down to about 206 bones. Bones provide support and protection for other systems of the body and for attachments of the muscles through which movement is produced. The **skeletal system** is composed of two regions: the appendicular skeleton and the axial skeleton. Figure 1.5 shows anterior and posterior views of the skeletal system. The green represents the appendicular skeleton, and the brown represents the axial skeleton. The appendicular skeleton is

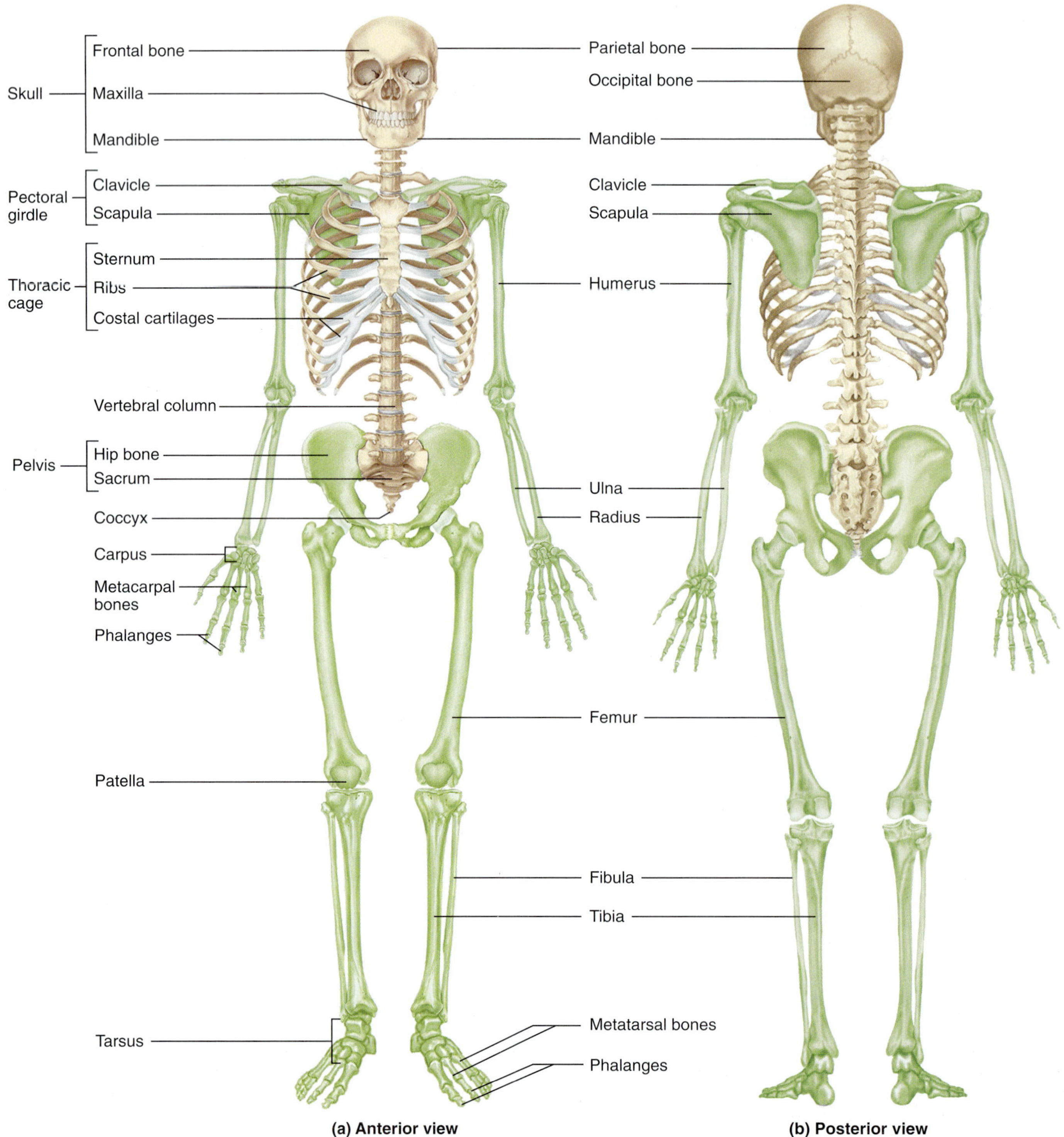

FIGURE 1.5 The adult skeleton

composed of the appendages, or the upper and lower extremities, and the shoulder and pelvic girdles; the axial skeleton consists of the skull, vertebral column, ribs, and sternum. Figure 1.6 shows surface features of bones, or *bony landmarks,* which are helpful to understand when studying kinesiology. Subsequent chapters in this text provide additional information and more detailed illustrations of specific bones.

SKELETAL FUNCTIONS

The skeleton has five major functions:

1. Protects vital soft tissues such as the heart, lungs, and brain.
2. Offers support to maintain posture.
3. Facilitates movement by serving as points of attachment for muscles and acting as levers.
4. Stores minerals such as calcium and phosphorus.
5. Enables hemopoiesis, which is the process of blood formation that occurs in the red bone marrow located in the vertebral bodies, femur, humerus, ribs, and sternum.

Types of Joints

The **articulation** of two or more bones allows various types of movement. The extent and type of movement determine the name applied to the joint. Bone structure limits the type and amount of movement in each joint. Some joints, or **arthroses**, have no movement, others are only very slightly movable, and others are freely movable with a variety of movement ranges. The type and range of movements are similar in all humans, but the freedom, range, and vigor of movements are limited by ligaments and muscles.

Articulations may be classified according to the structure or function. Classification by structure places joints into one of three categories: fibrous, cartilaginous, or synovial. Functional classification also results in three categories: synarthrosis (synarthrodial), amphiarthrosis (amphiarthrodial), and diarthrosis (diarthrodial). There are also subcategories in each classification, and due to the strong relationship between structure and function, significant overlap exists between the classification systems. That

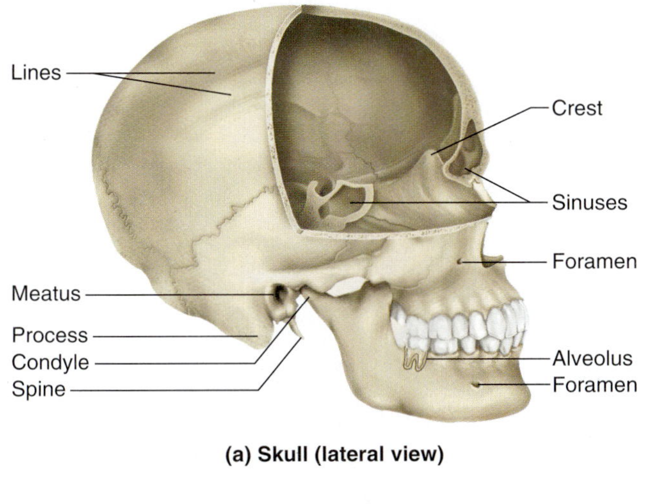

(a) Skull (lateral view)

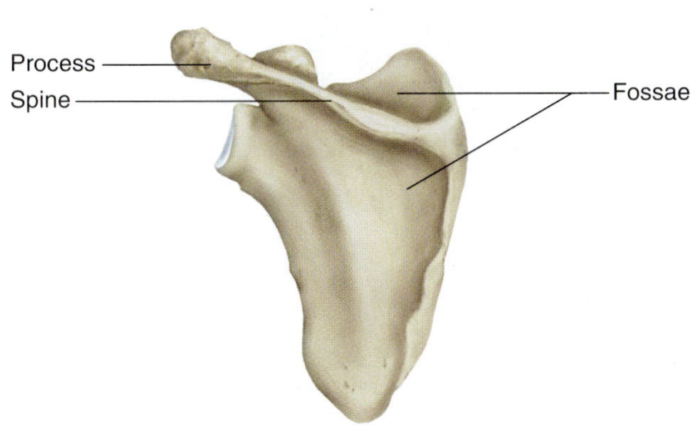

(b) Scapula (posterior view)

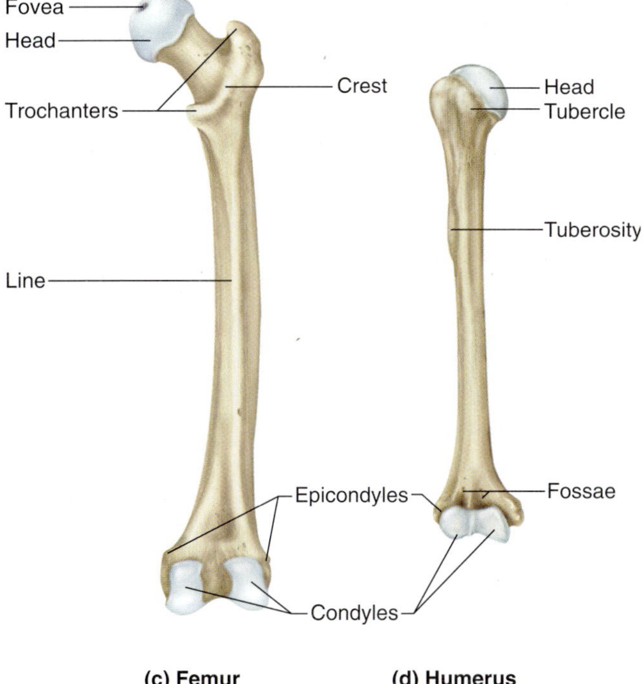

(c) Femur (posterior view)

(d) Humerus (anterior view)

FIGURE 1.6 Surface features of some representative bones

is, there is more similarity than difference between the two members in each of the following pairs: fibrous and **synarthrodial joints;** cartilaginous and **amphiarthrodial joints;** and synovial and diarthrodial joints. However, not all joints fit neatly into both systems. Since this text is concerned primarily with movement, the more functional system (synarthrodial, amphiarthrodial, and diarthrodial joints) is used throughout, following a brief explanation of structural classification.

Fibrous joints are joined together by connective tissue fibers and are generally immovable. Subcategories are **sutures** and **gomphoses,** which are immovable, and **syndesmoses,** which allow a slight amount of movement. Cartilaginous joints are joined together by hyaline cartilage or fibrocartilage, which allows very slight movement. Subcategories include synchondroses and symphyses. Synovial joints are freely movable and generally are diarthrodial. Their structure and subcategories are discussed in detail in the section on diarthrodial joints, below.

The articulations are grouped into three classes based primarily on the amount of movement possible, with consideration given to their structure.

SYNARTHRODIAL (IMMOVABLE FIBROUS) JOINTS

Structurally, synarthrodial articulations are divided into three types: suture, gomphosis, and syndesmosis (see figures below).

Suture

Figure 1.7 shows sutures of the cranial bones. The sutures of the skull are immovable after infancy.

Syndesmosis

A syndesmosis is a type of joint held together by strong ligamentous structures that allow minimal movement between the bones. Examples are the coracoclavicular joint and the inferior tibiofibular joint (figure 1.8).

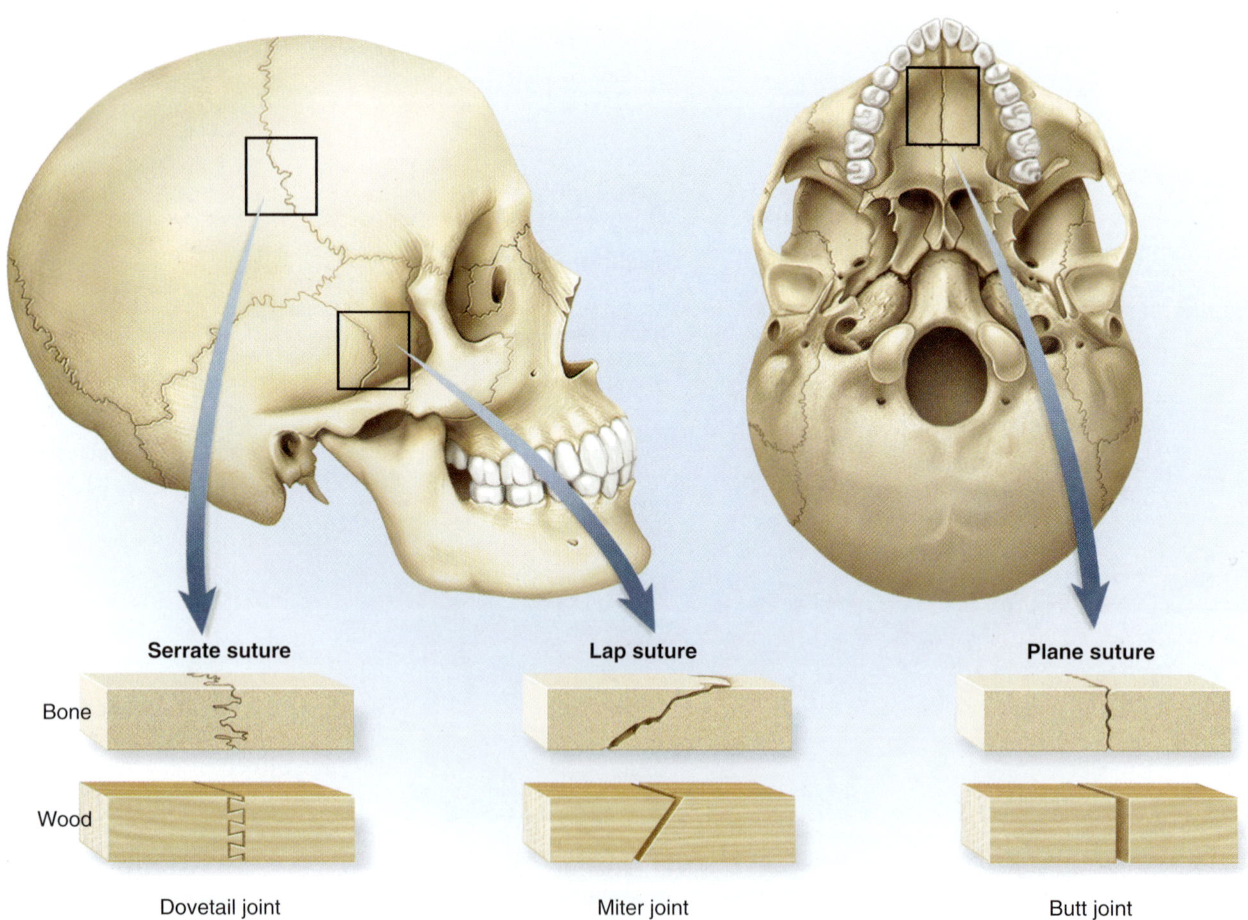

FIGURE 1.7 Sutures

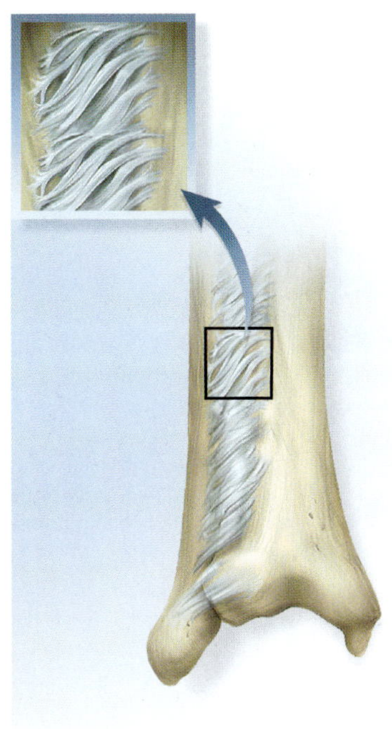

FIGURE 1.8 A syndesmosis between the tibia and the fibia

Gomphosis

Gomphoses are found in the sockets of the teeth (figure 1.9). The tooth socket is often referred to as a gomphosis (type of joint in which a conical peg fits into a socket). Normally, there should be a minimal amount of movement of the teeth in the mandible or maxilla.

AMPHIARTHRODIAL (SLIGHTLY MOVABLE CARTILAGINOUS) JOINTS

Structurally, amphiarthrodial articulations are divided into two types (figure 1.10a, b, and c).

Symphysis

A **symphysis** is a type of joint separated by a fibrocartilage pad that allows very slight movement between the bones. An example is the symphysis pubis, where the right and left pubic bones are joined by the cartilaginous interpubic disk.

Synchondrosis

A **synchondrosis** is a type of joint separated by hyaline cartilage that allows very slight movement between the bones. An example is the attachment of the first rib to the sternum by hyaline costal cartilage.

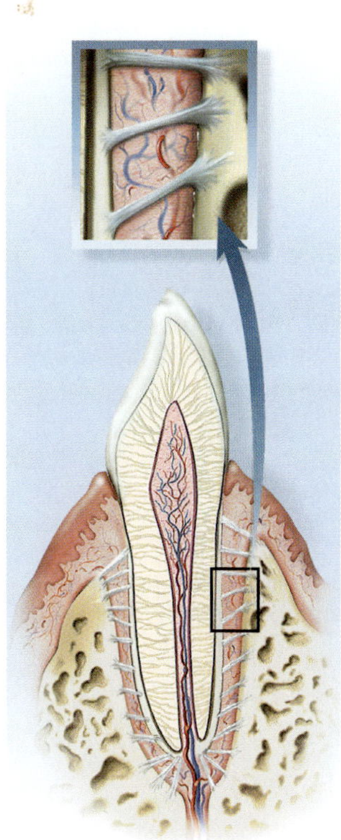

FIGURE 1.9 A gomphosis between a tooth and the jaw

DIARTHRODIAL (FREELY MOVABLE SYNOVIAL) JOINTS

Diarthrodial joints, also known as *synovial joints,* are freely movable (see figure 1.11). A sleevelike covering of ligamentous tissue, known as the **joint capsule,** surrounds the bony ends forming the joints. This ligamentous capsule is lined with a thin vascular synovial capsule that secretes synovial fluid to lubricate the area inside the joint capsule, known as the *joint cavity.* Synovial fluid contains the nutrient-rich elements albumin and hyaluronic acid, which lubricate the joint and help flush away toxins. In certain areas, the capsule is thickened to form tough, nonelastic ligaments that provide additional support against abnormal movement or joint opening. These ligaments vary in location, size, and strength depending on the particular joint.

In many cases, additional ligaments, not continuous with the joint capsule, provide further support. In some cases, the additional ligaments are interarticular (contained entirely within the joint capsule), such as the anterior cruciate ligament in the knee; in other cases, these ligaments are extra-articular (outside the joint), such as the fibular collateral ligament of the knee. The articular surfaces on the ends of the bones inside the joint cavity are covered with layers of articular cartilage, or *hyaline cartilage*. This

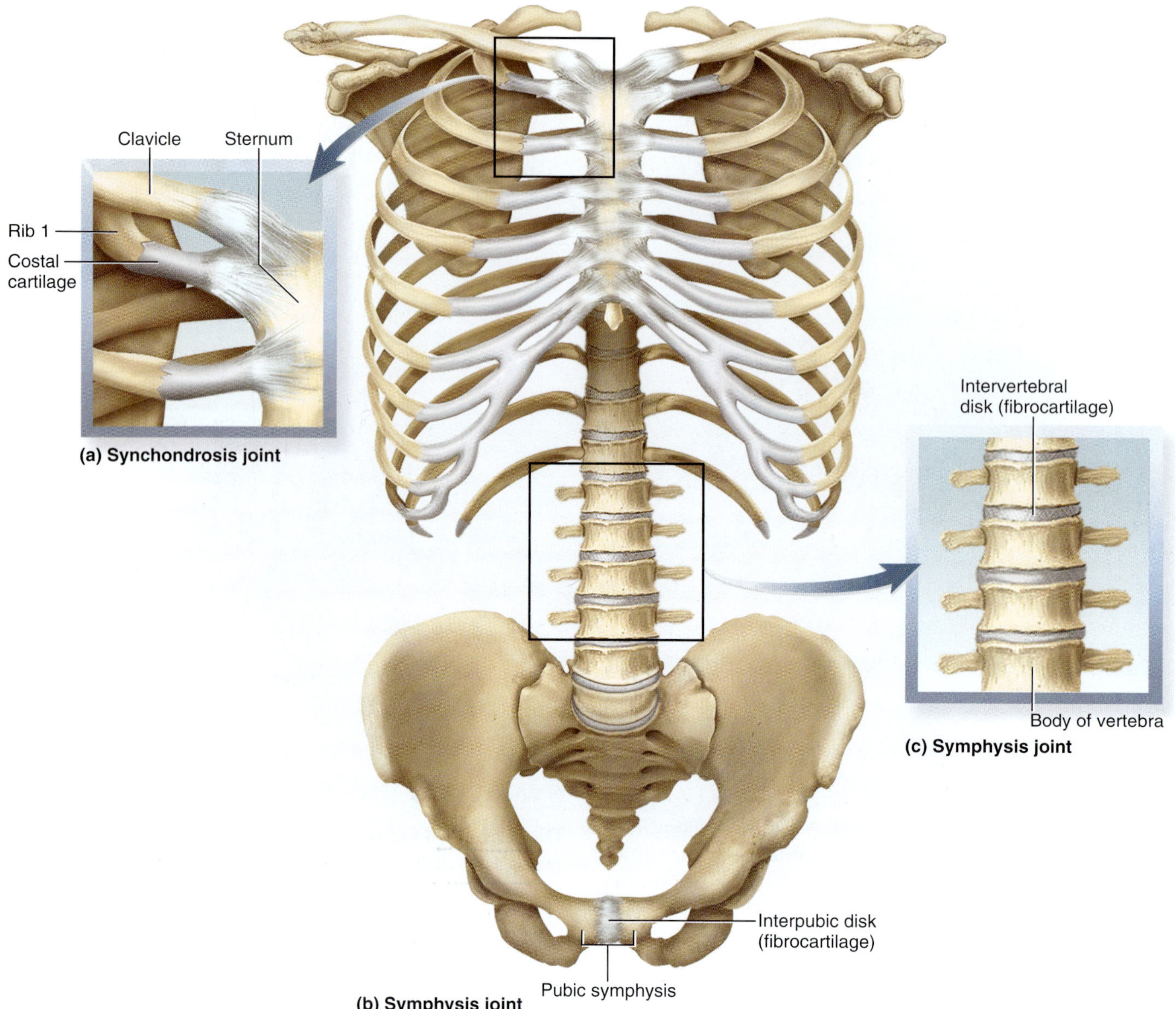

FIGURE 1.10 Amphiarthrodial (slightly movable cartilaginous) joints

resilient cartilage absorbs shock to protect the bone it covers. When the joint surfaces are unloaded or distracted, the articular cartilage slowly absorbs a slight amount of the joint synovial fluid, only to slowly secrete it during subsequent weight bearing and compression. Additionally, some diarthrodial joints have a fibrocartilage disk between their articular surfaces. Structurally, this type of articulation can be divided into six groups, as shown in figure 1.12.

Diarthrodial joints can have motion in one or more planes. Joints having motion in one plane are said to have one degree of freedom of motion, whereas joints having motion in two or three planes are described as having two and three degrees of freedom of motion, respectively.

Arthrodial (Gliding, Plane) Joint

The **arthrodial joint** type is characterized by two flat, or plane, bony surfaces that butt against each other. This type of joint permits limited gliding movement. Examples are the carpal bones of the wrist and the tarsometatarsal joints of the foot.

Condyloid (Ellipsoid, Ovoid, Biaxial Ball-and-Socket) Joint

The **condyloid joint** is a type of joint in which the bones permit movement in two planes without rotation. Examples are the wrist between the radius and the proximal row of the carpal bones or the second, third, fourth, and fifth metacarpophalangeal joints.

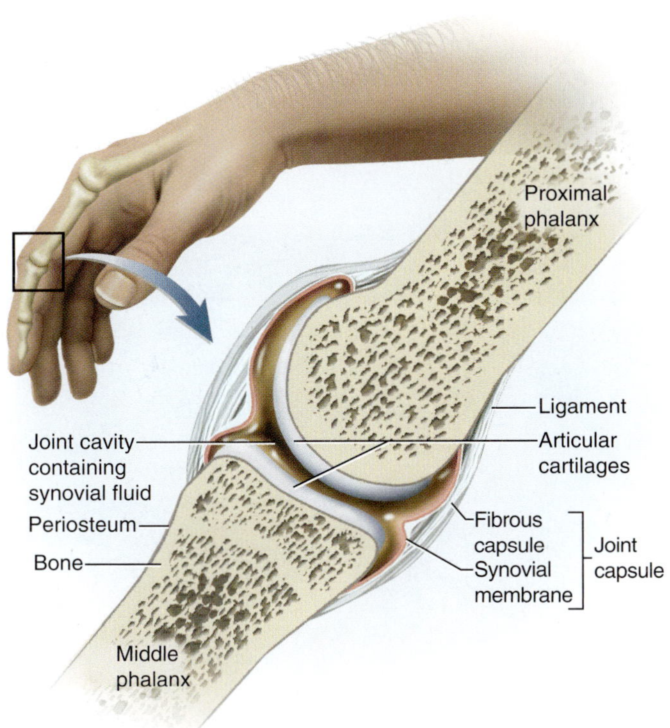

FIGURE 1.11 Structure of a simple synovial joint

Enarthrodial (Spheroidal, Multiaxial Ball-and-Socket) Joint

The **enarthrodial joint** is a type of joint that permits movement in all planes. Examples are the shoulder (glenohumeral) and hip joints.

Ginglymus (Hinge) Joint

The **ginglymus joint** is a type of joint that permits a wide range of movement in only one plane. Examples are the elbow, ankle, and knee joints.

Sellar (Saddle) Joint

The **sellar joint** is a type of reciprocal reception found only in the thumb at the carpometacarpal joint. It permits ball-and-socket movement, with the exception of slight rotation.

Trochoid (Pivot, Screw) Joint

The **trochoid joint** is a type of joint with a rotational movement around a long axis. An example is the rotation of the radius at the radioulnar joint.

Movements in Joints

Many joints are able to perform several different movements. Some joints permit only flexion and extension; others permit a wide range of movements, depending largely on the joint structure. The area through which a joint may normally, freely, and painlessly move is the **range of motion**. When measurements are required in a clinical setting, a **goniometer** may be used to measure the specific amount of possible movement in a joint or the range of motion and to compare changes in joint angles.

The goniometer axis, or hinge point, is placed even with the axis of rotation at the joint line. As the joint is moved, both arms of the goniometer are held in place either along or parallel to the long axis of the bones on either side of the joint. The joint angle can then be read from the goniometer. For example, a clinician could measure the angle between the femur and tibia in full knee extension (which would usually be zero) and then have the person flex the knee as far as possible. If the clinician measured the angle again on reaching full knee flexion, he or she would find a goniometer reading of around 140 degrees.

Range of motion can also be measured visually: The clinician measures joint movement in degrees by approximating degree increments. Normal range of motion for a particular joint can vary to some degree from person to person, due to dysfunctions, limited muscle tissue, and the presence of surgical pins. Appendixes A and B provide average normal ranges of motion for all joints; these measurements are helpful in assessing limited joint movement.

It is important to understand that movement terminology is used to describe an actual change in position of the bones relative to each other. Thus, angles between bones change, but movement occurs between the articular surfaces of the joint. Hence, in describing knee movement, a clinician might instruct a person to "flex the knee," which results in the leg moving closer to the thigh. But some clinicians might instead describe this as leg flexion occurring at the knee joint and therefore instruct the person to "flex the leg," when what the clinician actually means is that the person should flex the knee.

Movement terms are also used to describe movement occurring throughout the full range of motion or through a very small range. Using the above example, one may flex the knee through the full range by beginning in full knee extension (zero degrees of knee flexion) and flexing it fully so that the heel comes in contact with the buttocks; this would be approximately 140 degrees of flexion. The movement may also be done by beginning with the knee in 90 degrees of flexion and then flexing it 30 degrees more; this movement results in a knee flexion angle of 120 degrees, even though the knee flexed only 30 degrees. In both examples, the knee is in different degrees of flexion. The movement may also begin by having the knee in 90 degrees of flexion and then extending it 40 degrees,

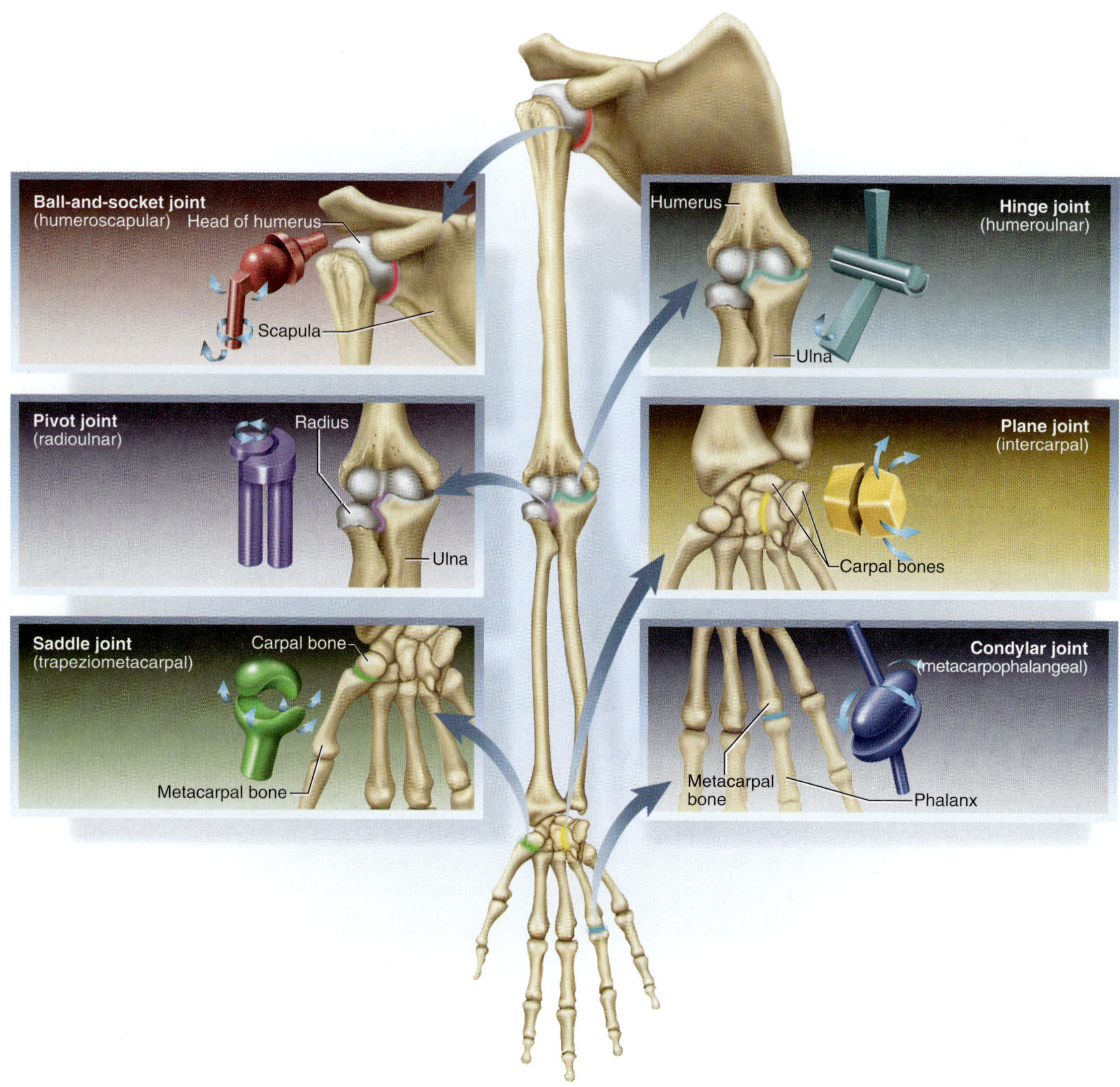

FIGURE 1.12 The six types of synovial joints

which would result in a flexion angle of 50 degrees. Even though the knee is extended, it is still flexed, only less so than before.

Some movement terms may be used to describe motion at several joints throughout the body, whereas other terms are relatively specific to a joint or group of joints. In the sections below, rather than being listed alphabetically, the terms are grouped according to body area and paired with opposite terms where applicable. Additionally, prefixes such as *hyper-* or *hypo-* are sometimes combined with these terms to emphasize motion beyond or below normal, respectively. Of these combined terms, *hyperextension* is the most commonly used.

TERMS DESCRIBING GENERAL MOVEMENTS

Abduction

Abduction is lateral movement away from the midline of the trunk in the frontal plane. An example is raising the arms or legs to the side horizontally.

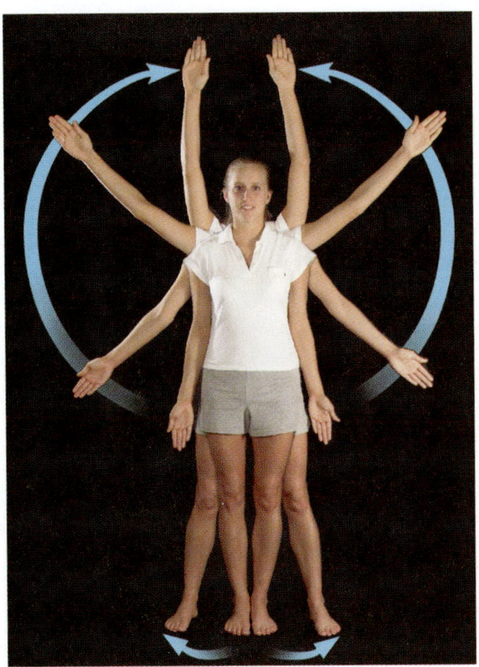

Adduction

Adduction is movement medially toward the midline of the trunk in the frontal plane. Examples are lowering the arm to the side and lowering the thigh back to the anatomical position.

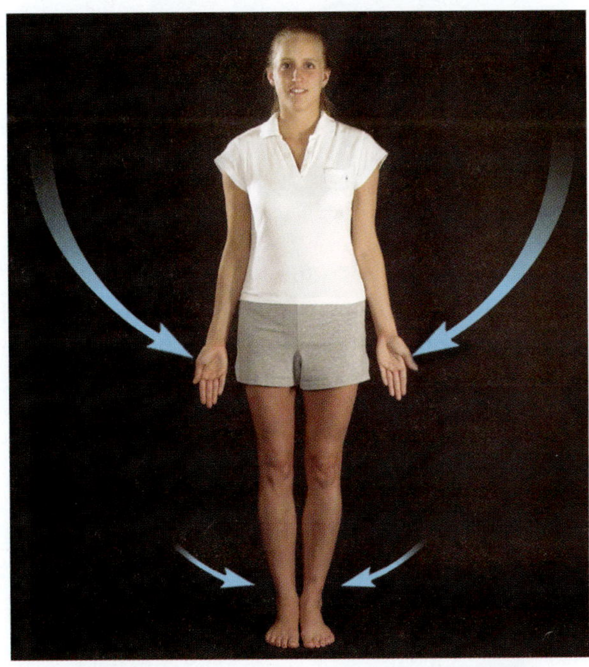

Flexion

Flexion is a bending movement that results in a decrease of the angle in a joint by bringing bones together, usually in the sagittal plane. An example is when the hand is drawn to the shoulder.

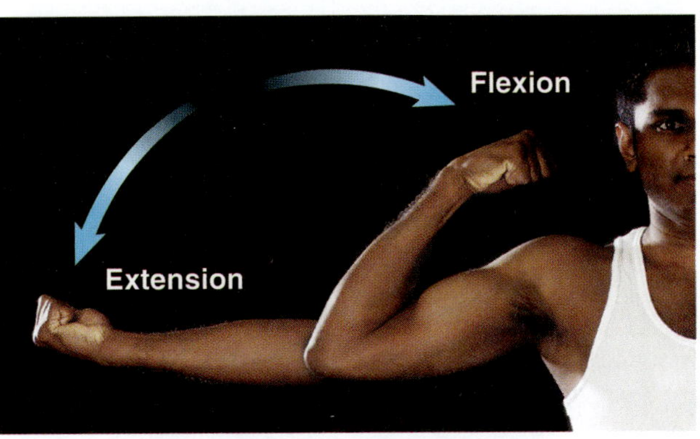

Extension

Extension is a straightening movement that results in an increase of the angle in a joint by moving bones apart, usually in the sagittal plane. An example is the movement in the elbow joint when the hand moves away from the shoulder.

Circumduction

Circumduction is a circular movement of a limb that delineates an arc or a cone. It is a combination of flexion, extension, abduction, and adduction; sometimes it is referred to as *circumflexion*. An example occurs when the shoulder joint and the hip joint move in a circular fashion around a fixed point, either clockwise or counterclockwise.

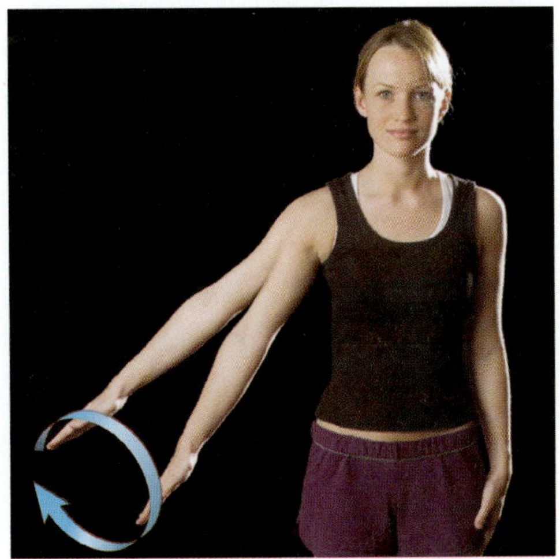

External Rotation

External rotation is a rotary movement around the longitudinal axis of a bone away from the midline of the body. It occurs in the transverse plane and is also known as *rotation laterally, outward rotation,* and *lateral rotation*. The femur is rotated externally if a person turns the feet out while walking.

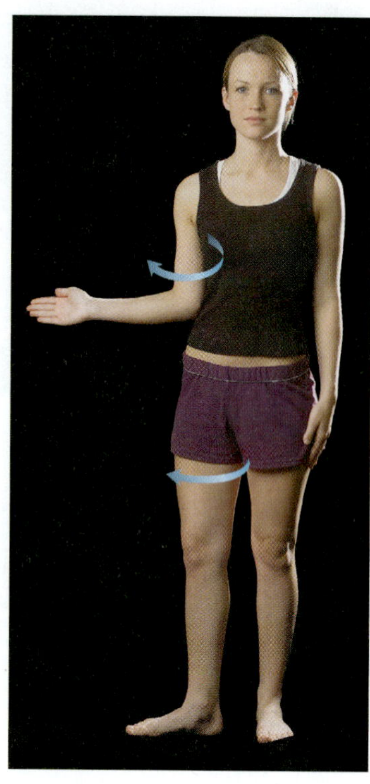

Internal Rotation

Internal rotation is a rotary movement around the longitudinal axis of a bone toward the midline of the body. It occurs in the transverse plane and is also known as *rotation medially, inward rotation,* and *medial rotation.* The femur is rotated internally if the feet are turned in while walking.

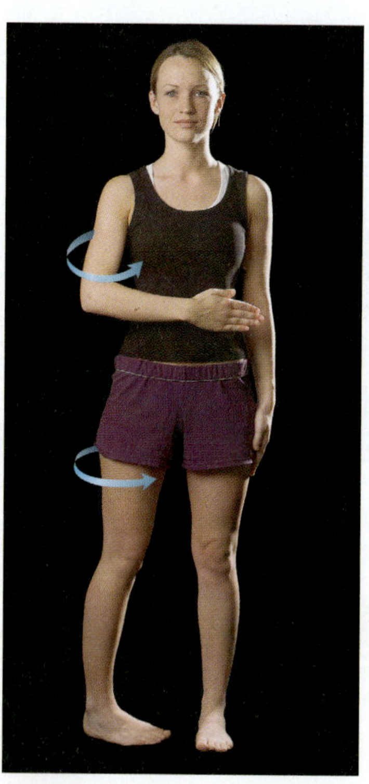

TERMS DESCRIBING ANKLE AND FOOT MOVEMENTS

Eversion

Eversion consists of turning the sole of the foot outward or laterally in the frontal plane; it is also known as abduction of the foot. An example is standing with the weight on the inner edge of the foot.

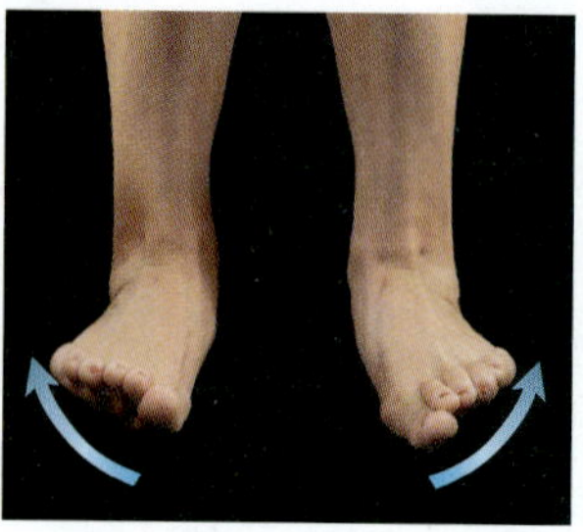

Inversion

Inversion consists of turning the sole of the foot inward or medially in the frontal plane; it is also known as adduction of the foot. An example is standing with the weight on the outer edge of the foot.

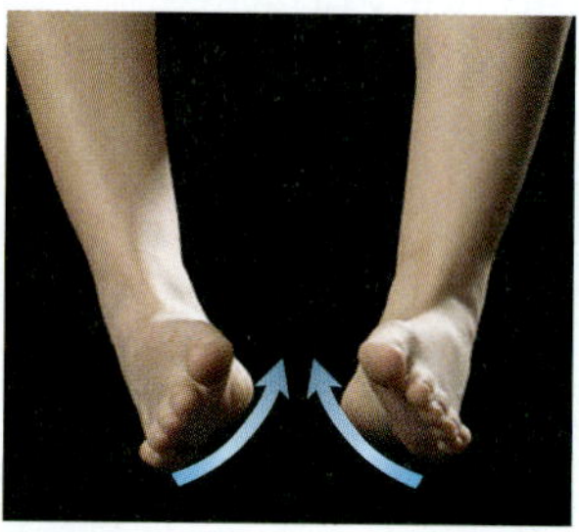

Dorsal Flexion (Dorsiflexion)

Dorsiflexion is a flexion movement of the ankle that results in the top of the foot moving toward the anterior tibia bone in the sagittal plane.

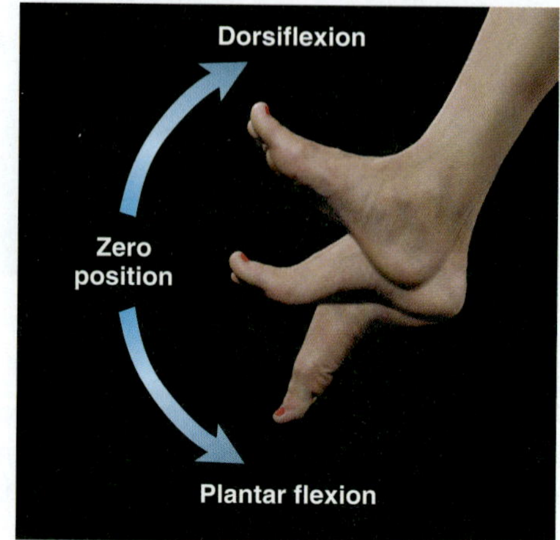

Plantar flexion

Plantar flexion is an extension movement of the ankle that results in the foot and/or toes moving away from the body in the sagittal plane.

Pronation

Pronation is a combination of ankle dorsiflexion, subtalar eversion, and forefoot abduction (toe-out).

Supination

Supination is a combination of ankle plantar flexion, subtalar inversion, and forefoot adduction (toe-in).

TERMS DESCRIBING RADIOULNAR JOINT MOVEMENTS

Pronation (Radial Rotation)

Pronation consists of internally rotating the radius in the transverse plane so that it lies diagonally across the ulna, resulting in the palm-down position of the forearm. Also known as *radial rotation*.

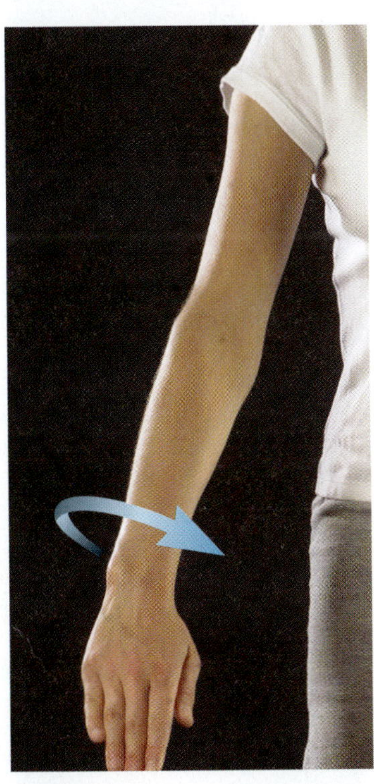

Supination (Ulnar Rotation)

Supination consists of externally rotating the radius in the transverse plane so that it lies parallel to the ulna, resulting in the palm-up position of the forearm. It is also known as *ulnar rotation*.

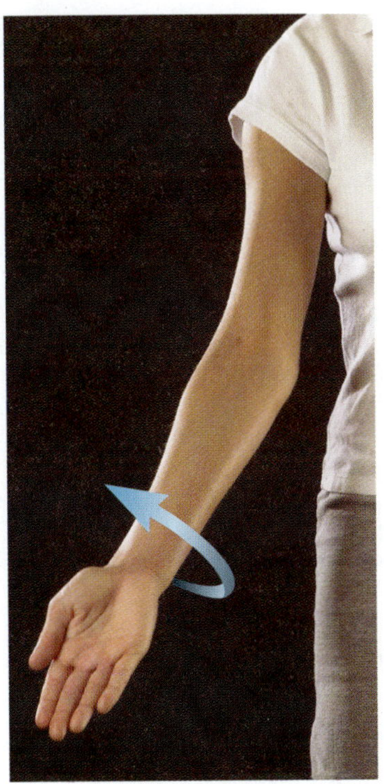

TERMS DESCRIBING SHOULDER GIRDLE MOVEMENTS

Elevation

Elevation is a superior movement of the shoulder girdle in the frontal plane. An example is shrugging the shoulders.

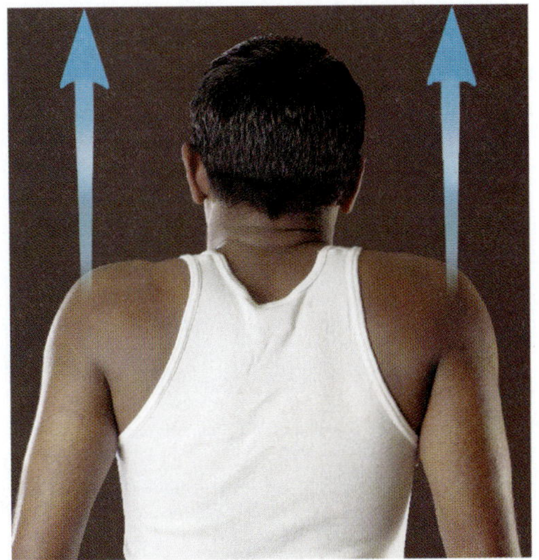

Depression

Depression is an inferior movement of the shoulder girdle in the frontal plane. An example is returning to the normal position from a shoulder shrug.

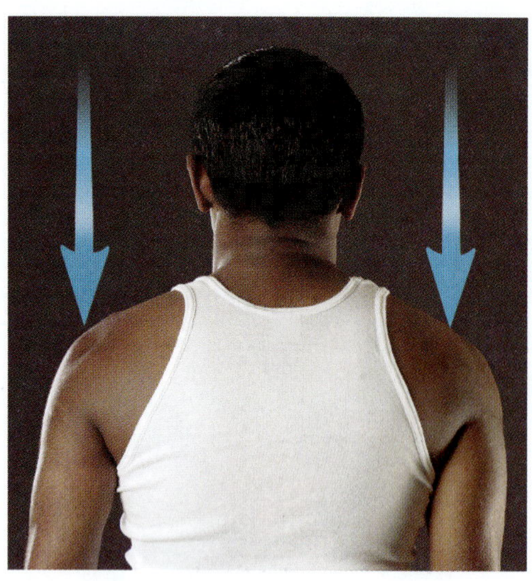

Rotation Upward

Rotation upward is a rotary movement of the scapula in the frontal plane with the inferior angle of the scapula moving laterally and upward.

Rotation Downward

Rotation downward is a rotary movement of the scapula in the frontal plane with the inferior angle of the scapula moving medially and downward. It occurs primarily in the return from upward rotation. The inferior angle may actually move upward slightly as the scapula continues in extreme downward rotation.

Protraction (Abduction)

Protraction is a forward movement of the shoulder girdle in the horizontal plane, away from the spine. It is also known as *abduction of the scapula.*

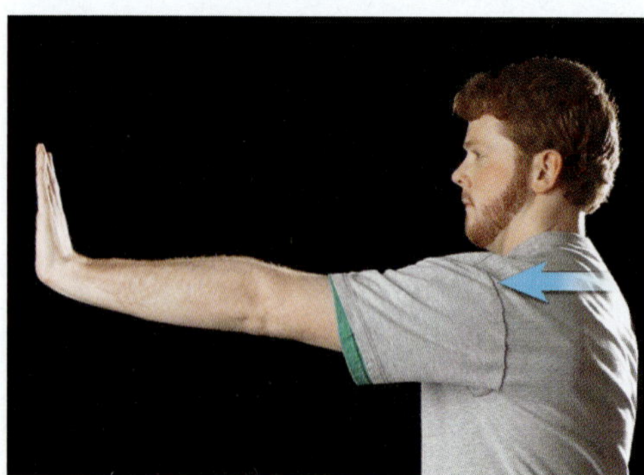

Retraction (Adduction)

Retraction is a backward movement of the shoulder girdle in the horizontal plane, toward the spine. It is also known as *adduction of the scapula*.

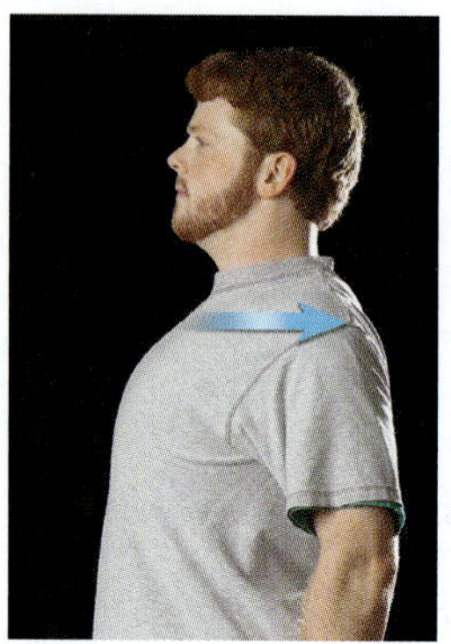

TERMS DESCRIBING SHOULDER JOINT MOVEMENTS

Horizontal Abduction

Horizontal abduction is a movement of the humerus in the horizontal plane away from the midline of the body. It is also known as *horizontal extension* or *transverse abduction.*

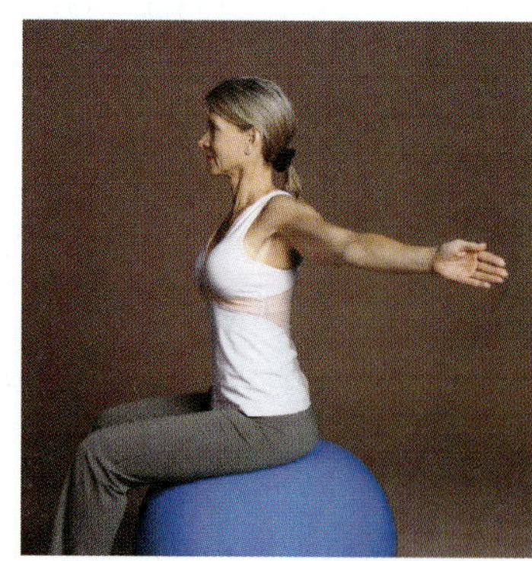

Horizontal Adduction

Horizontal adduction is a movement of the humerus in the horizontal plane toward the midline of the body. It is also known as *horizontal flexion* or *transverse adduction.*

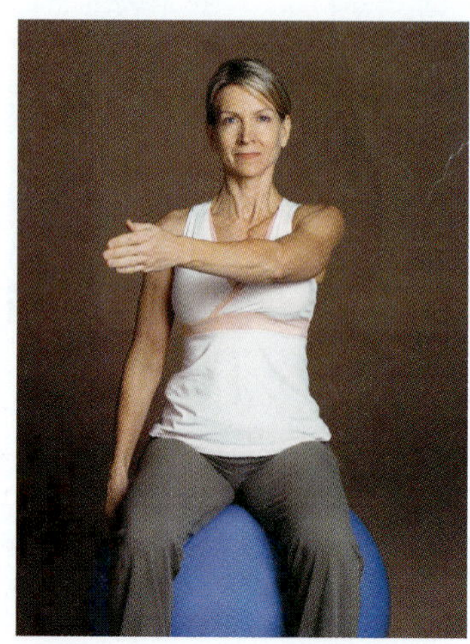

TERMS DESCRIBING SPINE MOVEMENTS

Lateral Flexion (Side Bending)

Lateral flexion is a movement of the head and/or trunk in the frontal plane laterally away from the midline. It is also known as *abduction of the spine.*

Extension (Reduction)

Extension is the return of the spinal column in the frontal plane to the anatomical position from lateral flexion. It is also known as *adduction of the spine.* Hyperextension of the spine [panel (b), below] occurs when the spine goes beyond neutral extension.

Rotation

Rotation is a movement in the transverse plane; the spine can rotate 90 degrees.

TERMS DESCRIBING WRIST AND HAND MOVEMENTS

Dorsal Flexion (Dorsiflexion)

Dorsal flexion is an extension movement of the wrist in the sagittal plane with the dorsal, or posterior, side of the hand moving toward the posterior side of the lateral forearm.

Palmar Flexion

Palmar flexion is a flexion movement of the wrist in the sagittal plane with the volar, or anterior, side of the hand moving toward the anterior side of the forearm.

Radial Flexion (Radial Deviation)

Radial flexion is an abduction movement at the wrist in the frontal plane of the thumb side of the hand toward the lateral forearm.

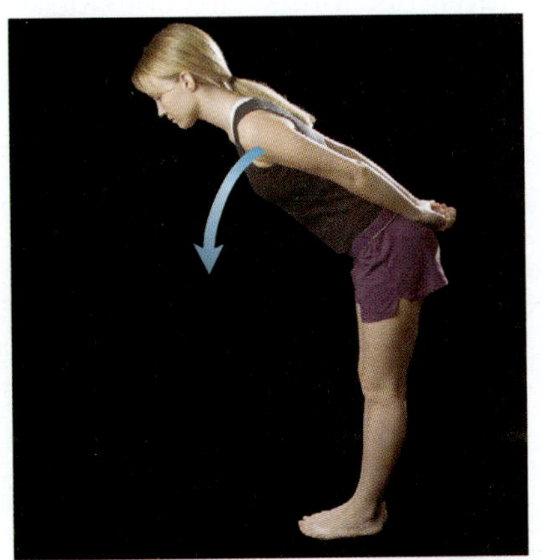

(a) Flexion

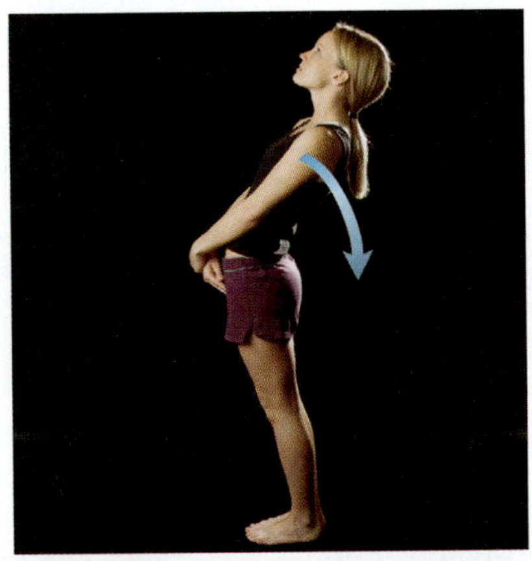

(b) Hyperextension

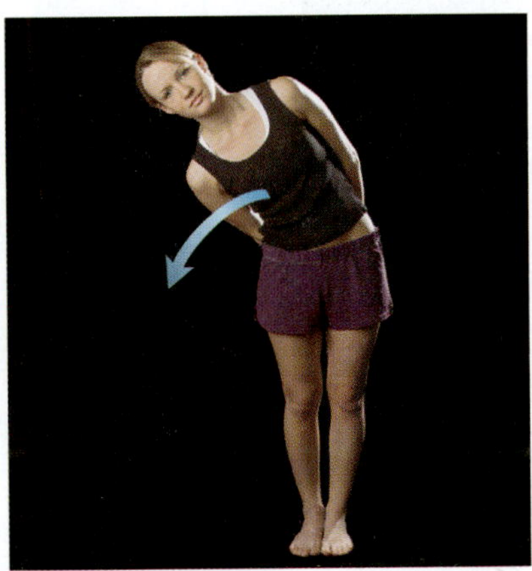

(c) Lateral flexion

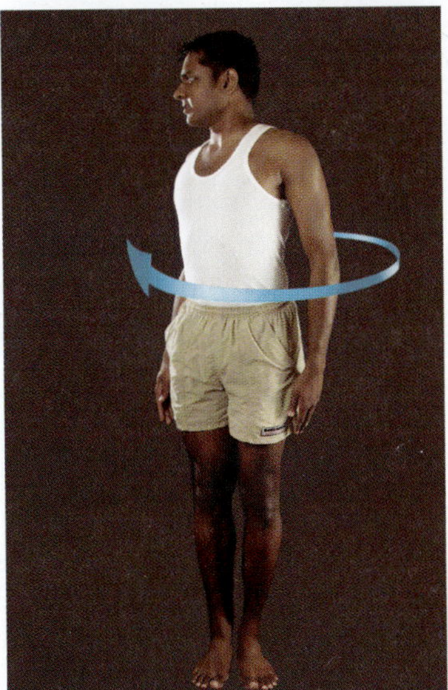

(d) Right rotation

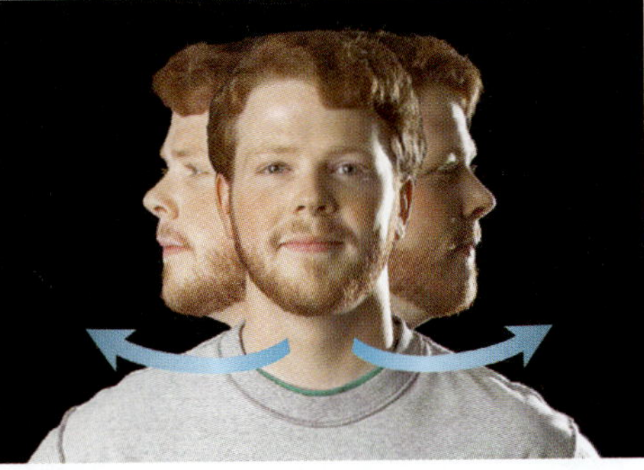

(e) Rotation

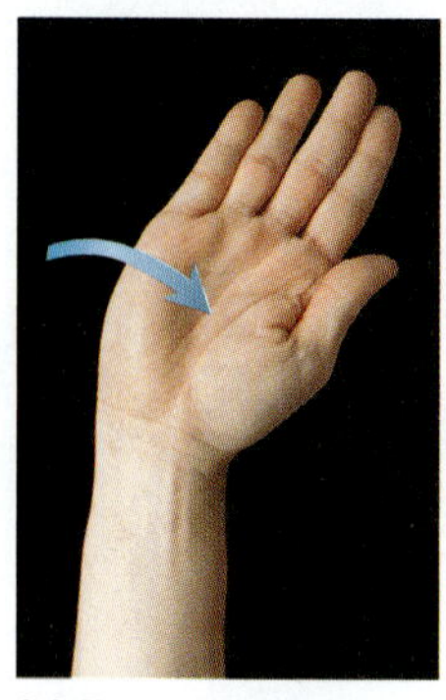
(a) Radial flexion

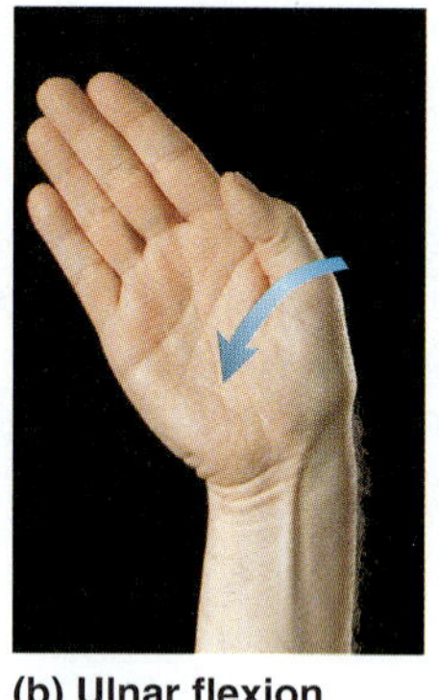
(b) Ulnar flexion

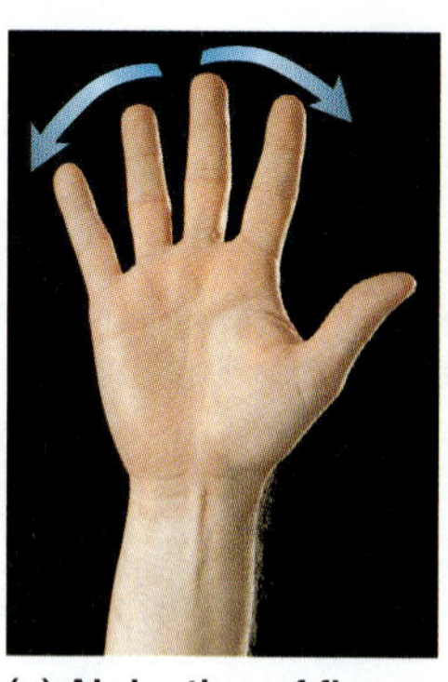
(c) Abduction of fingers

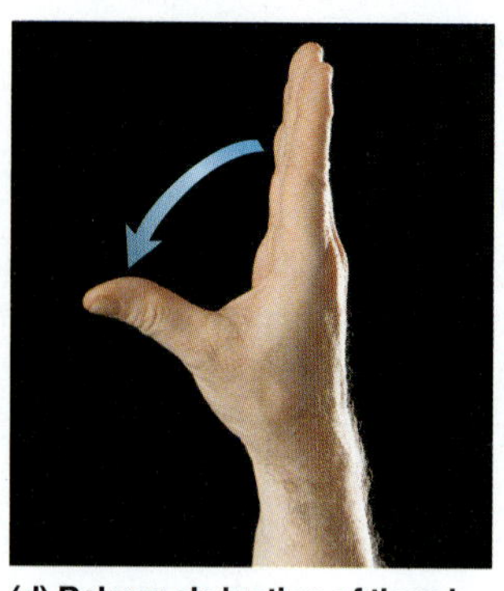
(d) Palmar abduction of thumb

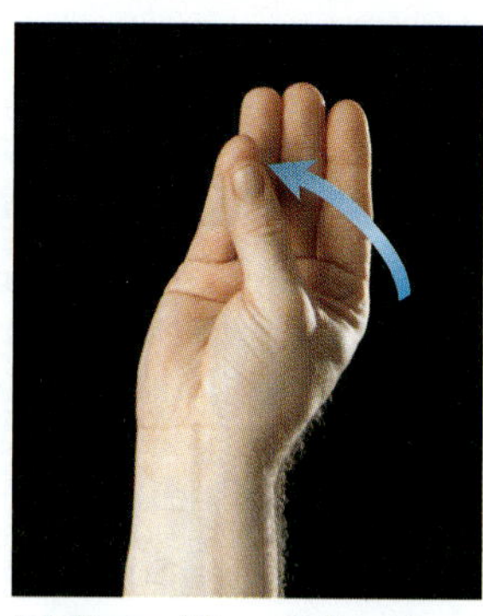
(e) Opposition of thumb

Ulnar Flexion (Ulnar Deviation)

Ulnar flexion is an adduction movement at the wrist in the frontal plane of the little-finger side of the hand toward the medial forearm.

Opposition of the Thumb

Opposition of the thumb is a diagonal movement of the thumb across the palmar surface of the hand to make contact with the fingers.

Reposition of the Thumb

Reposition of the thumb is a diagonal movement of the thumb as it returns to the anatomical position from opposition with the hand and/or fingers.

Also, combinations of wrist and hand movements can occur. Flexion or extension can occur with abduction, adduction, or rotation. These movements, as they apply to individual joints, are considered in more detail in the chapters that follow.

CHAPTER *summary*

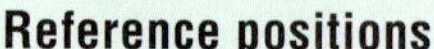

Reference positions

- ✔ To better understand the musculoskeletal system, planes of motion, joint classification, and joint movement terminology, it is crucial for kinesiology students to begin with a reference point.

Anatomical directional terminology

- ✔ In order to study the human body, students must understand the directional terminology applied to it. Because students often get confused by the multiple terms used to describe areas of the body, it is important and necessary to start with the basics.

Body regions

- ✔ The body can be divided into axial and appendicular regions. Each of these regions may be further divided into different regions such as the cephalic, cervical, trunk, upper limbs, and lower limbs. Within each of these regions are many specific subregions.

Planes of motion

- ✔ For the clinician to analyze human movement, it is necessary to understand the planes of motion. A plane of motion may be defined as an imaginary two-dimensional surface through which a limb or body segment moves.
- ✔ There are three specific, or cardinal, planes of motion into which the various joint movements can be classified; they are the sagittal, frontal, and transverse planes, and each divides a segment of the body into halves.

Axes of rotation

- ✔ As movement occurs in a given plane, the joint moves or turns around an axis of rotation that has a 90-degree relationship to that plane. The axes are named in relation to their orientations to planes of motion.

Skeletal system

- ✔ The skeletal system is divided into two distinct parts: the central axial skeleton (skull, vertebral column, and thoracic cage) and the appendicular skeleton (bones of the upper and lower limbs). There are typically 206 bones in the adult skeleton, but the actual number differs from person to person. A newborn has more bones, and the number increases into adolescence before decreasing as the bones fuse.

✔ Bones have specific markings that assist muscles, ligaments, and tendons in their functions. Many markings serve as bony landmarks for muscle attachments and joint function. These bone markings include processes and cavities.

Types of joints

✔ The articulation of two or more bones allows various types of movements. The extent of the movement, or range of motion, is determined by the type of joint. Some joints are slightly movable, some move freely, and some do not move at all. The three structural classifications of joints are synarthrodial, amphiarthrodial, and diarthrodial.

Movements in joints

✔ Joints have a wide range of movements, and range of motion can be measured on the human body via a goniometer. Since every joint has a specific range of motion, it is important to establish a baseline so that the clinician can compare changes within the movements.

CHAPTER *review*

True or False

Write true *or* false *after each statement.*

1. The synovial joints of the body are diarthrodial joints. T
2. A good example of a gomphosis joint is the thumb joint. F
3. Humans are born with exactly 206 bones. F
4. The term *ipsilateral* describes a movement, position, or landmark location that is on the same side as the reference point. T
5. The tensor fascia latae is located on the anterolateral femur. T
6. Range of motion can be measured only by a measuring tape. F
7. Hyaline cartilage offers support and reduces friction in joints. T
8. Diarthrodial joints can have motion in one or more planes. T
9. A joint moves or turns around an axis that has a 90-degree relationship to a plane. T
10. The skeletal system is composed of two regions: the appendicular skeleton and the cervical skeleton. F

Short Answers

Write your answers on the lines provided.

1. Why is the anatomical (or fundamental) position so important in understanding anatomy and joint movements?
   It is set point for Measuring range of motion
2. Why is it important to understand functional anatomy as well as structural anatomy?
   So, the bodys movement can be analyzed
3. Why are synovial joints so important?
   freely movable joints
4. What is a good example of a gomphosis joint?
   Teeth sockets
5. In which plane does the movement of a golf swing take place?
   Mostly Frontal
6. A patient presents with sciatic pain and has great difficulty getting out of a chair. How can understanding functional anatomy help a clinician assess this patient?
   locate weak muscles & better assess movement

7. Describe the agonist and antagonist in hip abduction.

Agonist – Gluteus medius, TFL
Antagonist – Adductors

8. What covers the ends of the bones located in the joint cavities?

Hyaline cartilage

9. How would poor hip range of motion affect gait?

Limited ROM hinders gait.

10. In which plane does radioulnar rotation (supination and pronation) take place?

Transverse

Multiple Choice

Circle the correct answers.

1. A biceps curl occurs in which plane?
   a. sagittal
   b. frontal
   c. transverse
   d. diagonal

2. Understanding movement in planes helps the professional:
   a. locate muscle attachments
   b. analyze movements more precisely
   c. heal muscle strains
   d. prevent faulty gait issues

3. The humerus is part of the:
   a. rib cage
   b. appendicular skeleton
   c. scapulae
   d. axial skeleton

4. Diarthrodial joints are best described as:
   a. joint capsules
   b. partially movable
   c. fixed
   d. freely movable

5. Range of motion is defined as:
   a. the speed at which a joint moves
   b. eccentric contraction of muscles
   c. how far a joint moves freely and painlessly
   d. a measurement of muscle length

6. Circumduction is a combination of:
   a. adduction and abduction
   b. internal and external rotation
   c. flexion and extension
   d. all of the above

7. The iliopsoas flexes the hip in which plane?
   a. frontal
   b. sagittal
   c. transverse
   d. oblique

8. Elevation of the shoulder is an important movement for:
   a. playing tennis
   b. reaching for a glass on the top shelf
   c. lifting a child
   d. all of the above

9. Supination of the radius occurs in which plane?
   a. frontal
   b. sagittal
   c. horizontal
   d. coronal

10. To help with assessment, muscle attachments and functional movements should:
    a. be applied to real-life situations
    b. never be considered
    c. be calculated with a goniometer
    d. be assessed by a physician

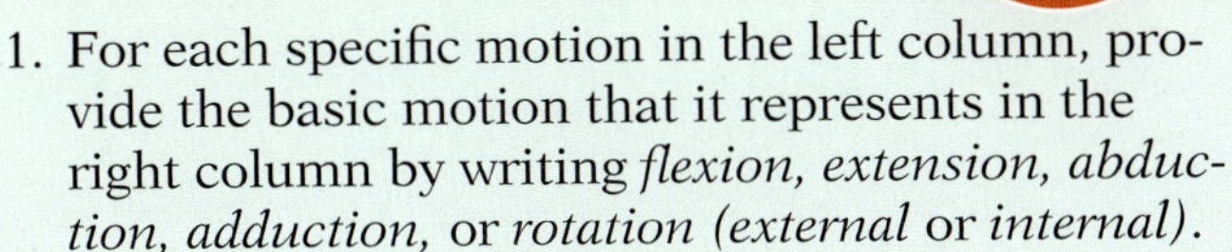

1. For each specific motion in the left column, provide the basic motion that it represents in the right column by writing *flexion, extension, abduction, adduction,* or *rotation (external* or *internal)*.

Specific Motion	Basic Motion
Eversion	Abduction
Inversion	adduction
Dorsal flexion	Flexion
Plantar flexion	extension
Pronation	internal rotation
Supination	external rotation
Lateral flexion	abduction
Radial flexion	abduction
Ulnar flexion	adduction

2. For each diarthrodial classification, give a joint example, the plane in which it moves, and its type of movement.

Classification	Joint Example	Plane	Movement
Ginglymus	Elbow, Knee, ankle	Saggital	Flexion, Extension
Trochoid	Radio ulnar, atlanto axial	Transverse	Rotation
Condyloid	2–5th, Metacarpophalangeal metatarsophalangeal	Saggital, Frontal	Flex, Ext, abd, add
Arthrodial	Transverse tarsal C2–S1	" , transv.	Flex, ext, add, abd, rot.
Enarthrodial	Glenohumeral acetabularfemoral	" "	Flex, ext, add, abd, rot.
Sellar	1st Carpometacarpal	" "	Flex, ext, add

chapter 2

Neuromuscular Fundamentals

LEARNING OUTCOMES

After completing this chapter, you should be able to:

2-1 Review the basic anatomy and function of the muscular and nervous systems.

2-2 Identify terminology used to describe muscular locations, arrangements, characteristics, and roles, as well as neuromuscular functions.

2-3 List the different types of muscle contractions and the factors involved in each.

2-4 Define neuromuscular concepts in relation to how muscles function in joint movement and work together to achieve motion.

2-5 Describe the neural control mechanisms for movement.

KEY TERMS

Action
Aggregate muscle action
Agonists
All-or-none principle
Amplitude
Angle of pull
Antagonists
Biarticular
Concentric contractions
Contractibility
Dermatome
Eccentric contractions
Elasticity
Extensibility
Extrinsic
Gaster
Golgi tendon organ (GTO)
Innervation
Insertion
Intrinsic
Isokinetics
Isometric contractions
Isotonic contractions
Kinesthesis
Line of pull
Multiarticular
Muscle spindle
Myotome
Neurons
Neutralizers
Origin
Proprioceptors
Reciprocal innervation
Sliding-filament theory
Stabilizers
Stretch reflex
Synergists
Tendon
Treppe
Uniarticular

Introduction

When the human body begins a movement, myriad actions are involved that people usually never consider. The brain sends nerve signals to the skeletal muscles, and chemicals are released to contract those muscles; then the joints move with the cooperation of all of these elements. Since there are hundreds of muscles in the human body, it is necessary to have knowledge about their shapes, locations, and functions, as well as their neuromuscular principles. Joint movements are possible because of the combined efforts of nerves and muscles, and the precision of the body's movements is driven by thousands of contractions and nerve innervations. Humans have the capacity to generate great force with their arms and hands, and yet they are able to switch in a split second to a task as precise as playing a piano. Governing such movements is the fascinating world of neuromuscular fundamentals.

Muscle contraction produces the force that causes joint movement. In addition to contributing to movement, muscles also provide protection, contribute to posture and support, and produce a major portion of total body heat. There are more than 600 skeletal muscles, which constitute approximately 40 to 50 percent of the body's weight. Of these, there are 215 pairs of skeletal muscles. These pairs of muscles usually work in cooperation with each other to perform opposite actions at the joints they cross. In most cases, muscles work in groups rather than independently to achieve a particular joint motion. This is known as **aggregate muscle action.**

Muscle Nomenclature

In attempting to learn the skeletal muscles, it is helpful to study how they are named. For example, a rotary-shaped muscle such as the gluteus maximus has a powerful action because of its quadrilateral shape. The functional action can be assessed by the muscle shape. In addition to being named for their shape, muscles are usually named because of one or more distinctive characteristics, such as their anatomical location or their function. Examples of skeletal muscle naming are as follows:

Shape: deltoid, rhomboid

Size: gluteus maximus, teres minor

Number of divisions: triceps brachii

Direction of its fibers: external oblique

Location: rectus femoris, palmaris longus

Points of attachment: coracobrachialis, extensor hallucis longus, flexor digitorum longus

Action: erector spinae, supinator, extensor digiti minimi

Action and shape: pronator quadratus

Action and size: adductor magnus

Shape and location: serratus anterior

Location and attachment: brachioradialis

Location and number of divisions: biceps femoris

When discussing the muscles, educators often group them together for brevity of conversation and clearer understanding. In this text, later chapters group muscles as they best suit the techniques. The naming of muscle groups follows a pattern similar to the naming of individual muscles. Below are some muscle groups according to different naming rationales:

Shape: hamstrings

Number of divisions: quadriceps, triceps surae

Location: peroneals, abdominal, shoulder girdle

Action: hip flexors, rotator cuff

Figure 2.1 depicts the muscular system from a superficial point of view. Not shown in these diagrams are the deep muscles. The muscles shown in figure 2.1, and many other muscles, are studied in more detail as each joint of the body is considered in other chapters of this book.

Shape of Muscles and Fascicle (Fiber Bundle) Arrangement

Various muscles have different shapes, and their fibers may be arranged differently in relation to each other and to the tendons to which they join. Figure 2.2 shows the classification of muscles according to fascicle orientation. As mentioned about the gluteus maximus muscle, the shape and fiber arrangement play a role in the muscle's ability to exert force. These factors also affect the range through which a muscle can effectively exert force. One factor in the muscle's ability to exert force is its cross-section diameter. Keeping all other factors constant, a muscle with a greater cross-section diameter will be able to exert a greater force. Another factor relative to a muscle's ability to move a joint through a large range of motion is its ability to shorten. Generally, longer muscles can shorten through a greater range and therefore are more effective in moving joints through large ranges of motion.

Essentially, all skeletal muscles may be grouped into two major types of fiber arrangements: parallel and pennate. Each may be subdivided further according to shape.

Parallel muscles have their fibers arranged parallel to the length of the muscle. Generally, parallel muscles produce a greater range of movement than similar-size muscles with a pennate arrangement. Parallel muscles are categorized into the shapes listed below:

- *Flat* muscles are usually thin and broad, originating from broad, fibrous, sheetlike aponeuroses that allow them to spread their forces over a broad area. Examples include the rectus abdominis and external oblique.
- *Fusiform* muscles are spindle-shaped with a central belly that tapers to tendons on each end; this allows them to focus their power onto small, bony targets. Examples are the brachialis and the brachioradialis.

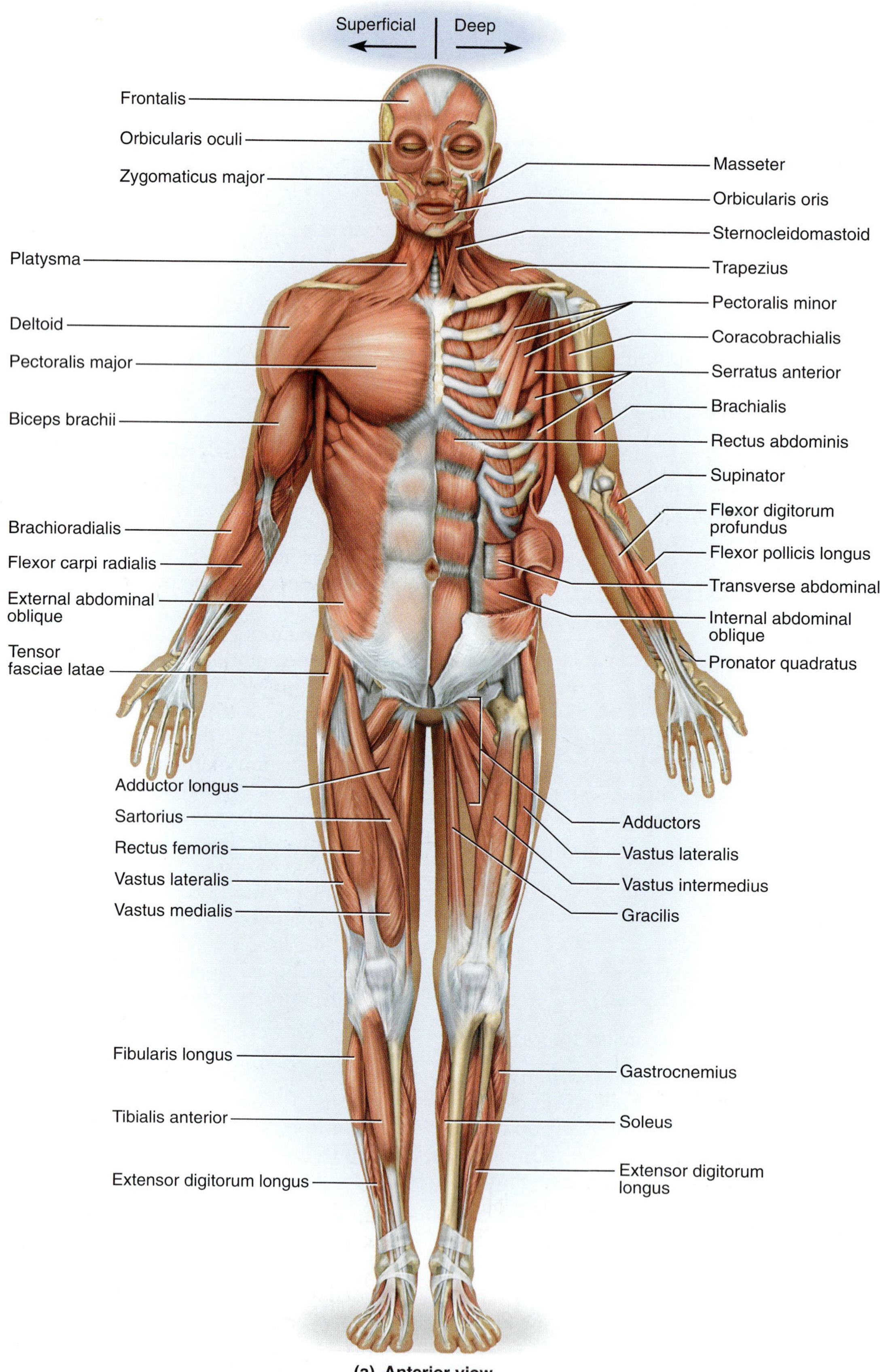

(a) Anterior view

FIGURE 2.1 The muscular system

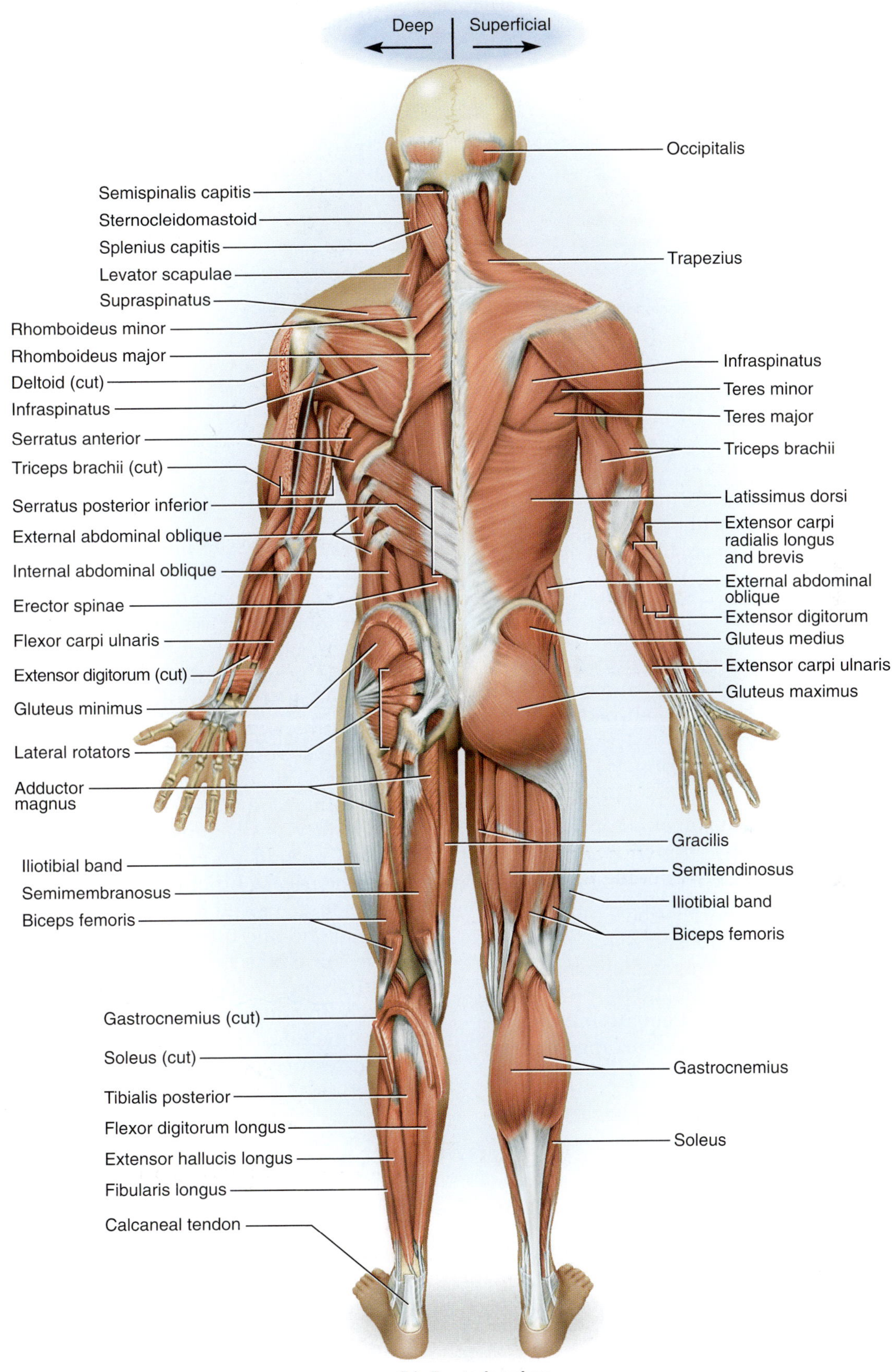

(b) Posterior view

FIGURE 2.1 *(Continued)*

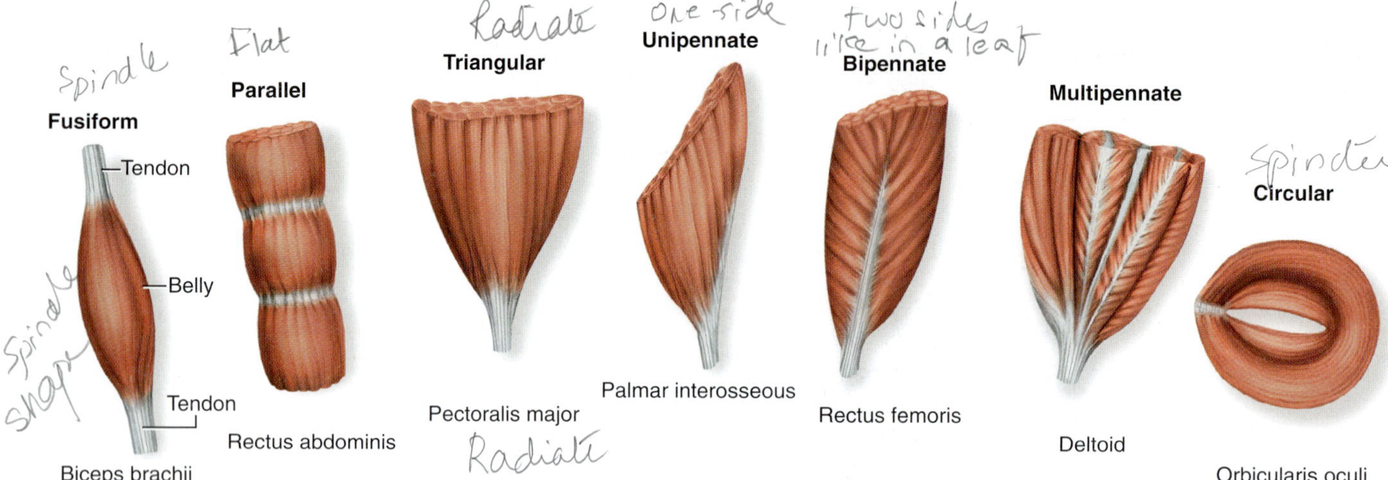

FIGURE 2.2 Classification of muscles

- *Strap muscles* are more uniform in diameter, with essentially all of their fibers arranged in a long parallel manner. This enables a focusing of power onto small, bony targets. The sartorius is an example.
- *Radiate* muscles are sometimes described as being triangular, fan-shaped, or convergent. They have the combined arrangement of flat and fusiform muscles, in that they originate on broad aponeuroses and converge onto a tendon. Examples are the pectoralis major and trapezius.
- *Sphincter,* or circular, muscles are technically endless strap muscles that surround openings and function to close them on contraction. An example is the orbicularis oris surrounding the mouth.

Pennate muscles have shorter fibers that are arranged obliquely to their tendons in a structure similar to that of a feather. This arrangement increases the cross-sectional area of the muscle, thereby increasing its force production capability. Pennate muscles are categorized on the basis of the exact arrangement between the fibers and the tendon:

- *Unipennate* muscle fibers run obliquely from a tendon on one side only. Examples are seen in the biceps femoris, extensor digitorum longus, and tibialis posterior.
- *Bipennate* muscle fibers run obliquely on both sides from a central tendon, as in the rectus femoris and flexor hallucis longus.
- *Multipennate* muscles have several tendons with fibers running diagonally between them, as in the deltoid.

Bipennate and unipennate produce the strongest contraction.

Muscle-Tissue Properties

Skeletal muscle tissue has four properties related to its ability to produce force and movement about the joints. *Irritability* or *excitability* is the muscle property of being sensitive or responsive to chemical, electrical, and mechanical stimuli. When an appropriate stimulus is provided, the muscle responds by developing tension. **Contractibility** is the muscle's ability to contract and develop tension or an internal force against resistance when stimulated. The ability of muscle tissue to develop tension or contract is unique; other body tissues do not have this property. **Extensibility** is the muscle's ability to be passively stretched beyond its normal resting length. For example, the triceps brachii displays extensibility when it is stretched beyond its normal resting length by the biceps brachii and other elbow flexors contracting to achieve full elbow flexion. **Elasticity** is the muscle's ability to return to its original resting length following a stretch. In continuing with the elbow example, the triceps brachii displays elasticity by returning to its original resting length when the elbow flexors cease contracting and relax.

Muscle Terminology

Locating the muscles, their proximal and distal attachments, and their relationships to the joints they cross is critical in determining the effects that muscles have on the joints. The following terms are necessary to consider in the study of body movement:

Intrinsic: a term pertaining, usually, to muscles that are within or belong solely to the body part on which they act. Examples are the small intrinsic muscles found entirely within the hand.

Extrinsic: a term pertaining, usually, to muscles that arise or originate outside (proximal to) the body part on which they act. Examples are the forearm muscles that attach proximally on the distal humerus and insert on the fingers.

Action: the specific movement of a joint that results from a concentric contraction of a muscle that crosses the joint. An example is the biceps brachii, which has the action of flexion at the elbow. In most cases, a particular action is caused by a group of muscles working together. Any of the muscles in the group can be said to cause the action (be the primary mover), even though the action is usually an effort of the entire group. A particular muscle may cause more than one action either at the same joint or at different joints, depending on the characteristics of the joints crossed by the muscle and the exact location of the muscle and its attachments in relation to the joint(s).

Innervation: the segment of the nervous system defined as being responsible for providing a stimulus to muscle fibers within a specific muscle or portion of a muscle. A particular muscle may be innervated by more than one nerve, and a particular nerve may innervate more than one muscle or portion of a muscle.

Amplitude: the range of muscle-fiber length between maximal and minimal lengthening.

Gaster (belly or body): the central, fleshy portion of the muscle that generally increases in diameter as the muscle contracts. The gaster is the contractile portion of the muscle. When a particular muscle contracts, it tends to pull both ends toward the gaster, or middle, of the muscle. Consequently, if neither of the bones to which a muscle is attached were stabilized, both bones would move toward each other on contraction. The more common case, however, is that one bone is more stabilized by a variety of factors, and, as a result, the less stabilized bone usually moves toward the more stabilized bone on contraction.

Tendon: the fibrous connective tissue, often cordlike in appearance, that connects muscles to bones and other structures. In some cases, two muscles may share a common tendon, such as the Achilles tendon of the gastrocnemius and soleus muscles. In other cases, a muscle may have multiple tendons connecting it to one or more bones, such as the three proximal attachments of the triceps brachii.

Origin: from a structural perspective, the proximal attachment of a muscle, or the part that attaches closest to the midline or center of the body. From a functional and historical perspective, the least movable part or attachment of the muscle has generally been considered to be the origin.

Insertion: structurally, the distal attachment of a muscle, or the part that attaches farthest from the midline or center of the body. Functionally and historically, the most movable part is generally considered the insertion.

As an example, in the biceps curl exercise, the biceps brachii muscle in the arm has its origin on the scapula (least movable bone) and its insertion on the radius (most movable bone). In some movements this process can be reversed. An example of this reversal can be seen in the pull-up, in which the radius is relatively stable and the scapula moves up. Even though in this example the most movable bone is reversed, the proximal attachment of the biceps brachii is always on the scapula and still considered to be the origin, while the insertion is still on the radius. The biceps brachii would be an extrinsic muscle of the elbow, whereas the brachialis would be intrinsic to the elbow. For each muscle studied in this text, the origin and insertion are indicated.

Contraction: The Sliding-Filament Theory

While this book will not delve into the minute anatomy of skeletal muscle (which can be studied in a good physiology text), it is important to understand the principle of contraction. When tension develops in a muscle as a result of a stimulus, the muscle may shorten. This is known as a *contraction.* (Muscles can develop tension without shortening, but this will be discussed later.) Just how a muscle shortens was a puzzle until electron microscopy allowed cytologists to view the molecular organization of muscle fibers. In 1954, Hugh Huxley and Jean Hanson, two researchers at the Massachusetts Institute of Technology, developed a model called the **sliding-filament theory.** Their assumption, or model, was that the myofilaments in muscle do not shorten during a contraction but, rather, that the thin filaments (actin) slide over the thick ones (myosin) and pull the Z disks behind them. This causes each sarcomere as a unit to shorten. A muscle fiber can shorten as much as 40 percent of its resting length. Figure 2.3 shows the entire process, as well as the muscle striations and the location of the Z disks and sarcomere. It should be remembered that even though the muscle fiber contracts to produce force, such as flexion during an elbow curl, the myofilaments do not become shorter. The contraction is a result of a shortening of the sarcomere and the sliding mechanism of the thin and thick filaments. When

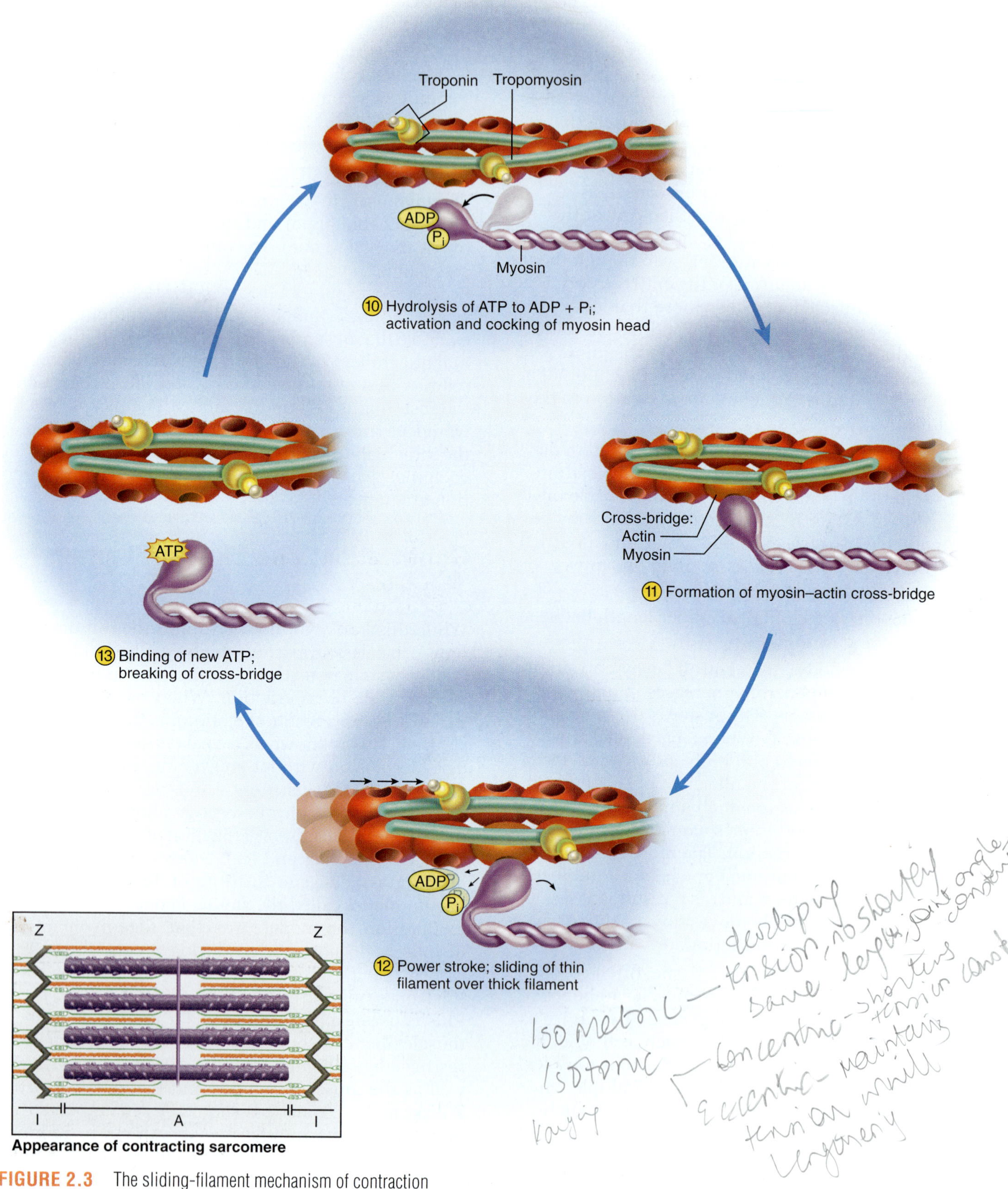

FIGURE 2.3 The sliding-filament mechanism of contraction

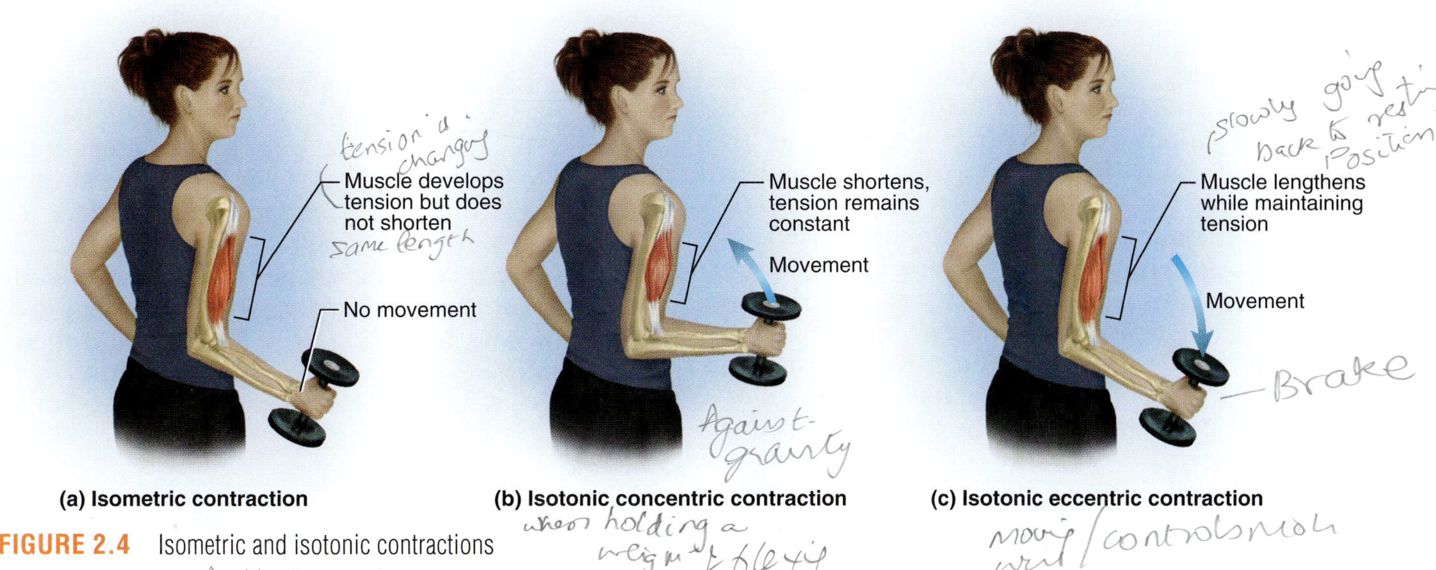

FIGURE 2.4 Isometric and isotonic contractions

a muscle's work is complete—for example, after lifting a dumbbell—the muscle fiber relaxes and returns to its resting length.

Types of Muscle Contractions (Actions)

The term *muscle contraction* may be confusing, because in some types of contractions the muscle does not shorten in length as the term *contraction* indicates. As a result, it is becoming increasingly common to refer to the various types of muscle contractions as *muscle actions* instead.

Muscle contractions can be used to cause, control, or prevent joint movement. To elaborate, muscle contractions can be used to initiate or accelerate the movement of a body segment, to slow down or decelerate the movement of a body segment, or to prevent movement of a body segment by external forces. All muscle contractions or actions can be classified as being either isometric or isotonic. An **isometric contraction** occurs when tension develops within the muscle but the joint angles remain constant. Isometric contractions may be thought of as static contractions, because a significant amount of tension may be developed in the muscle to maintain the joint angle in a relatively static or stable position, without an actual shortening of muscle fibers. Isometric contractions may be used to stabilize a body segment to prevent it from being moved by external forces.

Isotonic contractions occur when the muscle develops tension to either cause or control joint movement. They may be thought of as dynamic contractions, because the varying degrees of tension in the muscles are causing the joint angles to change. The isotonic type of muscle contraction is classified further as being either concentric or eccentric on the basis of whether shortening or lengthening occurs. **Concentric contractions** occur when the muscle develops tension as it shortens, whereas **eccentric contractions** occur when the muscle lengthens under tension. Figure 2.4 illustrates isometric contractions and isotonic concentric and eccentric contractions.

It is also important to note that movement may occur at any given joint without any muscle contraction whatsoever. This movement is referred to as *passive* and is solely due to external forces such as force applied by another person, object, or resistance or the force of gravity in the presence of muscle relaxation. An example of passive movement occurs when the femur is being moved manually into abduction by a therapist.

CONCENTRIC CONTRACTION

Concentric contraction involves the muscle developing tension as it shortens; it occurs when the muscle develops enough force to overcome applied resistance. Concentric contractions may be thought of as causing movement against gravity or resistance; they are described as *positive contractions*. The force developed by the muscle is greater than that of the resistance. This results in the joint angle being changed in the direction of the applied muscular force and causes the body part to move against gravity or external forces. Flexing a dumbbell with the biceps is an example of a concentric contraction; the biceps shortens to overcome the resistance.

ECCENTRIC CONTRACTION (MUSCLE ACTION)

Eccentric contraction involves the muscle lengthening under tension; it occurs when the muscle gradually lessens in tension to control the descent of the resistance. The weight or resistance may be thought of as overcoming the muscle contraction, but not to the point that the muscle cannot control the descending movement. Eccentric muscle actions control movement with gravity or resistance; they are described as *negative contractions*. If a dumbbell is curled using the biceps and then slowly returned to the starting position, the return phase is an eccentric contraction. The resistance is greater than the force developed by the biceps. Yet the biceps is able to control the down phase by "braking" as the weight is slowly lowered. Eccentric contractions are used to decelerate the movement of a body segment from a higher speed to a slower speed or to stop the movement of a joint already in motion. Since the muscle is lengthening as opposed to shortening, the relatively recent change in terminology from *muscle contraction* to *muscle action* is becoming more commonly accepted.

Table 2.1 explains the various types of contraction and resultant joint movements. The terminology used in defining and describing these actions is included.

Various exercises may use any one or all of these contraction types for muscle development. Development

TABLE 2.1 Muscle Contraction and Movement Matrix

Definitive and descriptive factors	Type of contraction (muscle action)			Movement without contraction
		Isotonic		
	Isometric	Concentric	Eccentric	
Agonist muscle length	No appreciable change	Shortening →←	Lengthening ←→	Dictated solely by gravity and/or external forces
Antagonist muscle length	No appreciable change	Lengthening ←→	Shortening →←	Dictated solely by gravity and/or external forces
Joint angle changes	No appreciable change	In direction of applied muscular force	In direction of external force (resistance)	Dictated solely by gravity and/or external forces
Direction of body part	Against immovable object or matched external force (resistance)	Against gravity and/or other external force (resistance)	With gravity and/or other external force (resistance)	Consistent with gravity and/or other external forces
Motion	Prevents motion; pressure (force) applied, but no resulting motion	Causes motion	Controls motion	Either no motion or passive motion occurs as a result of gravity and/or other external forces
Description	Static; fixating	Dynamic shortening; positive work	Dynamic lengthening: negative work	Passive; relaxation
Applied muscle force versus resistance	Force = resistance	Force > resistance	Force < resistance	No force, all resistance
Speed relative to gravity or applied resistance including inertial forces	Equal to speed of applied resistance	Faster than the inertia of the resistance	Slower than the speed of gravity or applied inertial forces	Consistent with inertia of applied external forces or the speed of gravity
Acceleration/ deceleration	Zero acceleration	Acceleration ↗	Deceleration ↘	Either zero or acceleration consistent with applied external forces
Descriptive symbol	(=)	(+)	(–)	(0)
Practical application	Prevents external forces from causing movement	Initiates movement or speeds up the rate of movement	Slows down the rate of movement or stops movement, "braking action"	Passive motion by force from gravity and/or other external forces

of exercise machines has resulted in another type of muscle exercise known as **isokinetics.** Isokinetics is not another type of contraction, as some authorities have mistakenly described; rather, it is a specific technique that may use any or all of the different types of contractions. Isokinetics is a type of dynamic exercise usually using concentric and/or eccentric muscle contractions in which the speed (or velocity) of movement is constant and muscular contraction (ideally, maximum contraction) occurs throughout the movement. Biodex, Cybex, Gow, and other new types of apparatuses are engineered to allow this type of exercise.

Students well educated in kinesiology should be able to read the description of an exercise or observe an exercise and immediately know the most important muscles being used. If it is within the student's scope of practice, she should be able to prescribe exercises and activities for the development of muscles and muscle groups in the human body. Descriptive terms of how muscles function in joint movements follow.

ROLE OF MUSCLES

Agonists: muscles that, when contracting concentrically, cause joint motion through a specified plane of motion. They are known as *primary* or *prime movers,* or the muscles most involved.

Antagonists: muscles that are usually located on the opposite side of the joint from the agonist and have the opposite concentric action. Known as *contralateral muscles,* they work in cooperation with agonist muscles by relaxing and allowing movement, but when contracting concentrically, they perform the joint motion opposite that of the agonist.

Stabilizers: muscles that surround the joint or body part and contract to fixate or stabilize the area to enable another limb or body segment to exert force and move. Known as *fixators,* they are essential in establishing a relatively firm base for the more distal joints to work from when carrying out movements.

Synergists: muscles that assist in the action of agonists but are not necessarily prime movers for the action. Known as *guiding muscles,* they assist in refined movement and rule out undesired motions.

Neutralizers: muscles that counteract or neutralize the action of other muscles to prevent undesirable movements such as inappropriate muscle substitutions. Referred to as *neutralizing,* they contract to resist specific actions of other muscles.

Tying Roles of Muscles All Together

When a muscle with multiple agonist actions contracts, it attempts to perform all of its actions. Muscles cannot determine which of their actions are appropriate for the task at hand. The resulting actions actually performed depend on several factors, such as the motor units activated, joint position, muscle length, and relative contraction or relaxation of other muscles acting on the joint. A surgeon might require the delicate preciseness of the fingers and hand to perform a surgery, or he might need the larger muscle groups of the shoulders and arms to split wood outside his house. In certain instances, two muscles may work in synergy by counteracting their opposing actions to accomplish a common action.

As discussed, agonist muscles are primarily responsible for a given movement, such as that of hip flexion and knee extension while a person is kicking a ball. In this example, the hamstrings are antagonistic and relax to allow the kick to occur. This does not mean all other muscles in the hip area are uninvolved. The preciseness of the kick depends on the involvement of many other muscles and the number of motor units innervated. As the lower extremity swings forward, its route and subsequent angle at the point of contact depend on a certain amount of relative contraction or relaxation in the hip abductors, adductors, internal rotators, and external rotators. These muscles act in a synergistic fashion to guide the lower extremity in a precise manner. That is, they are not primarily responsible for knee extension and hip flexion, but they do contribute to the accuracy of the total movement. These guiding muscles assist in refining the kick and preventing extraneous motions. Additionally, the muscles in the contralateral hip and pelvic area must be under relative tension to help fixate or stabilize the pelvis on that side in order to provide a relatively stable pelvis for the hip flexors on the involved side to contract against. In kicking the ball, the pectineus and tensor fascia latae are adductors and abductors, respectively, in addition to flexors. The actions of abduction and adduction are neutralized by each other, and the common action of the two muscles results in hip flexion.

From a practical point of view, it is not essential that one know the exact force exerted by each of the elbow flexors—biceps, brachialis, and brachioradialis—in a biceps curl. It is important to understand that this muscle group is the agonist or primary mover responsible for elbow joint flexion. Similarly, one must know that these muscles contract concentrically when the weight is pulled up and that they contract eccentrically when the weight is lowered slowly. Antagonist muscles produce actions opposite those of the agonist. For example, the muscles that produce extension of the elbow joint are antagonistic to the muscles that produce flexion of the elbow joint. It is important to recognize that specific exercises need to be given for the development of each agonist and antagonist muscle group; they should be thought of together whenever exercise is implemented. (Later chapters reiterate this point with examples.) The return movement of the weight at the elbow joint is elbow joint extension, but the triceps and anconeus are not being strengthened. A concentric contraction of the elbow joint flexors occurs during the lifting of the weight, followed by an eccentric contraction of the same muscles as the weight is returned. Both contractions are important in hypertrophy of muscle fibers, but the eccentric phase challenges the muscles for growth, especially if the movement is slow and controlled.

REVERSAL OF MUSCLE FUNCTION

One example of agonist and antagonist muscles that contract to control their opposite motion is the biceps and triceps (figure 2.5). If the biceps contracts concentrically, it acts as an agonist to flex the elbow.

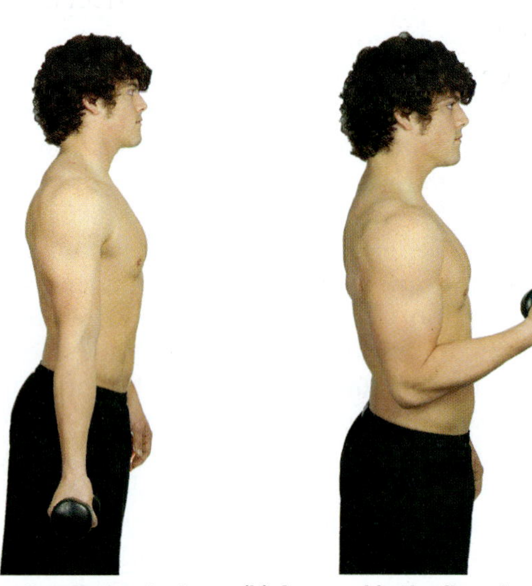

(a) Arm curl at the beginning position in extension (b) Arm curl in the flexed position

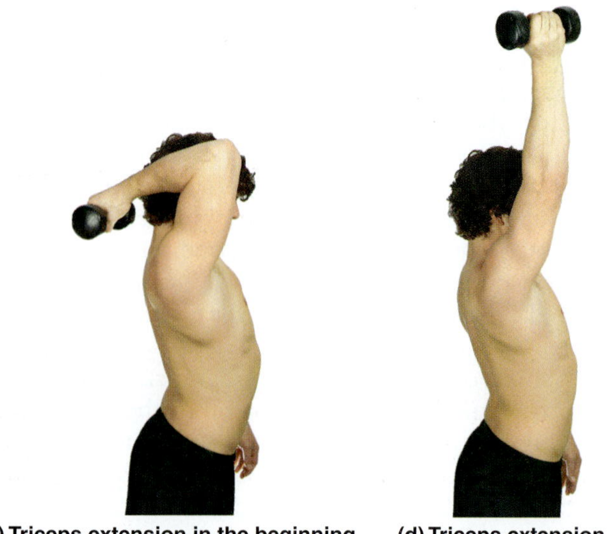

(c) Triceps extension in the beginning position in flexion (d) Triceps extension in extended position

FIGURE 2.5 Synergistic and antagonistic muscles

The triceps is an antagonist to elbow flexion, and the pronator teres is considered a synergist to the biceps in this example. If, when a person is holding a dumbbell, the biceps were to slowly lengthen and control elbow extension, the biceps would still be the agonist, but it would be contracting *eccentrically*. If the elbow was extended against gravity, with the weight overhead, the triceps becomes an agonist by contracting concentrically to extend the elbow. The biceps is an antagonist to elbow extension in this example. On the return phase of triceps extension, the triceps lengthens and controls elbow flexion and is *eccentrically* contracting. In both of these examples, the deltoid, trapezius, and various other shoulder muscles are serving as stabilizers of the shoulder area. These two muscle-group examples, biceps brachii and triceps, should serve as a template for how the focus of an exercise should be performed. For every muscle group—hamstrings, quadriceps, tensor fascia latae, adductor magnus—the agonist and antagonist are strengthened or stretched together so that a balance is maintained between the groups during joint movement.

Determination of Muscle Action

The specific action of a muscle may be determined through a variety of methods. These include reasoning in consideration of anatomical lines of pull, anatomical dissection, palpation, models, electromyography, and electrical stimulation. Studying a muscle's line of pull against forces such as gravity and resistance is vital in a clinical setting.

A muscle's action at the joint is predicted by determining the muscle's line of pull (see "Lines of Pull" below). While not available to all students, seminars specializing in cadaver dissection of muscles and joints are an excellent way to further learn muscle action.

For most of the skeletal muscles, palpation is a very useful way to determine muscle action. This is done through using the sense of touch to feel or examine a muscle as it is contracted. Palpation is limited to superficial muscles, but it is helpful in furthering one's study of joint mechanics. Models such as long rubber bands may be used to study lines of pull and muscle lengthening or shortening as joints move through various ranges of motion.

Electromyography (EMG) utilizes either surface electrodes that are placed over the muscle or fine wire or needle electrodes placed into the muscle. As the subject moves the joint and contracts the muscles, the EMG unit detects the action potentials of muscles and provides an electronic readout of the contraction intensity and duration. EMG is the most accurate way of detecting the presence and extent of muscle activity.

Electrical muscle stimulation is somewhat a reverse approach of electromyography. Instead of electricity being used to detect muscle action, it is used to cause muscle activity. Surface electrodes are placed over a muscle, and then the stimulator causes the muscle to contract. The joint's actions may then be observed to see the effect of the muscle's contraction on the joint.

LINES OF PULL

Combining the knowledge of a particular joint's functional design and the specific location of a musculotendinous unit as it crosses a joint is extremely helpful in understanding the muscle's action on the joint. For example, knowing that the rectus femoris has its origin on the anterior inferior iliac spine and its insertion on the tibial tuberosity via the patella, a therapist can then determine that the muscle must have an anterior relationship to the knee and hip. Since its fibers run vertically along the shaft of the femur, its **line of pull** must be in the sagittal plane. Knowing that both joints are capable of sagittal plane movements such as flexion and extension, the therapist can then determine that when the rectus femoris contracts concentrically, it should cause the knee to extend and the hip to flex. An exercise to strengthen or stretch this muscle should be designed with these things in mind.

The origin of the semitendinosus, semimembranosus, and biceps femoris on the ischial tuberosity helps define the joint actions of the hamstring group. For the distal attachments, the semitendinosus and semimembranosus cross the knee posteromedially before inserting on the tibia; the biceps femoris crosses the knee posterolaterally before inserting on the tibia and fibula head. All of this helps determine that all three muscles have posterior relationships to the hip and knee, which would enable them to be hip extensors and knee flexors on concentric contraction. The specific knowledge related to their distal attachments and the knee's ability to rotate when flexed would allow the therapist to determine that the semitendinosus and semimembranosus would cause internal rotation, whereas the biceps femoris would cause external rotation. Knowing that the knee's axes of rotation are only frontal and vertical, but not sagittal, enables practitioners to determine that—although the semitendinosus and semimembranosus have a posteromedial line of pull and the biceps femoris has a posterolateral line of pull—these muscles are not capable of causing knee adduction and abduction, respectively.

The reverse can be true for this concept. For example, if the only action of a muscle, such as the brachialis, is known to be elbow flexion, it could then be determined that its line of pull must be anterior to the joint. Additionally, it seems logical that the origin of the brachialis must be located somewhere on the anterior humerus and the insertion must be somewhere on the anterior ulna.

Students must consider all the following factors and their relationships as they study movements of the body:

- Exact locations of bony landmarks to which muscles attach proximally and distally and their relationship to joints.
- The planes of motion through which a joint is capable of moving.
- The muscle's relationship or line of pull relative to the joint's axes of rotation.
- As a joint moves through a particular range of motion, the ability of the line of pull to change so that the muscle has a different or opposite action than it had in the original position.
- The potential effect of other muscles' relative contraction or relaxation on a particular muscle's ability to cause motion.
- The effect of a muscle's relative length on its ability to generate force. (See "Muscle Length-Tension Relationship" and "Active and Passive Insufficiency," below.)
- The effect of the position of other joints on the ability of a biarticular or multiarticular muscle to generate force or allow lengthening. (See "Uniarticular, Biarticular, and Multiarticular Muscles," below.)
- The direction that the fibers of a muscle run. For example, the biceps brachii's fibers run longitudinal along the humerus; thus, line of pull would cause movement in the sagittal plane.

Neural Control of Voluntary Movement

When discussing muscular activity, one should really refer to it as *neuromuscular activity,* since muscle cannot be active without nervous *innervation.* All voluntary movement is a result of both the muscular and nervous systems working together. All muscle contraction occurs as a result of stimulation from the nervous system. Ultimately, every muscle fiber is innervated by a somatic motor neuron, which, when an appropriate stimulus is provided, results in a muscle contraction. Depending on a variety of factors, this stimulus may be processed in varying degrees at different levels of the central nervous system (CNS), which, for the purposes of this discussion, may be divided into five levels of control. This listing, in order from the most general level of control and the most superiorly located to the most specific level of control and the most inferiorly located, includes the cerebral cortex, the basal ganglia, the cerebellum, the brainstem, and the spinal cord.

- The *cerebral cortex* is the highest level of control. It provides for the creation of voluntary movement as aggregate muscle action but not as specific muscle activity. Sensory stimuli from the body also are interpreted here to a degree for the determination of needed responses.
- The *basal ganglia* is the next level. It controls the maintenance of postures and equilibrium and learned movements such as driving a car. Sensory integration for balance and rhythmic activities is controlled here.
- The *cerebellum* is a major integrator of sensory impulses and provides feedback relative to motion. It controls the timing and intensity of muscle activity to assist in the refinement of movements.
- The *brainstem* integrates all CNS activity through excitation and inhibition of desired neuromuscular actions, and it functions in arousal or maintaining a wakeful state.
- The *spinal cord* is the common pathway between the CNS and the peripheral nervous system (PNS), which contains all the remaining nerves throughout the body. It has the most specific control and integrates various simple and complex spinal reflexes, as well as cortical and basal ganglia activity, with various classifications of spinal reflexes.

Functionally, the PNS can be divided into *sensory* and *motor* divisions. The sensory, or *afferent,* nerves bring impulses from receptors in the skin, joints, muscles, and other peripheral aspects of the body to the CNS, while the motor, or *efferent,* nerves carry impulses to the outlying regions of the body.

The *spinal nerves,* illustrated in figure 2.6, also provide both motor and sensory function for their respective portions of the body and are named for the locations from which they exit the vertebral column. From each side of the spinal column, there are 8 cervical nerves, 12 thoracic nerves, 5 lumbar nerves,

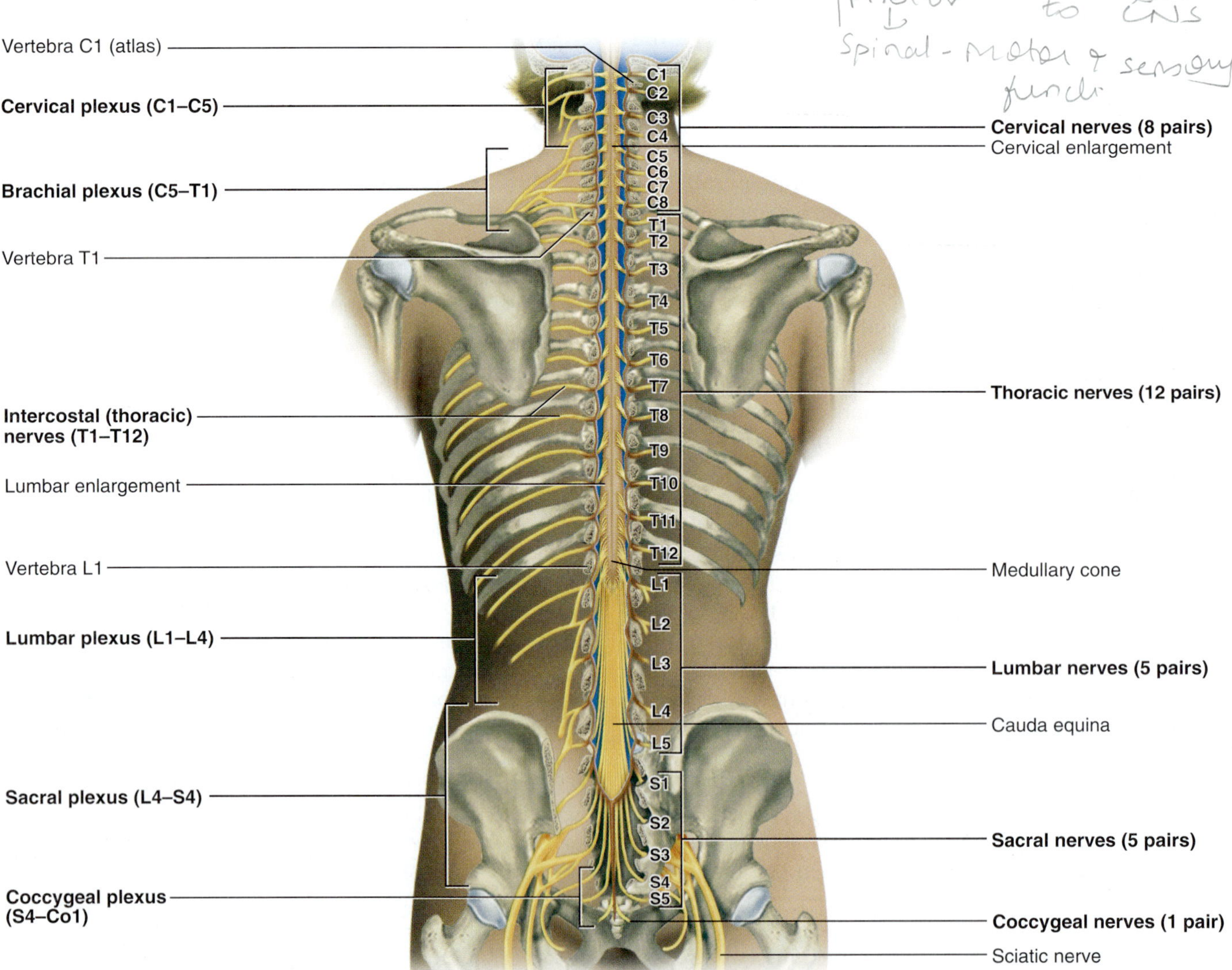

FIGURE 2.6 The spinal nerve roots and plexuses

5 sacral nerves, and 1 coccygeal nerve. Cervical nerves 1 through 4 form the cervical plexus, which is generally responsible for sensation from the upper part of the shoulders to the back of the head and front of the neck. The cervical plexus supplies motor innervation to several muscles of the neck. Cervical nerves 5 through 8, along with thoracic nerve 1, form the brachial plexus, which supplies motor and sensory function to the upper extremity and most of the scapula. Thoracic nerves 2 through 12 run directly to specific anatomical locations in the thorax. All the lumbar, sacral, and coccygeal nerves form the lumbosacral plexus, which supplies sensation and motor function to the lower trunk and the entire lower extremity and perineum.

One aspect of the sensory function of spinal nerves is to provide feedback to the CNS regarding skin sensation. A defined area of skin supplied by a specific spinal nerve is known as a **dermatome.** Regarding motor function of spinal nerves, a **myotome** is defined as a muscle or group of muscles supplied by a specific spinal nerve. Certain spinal nerves are also responsible for reflexes. See table 2.2 regarding the specific spinal nerve functions.

TABLE 2.2 Spinal Nerve Root Dermatomes, Myotomes, Reflexes, and Functional Application

	Nerve root	Dermatome afferent (sensory)	Myotome efferent (motor)	Reflexes	Functional application
Cervical plexus	C1	Touch: Vertex of skull	Upper neck muscles	None	None
	C2	Touch: Temple, forehead, occiput	Upper neck muscles	None	None
	C3	Touch: Entire neck, posterior cheek, temporal area, under mandible	Trapezius, splenius, capitis	None	Scapula retraction, neck extension Sensation to cheek and side of neck
	C4	Touch: Shoulder area, clavicular area, upper scapular area	Trapezius, levator scapulae	None	Scapula retraction and elevation Sensation to clavicle and upper scapula
Brachial plexus	C5	Touch: Deltoid area, anterior aspect of entire arm to base of thumb	Supraspinatus, infraspinatus, deltoid, biceps brachii	Biceps brachii	Shoulder abduction Sensation to lateral side of arm and elbow
	C6	Touch: Anterior arm, radial side of hand to thumb and index finger	Biceps, supinator, wrist extensors	Biceps brachii, brachioradialis	Elbow flexion, wrist extension Sensation to lateral side of forearm including thumb and index finger
	C7	Touch: Lateral arm and forearm to index, long, and ring fingers	Triceps brachii, wrist flexors	Triceps brachii	Elbow extension, wrist flexion Sensation to middle of anterior forearm and long finger
	C8	Touch: Medial side of forearm to ring and little fingers	Ulnar deviators, thumb extensors, thumb adductors (rarely triceps)	None	Wrist ulnar deviation, thumb extension Sensation to posterior elbow and medial forearm to little finger
	T1	Touch: Medial arm and forearm to wrist	Intrinsic muscles of the hand except for opponens pollicis and abductor pollicis brevis	None	Abduction and adduction of fingers Sensation to medial arm and elbow
	T2	Touch: Medial side of upper arm to medial elbow, pectoral and midscapular areas	Intercostal muscles	None	Sensation to medial upper arm, upper chest, and midscapular area
	T3–T12	Touch: T3–T6, upper thorax; T5–T7, costal margin; T8–T12, abdomen and lumbar region	Intercostal muscles, abdominal muscles	None	Sensation to chest, abdomen, and low back

(*Continued*)

TABLE 2.2 (*Continued*)

	Nerve root	Dermatome afferent (sensory)	Myotome efferent (motor)	Reflexes	Functional application
Lumbosacral plexus	LI	Touch: Lower abdomen, groin, lumbar region from 2nd to 4th vertebrae, upper and outer aspect of buttocks	Quadratus lumborum	None	Sensation to low back, over trochanter and groin
	L2	Touch: Lower lumbar region, upper buttock, anterior aspect of thigh	Iliopsoas, quadriceps	None	Hip flexion Sensation to back, front of thigh to knee
	L3	Touch: Medial aspect of thigh to knee, anterior aspect of lower 1/3 of the thigh to just below patella	Psoas, quadriceps	Patella or knee extensors	Hip flexion and knee extension Sensation to back, upper buttock, anterior thigh and knee, medial lower leg
	L4	Touch: Medial aspect of lower leg and foot, inner border of foot, great toe	Tibialis anterior, extensor hallucis and digitorum longus, peroneals	Patella or knee extensors	Ankle dorsiflexion, transverse tarsal/subtalar inversion Sensation to medial buttock, lateral thigh, medial leg, dorsum of foot, great toe
	L5	Touch: Lateral border of leg, anterior surface of the lower leg, top of foot to middle three toes	Extensor hallucis and digitorum longus, peroneals, gluteus maximus and medius, and dorsiflexors	None	Great toe extension, transverse talar/subtalar eversion Sensation to upper lateral leg, anterior surface of the lower leg, middle three toes
	S1	Touch: Posterior aspect of the lower 1/4 of the leg, posterior aspect of the foot, including the heel, lateral border of the foot and sole	Gastrocnemius, soleus, gluteus maximus and medius, hamstrings, peroneals	Achilles reflex	Ankle plantarflexion, knee flexion, transverse talar/subtalar eversion Sensation to lateral leg, lateral foot, lateral two toes, plantar aspect of foot
	S2	Touch: Posterior central strip of the leg from below the gluteal fold to 3/4 of the way down the leg	Gastrocnemius, soleus, gluteus maximus, hamstrings	None	Ankle plantar flexion and toe flexion Sensation to posterior thigh and upper posterior leg
	S3	Touch: Groin, medial thigh to knee	Intrinsic foot muscles	None	Sensation to groin and adductor region
	S4	Touch: Perineum, genitals, lower sacrum	Bladder, rectum	None	Urinary and bowel control Sensation to saddle area, genitals, anus

The basic functional units of the nervous system responsible for generating and transmitting impulses are nerve cells known as **neurons.** Neurons consist of a *neuron cell body;* one or more branching projections known as *dendrites,* which transmit impulses to the neuron and cell body; and an *axon,* which is an elongated projection that transmits impulses away from neuron cell bodies. Neurons are classified into three types, according to the direction in which they transmit impulses. *Sensory neurons* transmit impulses to the spinal cord and brain from all parts of the body, whereas *motor neurons* transmit impulses away from the brain and spinal cord to muscle and glandular tissue. *Interneurons* are central or connecting neurons that conduct impulses from sensory neurons to motor neurons.

Proprioception and Kinesthesis

The performance of various activities is significantly dependent on neurologic feedback from the body. More importantly, people could not survive without the ability to sense where they are in space or sense temperature and pressure to the skin. Very simply, humans use the various senses to determine responses to their environment, such as using sight to know when to lift the hand to catch a fly ball. All humans are familiar with the senses of smell, touch, sight, hearing, and taste, as well as other sensations, such as pain, pressure, heat, and cold; however, people often take for granted the sensory feedback provided by proprioceptors during neuromuscular activity. **Proprioceptors** are internal receptors located in the skin, joints, muscles, and tendons that provide feedback relative to the tension, length, and contraction state of muscles, the position of the body and limbs, and movements of the joints. These proprioceptors, in combination with the body's other sense organs, are vital in **kinesthesis,** which is the conscious awareness of the position and movement of the body in space. For example, when a person stands on one leg with the other knee flexed, he does not have to look at his non-weight-bearing leg to know the approximate number of degrees that he may have it flexed. The proprioceptors in and around the knee provide information so that he is kinesthetically aware of his knee position. Proprioceptors specific to the muscles are muscle spindles and Golgi tendon organs (GTOs), whereas Meissner's corpuscles, Ruffini's corpuscles, pacinian corpuscles, and Krause's end-bulbs are proprioceptors specific to the joints and skin.

While kinesthesis is concerned with the conscious awareness of the body's position, proprioception is the subconscious mechanism by which the body is able to regulate posture and movement by responding to stimuli originating in the proprioceptors embedded in the joints, tendons, muscles, and inner ear. When a person who has good proprioception unexpectedly steps on an unlevel or unstable surface, the muscles in and about the lower extremity may respond very quickly by contracting appropriately to prevent a fall or injury. This is a protective response of the body that occurs without the person having to take time to make a conscious decision about how to respond. Kinesthesis and proprioception have become important developmental components in exercise prescription, especially in the older population whose balance and muscle tissue are compromised. Everyone, young or old, athletic or not, will benefit from exercises that stress body awareness.

Muscle spindles (figure 2.7), concentrated primarily in the muscle belly between the fibers, are sensitive to stretch and rate of stretch. Specifically, they insert into the connective tissue within the muscle and run parallel with the muscle fibers. The number of spindles in a particular muscle varies depending on the level of control needed for the area. Consequently, the concentration of muscle spindles in the hands is much greater than that in the thigh.

When a rapid stretch occurs, an impulse is sent to the CNS. The CNS then activates the motor neurons of the muscle and causes it to contract. All muscles possess this myotatic, or stretch, reflex, but it is more remarkable in the extensor muscles of the extremities. The knee jerk, or patellar tendon reflex, can be used as an example, as shown in figure 2.8. When the reflex hammer strikes the patellar tendon, it causes a quick stretch to the musculotendinous unit of the quadriceps. In response, the quadriceps fires, and the knee extends. The power of this contraction is increased if the tap of the hammer is more intense. Consider, for example, what happens when a student begins to doze off in class. As the head starts to nod forward, there is a sudden stretch placed on the neck extensors, which activates the muscle spindles and ultimately results in a sudden jerk back to an extended position.

The **stretch reflex** provided by the muscle spindle may be utilized to facilitate a greater response, as in the case of a quick, short squat before attempting a jump. The quick stretch placed on the muscles in the squat enables the same muscles to generate more force when the body subsequently jumps off the floor. Athletes use this physiology when training in plyometrics, a type of exercise designed to make use of the myotatic reflex arc. As a muscle is lengthened while loaded, the contraction will produce a greater force because of stored elastic energy. Thus, a basketball player may jump higher and more powerfully. Yet the stretch reflex contraction can also be detrimental, especially during stretching exercises. Because the muscle spindles are triggered by a lengthened muscle, and the muscle has reached its length at a high velocity, the stretch reflex has the power to return a rapid concentric contraction in response. In a lengthened muscle that is already under stretch pressure, injury could result to the muscle-tendon units. This is discussed more in later chapters.

The **Golgi tendon organ (GTO),** serially located in the tendon close to the muscle-tendon junction (figure 2.9), are continuously sensitive to both muscle tension and active contraction. The GTO is much less sensitive to stretch than are muscle spindles and requires a greater stretch to be activated. Tension in tendons, and consequently in the GTO, increases as the muscle contracts, and this in turn activates the GTO. When the GTO stretch threshold is reached, an impulse is sent to the CNS, which in turn causes the muscle to relax and facilitates activation of the antagonists as a protective mechanism. That is, the GTO, through this inverse stretch reflex, protects the body

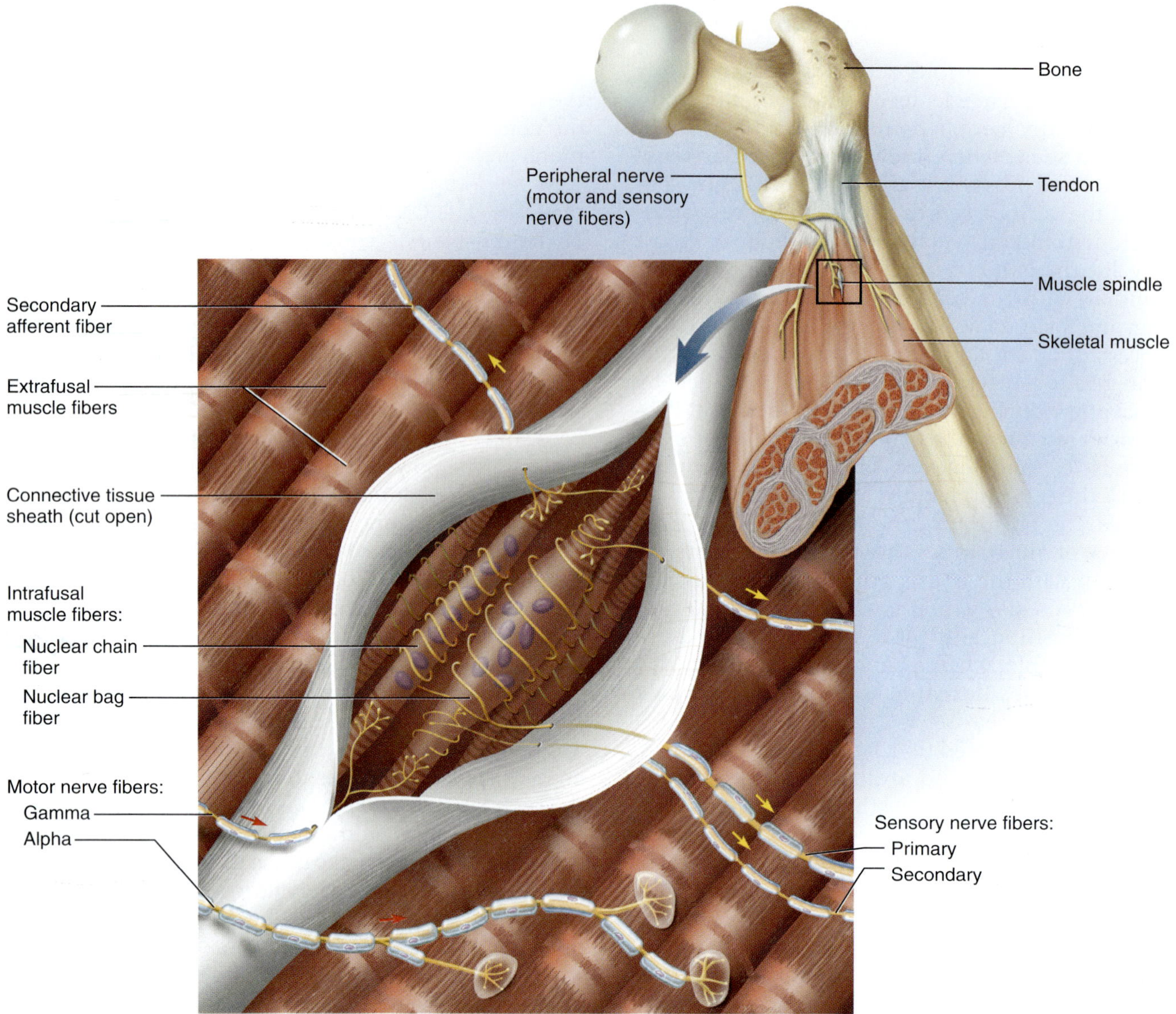

FIGURE 2.7 Muscle spindles

from an excessive contraction by causing the muscle it supplies to relax. For example, when a weight lifter attempts a very heavy resistance in the biceps curl and reaches the point of extreme overload, the GTO is activated, the biceps suddenly relaxes, and the triceps contracts, which is why it appears as if the lifter is throwing the weight down.

Pacinian corpuscles, concentrated around joint capsules, ligaments, and tendon sheaths and beneath the skin, are activated by rapid changes in the joint angle and by pressure changes affecting the capsule. This activation lasts only briefly and is not effective in detecting constant pressure. Pacinian corpuscles are helpful in providing feedback regarding the location of a body part in space after quick movements such as running or jumping.

Ruffini's corpuscles, located in deep layers of the skin and the joint capsule, are activated by strong and sudden joint movements as well as pressure changes. Unlike pacinian corpuscles, their reaction to pressure changes is slower to develop, but their activation is continued as long as pressure is maintained. They are essential in detecting even minute joint position changes and providing information as to the exact joint angle.

Meissner's corpuscles and *Krause's end-bulbs* are located in the skin and in subcutaneous tissues. While they are important in receiving stimuli from touch, they are not so relevant to a discussion about

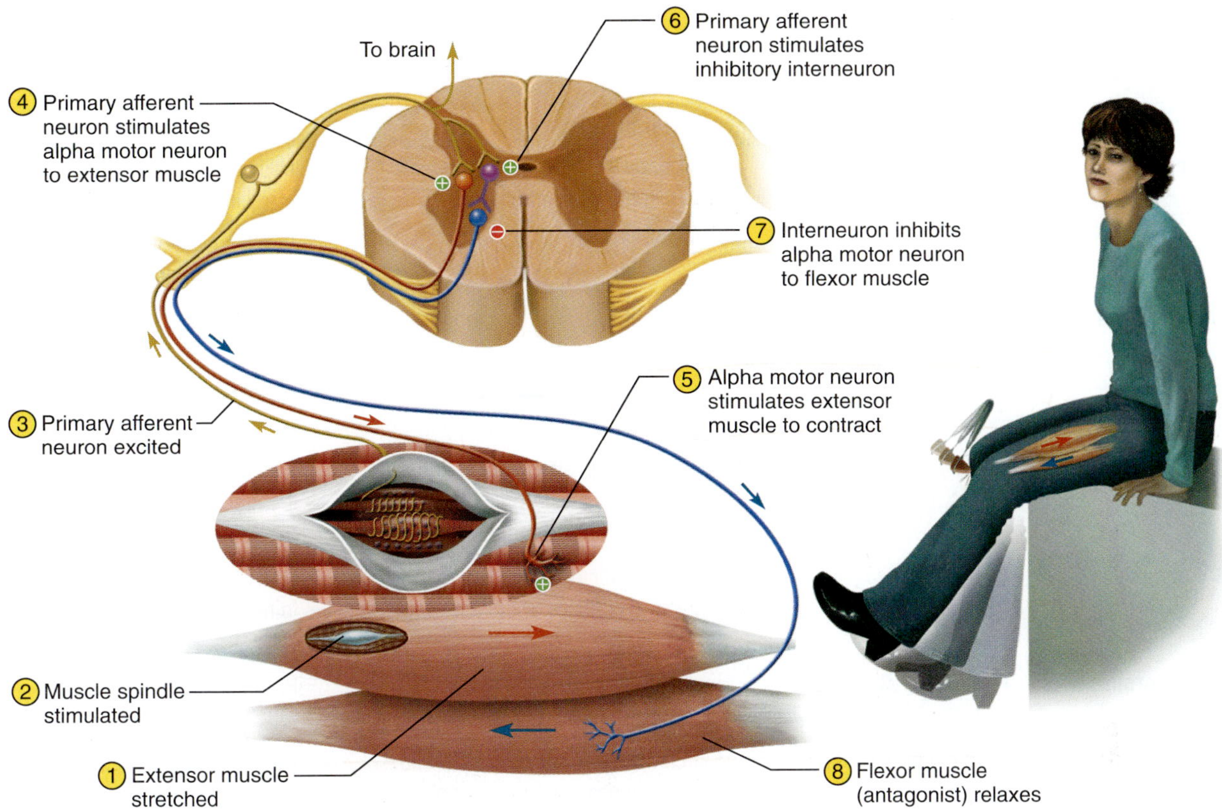

FIGURE 2.8 The patellar tendon reflex arc

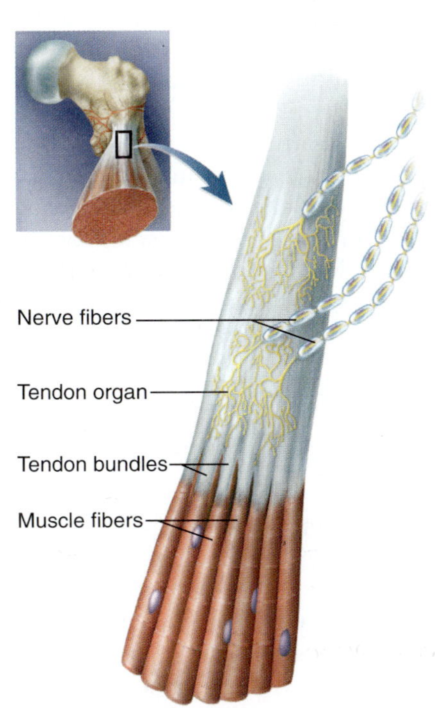

FIGURE 2.9 A Golgi tendon organ

kinesthesis. See table 2.3 for further comparisons of sensory receptors.

The quality of movement and how the body reacts to position change is significantly dependent on the proprioceptive feedback from the muscles and joints. Like the other factors involving body movement, proprioception may be enhanced through specific training that utilizes the proprioceptors to a high degree, such as martial arts and any activity that requires balance as the body moves through space. Attempting to maintain balance while seated on a physio ball, first with both feet down on a level surface, may serve as an initial low-level proprioceptive activity. Progressing to more difficult movements with just one foot down will help build proprioceptive skills. There are numerous additional proprioceptive training activities that are limited only by the imagination and the level of proprioception.

Neuromuscular Concepts

MOTOR UNITS AND THE ALL-OR-NONE PRINCIPLE

When a particular muscle contracts, the contraction actually occurs at the muscle-fiber level within a particular motor unit. A motor unit consists of a single

TABLE 2.3 Sensory Receptors

Receptors	Sensitivity	Location	Response
Muscle spindles	Subconscious muscle sense, muscle length changes	In skeletal muscles among muscle fibers in parallel with fibers	Initiate rapid contraction of stretched muscle Inhibits development of tension in antagonistic muscles
Golgi tendon organs	Subconscious muscle sense, muscle tension changes	In tendons, near muscle-tendon junction in series with muscle fibers	Inhibit development of tension in stretched muscles Initiates development of tension in antagonistic muscles
Pacinian corpuscles	Rapid changes in joint angles, pressure, vibration	Subcutaneous, submucosa, and subserous tissues around joints and external genitals, mammary glands	Provide feedback regarding location of body part in space following quick movements
Ruffini's corpuscles	Strong, sudden joint movements, touch, pressure	Skin and subcutaneous tissue of fingers, collagenous fibers of the joint capsule	Provide feedback as to exact joint angle
Meissner's corpuscles	Fine touch, vibration	In skin	Provide feedback regarding touch, two-point discrimination
Krause's end-bulbs	Touch, thermal change	Skin, subcutaneous tissue, lip and eyelid mucosa, external genitals	Provide feedback regarding touch

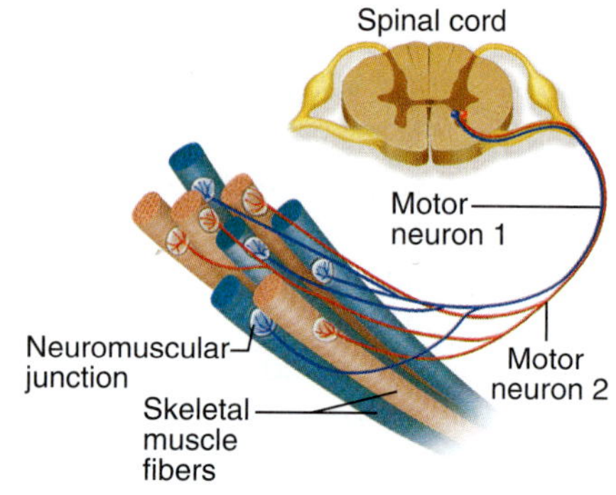

FIGURE 2.10 A motor unit

motor neuron and all the muscle fibers it innervates (figure 2.10). Motor units function as a single unit. In a typical muscle contraction, the number of motor units innervated and the number of muscle fibers contracting may vary significantly. Depending on the number of muscle fibers within each activated motor unit, and the number of motor units activated, muscle contractions may be powerful for doing sports movements or delicate for performing surgery. Regardless of the number involved, the individual muscle fibers within a given motor unit will fire and contract either maximally or not at all. This is referred to as the **all-or-none principle.**

FACTORS AFFECTING MUSCLE TENSION DEVELOPMENT

The difference between a particular muscle contracting to lift a minimal resistance and the same muscle contracting to lift a maximal resistance is the number of muscle fibers recruited. The number of muscle fibers recruited may be increased by activating the motor units that contain a greater number of muscle fibers, by activating more motor units, or by increasing the frequency of motor unit activation. The number of muscle fibers per motor unit varies significantly from fewer than 10 in muscles requiring a very precise and detailed response, such as the muscles of the eye, to as many as a few thousand in large muscle groups, such as the quadriceps that perform less complex activities.

For the muscle fibers in a particular motor unit to contract, the motor unit must first receive a stimulus via an electrical signal known as an *action potential* from the brain and spinal cord through its axons. If the stimulus is not strong enough to cause an action potential, it is known as a *subthreshold stimulus* and does not result in a contraction. When the stimulus becomes strong enough to produce an action potential in a single motor unit axon, it is known as a *threshold stimulus,* and all the muscle fibers in the motor unit contract. Stimuli that are stronger to the point of producing action potentials in additional motor units are

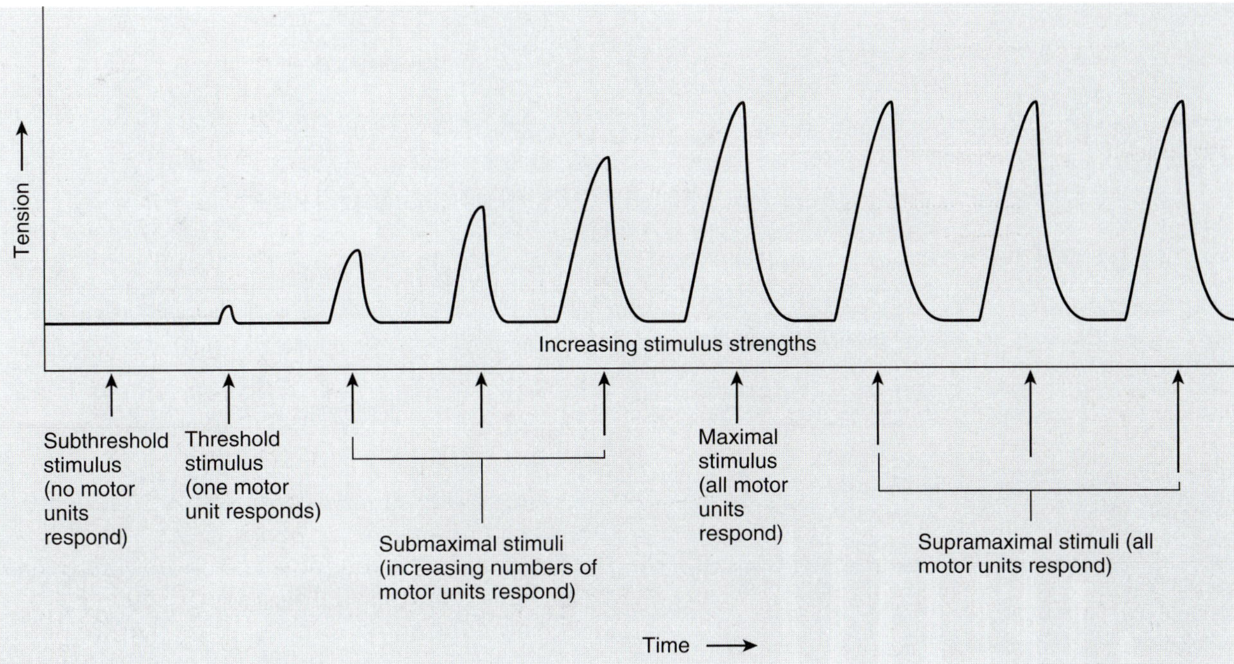

FIGURE 2.11 Achieving threshold stimulus and the effect of recruiting more motor units on increasing tension

known as *submaximal stimuli.* For action potentials to be produced in all the motor units of a particular muscle, a maximal stimulus would be required. As the strength of the stimulus increases from threshold up to maximal, more motor units are recruited and the overall force of the muscle contraction increases in a graded fashion. Increasing the stimulus beyond maximal has no effect. The effect of increasing the number of motor units activated is detailed in figure. 2.11.

Greater contraction forces may also be achieved by increasing the frequency of motor unit activation. To simplify the phases of a single muscle-fiber contraction or twitch, a stimulus is provided and followed by a brief latent period of a few milliseconds. Then the second phase, known as the *contraction phase,* begins, during which the muscle fiber begins shortening. The contraction phase lasts about 40 milliseconds and is followed by the *relaxation phase,* which lasts approximately 50 milliseconds. This is illustrated in figure 2.12. When successive stimuli are provided before the relaxation phase of the first twitch has completed, the subsequent twitches combine with the first to produce a sustained contraction. This summation of contractions generates a greater amount of tension than a single contraction would produce individually. As the frequency of stimuli increases, the resultant summation increases accordingly, producing increasingly greater total muscle tension. If the stimuli are provided at a frequency high enough that no relaxation can occur between contractions, tetanus results. Figure 2.13 illustrates the effect of increasing the rate of stimulation to gain increased muscle tension.

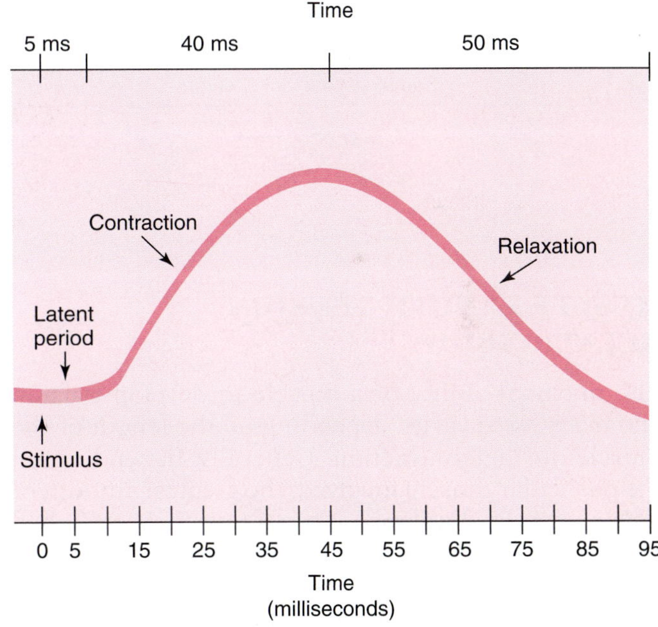

FIGURE 2.12 A recording of a simple twitch

Treppe is another type of muscle contraction that occurs when multiple maximal stimuli are provided at a low enough frequency to allow complete relaxation between contractions. Slightly greater tension is produced by the second stimulus than by the first. A third stimulus produces even greater tension than the second. This staircase effect, as illustrated in figure 2.14, occurs only with the first few stimuli, and the resultant contractions after the initial ones result in equal tension being produced.

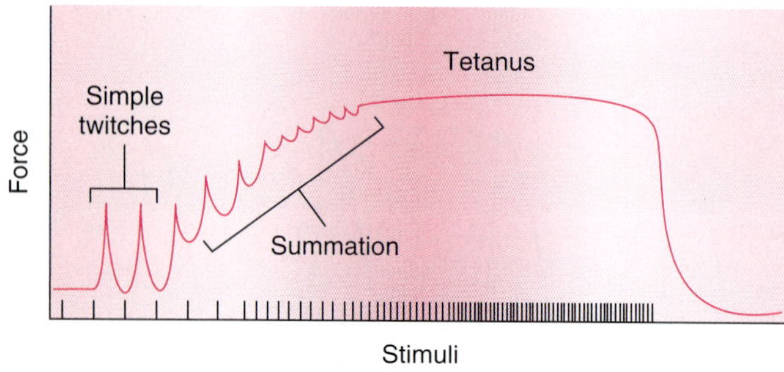

FIGURE 2.13 A recording showing the change from simple twitches to summation and finally tetanus

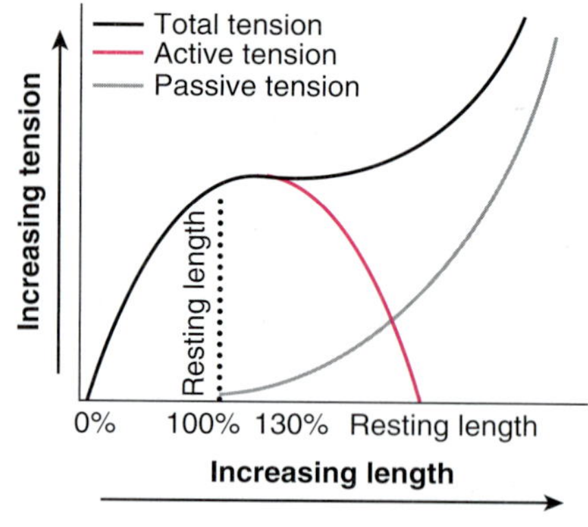

FIGURE 2.15 Muscle length-tension relationship

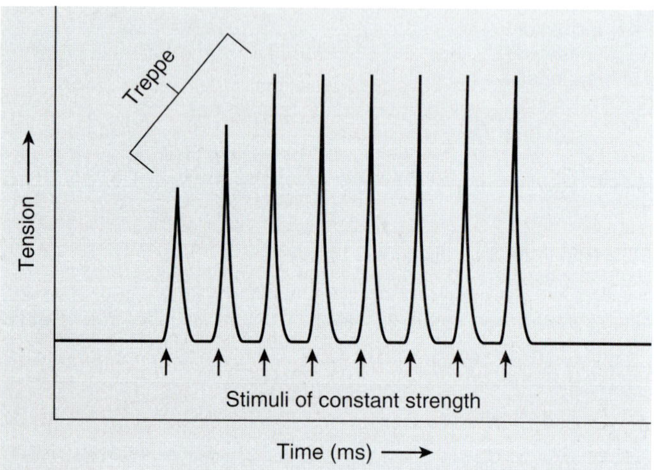

FIGURE 2.14 Treppe

MUSCLE LENGTH-TENSION RELATIONSHIP

The maximal ability of a muscle to develop tension and exert force varies depending on the length of the muscle during contraction. Generally, depending on the particular muscle involved, the greatest amount of tension can be developed when a muscle is stretched between 100 percent and 130 percent of its resting length. As a muscle is stretched beyond this point, the amount of force it can exert significantly decreases. Likewise, a proportional decrease in the ability to develop tension occurs as a muscle is shortened. When a muscle is shortened to around 50 percent to 60 percent of its resting length, its ability to develop contractile tension is essentially reduced to zero.

During the preparatory phase in most sporting activities, a person generally places the muscles in an optimum stretch that he intends to contract forcefully in the subsequent movement, or action, phase of the skill. The various phases of performing a movement skill are discussed in much greater detail in later chapters. This principle may be seen at work when a person squats slightly to stretch the calf, hamstrings, and quadriceps before contracting them concentrically to jump. If the muscles are not first lengthened through squatting slightly, they are unable to generate enough contractile force to jump very high. If, however, a person squats fully and lengthens the muscles too much, she loses the ability to generate as much force, and as a result, she cannot jump as high.

Manual therapists can take advantage of this principle by effectively reducing the contribution of some muscles in a group by placing them in a shortened state in order to isolate the work to the muscle(s) remaining in the lengthened state. For example, in hip extension, the therapist may isolate the work of the gluteus maximus as a hip extensor by maximally shortening the hamstrings with flexion of the knee to reduce their ability to act as hip extensors. See figures 2.15 and 2.16.

MUSCLE FORCE-VELOCITY RELATIONSHIP

When the muscle is either concentrically or eccentrically contracting, the rate of length change is significantly related to the amount of force potential. When contracting concentrically against a light resistance, the muscle is able to contract at a high velocity. As the resistance increases, the maximal velocity at which the muscle is able to contract decreases. Eventually, as the load increases, the velocity decreases to zero; this results in an isometric contraction.

As the load increases even further beyond that which the muscle can maintain with an isometric contraction, the muscle begins to lengthen, resulting in an eccentric contraction or action. A slight increase in the load will result in relatively low velocity of lengthening. As the load increases even further, the velocity of lengthening will increase as well. Eventually, the load may increase to the point where the muscle can no longer resist. This will result in uncontrollable lengthening or, more likely, dropping of the load.

(a) Muscles in a relatively shortened position
(b) Muscles in an optimally lengthened position
(c) Muscles are lengthened too much

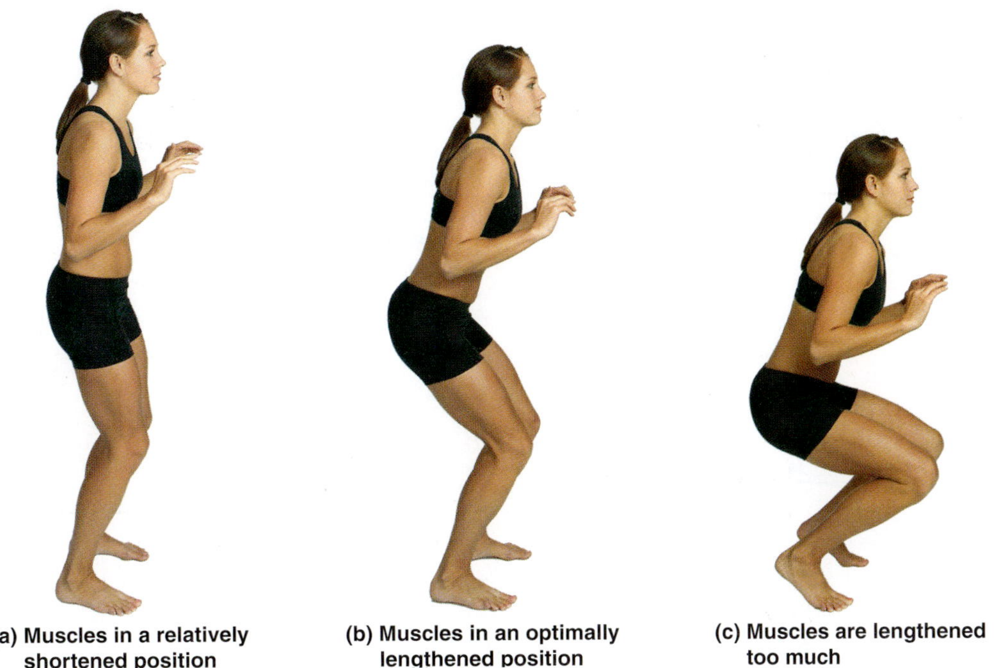

FIGURE 2.16 Practical application of muscle length

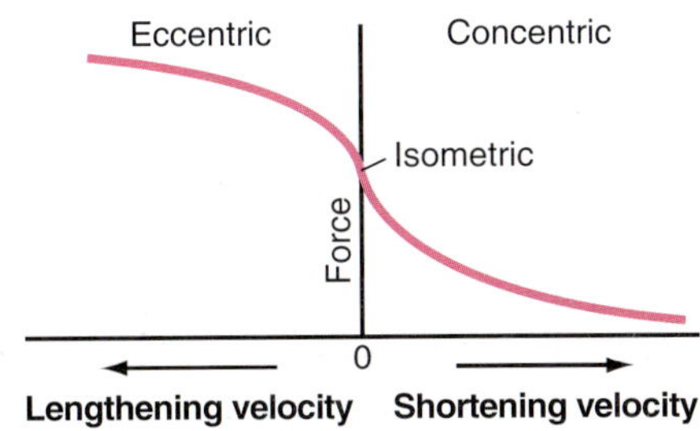

FIGURE 2.17 Muscle force-velocity relationship

From this explanation, it is easy to see that there is an inverse relationship between concentric velocity and force production. As the force needed to cause movement of an object increases, the velocity of concentric contraction decreases. Furthermore, there is a somewhat proportional relationship between eccentric velocity and force production. As the force needed to control the movement of an object increases, the velocity of eccentric lengthening increases, at least until the point at which control is lost. This is illustrated in figure 2.17.

ANGLE OF PULL

Another factor of considerable importance in using the leverage system is the angle of pull of the muscles on the bone. The **angle of pull** may be defined as the angle between the line of pull of the muscle and the bone on which it inserts. For the sake of clarity and consistency, it is necessary to specify that the actual angle referred to is the angle toward the joint. With every degree of joint motion, the angle of pull changes. Joint movements and insertion angles involve mostly small angles of pull. The angle of pull decreases as the bone moves away from its anatomical position through the contraction of the local muscle group. This range of movement depends on the type of joint and bony structure.

Most muscles work at a small angle of pull, generally less than 50 degrees. The amount of muscular force needed to cause joint movement is affected by the angle of pull. Two components of muscular force are involved. The *rotary component,* also referred to as the *vertical component,* is the component of muscular force that acts perpendicular to the long axis of the bone (lever). When the line of muscular force is at 90 degrees to the bone on which it attaches, all the muscular force is rotary force; therefore, 100 percent of the force is contributing to the movement. That is, all the force is being used to rotate the lever around its axis. The closer the angle of pull is to 90 degrees, the greater the rotary component. At all other degrees of the angle of pull, one of the other two components of force is operating in addition to the rotary component. The same rotary component is continuing, although with less force, to rotate the lever around its axis. The second force component is the *nonrotary component,* or *horizontal component,* and it is either a stabilizing component or a dislocating component, depending on whether the angle of pull is less than or greater than 90 degrees. If the angle is

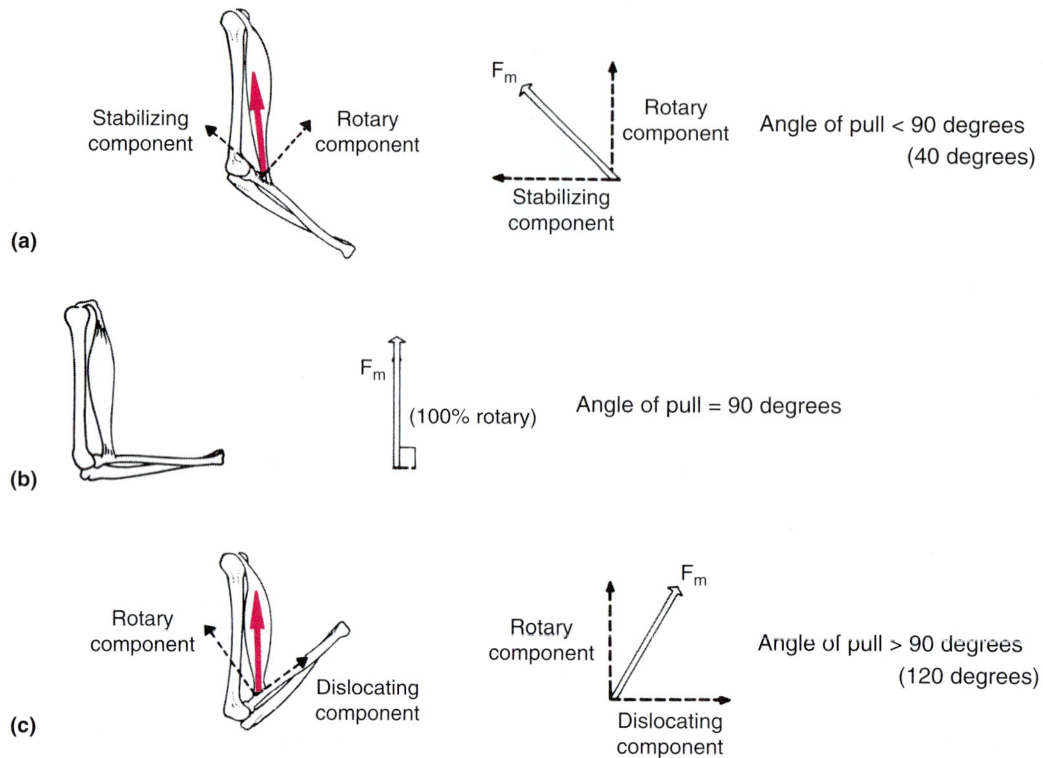

FIGURE 2.18 Components of force due to the angle of pull

less than 90 degrees, the force is a stabilizing force, because its pull directs the bone toward the joint axis. If the angle is greater than 90 degrees, the force is dislocating, because its pull directs the bone away from the joint axis (figure 2.18).

In some activities, it is desirable to have a person begin a movement when the angle of pull is at 90 degrees. Many people are unable to do a chin-up (pull-up) unless they start with the elbow in a position that allows the elbow flexor muscle group to approximate a 90-degree angle with the forearm.

This angle makes the chin-up easier because of the more advantageous angle of pull. The application of this fact can compensate for lack of sufficient strength. In its range of motion, a muscle pulls a lever through a range characteristic of itself, but it is most effective when approaching and going beyond 90 degrees. An increase in strength is the only solution for muscles that operate at disadvantageous angles of pull and require greater force to operate efficiently.

UNIARTICULAR, BIARTICULAR, AND MULTIARTICULAR MUSCLES

Uniarticular muscles are those that cross and act directly on only the joint that they cross. The brachialis of the elbow is one example in that it can only pull the humerus and ulna closer to each other on concentric contraction. When the humerus is relatively stabilized, as in an elbow curl, the brachialis contracts to flex the elbow and pulls the ulna closer to the humerus. However, when the ulna is relatively stabilized, as in a pull-up, the brachialis indirectly causes motion at the shoulder even though it does not cross it. In this example, the brachialis contracts and pulls the humerus closer to the ulna as an elbow flexor. Correspondingly, the shoulder has to move from flexion into extension for the pull-up to be accomplished.

Biarticular muscles are those that cross and act directly on two different joints. Depending on a variety of factors, a biarticular muscle may contract to cause, control, or prevent motion at either one or both of its joints. Biarticular muscles have two advantages over uniarticular muscles. They can cause, control, and/or prevent motion at more than one joint, and they may be able to maintain a relatively constant length due to "shortening" at one joint and "lengthening" at another joint. The muscle does not actually shorten at one joint and lengthen at the other; instead, the concentric shortening of the muscle to move one joint is offset by motion of the other joint, which moves its attachment of the muscle farther away. This maintenance of a relatively constant length results in the muscle's ability to continue its exertion of force. In the pull-up example, the biceps brachii acts as a flexor at the elbow. In the initial stage of the pull-up, the biceps brachii is in a relatively lengthened state at the elbow due to its extended position and is in a relatively shortened state at the shoulder due to its flexed position. To accomplish the pull-up, the biceps brachii contracts concentrically to flex the elbow so that it effectively "shortens" at the elbow. Simultaneously, the shoulder is extending during the pull-up, and this effectively "lengthens" the biceps brachii at the shoulder.

The biarticular muscles of the hip and knee provide excellent examples of two different patterns of action. An example of a concurrent movement pattern occurs when both the knee and the hip extend at the same time. If only the knee were to extend, the rectus femoris would shorten and lose tension as do the other quadriceps muscles, but its relative length and subsequent tension may be maintained due to its relative lengthening at the hip joint during extension. When a ball is kicked, an example of a countercurrent movement pattern may be observed. During the forward movement phase of the lower extremity, the rectus femoris is concentrically contracted to both flex the hip and extend the knee. These two movements, when combined, increase the tension or stretch on the hamstring muscles at both the knee and the hip.

Multiarticular muscles act on three or more joints due to the line of pull between their origin and insertion crossing multiple joints. The principles discussed relative to biarticular muscles apply in a similar fashion to multiarticular muscles.

RECIPROCAL INHIBITION OR INNERVATION

As stated earlier, antagonist muscle groups must relax and lengthen when the agonist muscle group contracts. This effect, **reciprocal innervation,** occurs through reciprocal inhibition of the antagonists. Activation of the motor units of the agonists causes a reciprocal neural inhibition of the motor units of the antagonists. This reduction in neural activity of the antagonists allows them to subsequently lengthen under less tension. This may be demonstrated by comparing the ease with which one can stretch the hamstrings when simultaneously contracting the quadriceps versus attempting to stretch the hamstrings without the quadriceps contracted. This concept is discussed more in Chapter 21.

ACTIVE AND PASSIVE INSUFFICIENCY

As discussed earlier, as a muscle shortens, its ability to exert force diminishes. When the muscle becomes shortened to the point at which it cannot generate or maintain active tension, *active insufficiency* is reached. If the opposing muscle becomes stretched to the point at which it can no longer lengthen and allow movement, *passive insufficiency* is reached. These principles are most easily observed in either biarticular or multiarticular muscles when the full range of motion is attempted in all the joints crossed by the muscle. A good example of active and passive insufficiency is seen in wrist movements. For active insufficiency, making a fist with the wrist extended is easier than doing so with the wrist flexed. The shortened flexor muscles are weaker as they attempt to make the fist. In the multijoint muscles of the extensors of the wrist and fingers, passive insufficiency limits finger and wrist flexion when they are performed together. A greater range of motion of wrist flexion is possible with the fingers extended.

CHAPTER *summary*

Introduction

- When the human body begins a movement, there are myriad actions involved that people usually never consider. The brain sends nerve signals to the skeletal muscles, and chemicals are released to contract those muscles; then the joints move with the cooperation of all these elements. Since there are hundreds of muscles in the human body, it is necessary to have knowledge about their shapes, locations, and functions, as well as their neuromuscular principles.

Muscle Nomenclature

- In attempting to learn the skeletal muscles, it is helpful to study how they are named. For example, a rotary-shaped muscle such as the gluteus maximus has a powerful action because of its quadrilateral shape. The functional action can be assessed by the muscle shape.

Shape of Muscles and Fascicle (Fiber Bundle) Arrangement

- Various muscles have different shapes, and their fibers may be arranged differently in relation to each other and to the tendons to which they join. As mentioned with the gluteus maximus muscle, the shape and fiber arrangement play a role in the muscle's ability to exert force. These factors also affect the range through which a muscle can effectively exert force. One factor in the muscle's ability to exert force is its cross-section diameter. Keeping all other factors constant, a muscle with a greater cross-section diameter will be able to exert a greater force.

Muscle-Tissue Properties

✔ Skeletal muscle tissue has four properties related to its ability to produce force and movement about the joints. *Irritability* or *excitability* is the muscle property of being sensitive or responsive to chemical, electrical, and mechanical stimuli. When an appropriate stimulus is provided, the muscle responds by developing tension. *Contractibility* is the muscle's ability to contract and develop tension or an internal force against resistance when stimulated. The ability of muscle tissue to develop tension or contract is unique; other body tissues do not have this property. *Extensibility* is the muscle's ability to be passively stretched beyond its normal resting length. *Elasticity* is the muscle's ability to return to its original resting length following a stretch.

Muscle Terminology

✔ Locating the muscles, their proximal and distal attachments, and their relationships to the joints they cross is critical to determining the effects that muscles have on the joints.

Contraction: The Sliding-Filament Theory

✔ In 1954, Hugh Huxley and Jean Hanson, two researchers at the Massachusetts Institute of Technology, developed a model called the *sliding-filament theory.* Their assumption, or model, was that the myofilaments in muscle do not shorten during a contraction but that the thin filaments (actin) slide over the thick ones (myosin) and pull the Z disks behind them.

Types of Muscle Contractions (Actions)

✔ The term *muscle contraction* may be confusing, because in some types of contractions the muscle does not shorten in length as the term *contraction* indicates. As a result, it has become increasingly common to refer to the various types of muscle contractions as *muscle actions* instead.

✔ Muscle contractions can be used to cause, control, or prevent joint movement. To elaborate, muscle contractions can be used to initiate or accelerate the movement of a body segment, to slow down or decelerate the movement of a body segment, or to prevent movement of a body segment by external forces. All muscle contractions or actions can be classified as being either isometric or isotonic.

Tying Roles of Muscles All Together

✔ When a muscle with multiple agonist actions contracts, it attempts to perform all of its actions. Muscles cannot determine which of their actions are appropriate for the task at hand. The resulting actions actually performed depend on several factors, such as the motor units activated, joint position, muscle length, and relative contraction or relaxation of other muscles acting on the joint.

Determination of Muscle Action

✔ The specific action of a muscle may be determined through a variety of methods. These include reasoning in consideration of anatomical lines of pull, anatomical dissection, palpation, models, electromyography, and electrical stimulation. Studying a muscle's line of pull against forces such as gravity and resistance is vital in a clinical setting.

✔ Combining the knowledge of a particular joint's functional design and the specific location of a musculotendinous unit as it crosses a joint is extremely helpful in understanding the muscle's action on the joint.

Neural Control of Voluntary Movement

✔ When discussing muscular activity, one should really refer to it as *neuromuscular activity,* since muscle cannot be active without nervous *innervation.* All voluntary movement is a result of both the muscular and nervous systems working together. All muscle contraction occurs as a result of stimulation from the nervous system. Ultimately, every muscle fiber is innervated by a somatic motor neuron, which, when an appropriate stimulus is provided, results in a muscle contraction.

Proprioception and Kinesthesis

✔ The performance of various activities is significantly dependent on neurologic feedback from the body. More importantly, people could not survive without the ability to sense where they are in space or sense temperature and pressure to the skin. Very simply, humans use the various senses to determine responses to their environment, such as using sight to know when to lift the hand to catch a fly ball.

Neuromuscular Concepts

✔ When a particular muscle contracts, the contraction actually occurs at the muscle-fiber level within a particular motor unit. A motor unit consists of a single motor neuron and all the muscle fibers it innervates. Motor units function as a single unit. In a typical muscle contraction, the number of motor units innervated and the number of muscle fibers contracting may vary significantly. This is known as the all-or-none principle.

✔ The difference between a particular muscle contracting to lift a minimal resistance and the same muscle contracting to lift a maximal resistance is the number of muscle fibers recruited. The number of muscle fibers recruited may be increased by activating the motor units that contain a greater number of muscle fibers, by activating more motor units, or by increasing the frequency of motor unit activation.

✔ The maximal ability of a muscle to develop tension and exert force varies depending on the length of the muscle during contraction. Generally, depending on the particular muscle involved, the greatest amount of tension can be developed when a muscle is stretched between 100 percent and 130 percent of its resting length.

✔ When the muscle is either concentrically or eccentrically contracting, the rate of length change is significantly related to the amount of force potential. When contracting concentrically against a light resistance, the muscle is able to contract at a high velocity.

CHAPTER *review*

True or False

Write true *or* false *after each statement.*

1. Under the definition of *reciprocal inhibition,* if the hamstrings flex the knee, then the quadriceps is lengthening to allow the movement. T
2. Angle of pull for skeletal muscles has no relationship to the planes of the body. F
3. After receiving innervations from the nerves, a muscle will contract. T
4. Kinesthesis is related to proprioceptors in the lower body. F
5. The stretch reflex is also known as a Golgi tendon reflex. T
6. Sensory neurons transmit impulses to the spinal cord and brain from all parts of the body.
7. Stabilizer muscles help primary mover muscles work effectively.
8. Eccentric muscle contraction is a *shortening* of muscle fibers.
9. A good example of a radiate muscle is the sartorius.
10. A good example of the myotatic reflex arc occurs when a person suddenly extends the head after being awakened from a chair.

Short Answers

Write your answers on the lines provided.

1. Describe how motor units and muscle fibers are affected by the all-or-none principle.

2. Describe reciprocal inhibition between the gastrocnemius and the anterior tibialis if the gastrocnemius is the agonist.

3. What functions does a Meissner's corpuscle have?

skin, stimuli

4. What are two factors that affect muscle tension development?

5. What affects the maximal ability of a muscle to develop tension and exert force?

6. The amount of muscular force needed to cause joint movement is greatly affected by what factor?

7. Explain the specific function uniarticular muscles have in joint movement.

8. Define active insufficiency in a muscle.

9. Define four properties related to a muscle's ability to produce force and movement.

10. Describe which muscle contractions an isokinetic exercise machine uses.

Multiple Choice

Circle the correct answers.

1. Reciprocal inhibition involves the agonist and antagonist so that:
   a. a muscle can contract
   b. cooperation occurs in joint movement
   c. more weight can be lifted
   d. the agonist and antagonist relax
2. Plyometrics uses what neuromuscular concept?
   a. all-or-none principle
   b. treppe
   c. pacinian corpuscles
   d. myotatic stretch reflex
3. Kinesthesis involves which of the following?
   a. pacinian corpuscles
   b. Ruffini's corpuscles
   c. Meissner's corpuscles
   d. all of the above
4. The highest level of neural control in the central nervous system is in the:
   a. cerebral cortex
   b. brainstem
   c. spinal cord
   d. cerebellum
5. Muscles that surround the joint or body part and contract to fixate on an area to allow another limb to move are considered:
   a. agonists
   b. synergists
   c. neutralizers
   d. stabilizers
6. A useful way to determine muscle action in the human body is by:
   a. palpation
   b. electromyography
   c. cadaver study
   d. all of the above
7. Sensory or afferent nerves are responsible for:
   a. carrying impulses to the outlying regions of the body
   b. spinal fluid circulation
   c. bringing impulses from receptors in skin, joints, and muscles to the CNS
   d. none of the above
8. During an extreme muscle stretch, muscle spindles react by:
   a. initiating the stretch reflex
   b. initiating the myotatic reflex arc
   c. doing both a and b
   d. sending pain signals to the medulla
9. Three components of muscular force are:
   a. transitory, synergistic, rotary
   b. nonrotary, dislocating, stabile
   c. angle of pull, insertion, velocity
   d. rotary, nonrotary, stabilizing
10. The rectus femoris contracting to flex the hip and extend the knee is a good example of:
    a. the stretch reflex
    b. active and passive insufficiency
    c. reciprocal stabilization
    d. angle of pull

EXPLORE & practice

1. Choose a particular sports skill and determine the type of muscle contractions that occur in various major muscle groups in the body at different phases of the skill.
2. Using a reflex hammer or the flexed knuckle of your long finger, compare the stretch reflex among several subjects.
3. Ask a partner to stand with eyes closed while you position the partner's arms in an odd position at the shoulders, elbows, and wrists. Ask your partner to describe the exact position of each joint while keeping his or her eyes closed. Then have your partner begin in the anatomical position, close the eyes, and subsequently reassume the position in which you had previously placed him or her. Explain the neuromechanisms involved in your partner's being able to both sense the joint position you placed him or her in and then reassume the same position.

4. On a flat surface, stand up straight on one leg with the other knee flexed slightly and not in contact with anything. Look straight ahead and attempt to maintain your balance in this position for up to 5 minutes. What do you notice happening to the muscles in your lower leg? Try this again with the knee of the leg you are standing on slightly flexed. What differences do you notice? Try it again standing on a piece of thick foam. Try it in the original position with your eyes closed. Elaborate on the differences between the various attempts.

5. While standing, hold a heavy book in your hand with your forearm supinated and elbow flexed approximately 90 degrees. Have a partner suddenly place another heavy book upon the one you are holding. What is the immediate result regarding the angle of flexion in your elbow? Explain why this result occurs.

6. Sit up very straight on a table with the knees flexed 90 degrees and the feet hanging free. Maintain this position while then flexing the right hip and attempting to cross your legs to place the right leg across the left knee. Is this difficult? What motion is occurring in the right leg or femur and why might it feel uncomfortable?

7. Determine your one-repetition maximum for a biceps curl, beginning in full extension and ending in full flexion. Carry out each of the following exercises with adequate periods for recovery in between:
   a. Begin with your elbow flexed 45 degrees, and have a partner hand you a weight slightly heavier than your one-repetition maximum (approximately 5 pounds). Attempt to lift it through the remaining range of flexion. Can you reach full flexion? Explain your results.
   b. Begin with your elbow in 90 degrees of flexion. Have your partner hand you a slightly heavier weight than described in 8a, above. Attempt to hold the elbow flexed in this position for 10 seconds. Can you do so? Explain.
   c. Begin with your elbow in full flexion. Have your partner hand you a slightly heavier weight than described in 8b. Attempt to slowly lower the weight under control until you reach full extension. Can you do this? Explain.

8. With the wrist in neutral, extend the fingers maximally and attempt to maintain the position and then extend the wrist maximally. What happens to the fingers and why?

9. Maximally flex your fingers around a pencil with your wrist in neutral. Maintain the maximal finger flexion while you allow a partner to grasp your forearm with one hand and use his or her other hand to push your wrist into maximal flexion. Can you maintain control of the pencil? Explain.

10. Observe on a fellow student some of the muscles found in figures 2.1 and 2.2.

11. With a partner, choose a diarthrodial joint on the body, and carry out each of the following exercises:
    a. Familiarize yourself with all of the joint's various movements, and list them.
    b. Determine which muscles or muscle groups are responsible for each of the movements you listed in 11a.
    c. For the muscles or muscle groups you listed for each movement in 11b, determine the type of contraction occurring.
    d. Determine how to change the parameters of gravity and/or resistance so that the opposite muscles contract to control the same movements noted in 11c. Name the type of contraction occurring.
    e. Determine how to change the parameters of movement, gravity, and/or resistance so that the same muscles listed in 11c contract differently to control the opposite movement.

12. *Muscle nomenclature chart:* Complete the chart by providing the characteristics of each muscle listed.

Muscle name	Distinctive characteristic(s) for which it is named
Adductor magnus	
Biceps brachii	
Biceps femoris	
Brachialis	
Brachioradialis	
Coracobrachialis	
Deltoid	
Extensor carpi radialis brevis	
Extensor carpi ulnaris	
Extensor digiti minimi	
Extensor digitorum	
Extensor hallucis longus	
Extensor indicis	
Extensor pollicis brevis	
External oblique	
Fibularis brevis	
Flexor carpi radialis	
Flexor digitorum longus	
Flexor digitorum profundus	
Flexor digitorum superficialis	

Muscle name	Distinctive characteristic(s) for which it is named
Flexor pollicus longus	
Gastrocnemius	
Gluteus maximus	
Gluteus medius	
Iliacus	
Iliocostalis thoracis	
Infraspinatus	
Latissimus dorsi	
Levator scapulae	
Longissimus lumborum	
Obturator externus	
Palmaris longus	
Pectoralis minor	
Peroneus tertius	
Plantaris	
Pronator quadratus	
Pronator teres	
Psoas major	
Rectus abdominis	
Rectus femoris	
Rhomboid	

(*Continued*)

Muscle name	Distinctive characteristic(s) for which it is named
Semimembranosus	
Semitendinosus	
Serratus anterior	
Spinalis cervicis	
Sternocleidomastoid	
Subclavius	
Subscapularis	
Supinator	
Supraspinatus	
Tensor fasciae latae	
Teres major	
Tibialis posterior	
Transversus abdominis	
Trapezius	
Triceps brachii	
Vastus intermedius	
Vastus lateralis	
Vastus medialis	

13. *Muscle shape and fiber arrangement chart:* Complete the chart by writing in *flat, fusiform, strap, radiate,* or *sphincter* for muscles classified as parallel. Write in *unipennate, bipennate,* or *multipennate* for those classified as pennate.

Muscle	Parallel	Pennate
Adductor longus		
Adductor magnus		
Brachioradialis		
Extensor digitorum		
Flexor carpi ulnaris		
Flexor digitorum longus		
Gastrocnemius		
Gluteus maximus		
Iliopsoas		
Infraspinatus		
Latissimus dorsi		
Levator scapulae		
Palmaris longus		
Pronator quadratus		
Pronator teres		
Rhomboid		
Serratus anterior		
Subscapularis		
Triceps brachii		
Vastus intermedius		
Vastus medialis		

14. *Muscle contraction typing chart:* Write the type of contraction, if any, in the cell of the muscle group that is contracting. Place a dash in the cell if no contraction is occurring.

Exercise	Quadriceps	Hamstrings
a. Lie prone on a table with your knee in full extension.		
Maintain your knee in full extension.		
Very slowly flex your knee maximally.		
Maintain your knee in full flexion.		
From the fully flexed position, extend your knee fully as fast as possible but stop immediately before reaching maximal extension.		
From the fully flexed position, very slowly extend your knee fully.		
b. Begin sitting on the edge of the table with your knee in full extension.		
Maintain your knee in full extension.		
Very slowly flex your knee maximally.		
Maintain your knee in full flexion.		
Maintain your knee in approximately 90 degrees of flexion.		
From the fully flexed position, slowly extend your knee fully.		
c. Stand on one leg and move the other knee as directed.		
Maintain your knee in full extension.		
Very slowly flex your knee maximally.		
From the fully flexed position, slowly extend your knee fully.		
From the fully flexed position, extend your knee fully as fast as possible.		

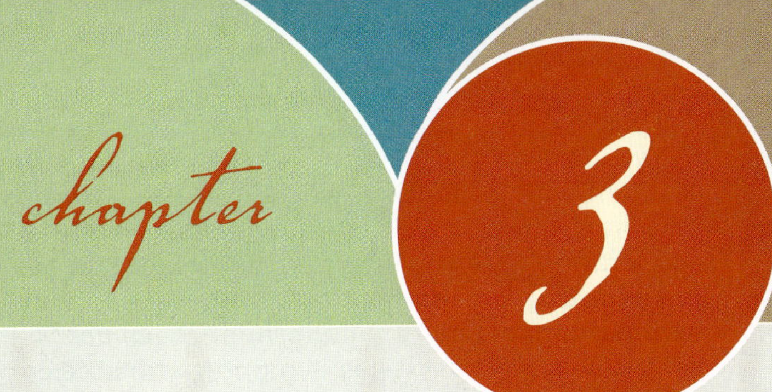

Basic Biomechanical Factors and Concepts

LEARNING OUTCOMES

After completing this chapter, you should be able to:

3-1 Differentiate between the levers and explain how they apply to physical performance.

3-2 Discuss how the musculoskeletal system functions as a series of simple machines.

3-3 Describe how knowledge of torque and lever arm lengths can help improve physical performance.

3-4 Recall Newton's laws of motion and cite examples of how the laws can apply to improving physical performance.

3-5 Compare balance, equilibrium, and stability and discuss how they can each help improve physical performance.

3-6 Define *force* and *momentum* and describe how they can help improve physical performance.

3-7 Analyze the basic effects of mechanical loading on the tissues of the body.

KEY TERMS

Acceleration
Angular motion
Axis
Balance
Biomechanics
Displacement
Distance
Eccentric force
Force
Force arm
Friction
Inertia
Kinematics
Kinetics
Law of acceleration
Law of inertia
Law of reaction
Linear motion
Mass
Mechanical advantage
Resistance arm
Sherrington's law
Speed
Torque
Velocity

Introduction

Human movement is often complex and beautiful. Consider, for example, a ballerina's pirouette—a movement that requires years of training. Yet behind the dancer's graceful movements are hundreds of laws, forces, and biomechanical principles at work. Motion cannot occur unless there is a force behind it; however, motion includes many levers, torque, and pulleys that all exist as force is applied. Studying movement requires analyzing all of these elements. This chapter introduces some of the basic biomechanical factors and concepts that help make the study of kinesiology more logical.

The study of mechanics as it relates to the functional and anatomical analysis of biological systems is known as **biomechanics.** Because the topic is so complex, students would benefit from a separate, concentrated study of biomechanics; however, to make recommendations for improving human movement, it is necessary to examine motion from a biomechanical perspective, both qualitatively and quantitatively.

Many students studying kinesiology have some knowledge, from a college or high school physics course, of the laws that affect motion. These principles and others are discussed briefly in this chapter, which should prepare students as they begin to apply them to motion in the human body. The more one can put these principles and concepts into practical application, the easier it will be to determine how they apply to actions.

Mechanics, the study of physical actions of forces, can be subdivided into statics and dynamics. *Statics* involves the study of systems that are in a constant state of motion, whether at rest with no motion or moving at a constant velocity without acceleration. Statics involves the balance of all forces acting on the body, resulting in the body maintaining a state of equilibrium. *Dynamics* involves the study of systems in motion with acceleration. A system in acceleration is unbalanced due to unequal forces acting on the body. Additional components of biomechanical study include kinematics and kinetics. **Kinematics** is concerned with the description of motion and includes consideration of time, displacement, velocity, acceleration, and space factors of a system's motion. **Kinetics** is the study of forces associated with the motion of a body.

Types of Machines Found in the Body

As discussed in Chapter 2, the body utilizes muscles to apply force to the bones on which they attach to cause, control, or prevent movement in the joints that they cross. As is often the case, humans utilize the bones, such as those in the hand, to either hold, push, or pull on an object while also using a series of bones and joints throughout the body to apply force via the muscles to affect the position of the object. In doing so, the body is using a series of simple machines to accomplish the tasks. Machines are used to increase or multiply the applied force in performing a task or to provide a mechanical advantage. The **mechanical advantage** provided by machines enables the body to apply a relatively small force, or effort, to move a much greater resistance. It is possible to determine mechanical advantage by dividing the load by the effort. The mechanical aspect of each component should be considered in analysis with respect to the components' machinelike function.

Another way of thinking about machines is that they convert smaller amounts of force over a longer distance to large amounts of force exerted over a shorter distance. This may be turned around so that a larger amount of force exerted over a shorter distance converts to a smaller amount of force over a greater distance.

Machines function in four ways:

1. To balance multiple forces.
2. To enhance force in an attempt to reduce the total force needed to overcome a resistance.
3. To enhance range of motion and speed of movement so that resistance may be moved farther or faster than the applied force.
4. To alter the resulting direction of the applied force.

Simple machines are the lever, wheel and axle, pulley, inclined plane, screw, and wedge. The arrangement of the musculoskeletal system provides three types of machines for producing movement: levers, wheels and axles, and pulleys. Each of these involves a balancing of rotational forces around an axis. The lever is the most common form of simple machine found in the human body.

Levers

While most people might not think of the body as a machine in a literal sense, human movement is possible through the organized use of a system of levers. The body's anatomical levers cannot be changed, but when the system is properly understood, they can be used more efficiently to maximize muscular efforts.

A *lever* is defined as a rigid bar that turns around an axis of rotation, or fulcrum. The **axis** is the point of rotation around which the lever moves.

The lever rotates around the axis as a result of the force (sometimes referred to as *effort*, or *E*) applied to it to cause its movement against a resistance or weight. In the body, the bones represent the lever bars, the joints are the axes, and the muscles contract to apply the force. The amount of resistance can vary from maximal to minimal. In fact, the bones themselves or the weight of the body segment may be the only resistance applied. All lever systems have each of these three components in one of three possible arrangements.

The arrangement of these three components in relation to one another determines the type of lever and the application for which it is best suited. Each component represents a location, or point. These points are the axis, the point of force application (usually

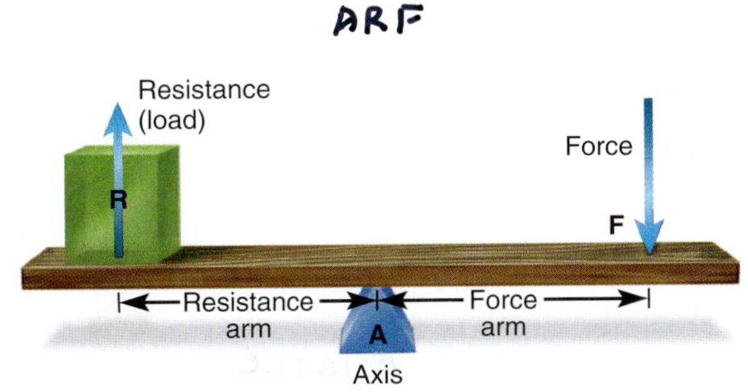

FIGURE 3.1 The basic components of a lever

the muscle insertion), and the point of resistance application (sometimes the center of gravity of the lever and sometimes the location of an external resistance). When the axis (*A*) is placed between the force (*F*) and the resistance (*R*), a first-class lever is produced (figure 3.1). In second-class levers, the resistance is between the axis and the force. If the force is placed between the axis and the resistance, a third-class lever is created (figure 3.2). Table 3.1 provides a summary of the three classes of levers and the characteristics of each.

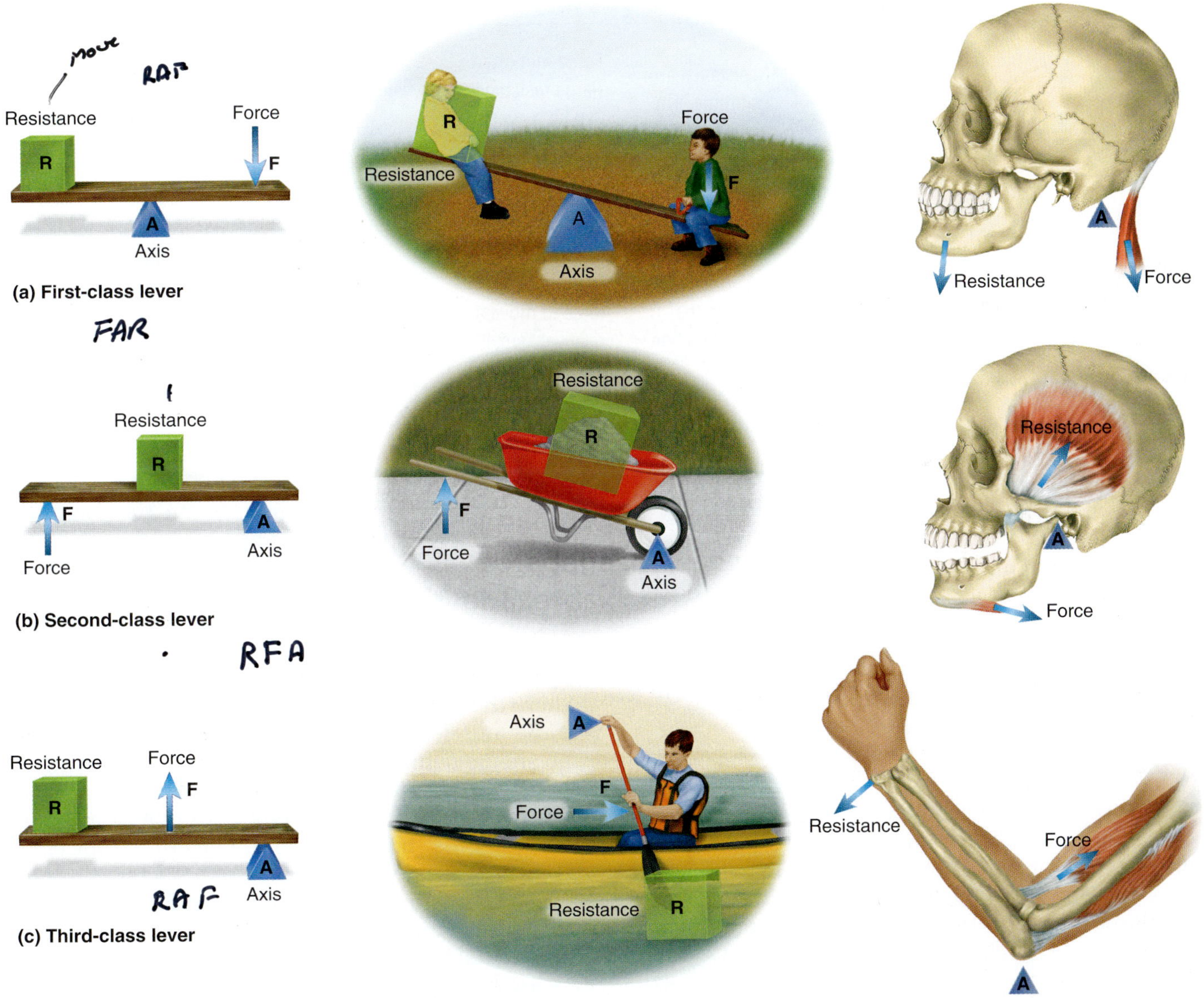

(a) First-class lever

(b) Second-class lever

(c) Third-class lever

FIGURE 3.2 The three classes of levers

TABLE 3.1 Classification of Levers and Characteristics of Each

Class	Illustration	Arrangement	Arm movement	Functional design	Relationship to axis	Practical example	Human example
1st	F R A	**F–A–R** Axis between force and resistance	Resistance arm and force arm move in opposite directions	Balanced movements	Axis near middle	Seesaw	Erector spinae extending the head on cervical spine
				Speed and range of motion	Axis near force	Scissors	Triceps brachii in extending the elbow
				Force motion	Axis near resistance	Crowbar	
2nd	R F A	**A–R–F** Resistance between axis and force	Resistance arm and force arm move in the same direction	Force motion (large resistance can be moved with relatively small force)	Axis near resistance	Wheelbarrow, nutcracker	Gastrocnemius and soleus in plantar flexing the foot to raise the body on the toes
3rd	F R A	**A–F–R** Force between axis and resistance	Resistance arm and force arm move in the same direction	Speed and range of motion (requires large force to move a relatively small resistance)	Axis near force	Shoveling dirt, catapult	Biceps brachii and brachialis in flexing the elbow

The mechanical advantage of levers may be determined using the following equations:

$$\text{Mechanical advantage} = \frac{\text{resistance}}{\text{force}}$$

or

$$\text{Mechanical advantage} = \frac{\text{length of force arm}}{\text{length of resistance arm}}$$

FIRST-CLASS LEVERS

Typical examples of a first-class lever are the crowbar, the seesaw, pliers, oars, and the triceps in overhead elbow extension. An example of this type of lever at work in the body is seen when the triceps is applying the force to the olecranon (*F*) in extending the nonsupported forearm (*R*) at the elbow (*A*). Other examples may be seen in the body when the agonist and antagonist muscle groups on either side of a joint axis are contracting simultaneously, with the agonist producing force and the antagonist supplying the resistance. A first-class lever is designed basically to produce balanced movements when the axis is midway between the force and the resistance (e.g., a seesaw). When the axis is close to the force, the lever produces speed and range of motion (e.g., the triceps in elbow extension). When the axis is close to the resistance, the lever produces force motion (e.g., a crowbar).

In applying the principle of levers to the body, it is important to remember that the force is applied where the muscle inserts in the bone, not in the belly of the muscle. For example, in elbow extension with the shoulder fully flexed and the arm beside the ear, the triceps applies the force to the olecranon of the ulna behind the axis of the elbow joint. As the applied force exceeds the amount of forearm resistance, the elbow extends.

The type of lever may be changed for a given joint and muscle, depending on whether the body segment is in contact with a surface, such as a floor or wall. For example, as previously mentioned, the triceps in elbow extension is a first-class lever with the hand free in space where the arm is pushed away from the body. By placing the hand in contact with the floor, as in performing a push-up to push the body away from the floor, the same muscle action at this joint now changes the lever to second class, because the axis is at the hand and the resistance is the body weight at the elbow joint.

SECOND-CLASS LEVERS

A second-class lever is designed to produce force movements, since a large resistance can be moved by a relatively small force. Examples of second-class levers include a bottle opener, wheelbarrow, and nutcracker. In addition to the previous example of the triceps extending the elbow in a push-up, a similar example of a second-class lever is plantar flexion of the ankle to raise the body up on the toes. The ball (*A*) of the foot serves as the axis of rotation as the ankle plantar flexors apply force to the calcaneus (*F*) to lift the resistance of the body at the tibiofibular articulation (*R*) with the talus. Opening the mouth against resistance provides another example of a second-class lever. There are relatively few other occurrences of second-class levers in the body.

THIRD-CLASS LEVERS

Third-class levers, with force applied between the axis and the resistance, are designed to produce speed and range-of-motion movements. Most of the levers in the human body are of this type and require a great deal of force to move even a small resistance. Examples include a catapult, a screen door operated by a short spring, and the application of a lifting force to a shovel handle with the lower hand while the upper hand on the shovel handle serves as the axis of rotation. The biceps brachii is a typical example in the body. Using the elbow joint (*A*) as the axis, the biceps brachii applies force at its insertion on the radial tuberosity (*F*) to rotate the forearm up, with its center of gravity (*R*) serving as the point of resistance application.

The brachialis is an example of true third-class leverage. It pulls on the ulna just below the elbow, and since the ulna cannot rotate, the pull is direct and true. The biceps brachii, in contrast, supinates the forearm as it flexes, so the third-class leverage applies to flexion only.

Other examples include the hamstrings contracting to flex the leg at the knee while in a standing position and the iliopsoas when it is used to flex the thigh at the hip.

Factors in the Use of Anatomical Levers

The body's anatomical leverage system can be used to gain a mechanical advantage that will improve simple or complex physical movements. Some individuals unconsciously develop habits of using human levers properly, but frequently this is not the case.

To understand the leverage system, therapists must be familiar with the concept of torque. **Torque,** or moment of force, is the turning effect of an eccentric force. **Eccentric force** is a force that is applied in a direction not in line with the center of rotation of an object with a fixed axis. In objects without a fixed axis, it is an applied force that is not in line with the object's center of gravity. For rotation to occur, an eccentric force must be applied. In the human body, the contracting muscle applies an eccentric force (not to be confused with eccentric contraction) to the bone on which it attaches and causes the bone to rotate around an axis at the joint. The amount of torque can be determined by multiplying the amount of force (force magnitude) by the force arm. An example is pushing on a door to open it. Force generated by the push causes the door to open, with the hinges rotating on an axis (pivot point). How much force the push must have to open the door depends on many things, such as how close the arm is to the hinges. The closer the push is to the hinges, the more difficult it becomes to open the door. The perpendicular distance between the location of force application and the axis is known as the **force arm,** *moment arm,* or *torque arm.* The force arm may be best defined as the shortest distance from the axis of rotation to the line of action of the force. The greater the distance of the force arm, the more torque produced by the force. A frequent practical application of torque and levers occurs when a person purposely increases the force-arm length in order to increase the torque so that she can more easily move a relatively large resistance. This is commonly referred to as *increasing leverage.*

TORQUE AND LENGTH OF LEVER ARMS

It is also important to note the **resistance arm,** which may be defined as the distance between the axis and the point of resistance application. In discussing the application of levers, it is necessary to study the length relationship between the two lever arms. There is an inverse relationship between force and the force arm, just as there is between resistance and the resistance arm. The longer the force arm, the less force required to move the lever if the resistance and resistance arm remain constant, as shown graphically in figure 3.3. In addition, if the force and force arm remain constant, a greater resistance may be moved by shortening the resistance arm.

There also is a proportional relationship between the force components and the resistance components. That is, for movement to occur when either of the resistance components increases, there must be an increase in one or both of the force components.

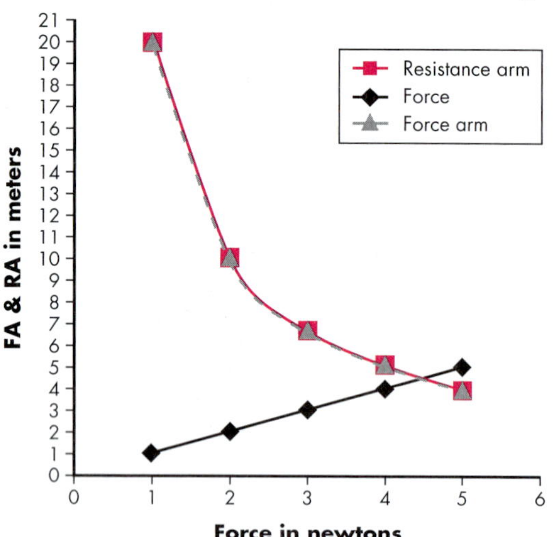

FIGURE 3.3 Relationships among forces

Lever equation for a child performing biceps curls

Lever equation

F	x	FA	=	R	x	RA
(Force)	x	(Force arm)	=	(Resistance)	x	(Resistance arm)

Initial Example

F x 0.1 = 45 newtons x 0.25 meter
F x 0.1 = 11.25 newton-meters
F = 112.5 newtons

Example A – Lengthening the force arm

Increase FA by moving the insertion distally 0.05 meter:

F x 0.15 = 45 newtons x 0.25 meter
F x 0.15 = 11.25 newton-meters
F = 75 newtons

An increase in the insertion from the axis by 0.05 meter results in a substantial reduction in the force necessary to move the resistance.

Example B – Shortening the resistance arm

Reduce RA by moving the point of resistance application proximally by 0.05 meter:

F x 0.1 = 45 newtons x 0.2 meter
F x 0.1 = 9 newton-meters
F = 90 newtons

A decrease in the resistance application from the axis by 0.05 meter results in a considerable reduction in the force necessary to move the resistance.

Example C – Reducing the resistance

Reduce R by reducing the resistance 1 newton:

F x 0.1 = 44 newtons x 0.25 meter
F x 0.1 = 11 newton-meters
F = 110 newtons

Decreasing the amount of resistance can decrease the amount of force needed to move the lever.

FIGURE 3.4 Torque calculations with examples of modifications in force arms

See figure 3.2, which shows how these components relate to first-, second-, and, third-class levers.

Even slight variations in the location of the force and the resistance are important in determining the mechanical advantage and the effective force of the muscle. This point is illustrated through a simple formula, using the biceps brachii muscle in each example, as shown in figure 3.4.

In example A, only surgery can move the insertion of the biceps brachii, so this is not practical. In some orthopedic conditions, the attachments of tendons are surgically relocated in an attempt to change the dynamic forces of the muscles on the joints. In example B, a person can and often does shorten the resistance arm to enhance his ability to move an object. When attempting to lift a maximal weight in a biceps curl exercise, the person may flex his wrist to move the weight just a little closer, thereby shortening the resistance arm. Example C is straightforward in that a person can obviously reduce the force needed by reducing the resistance.

The human body's system of leverage is built for speed and range of movement at the expense of force. Short-force arms and long-resistance arms require great muscular strength to produce movement. In the forearm, the attachments of the biceps and triceps muscles clearly illustrate this point, since the force arm of the biceps is 1 to 2 inches and the force arm of the triceps less than 1 inch. Many similar examples are found all over the body. From a practical point of view, this means that the muscular system should be strong to supply the necessary force for body movements, especially in strenuous sports activities.

When people speak of human leverage in relation to athletic skills, they are generally referring to several levers. For example, in throwing a ball, there are levers at the shoulder, elbow, and wrist joints, as well as from the ground up through the lower extremities and the trunk. In fact, it can be said that there is one long lever from the feet to the hands.

The longer the lever, the more effective it is in imparting velocity. A tennis player can hit a tennis ball harder (deliver more force to it) with a straight-arm drive than with a bent-elbow drive because the lever (including the racket) is longer and moves at a faster speed.

Figure 3.5 indicates that a longer lever (Z_1) travels faster than a shorter lever (S_1) in traveling the same number of degrees. In sports activities in which it is

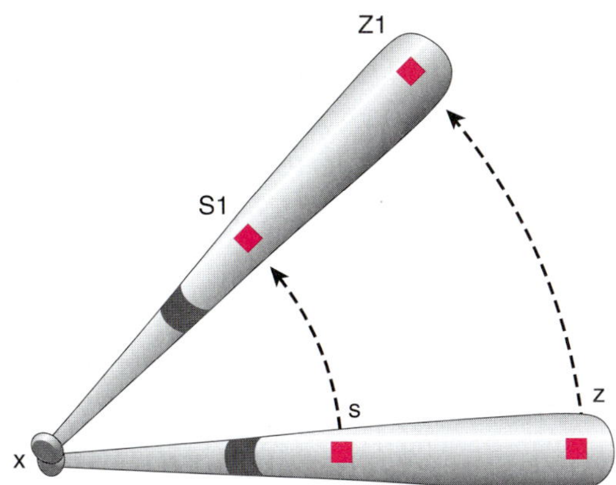

FIGURE 3.5 Length of levers

possible to increase the length of a lever with a racket or bat, the same principle applies.

In baseball, hockey, golf, field hockey, and other sports, long levers similarly produce more linear force and thus better performance. However, to fully execute the movement in as short a time as possible, it is sometimes desirable to have a short lever arm. For example, a baseball catcher attempting to throw a runner out at second base does not have to throw the ball so that it travels as fast as it may when the pitcher is attempting to throw a strike. In the catcher's case, it is more important to initiate and complete the throw as soon as possible rather than to deliver as much velocity to the ball as possible. The pitcher, when attempting to throw a ball at 90-plus miles per hour, will utilize his body as a much longer lever system throughout a greater range of motion to impart velocity to the ball.

WHEELS AND AXLES

Wheels and axles are used primarily to enhance range of motion and speed of movement in the musculoskeletal system. A wheel and an axle essentially function as a form of lever. When either the wheel or the axle turns, the other must turn as well. Both complete one turn at the same time. The center of the wheel and the axle both correspond to the fulcrum. Both the radius of the wheel and the radius of the axle correspond to the force arms. If the radius of the wheel is greater than the radius of the axle, then, due to the longer force arm, the wheel has a mechanical advantage over the axle. That is, a relatively smaller force may be applied to the wheel to move a relatively greater resistance applied to the axle. Very simply, if the radius of the wheel is five times the radius of the axle, the wheel has a 5-to-1 mechanical advantage over the axle, as shown in figure 3.6. The mechanical advantage of a wheel and axle for this scenario may be calculated

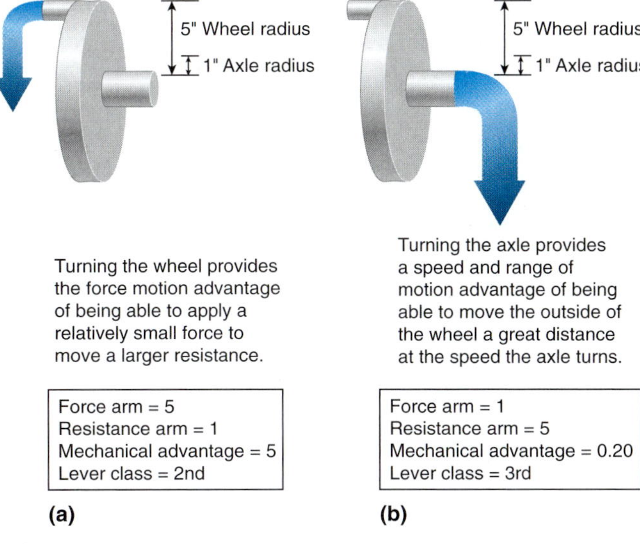

FIGURE 3.6 Wheel and axle

by dividing the radius of the wheel by that of the axle:

$$\text{Mechanical advantage} = \frac{\text{radius of wheel}}{\text{radius of axle}}$$

In this case, the mechanical advantage is always more than 1. An application of this example is using the outer portion of an automobile steering wheel to turn the steering mechanism. Before the development of power steering, steering wheels had a much larger diameter than they do today in order to enable the driver to have more of a mechanical advantage. An example of applying force to a wheel in the body occurs when one person attempts to manually force another person's shoulder into internal rotation while the latter person holds it in external rotation isometrically. The humerus acts as the axle, and the person applies the force to the humerus with the hand and wrist located near the outside of the wheel. To help create a better lever, the elbow, or axle, is flexed approximately 90 degrees. If the person applying the force at the midforearm unsuccessfully breaks the opposite force of the contraction of the external rotators by pushing internally, he can increase leverage, or mechanical advantage, by applying force nearer to the hand and wrist. Doing so, he has a better chance of overcoming the resistant force.

If the application of force is reversed so that it is applied to the axle, the mechanical advantage results from the wheel's turning a greater distance and speed. Using the same example, if the wheel radius is five times greater than the radius of the axle, the outside of the wheel will turn at a speed five times that of the axle. Additionally, the distance that the outside of the wheel turns will be five times the distance that the outside of the axle turns. The mechanical advantage of a wheel and axle for this scenario may be calculated by dividing the radius of the axle by the radius of the wheel:

$$\text{Mechanical advantage} = \frac{\text{radius of the axle}}{\text{radius of the wheel}}$$

In this case, the mechanical advantage is always less than 1. This is the principle utilized in the drive train of an automobile to turn the axle, which subsequently turns the tire around one revolution for every turn of the axle. Humans use the powerful engine of the automobile to supply the force to increase the speed of the tire and subsequently carry them great distances. An example of the muscles applying force to the axle to result in greater range of motion and speed may again be seen in the upper extremity, in the case of the internal rotators attaching to the humerus. With the humerus acting as the axle and the hand and wrist located at the outside of the wheel (when the elbow is flexed approximately 90 degrees), the internal rotators apply force to the humerus. With the internal rotators concentrically internally rotating the humerus a relatively small amount, the hand and wrist travel a great distance. Using the wheel and axle in this manner allows a person to significantly increase the speed at which she can throw objects.

PULLEYS

Single pulleys have a fixed axle and function to change the effective direction of force application. Single pulleys have a mechanical advantage of 1, as shown in figure 3.7. Numerous weight machines utilize pulleys to alter the direction of the resistive force. Pulleys may be movable and be combined to form compound pulleys to further increase the mechanical advantage. Every additional rope connecting to movable pulleys increases the mechanical advantage by 1, as shown in figure 3.8.

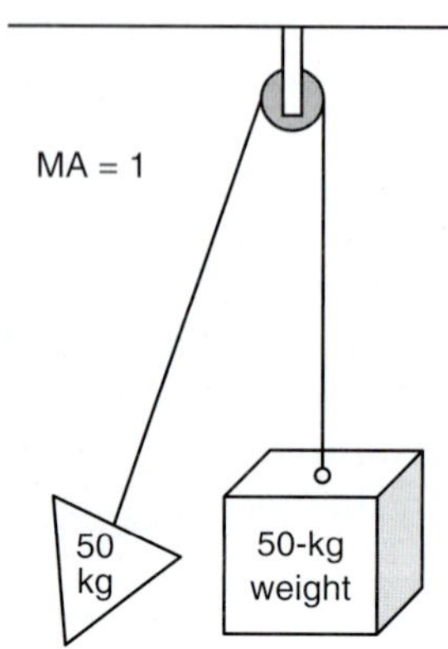

FIGURE 3.7 Single pulley

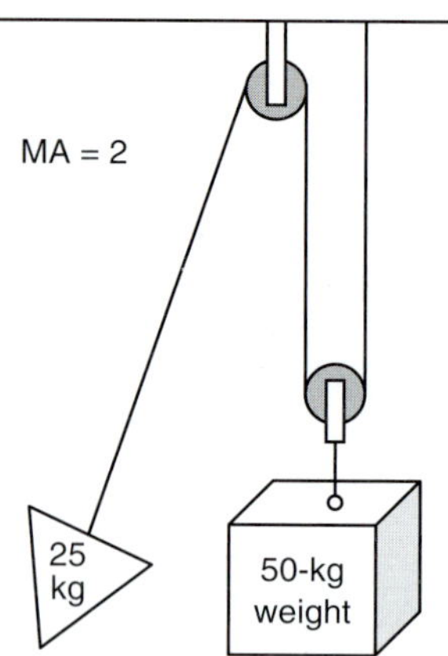

FIGURE 3.8 Compound pulley

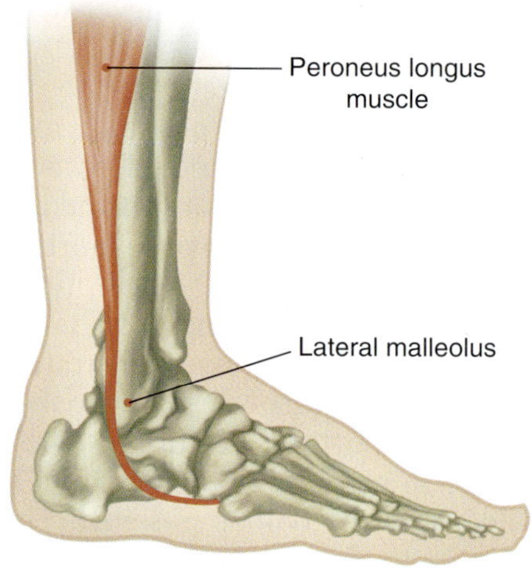

FIGURE 3.9 Force of pulley

In the human body, an excellent example is provided by the lateral malleolus, which acts as a pulley around which the tendon of the peroneus longus runs. As the peroneus longus muscle contracts, it pulls toward its belly, which is toward the knee. Due to its use of the lateral malleolus as a pulley (figure 3.9), the force is transmitted to the plantar aspect of the foot; this results in downward and outward movement of the foot. Other examples in the human body include pulleys on the volar aspect of the phalanges to redirect the force of the flexor tendons and pulleys on the patellofemoral joint to redirect the force of the quadriceps.

Laws of Motion and Physical Activities

Motion is fundamental in physical education and sports activity. Body motion is generally produced, or at least started, by some action of the muscular system. Motion cannot occur without a force, and the muscular system is the source of force in the human body. Thus, development of the muscular system is indispensable to movement.

Basically, there are two types of motion: linear motion and angular motion. **Linear motion,** also referred to as *translatory motion,* is motion along a line. If the motion is along a straight line, it is *rectilinear motion,* whereas motion along a curved line is known as *curvilinear motion.* **Angular motion,** also known as *rotary motion,* involves rotation around an axis. In the human body, the axis of rotation is provided by the various joints. In a sense, these two types of motion are related, since angular motion of the joints can produce the linear motion of walking. For example, in many sports activities, the cumulative angular motion of the joints of the body imparts linear motion to a thrown object (ball, shot) or to an object struck with an instrument (bat, racket).

Displacement is a change in the position or location of an object from its original point of reference, whereas **distance,** or the path of movement, is the actual sum length of measurement traveled. A vector quantity such as displacement is direction-aware, meaning that when an object changes direction of motion, displacement takes this change into consideration. An object going in an opposite direction effectively begins to cancel whatever displacement there once was. If a high school cross-country runner begins at the school, runs 10 miles, and then stops and runs back to the school, the displacement would be zero. Because he went the 10 miles and then reversed his direction, the original displacement was canceled. In figure 3.10, if the path of movement is from *A* to *B* and then *B* to *C,* the distance covered is $AB + BC$, but the displacement is the distance from *A* to *C,* or *AC.* If each cell is 1 square meter, then *AB* is 3 meters and *BC* is 3 meters, so the distance covered is 6 meters. Using the Pythagorean theorem (in a right triangle, the square of the measure of the hypotenuse is equal to the sum of the squares of the measures of the legs, or $a^2 + b^2 = c^2$), the displacement (*AC*) is determined to be 2.24 meters with $AB^2 + BC^2 = AC^2$.

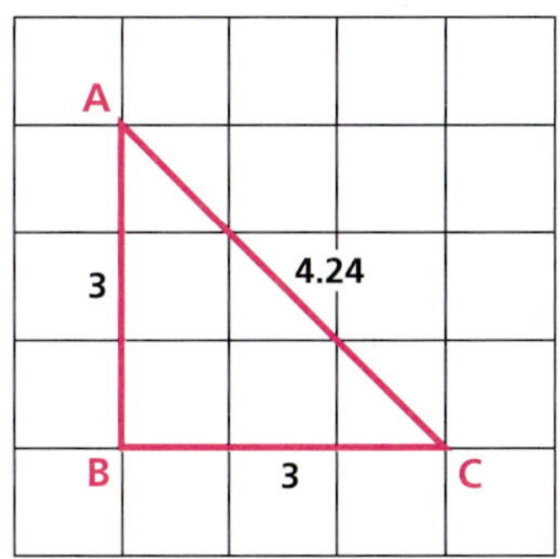

FIGURE 3.10 Displacement

Angular displacement is the change in location of a rotating body. Linear displacement is the distance that a system moves in a straight line.

The time it takes for displacement to occur is sometimes a concern. **Speed** is how fast an object is moving, or the distance an object travels in a specific amount of time. **Velocity** includes the direction and describes the rate of displacement.

A brief review of Newton's laws of motion will indicate the many applications of these laws to physical activities and sports. Newton's laws explain all the characteristics of motion, and they are fundamental to understanding human movement.

LAW OF INERTIA

According to the **law of inertia,** *a body in motion tends to remain in motion at the same speed in a straight line unless acted on by a force; a body at rest tends to remain at rest unless acted on by a force.*

Inertia may be described as the resistance to action or change. In terms of human movement, inertia is resistance to acceleration or deceleration. Inertia is the tendency for the current state of motion to be maintained, regardless of whether the body segment is moving at a particular velocity or is motionless.

Muscles produce the force necessary to start motion, stop motion, accelerate motion, decelerate motion, or change the direction of motion. Put another way, inertia is the reluctance to change status; only force can do that. The greater the mass of an object, the greater its inertia. Therefore, the greater the mass, the more force needed to significantly change an object's inertia. Numerous examples of this law are found in physical education activities. A sprinter in the starting blocks must apply considerable force to overcome resting inertia. A runner on an indoor track must apply considerable force to overcome moving inertia and stop before hitting the wall. Figure 3.11

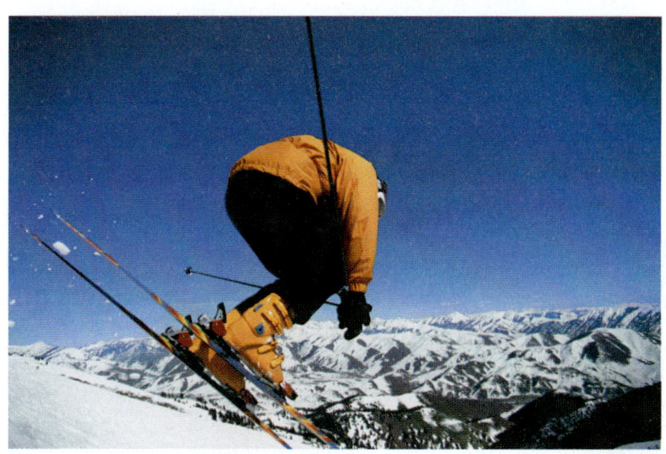

FIGURE 3.11 Skier on mountain

provides an example of how a skier in motion remains in motion even though airborne after skiing off a hill. Balls and other objects that are thrown or struck require force to stop them. Starting, stopping, and changing direction—a part of many physical activities—provide many other examples of the law of inertia applied to body motion.

Since force is required to change inertia, it is obvious that any activity that is carried out at a steady pace in a consistent direction will conserve energy and that any irregularly paced or directed activity will be very costly to energy reserves. This explains, in part, why activities such as handball and basketball are so much more fatiguing than jogging or dancing.

LAW OF ACCELERATION

The **law of acceleration** is as follows: *A change in the acceleration of a body occurs in the same direction as the force that caused it. The change in acceleration is directly proportional to the force causing it and inversely proportional to the mass of the body.*

Acceleration may be defined as the rate of change in velocity. To attain speed in moving the body, a strong muscular force is generally necessary. **Mass,** the amount of matter in a body, affects the speed and acceleration in physical movements. A much greater force is required from the muscles to accelerate an 80-kilogram man than to accelerate a 58-kilogram man to the same running speed. Also, it is possible to accelerate a baseball faster than a shot because of the difference in weight. The force required to run at half speed is less than the force required to run at top speed. To impart speed to a ball or an object, it is necessary to rapidly accelerate the part of the body holding the object. Football, basketball, track, and field hockey are a few sports that demand speed and acceleration.

LAW OF REACTION

The **law of reaction** states that *for every action there is an opposite and equal reaction.*

As a person places force on a supporting surface by walking over it, the surface provides an equal resistance back in the opposite direction to the soles of the feet. The feet push down and back, while the surface pushes up and forward. The force of the surface reacting to the force placed on it is referred to as *ground reaction force.* A person provides the action force, while the surface provides the reaction force. It is easier to run on a hard track than it is on a sandy beach because of the difference in the ground reaction forces of the two surfaces. The track resists the runner's propulsion force, and the reaction drives the runner ahead. The sand dissipates the runner's force, and the reaction force is correspondingly reduced, with the apparent loss in forward force and speed (figure 3.12). A sprinter applies a force in excess of 1,335 newtons on the starting blocks, which resist with an equal force. When a body is in flight, as it is in jumping, movement of one part of the body produces a reaction in another part. This occurs because there is no resistive surface to supply a reaction force.

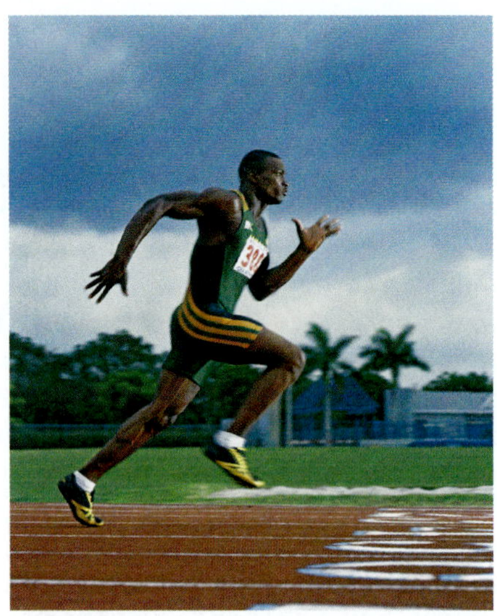

FIGURE 3.12 Runner

SHERRINGTON'S LAW

Sherrington's law is the law of reciprocal innervation (discussed in Chapter 2). It essentially states that for every neural activation of a muscle, there is a corresponding inhibition of the opposing muscle. When contraction of the agonist is stimulated, there is a simultaneous inhibition of its antagonist. For example, when the biceps brachii contracts, the triceps muscle relaxes, allowing the action to occur. This action is essential for coordinated movement; it is discussed more in Chapter 4, in the sections on clinical flexibility.

Friction

Friction is the force that results from the resistance between the surfaces of two objects moving against one another. Depending on the activity involved, one may desire increased or decreased friction. In running, a person depends on friction forces between the feet and the ground so that she may exert force against the ground and propel herself forward. When friction is reduced due to a slick ground or shoe surface, a person is more likely to slip. In skating, a person desires decreased friction so that he may slide across the ice with less resistance. Friction may be further characterized as either static friction or kinetic friction. *Static friction* is the amount of friction between two objects that have not yet begun to move, whereas *kinetic friction* is the friction that occurs between two objects sliding against one another. Static friction is always greater than kinetic friction. As a result, it is always more difficult to initiate dragging an object across a surface than it is to continue the movement. Static friction may be increased by increasing the normal or perpendicular forces pressing the two objects together, as in adding more weight to one object sitting on the other object. To determine the amount of friction forces, it is necessary to consider both of the forces pressing the two objects together and the coefficient of friction, which depends on the hardness and roughness of the surface textures. The coefficient of friction is the ratio of the force needed to overcome the friction to the force holding the surfaces together. Another type of friction, *rolling friction*, is the resistance to an object rolling across a surface, such as a ball rolling across a court or a tire rolling across the ground. Rolling friction is always much less than static or kinetic friction.

Balance, Equilibrium, and Stability

Balance is the ability to control equilibrium. In relation to human movement, the term *equilibrium* refers to a state of zero acceleration in which there is no change in the speed or direction of the body. Equilibrium may be either static or dynamic. In *static equilibrium*, the body is at rest or completely motionless. *Dynamic equilibrium* occurs when all the applied and inertial forces acting on the moving body are in balance, resulting in movement with unchanging speed or direction. For a person to control equilibrium and, hence, achieve balance, he needs to maximize stability. *Stability* is the resistance to a change in the body's acceleration, or, more appropriately, it is the resistance to a disturbance of the body's equilibrium. Stability may be enhanced by determining the body's center of gravity and changing it appropriately. The center of gravity is the point at which all of the body's mass and weight is equally balanced or equally distributed in all directions.

Balance is important for the resting body, as well as for the moving body. Generally, balance is desirable, but there are circumstances in which movement is improved when the body is unbalanced. Balance relates to many activities—not just to athletics. If a person picks up an object off the ground away from the body and the center of gravity, there is not enough balance to give stability to the action. The result is often injury and pain. These concepts are important to the manual therapist. To work around a massage table, the therapist must use information about balance for good body mechanics. Realizing where the center of gravity is and lowering the body to encourage better balance will enhance stability and support more momentum and force. If the table is too high, the therapist will not be able to utilize body weight and balance and will, therefore, be unstable. With a high table, the therapist often uses compensatory actions such as elevating the shoulders to try to rectify balance; this could lead to injury over a period of time.

The following general factors apply to enhancing equilibrium, maximizing stability, and ultimately achieving balance:

1. A person has balance when the center of gravity falls within the base of support.
2. A person has balance in direct proportion to the size of the base. The larger the base of support, the more balance.
3. A person has balance depending on the weight (mass). The greater the weight, the more balance.
4. A person has balance depending on the height of the center of gravity. The lower the center of gravity, the more balance.
5. A person has balance depending on where the center of gravity is in relation to the base of support. The balance is less if the center of gravity is near the edge of the base. However, when anticipating an oncoming force, a person can improve stability by placing the center of gravity nearer to the side of the base of support that is expected to receive the force.
6. In anticipation of an oncoming force, stability may be increased by enlarging the size of the base of support in the direction of the anticipated force.
7. Equilibrium may be enhanced by increasing the friction between the body and the surfaces it contacts.
8. Rotation around an axis aids balance. A moving bike is easier to balance than a stationary bike.
9. Kinesthetic physiologic functions contribute to balance. The semicircular canals of the inner ear, vision, touch (pressure), and kinesthetic sense all provide balance information to the performer. Balance and its components of equilibrium and stability are essential in all movements. They are all affected by the constant force of gravity, as well as by inertia. Walking has been described as an activity in which a person throws the body in and out of balance with each step. In rapid running movements in which moving inertia is high,

the individual has to lower the center of gravity to maintain balance when stopping or changing direction. Conversely, in jumping activities, the individual attempts to raise the center of gravity as high as possible.

10. The principles of balance, stability, and center of gravity can be applied to enhance sports performance, prevent injury in the older population, and achieve good body mechanics for the manual therapist.

Force

Muscles are the main source of force that produces or changes the movement of a body segment or the entire body or of an object thrown, struck, or stopped. Strong muscles are able to produce more force than weak muscles. This applies to both maximum and sustained exertion over a period of time.

Forces either push or pull on an object in an attempt to affect motion or shape. Without forces acting on an object, there is no motion. **Force** is the product of mass times acceleration. The mass of a body segment or the entire body times the speed of acceleration determines the force. Obviously, in football this is very important. Yet it is just as important in other activities that use only a part of the human body. When one throws a ball, the force applied to the ball is equal to the mass of the arm times the arm's speed of acceleration. Also, as previously discussed, leverage is important.

$$\text{Force} = \text{mass} \times \text{acceleration}$$

$$F = m \times a$$

The quantity of motion or, more scientifically stated, the momentum—which is equal to mass times velocity—is important in skill activities. The greater the momentum, the greater the resistance to change in the inertia or state of motion.

It is not necessary to apply maximum force and thus increase the momentum of a ball or an object being struck in all situations. In skillful performance, regulation of the amount of force is necessary. Judgment regarding the amount of force required to throw a softball a given distance, hit a golf ball 200 yards, or hit a tennis ball across the net and into the court is important.

In activities involving movement of various joints, as in throwing a ball or putting a shot, there should be a summation of forces from the beginning of movement in the lower segment of the body to the twisting of the trunk and movement at the shoulder, elbow, and wrist joints. The speed at which a golf club strikes the ball is the result of a summation of forces of the lower extremities, trunk, shoulders, arms, and wrists. Shot putting and discus and javelin throwing are other good examples that demonstrate how the summation of forces is essential.

Mechanical-Loading Basics

As one utilizes the musculoskeletal system to exert force on the body to move and to interact with the ground and other objects or people, significant mechanical loads are generated and absorbed by the tissues of the body. The forces causing these loads may be internal or external. Only muscles can actively generate internal force, but tension in tendons, connective tissues, ligaments, and joint capsules may generate passive internal forces. External forces are produced from outside the body and originate from gravity, inertia, or direct contact. All tissues, in varying degrees, resist changes in their shape. Obviously, tissue deformation may result from external forces, but it must be realized that the body also has the ability to generate internal forces large enough to fracture bones, dislocate joints, and disrupt muscles and connective tissues. To prevent injury or damage from tissue deformation, it is important to use the body to absorb energy from both internal and external forces. Along this line, it is to one's advantage to absorb this force over larger aspects of the body rather than smaller ones and to spread the absorption rate over a greater period of time. Additionally, the stronger and healthier a person is, the more likely that she is able to withstand excessive mechanical loading and the resultant excessive tissue deformation. Tension (stretching or strain), compression, shear, bending, and torsion (twisting) are all forces that act individually or in combination to provide mechanical loading that may result in excessive tissue deformation. Figure 3.13 illustrates the mechanical forces that act on tissues of the body.

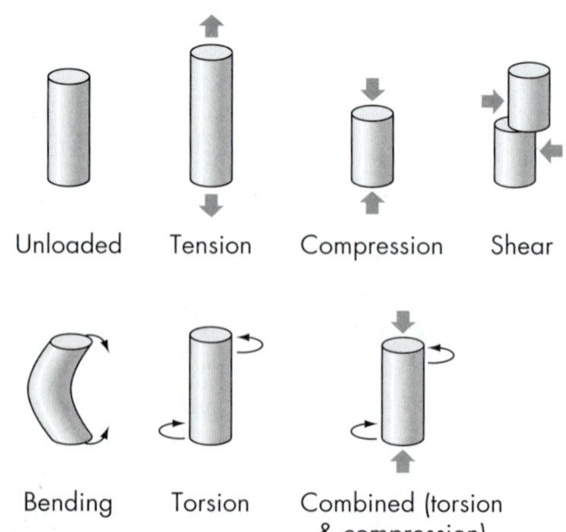

FIGURE 3.13 Mechanical forces

Functional Application of Throwing

Many applications of the laws of leverage, motion, and balance are found in the performance of various sports and athletic activities. One common skill is throwing. The object thrown may be a type of ball, but it is frequently an object of another size or shape, such as a rock, beanbag, Frisbee, discus, or javelin. A brief analysis of some of the basic mechanical principles involved in the skill of throwing will help demonstrate the importance of understanding the applications of these principles. Many activities involve these and other mechanical principles. Motion is basic to throwing when the angular motion (figure 3.14) of the levers (bones) of the body (trunk, shoulder, elbow, and wrist) is used to give linear motion to the ball when it is released.

Newton's laws of motion apply in throwing because the individual's inertia and the ball's inertia must be overcome by the application of force. The body's muscles provide the force to move the body parts and the ball held in the hand. The law of acceleration (Newton's second law) comes into operation with the muscular force necessary to accelerate the arm, wrist, and hand. The greater the force (mass times acceleration) that a person can produce, the faster the arm will move and, thus, the greater the speed that will be imparted to the ball. The reaction of the feet against the surface on which the person stands indicates the application of the law of reaction.

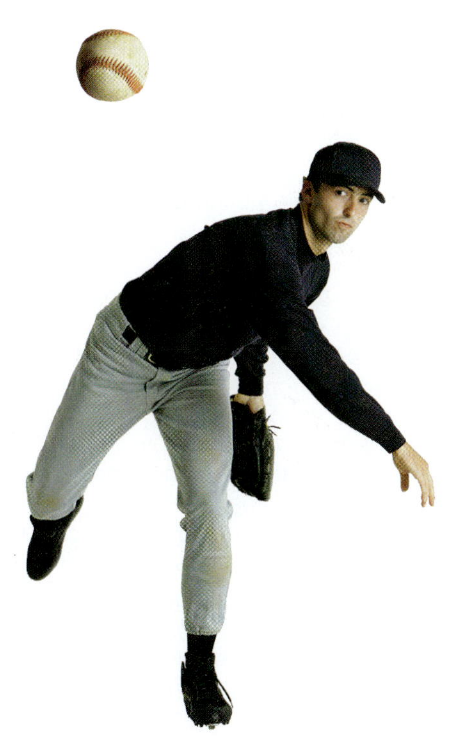

FIGURE 3.14 Throwing a ball

The leverage factor is very important in throwing a ball or an object. The longer the lever, the greater the speed that can be imparted to the ball. For all practical purposes, the body, from the feet to the fingers, can be considered one long lever. The longer the lever, either from natural body length or from the movements of the body to the extended backward position (as in throwing a softball, with extension of the shoulder and the elbow joints), the greater the arc through which it accelerates and thus the greater the speed imparted to the thrown object.

In certain circumstances, when the ball is to be thrown only a short distance, such as when a baseball is thrown by the catcher to the bases, the short lever is advantageous because it takes less total time to release the ball.

Balance, or equilibrium, is a factor in throwing when the body is rotated to the rear in the beginning of the throw. This motion moves the body nearly out of balance to the rear, and then balance changes again in the body with the forward movement. Balance is again established with the follow-through, when the feet are spread and the knees and trunk are flexed to lower the center of gravity.

The preceding discussion has been a brief overview of some of the factors affecting motion. Analysis of human motion in light of the laws of physics poses a problem: How comprehensive is the analysis to be? It can become very complex, particularly when body motion is combined with the manipulation of an object in the hand involved in throwing, kicking, striking, or catching.

These factors become involved when an analysis is attempted of the activities common to physical education programs and athletics—football, baseball, basketball, track and field, martial arts, and swimming, to mention a few. However, to have a complete view of which factors control human movement, one must have a working knowledge of both the physiologic and biomechanical principles of kinesiology.

It is beyond the scope of this book to make a detailed analysis of other activities. Some sources that consider these problems in detail are listed in Appendix A at the end of the book.

CHAPTER *summary*

Introduction

- Human movement is often complex and beautiful. Consider, for example, a ballerina's pirouette—a movement that requires years of training. Yet behind the dancer's graceful movements are hundreds of laws, forces, and biomechanical principles at work. Motion cannot occur unless there is a force behind it; however, motion includes many levers, torque, and pulleys that all exist as force is applied. Studying movement requires analyzing all of these elements.
- The study of mechanics as it relates to the functional and anatomical analysis of biological systems is known as *biomechanics*.
- Mechanics, the study of physical actions of forces, can be subdivided into statics and dynamics. Statics involves the study of systems that are in a constant state of motion, whether at rest with no motion or moving at a constant velocity without acceleration. Dynamics involves the study of systems in motion with acceleration.

Types of Machines Found in the Body

- As discussed in Chapter 2, the body utilizes muscles to apply force to the bones on which they attach to cause, control, or prevent movement in the joints that they cross. As is often the case, humans utilize the bones, such as those in the hand, to either hold, push, or pull on an object while also using a series of bones and joints throughout the body to apply force via the muscles to affect the position of the object. In doing so, the body is using a series of simple machines to accomplish the tasks.

Levers

- Human movement occurs through the organized use of a system of levers. The anatomical levers of the body cannot be changed, but when the system is properly understood, it can be used more efficiently to maximize the muscular efforts of the body.
- The lever rotates around the axis as a result of the force (sometimes referred to as *effort*, or *E*) applied to it to cause its movement against a resistance or weight. In the body, the bones represent the lever bars, the joints are the axes, and the muscles contract to apply the force.

Factors in the Use of Anatomical Levers

- The body's anatomical leverage system can be used to gain a mechanical advantage that will improve simple or complex physical movements. Some individuals unconsciously develop habits of using human levers properly, but frequently this is not the case.
- Torque, or moment of force, is the turning effect of an eccentric force. Eccentric force is a force that is applied in a direction not in line with the center of rotation of an object with a fixed axis. In objects without a fixed axis, it is an applied force that is not in line with the object's center of gravity.
- The perpendicular distance between the location of force application and the axis is known as the *force arm, moment arm,* or *torque arm.* The resistance arm is the distance between the axis and the point of resistance application.

Laws of Motion and Physical Activities

- Motion is fundamental in physical education and sports activity. Body motion is generally produced, or at least started, by some action of the muscular system. Motion cannot occur without a force, and the muscular system is the source of force in the human body.
- There are two types of motion: linear motion and angular motion. Linear motion, or translatory motion, is motion along a line. If the motion is along a straight line, it is rectilinear motion, whereas motion along a curved line is curvilinear motion. Angular motion, or rotary motion, involves rotation around an axis.
- Displacement is a change in the position or location of an object from its original point of reference, whereas distance, or the path of movement, is the actual sum length of measurement traveled.
- Speed is how fast an object is moving or the distance an object travels in a specific amount of time. Velocity includes the direction and describes the rate of displacement.
- Newton's laws explain all the characteristics of motion, and they are fundamental to understanding human movement.
- Law of inertia: *A body in motion tends to remain in motion at the same speed in a straight line unless acted on by a force; a body at rest tends to remain at rest unless acted on by a force.* Inertia may be described as the resistance to action or change. In terms of human movement, inertia is resistance to acceleration or deceleration. Inertia is the tendency for the current state of motion to be maintained, regardless of whether the body segment is moving at a particular velocity or is motionless.
- Law of acceleration: *A change in the acceleration of a body occurs in the same direction as the force that caused it. The change in acceleration is directly proportional to the force causing it and inversely proportional to the mass of the body.* Acceleration may be defined as the rate of change in velocity. To attain speed in moving the body, a strong muscular force is generally necessary. Mass, the amount of matter in a body, affects the speed and acceleration in physical movements.
- Law of reaction: *For every action there is an opposite and equal reaction.* As a person places force on a supporting surface by walking over it, the surface provides

an equal resistance back in the opposite direction to the soles of the feet. The feet push down and back, while the surface pushes up and forward. The force of the surface reacting to the force placed on it is referred to as *ground reaction force.* A person provides the action force, while the surface provides the reaction force.

- ✔ Sherrington's law is the law of reciprocal innervation (discussed in Chapter 2). When contraction of a muscle is stimulated, there is a simultaneous inhibition of its antagonist. For example, when the biceps brachii contracts, the triceps muscle relaxes, allowing the action to occur.

Friction

- ✔ Friction is the force that results from the resistance between the surfaces of two objects moving against one another. Depending on the activity involved, one may desire increased or decreased friction. In running, a person depends on friction forces between the feet and the ground so that he may exert force against the ground and propel himself forward. When friction is reduced due to a slick ground or shoe surface, a person is more likely to slip. In skating, a person desires decreased friction so that she may slide across the ice with less resistance. Friction may be further characterized as either static friction or kinetic friction.

Balance, Equilibrium, and Stability

- ✔ Balance is the ability to control equilibrium. In relation to human movement, equilibrium is a state of zero acceleration in which there is no change in the speed or direction of the body. Equilibrium may be either static or dynamic. If the body is at rest or completely motionless, it is in static equilibrium. Dynamic equilibrium occurs when all the applied and inertial forces acting on the moving body are in balance, resulting in movement with unchanging speed or direction.

Force

- ✔ Muscles are the main source of force that produces or changes the movement of a body segment or the entire body or of an object thrown, struck, or stopped. Strong muscles are able to produce more force than weak muscles. This applies to both maximum and sustained exertion over a period of time.

Mechanical-Loading Basics

- ✔ As one utilizes the musculoskeletal system to exert force on the body to move and to interact with the ground and other objects or people, significant mechanical loads are generated and absorbed by the tissues of the body. The forces causing these loads may be internal or external. Only muscles can actively generate internal force, but tension in tendons, connective tissues, ligaments, and joint capsules may generate passive internal forces.

Functional Application of Throwing

- ✔ Many applications of the laws of leverage, motion, and balance are found in the performance of various sports and athletic activities. One common skill is throwing. The object thrown may be a type of ball, but it is frequently an object of another size or shape, such as a rock, beanbag, Frisbee, discus, or javelin. A brief analysis of some of the basic mechanical principles involved in the skill of throwing will help demonstrate the importance of understanding the applications of these principles.

CHAPTER *review*

True or False

Write true *or* false *after each statement.*

1. Sherrington's law involves the agonist and antagonist of a joint.
2. Inertia is defined as high-velocity movement in a given plane.
3. Newton's laws explain all the characteristics of motion, but they are not fundamental in understanding human movement.
4. Acceleration may be defined as the rate of change of velocity.
5. Sports that involve throwing objects are good examples of the laws of leverage, motion, and balance.
6. The human body can be defined as a machine because it has the capacity to convert smaller amounts of force over a longer distance.
7. A lever can operate without a fulcrum or force.
8. A good example of a first-class lever is a seesaw.
9. Kinetic friction is defined as the friction occurring between two objects that have not yet begun to move.
10. A short lever can be advantageous in certain athletic circumstances.
11. To understand the leverage system, therapists must be familiar with the concept of torque.
12. A good example of a pulley in the human body is the lateral malleolus, which serves as a pulley for the peroneus longus tendon.

Short Answers

Write your answers on the lines provided.

1. Describe a practical example of Newton's law of inertia.

2. Anatomical levers can improve physical performance. Explain how this occurs, using the information you have learned in relation to throwing.

3. What term means the measurement of how much force it takes to cause an object to rotate?

4. Identify a practical example of Newton's law of acceleration. Explain how the example illustrates the law.

5. What equation is used to determine the mechanical advantage of levers?

6. What is the amount of force needed to lift an object in a pulley system if the weight of the object is 200 kilograms and the number of supporting ropes is four?

7. If a baseball player hit a triple and ran around the bases to third base, what was his displacement if the distance between each base was 90 feet?

8. What is a good example of a pulley in the human body?

9. If a pulley setup has four supporting ropes, what is the mechanical advantage of the setup?

10. Identify a practical example of Newton's law of reaction.

Multiple Choice

Circle the correct answers.

1. The law of reaction states:
   a. that a change in acceleration occurs
   b. that for every action there is an opposite and equal reaction
   c. that for every action the change of acceleration is directly proportional to the force causing it
   d. none of the above

2. Stability in the body may be enhanced by determining the body's:
   a. core strength limits
   b. lean muscle mass
   c. mean strength
   d. center of gravity

3. *Displacement* refers to:
   a. a change in the position or location of an object from its original point
   b. the actual sum length of measurement traveled
   c. both a and b
   d. none of the above
4. The system of leverage in the human body is designed for:
   a. force
   b. mechanical disadvantage
   c. friction
   d. speed and range of movement at the expense of force
5. Examples of levers include:
   a. wheels
   b. pulleys
   c. pliers
   d. all of the above
6. Single pulleys have a mechanical advantage of:
   a. 3
   b. 4
   c. 2
   d. 1
7. Momentum is equal to:
   a. friction times force
   b. displacement times distance
   c. mass times velocity
   d. none of the above
8. *Kinetics* is defined as the:
   a. description of motion that includes time, displacement, and velocity
   b. study of forces associated with the motion of a body
   c. study of gravity on a body
   d. study of athletic performance
9. The amount of torque can be determined by multiplying:
   a. the amount of force by the force arm
   b. the amount of force magnitude by the force arm
   c. both a and b
   d. the amount of velocity by the force arm
10. In essence, the human body is made up of a complex system of:
   a. mechanical forces
   b. lever arms
   c. levers
   d. machines

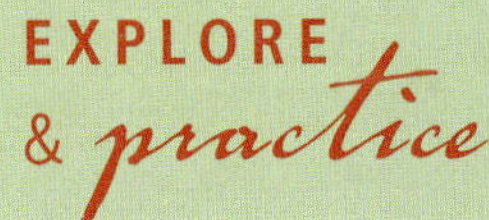

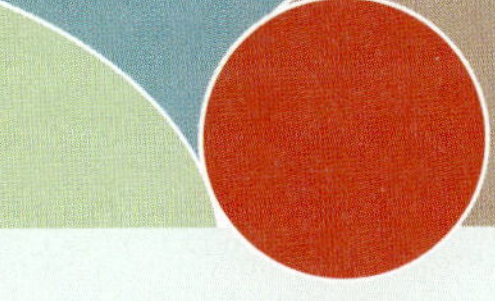

1. Select a sporting activity and explain how the presence of too much friction becomes a problem in the activity.
2. Select a sporting activity and explain how the presence of too little friction becomes a problem in the activity.
3. Using the mechanical-loading basic forces of compression, torsion, and shear, describe each force by giving examples from soccer or volleyball.
4. Explain the mechanical analysis of all the skills involved in each of the following:

a. Basketball	g. Golf
b. Baseball	h. Gymnastics
c. Dancing	i. Soccer
d. Diving	j. Swimming
e. Football	k. Tennis
f. Field hockey	l. Wrestling

5. Choose five or more of the following factors in motion and write a one-page report on how they are related to human movement:

a. Balance	m. Spin
b. Force	n. Rebound angle
c. Gravity	o. Momentum
d. Motion	p. Center of gravity
e. Torque	q. Equilibrium
f. Leverage	r. Stability
g. Projectiles	s. Base of support
h. Friction	t. Inertia
i. Buoyancy	u. Linear displacement
j. Aerodynamics	v. Angular displacement
k. Hydrodynamics	w. Speed
l. Restitution	x. Velocity

6. *Lever component identification chart:* List two levers for each class other than those illustrated in this chapter. Identify the force, axis, and resistance for each. Also explain the advantage of using each lever in terms of whether it is used to achieve balance, force motion, speed, or range of motion.

Lever class	Example	Force	Axis	Resistance	Advantage provided
1st					
1st					
2nd					
2nd					
3rd					
3rd					

7. *Laws-of-motion task comparison chart:* Assume that you possess the skill, strength, and so on, to be able to perform each of the paired tasks below. For each pair, circle the task that would be easiest to accomplish on the basis of Newton's laws of motion, and explain why.

	Paired tasks	Explanation
a.	Throw a baseball 60 mph OR Throw a shot put 60 mph.	
b.	Kick a bowling ball 40 yards OR Kick a soccer ball 40 yards.	
c.	Bat a whiffle ball over a 320-yard fence OR Bat a baseball over a 320-yard fence.	
d.	Catch a shotput that was thrown 60 mph OR Catch a softball that was thrown 60 mph.	
e.	Tackle a 240-pound running back sprinting toward you full speed OR Tackle a 200-pound running back sprinting toward you full speed.	
f.	Run a 40-yard dash in 4.5 seconds on a wet field OR Run a 40-yard dash in 4.5 seconds on a dry field.	

part 2

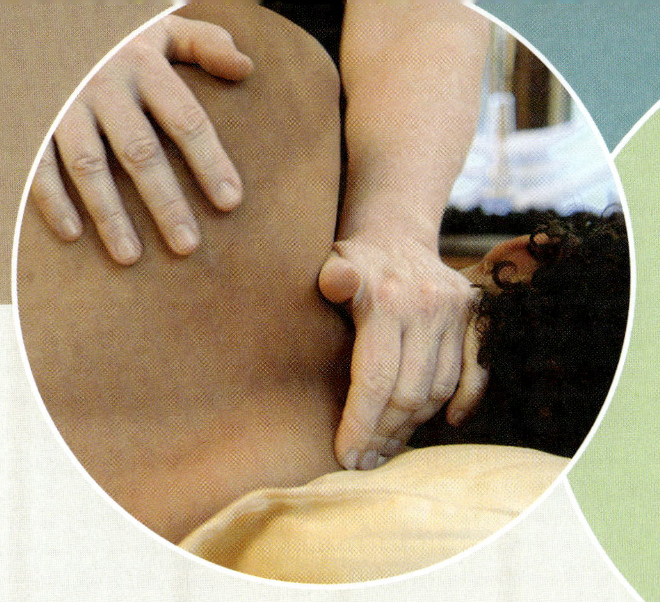

UPPER EXTREMITIES

chapter 4

The Shoulder Girdle—Dynamic Stability for the Shoulder Joint

LEARNING OUTCOMES

After completing this chapter, you should be able to:

- **4-1** Define key terms.
- **4-2** Identify on the skeleton all bony landmarks of the shoulder girdle.
- **4-3** Label on a skeletal chart all bony landmarks of the shoulder girdle.
- **4-4** Draw on a skeletal chart the muscles of the shoulder girdle and indicate shoulder girdle movements using arrows.
- **4-5** Demonstrate all the movements of the shoulder girdle using a partner.
- **4-6** Palpate the bony landmarks of the shoulder girdle on a partner.
- **4-7** Give examples of agonists, antagonists, stabilizers, and synergists of the shoulder girdle muscles.
- **4-8** Explore the origins and insertions of shoulder girdle muscles on a partner.
- **4-9** Discuss the principles of different forms of stretching.
- **4-10** Practice basic stretching and strengthening appropriate for the shoulder girdle.

KEY TERMS

Acromioclavicular
Active Isolated Stretching (AIS)
Brachial plexus
Cervical plexus
Clavicle
Clinical flexibility
Clinical Flexibility and Therapeutic Exercise (CFTE)
Flexibility
Levator scapulae
Myotatic reflex arc
Nerve compression
Nerve entrapment
Nerve impingements
Pectoralis minor
PNF stretching
Rhomboid
Scapula
Scapulothoracic
Serratus anterior
Shoulder girdle
Sternoclavicular
Stretching
Subclavius
Trapezius

Introduction

Although the statement "He carries the weight of the world on his shoulders" is best understood metaphorically as a means of describing someone who assumes an enormous burden or level of responsibility, it certainly reflects the understanding that the shoulders have a fundamental purpose in the body—to support the spine, neck, and head, as well as to provide a place for the upper extremities to attach. It is no wonder, then, that the shoulder girdle muscles often house chronic tension brought on by "the weight of the world."

As its name indicates, the shoulder girdle surrounds the trunk and provides dynamic stability for the upper extremity to utilize its ball-and-socket joint. Simple actions such as waving or fastening a seat belt would be impossible without the cooperation of the many shoulder girdle muscles. In addition to being the foundation of the shoulder joint, the shoulder girdle muscles all act independently to facilitate movements such as reaching for a glass or turning the wheel of a car. To perform these movements, the scapula must elevate and move in upward rotation, assisted by the contractions of the trapezius, serratus anterior, levator scapulae, and rhomboids. Without scapular movement, the shoulder's dynamic range would be extremely limited.

The posture of a kyphotic thoracic spine (rounded or extreme protraction of the shoulders) is common in the general population, as well as in massage therapists and Parkinson patients. The shoulder's antigravity muscles, particularly the rhomboids and trapezius, are designed to hold the shoulders in retraction as the body stands or sits in gravitational space. Unfortunately, these muscles often become lengthened and atrophied, unable to adequately perform scapular retraction. This is promoted by the additional workload that the body routinely places on their antagonists, the shoulder girdle protractors, which become disproportionately tighter and stronger. This uneven balance in the shoulder girdle muscles promotes poor posture and often affects the position of the head on the neck. Repetitive actions performed by the upper extremities, such as computer-related work, exhaust the shoulder girdle muscles, leading to fatigued and sore soft tissue.

Brief descriptions of the most important bones in the shoulder region will help students understand the skeletal structure and its relationship to the muscular system.

Bones

The two bones primarily involved in movements of the **shoulder girdle** (figures 4.1 and 4.2) are the **scapula** and the **clavicle,** which together move as a unit. Their only bony link to the axial skeleton is provided by the clavicle's articulation with the sternum. Key bony landmarks for studying the shoulder girdle are the manubrium, clavicle, coracoid process, acromion process, glenoid fossa, lateral border, inferior angle, medial border, superior angle, and spine of the scapula.

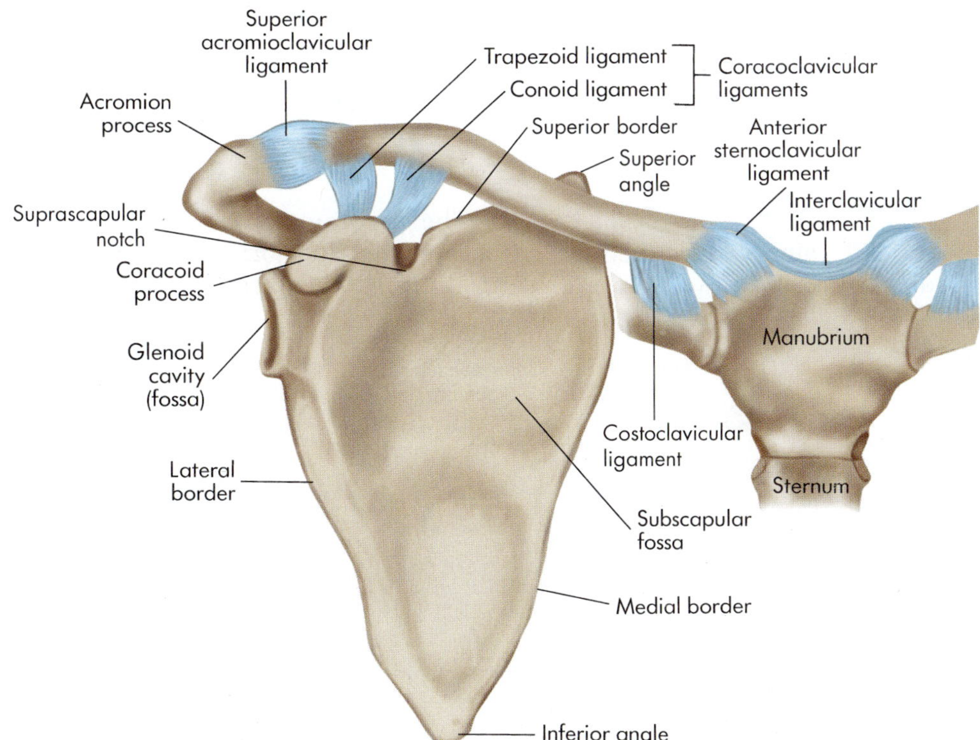

FIGURE 4.1 Right shoulder girdle, anterior view

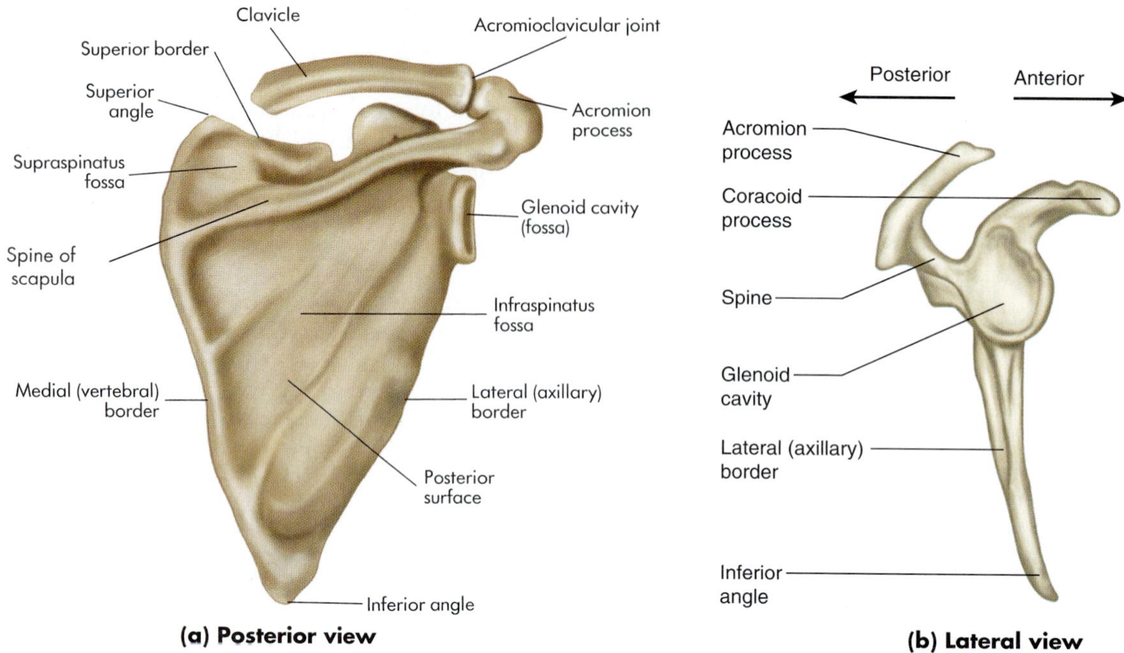

FIGURE 4.2 Right scapula

Joints

The scapula is actually embedded in muscles and is not physically attached to the rib cage. The movements of the shoulder girdle as the scapula moves in a variety of directions over the rib cage are described as **scapulothoracic** actions. The only two synovial joints are the *arthrodial* (gliding) **sternoclavicular** joint and the less mobile **acromioclavicular** joint. The scapula depends on the gliding actions of the sternoclavicular joint and acromioclavicular joint for its ability to move. (See figures 4.3 and 4.4.)

STERNOCLAVICULAR

The sternoclavicular (SC) joint is classified as a (multiaxial) arthrodial joint. It moves anteriorly 15 degrees with protraction and posteriorly 15 degrees with retraction. It moves superiorly 45 degrees with elevation and inferiorly 5 degrees with depression. Some clavicle rotation along its axis during various shoulder girdle movements results in a slight rotary gliding movement at the sternoclavicular joint. It is supported anteriorly by the anterior sternoclavicular ligament and posteriorly by the posterior ligament. Additionally, the costoclavicular and interclavicular ligaments provide stability against superior displacement.

ACROMIOCLAVICULAR

The acromioclavicular (AC) joint is classified as an arthrodial joint. It has a 20- to 30-degree total gliding and rotational motion accompanying other

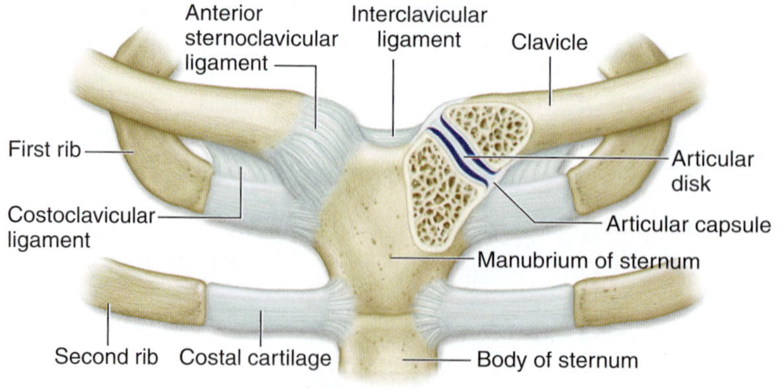

FIGURE 4.3 Sternoclavicular joint

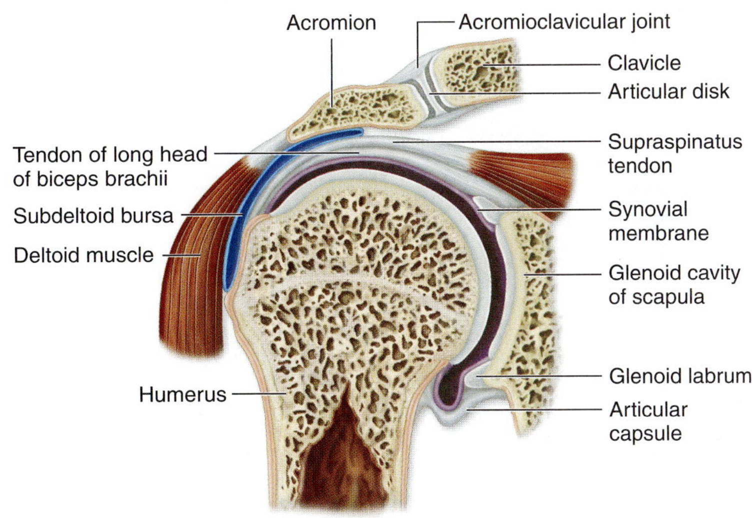

FIGURE 4.4 Acromioclavicular joint

shoulder girdle and shoulder joint motions. In addition to the strong support provided by the coracoclavicular ligaments (trapezoid and conoid), the superior and inferior acromioclavicular ligaments provide stability to this often injured joint. The coracoclavicular joint, classified as a syndesmotic-type joint, functions through its ligaments to greatly increase the stability of the acromioclavicular joint.

SCAPULOTHORACIC

The scapulothoracic joint is not a true synovial joint and does not have regular synovial features; its movement is totally dependent on the sternoclavicular and acromioclavicular joints. Even though scapula movement occurs as a result of motion at the SC and AC joints, the scapula has a total range of 25-degree abduction-adduction movement, 60-degree upward-downward rotation, and 55-degree elevation-depression. The scapulothoracic joint is supported dynamically by its muscles and lacks ligamentous support, since it has no synovial features.

There is no typical articulation between the anterior scapula and the posterior rib cage. Between these two osseous structures is the serratus anterior muscle, which originates off the upper nine ribs laterally and runs just behind the rib cage posteriorly to insert on the medial border of the scapula. Immediately posterior to the serratus anterior is the subscapularis muscle (see Chapter 6) on the anterior scapula.

CLINICAL NOTES **Scapulohumeral Rhythm**

The scapulothoracic joint and its ability to move may be affected by the glenohumeral joint's free range of movement. For example, if the ball-and-socket joint is restricted in abduction, the glenohumeral adductors may develop shortened fibers and the scapulothoracic elevators and upward rotators may compensate with additional activity to assist in total overhead motion of the extremity. Similarly, if the scapulothoracic joint is restricted in movement such as retraction, the glenohumeral joint external rotators may become stretched to assist in moving the entire upper extremity behind the body. This synergistic movement of the scapulothoracic joint with the shoulder joint is known as the *scapulohumeral rhythm*. The scapulohumeral rhythm can be examined by observing the scapula's position as a person lifts the arm into abduction and flexion. This is discussed more later in the chapter.

Movements

In analyzing shoulder girdle movements (figure 4.5), it is often helpful to focus on a specific scapular bony landmark, such as the inferior angle (posteriorly), the glenoid fossa (laterally), and the acromion process (anteriorly). All these movements have their pivotal point where the clavicle joins the sternum at the sternoclavicular joint. For palpation purposes, place two fingers on the sternoclavicular joint and repeat the movements; the gliding motion of the joint will be obvious.

Movements of the shoulder girdle can be described as movements of the scapula.

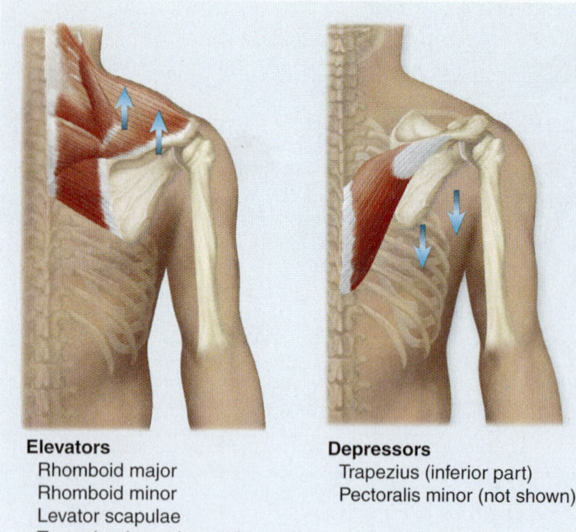

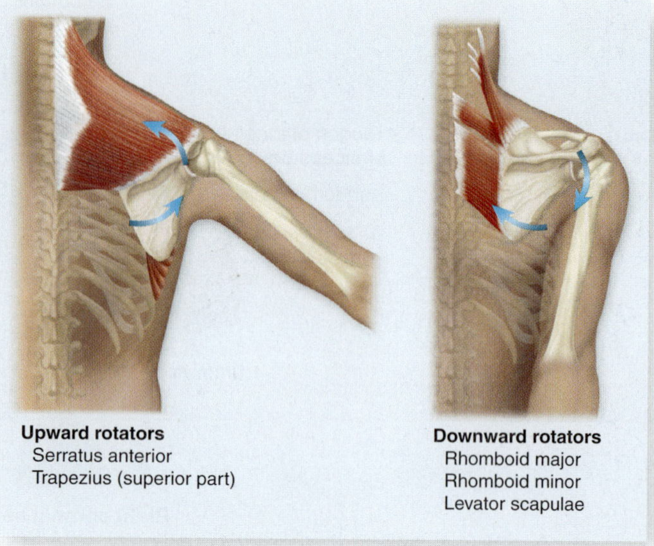

FIGURE 4.5 Movements of shoulder girdle muscles

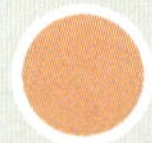

FLEXIBILITY AND STRENGTH

Movements of the Shoulder Girdle

Abduction (protraction)
Movement of the scapula laterally away from the spinal column, as in reaching for an object in front of the body.

Adduction (retraction)
Movement of the scapula medially toward the spinal column, as in pinching the shoulder blades together.

Upward rotation
Moving the inferior angle superiorly and laterally away from the spinal column and tipping the glenoid fossa upward, as in reaching overhead out to the side.

Downward rotation
Returning the inferior angle medially and inferiorly toward the spinal column and the glenoid fossa to its normal position. (Once the scapula has returned to its anatomical position, further downward rotation actually results in the superior angle moving slightly superomedial.)

Elevation
Upward or superior movement, as in shrugging the shoulders.

Depression
Downward or inferior movement, as in returning to a normal position from a shoulder shrug.

To accomplish some of the above-listed shoulder girdle movements, the scapula must rotate or tilt on its axis. Although they are not primary shoulder girdle movements, these accessory movements are necessary for the scapula to move normally throughout its *range of motion (ROM)* during the movements.

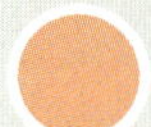

FLEXIBILITY AND STRENGTH

Accessory Movements of the Scapula

Lateral tilt (outward tilt)
Consequential movement during abduction in which the scapula rotates around its vertical axis, resulting in posterior movement of the medial border and anterior movement of the lateral border (also known as "winging" of the scapula).

Medial tilt (inward tilt)
Return from lateral tilt; consequential movement during extreme adduction in which the scapula rotates around its vertical axis, resulting in anterior movement of the medial border and posterior movement of the lateral border.

Anterior tilt (upward tilt)
Consequential rotational movement of the scapula around the frontal axis that occurs during hyperextension of the glenohumeral joint, resulting in the superior border moving anteroinferiorly and the inferior angle moving posterosuperiorly.

Posterior tilt (downward tilt)
Consequential rotational movement of the scapula around the frontal axis that occurs during hyperflexion of the glenohumeral joint, resulting in the superior border moving posteroinferiorly and the inferior angle moving anterosuperiorly.

SYNERGY WITH THE MUSCLES OF THE GLENOHUMERAL JOINT

The shoulder joint and shoulder girdle work together in performing upper-extremity activities. It is critical to understand that movement of the shoulder girdle is not dependent on the shoulder joint and its muscles. However, the shoulder girdle muscles are essential to providing a scapula-stabilizing effect; muscles of the shoulder joint must have a stable base from which to exert force for powerful movement involving the humerus. Consequently, the shoulder girdle muscles contract to maintain the scapula in a relatively static position during many shoulder joint actions.

As the shoulder joint goes through more extreme ranges of motion, the scapular muscles contract to move the shoulder girdle so that its glenoid fossa will be in a more appropriate position from which the humerus can move. Without the accompanying movement of the scapula, the humerus can raise only into approximately 90 degrees of total shoulder abduction and flexion. This scapulohumeral rhythm (see Clinical Notes, above) should work in a 2-to-1 ratio; for every 2 degrees of glenohumeral joint abduction or flexion, there is 1 degree of upward rotation at the scapulothoracic joint. Without this rhythm, the shoulder cannot move correctly. The appropriate muscles of both joints work cooperatively in synergy to accomplish the desired action of the entire upper extremity. For example, if a person abducts her hand out to the side laterally as high as possible, the serratus anterior and trapezius (middle and lower fibers) muscles upwardly rotate the scapula as the supraspinatus and deltoid initiate glenohumeral abduction. This synergy between the scapula and shoulder joint muscles enhances the movement of the entire upper extremity. If the shoulder joint muscles are not functioning to full capacity because of capsule inflammation, injury, or pathologic conditions, the shoulder girdle muscles are likely to shorten and further inhibit the movement of the scapula on the rib cage. Further discussion of the interaction and teamwork between these joints is provided at the beginning of Chapter 6, in Table 6.1, which lists the shoulder girdle movements that usually accompany shoulder joint movements.

CLINICAL NOTES **Possible Impingement**

Even when the scapula has free range of motion, sometimes the head of the humerus comes into contact with the acromion. This can occur if arthritic conditions exist on the acromion and the already tight space becomes narrower. With the humerus in about 90 degrees of abduction, this extreme position forces the head into the glenoid fossa. Impingement of the rotator cuff often occurs when the tendons of these muscles become inflamed. See Chapter 6 on the shoulder joint and rotator cuff for further details.

Muscles

There are five muscles (figure 4.6) primarily involved in shoulder girdle movements. These muscles insert on the scapula and clavicle; all have origins on the axial skeleton. Shoulder girdle muscles do not attach to the humerus, nor do they cause actions of the shoulder joint, a key point for understanding the actions of either the shoulder girdle or the shoulder joint. The only shoulder joint muscles that insert on the humerus are those that initiate and complete actions with the humerus. Shoulder joint actions, however, impact the position of the scapula. As the humerus abducts, the scapula upwardly rotates so that the humerus can operate optimally in full range of motion. When the humerus adducts, the scapula rotates down into its anatomical position.

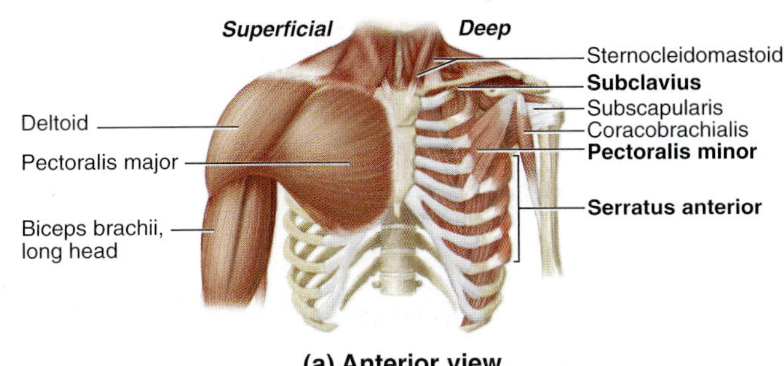

(a) Anterior view

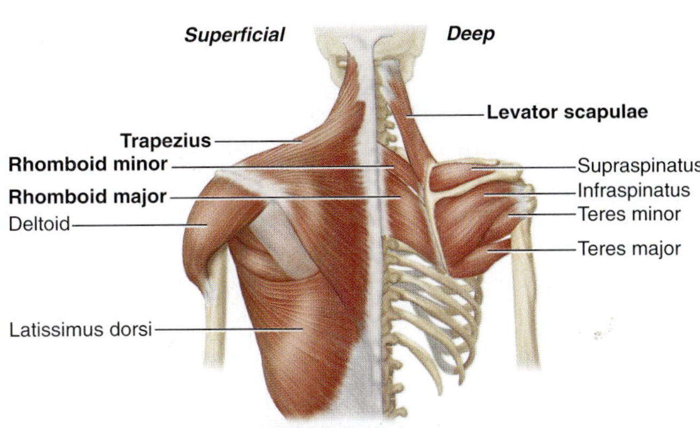

(b) Posterior view

FIGURE 4.6 Muscles that move the shoulder girdle, anterior and posterior views

The **pectoralis minor** and **subclavius** are located anteriorly in relation to the trunk. The subclavius muscle is a stabilizer and is not regarded as a primary mover in any shoulder girdle actions. The **serratus anterior** is located anteriorly to the scapula but posteriorly and laterally to the trunk. The **trapezius** (superficial), **rhomboid,** and **levator scapulae** are located posteriorly to the trunk.

The shoulder girdle muscles are essential in providing dynamic stability of the scapula and providing foundational support to all shoulder joint activities such as throwing a Frisbee, hitting a golf ball, shoveling snow, or raking leaves.

Shoulder Girdle Muscles—Location and Action

MUSCLE SPECIFIC

Anterior

Pectoralis minor: abduction, downward rotation, and depression

Subclavius: stabilization of the sternoclavicular joint, depression; draws the clavicle forward as the scapula abducts

Posterior and laterally

Serratus anterior: abduction and upward rotation, stabilization of the scapula

Posterior

Trapezius:

Upper fibers: elevation and extension of the head, stabilization of the scapula

Middle fibers: elevation, adduction, and upward rotation, stabilization of the scapula

Lower fibers: adduction, depression, and upward rotation, stabilization of the scapula

Rhomboid: adduction and slight elevation as it adducts, downward rotation, stabilization of the scapula

Levator scapulae: elevation, stabilization of the scapula

It is important to understand that muscles may not necessarily be active throughout the full range of motion for which they are noted as agonists.

Table 4.1 provides a detailed breakdown of the muscles responsible for primary shoulder girdle movements.

Nerves

The shoulder girdle muscles are innervated primarily from the nerves of the **cervical plexus** and **brachial plexus,** as illustrated in figures 4.7 and 4.8. The trapezius is innervated by the spinal accessory nerve and from branches of C3 and C4. In addition to supplying the trapezius, C3 and C4 also innervate the levator scapulae. The levator scapulae receives further innervation from the dorsal scapula nerve originating from C5. The dorsal scapula nerve also innervates the rhomboid. The long thoracic nerve originates from C5, C6, and C7 and innervates the serratus anterior. The medial pectoral nerve arises from C8 and T1 to innervate the pectoralis minor.

CLINICAL NOTES

Possible Nerve Impingements

The brachial plexus is vulnerable to **nerve impingements,** or "pinched nerves," from several perspectives. The bundles of nerves exit the cervical vertebrae in very specific, small areas. Osteoarthritis, a pathologic condition causing abnormal bony growth, can press on the nerves and cause **nerve compression.** Soft-tissue structures can apply pressure to nerves and cause **nerve entrapment.** Nerves that are compressed or entrapped from the brachial plexus adversely affect actions, soft-tissue tone, and strength in the entire upper extremity.

Clinical Flexibility and Therapeutic Exercise

Since the muscular system is susceptible to various dysfunctions, it is important to maintain a healthy range of motion (ROM) within the joints, as well as optimal strength. When a joint has limited movement, other muscle groups usually compensate as the body attempts to correct the poor movement. For example, if the scapula cannot upwardly rotate with abduction and flexion of the shoulder, the upper trapezius will elevate the scapula in an attempt to move the humerus into abduction. **Clinical Flexibility and Therapeutic Exercise (CFTE)** is a modality composed of stretching and strengthening the muscles of the body. It is designed to improve human movement and prevent current or past dysfunctions from worsening. The discussion on CFTE exercises will start with the shoulder girdle muscles and will be interspersed throughout the remainder of the text. See Chapters 12 and 21 for upper- and lower-extremity exercises.

BASIC STRETCHING IDEAS

The shoulder has a dynamic range of motion, and it allows the body to perform complex movements in sports and in daily living. To maintain this dynamic range and help prevent injuries, the shoulder must be stretched and strengthened. Muscles should always be stretched before any resistance is applied so that the

TABLE 4.1 Agonist Muscles of the Shoulder Girdle

Name of Muscle	Origins	Insertion	Actions	Innervations
Trapezius	*Upper:* occiput, ligamentum nuchae *Middle:* spinous processes of C7, T1–T3 *Lower:* spinous processes of T4–T12	*Upper:* lateral clavicle *Middle:* spine of scapula, acromion *Lower:* root of spine of scapula	*Upper:* elevation, upward rotation of scapula *Middle:* adduction, elevation, upward rotation *Lower:* depression, upward rotation of scapula, and adduction bilateral extension of spine	Accessory nerve (CN XI), branches of C3, C4
Levator scapulae	C1–C4 transverse processes	Vertebral border of scapula (medial) from superior angle to root of spine	Elevation of scapula	Dorsal scapular nerve (C5, C4, and C3)
Rhomboid major	T2–T5 spinous processes	Vertebral border of scapula below root of spine	Adduction (retraction), elevation accompanying adduction, downward rotation of scapula	Dorsal scapular nerve (C5)
Rhomboid minor	C7, T1 spinous processes	Root of spine of scapula	Same	Same
Serratus anterior	Surface of the upper nine ribs at the side of the chest	Anterior aspect of the whole length of the medial border of scapula	Abduction, upward rotation	Long thoracic nerve (C5–C7)
Pectoralis minor	Anterior surfaces of the 3rd to 5th ribs	Coracoid process of scapula	Abduction, downward rotation as it abducts, depression from upward rotation	Medial pectoral nerve (C8–T1)
Subclavius	Superior aspect of 1st rib at its junction with its costal cartilage	Inferior groove in the midportion of clavicle	Stabilization of sternoclavicular joint, depression; draws clavicle down as shoulders abduct	Nerve fibers from C5 and C6

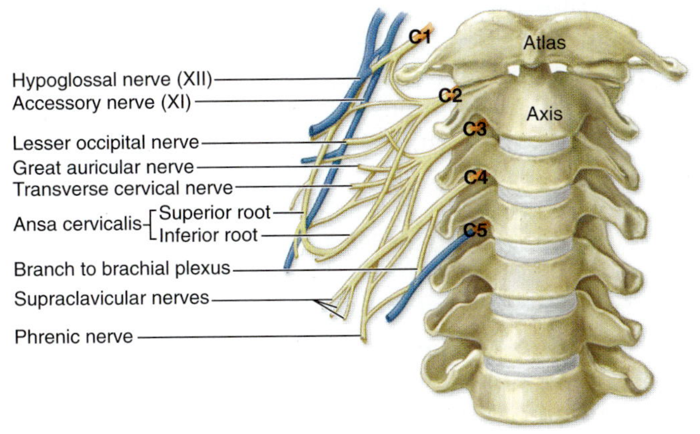

FIGURE 4.7 Cervical plexus

muscle fibers will perform optimally for the task. The shoulder area is often overlooked in both a flexibility focus and a strength focus. While it is important to strengthen the larger, prime movers of the shoulder, restoring the smaller antigravity muscles is also vital. For example, if an individual is strengthening his pectoralis major twice per week, he must also strengthen the rhomboids, serratus anterior, and trapezius. Because of the large fibers and powerful forward pull the pectoralis has on the shoulders, the opposite muscles of the posterior shoulder will become lengthened when an imbalance is present. Yet the pectoralis must also be stretched to allow the shoulders to return to a neutral position.

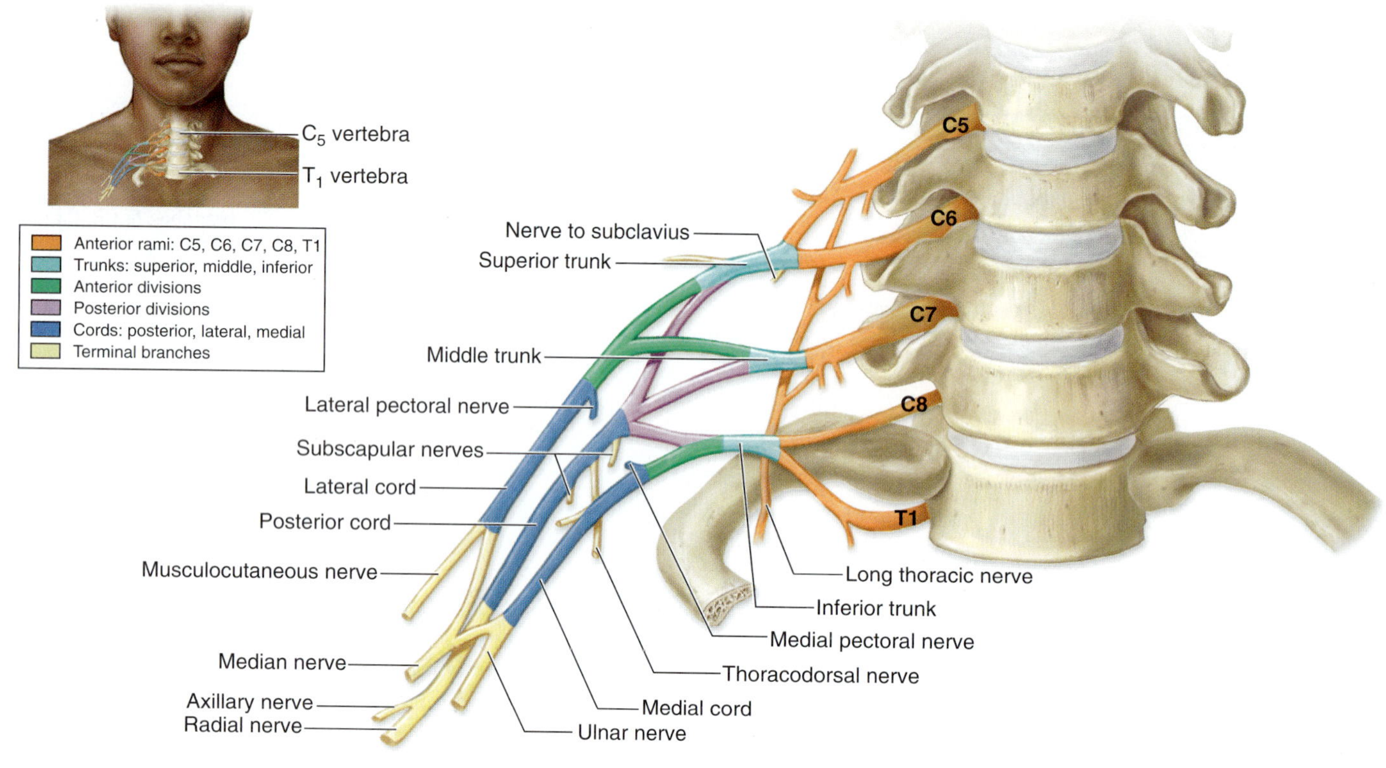

FIGURE 4.8 Brachial plexus

Understanding Flexibility

Flexibility is an important component in sports and general fitness, and it should not be overlooked in the study of kinesiology. Increasing proper range of motion—the total movement of which a joint is capable—by increasing flexibility has been shown to help improve poor posture, increase sports performance, and reduce wear and tear on the joints. **Flexibility** is defined as the end motion of a segment, and it can occur by active contraction of the *agonist* (active range of motion) or by motion of an external force (passive range of motion). **Stretching** is taking a muscle in its resting length and expanding it. Ligaments, in their supportive roles as joint protectors, restrict range of motion and flexibility at the end movement. Someone who is "double-jointed" in the knee joint (also known as *genu recurvatum*), for example, has ligaments with greater amounts of plasticity that allow for more range of motion. Many factors, such as obesity, muscle imbalance, and hypertrophy, contribute to poor flexibility, but muscle tissue has the ability to increase its resting length if the correct flexibility protocols are followed.

Two of the main influences on flexibility are the physical length of the *antagonist* muscle and the neurologic innervation of the muscle being stretched. When a muscle is stretched, so is the muscle spindle, which records the change in length and how fast the muscle is stretched. In a muscle stretch, there are two important neurologic properties to consider. To protect a muscle from being overstretched, a primary afferent neuron initiates a stretch reflex (**myotatic reflex arc,** see Chapter 2), which causes a contraction of the muscle being stretched. This mechanism fires in response to a stretch, and its response is proportional to the amount of force placed on the stretch. Because this reflex is so powerful, someone without adequate flexibility could easily cause injury to the muscle being stretched, especially if extreme force is applied into the stretch. This is one of the reasons ballistic stretching (see "Types of Flexibility," below) is precarious at best. While some research suggests that muscle spindles habituate to new muscle lengths with specific training (which explains why certain yoga postures are possible), the chance of injury for most individuals, especially those with existing conditions, is greater if long holds or ballistic-type motions are used.

Another factor with a stretched muscle is the *Golgi tendon organ,* or *GTO* (see Chapter 2). The GTO response occurs mostly in an active stretch—when the knee is extended and the hamstrings are being lengthened, for example—and when pressure is applied to tendons. The GTO initiates an inverse stretch reflex, which relaxes the muscle being stretched. Again, this component is a safety valve so that the muscle being stretched is not injured from excessive contraction of the myotatic reflex arc or lengthened muscle fibers.

Types of Flexibility

BALLISTIC STRETCHING

Ballistic stretching involves the use of bouncing or rhythmic motions to increase range of motion. It is sometimes employed in sports such as gymnastics and martial arts; however, it is rarely recommended in a health care setting because of its unsafe, forceful technique. Because of the nature of its forceful movement, the stretch reflex responds with dangerous contraction.

PASSIVE STRETCHING

Passive stretching is often used in the health care field, particularly with stroke or paralysis patients or those whose injury prevents the use of an extremity. The movement is usually assisted by a therapist, and the individual makes no contribution or active contraction in carrying out the stretch. The hold at the end movement is generally 30 seconds to 1 minute in duration.

STATIC STRETCHING

Static stretching is used in yoga and has been popularized by fitness programs. It is generally a slow stretch with holds of 10 to 30 seconds.

PROPRIOCEPTIVE NEUROMUSCULAR FACILITATION STRETCHING

Proprioceptive neuromuscular facilitation (PNF) stretching utilizes the components of muscle physiology to obtain an increased amount of flexibility in muscles. It also utilizes the fact that a muscle contraction is usually followed by relaxation of the opposite antagonistic muscle(s). Active PNF stretching involves taking a motion to its end point and then following that with a maximum isometric contraction of the counteracting muscles with resistance from a therapist. This is followed by a stretch that is usually held 10 to 30 seconds. Like many stretch protocols, PNF stretching techniques vary.

ACTIVE ISOLATED STRETCHING

Active Isolated Stretching (AIS) is used in this text as part of the *Clinical Flexibility and Therapeutic Exercise* modality. While active stretching has been in existence for some time, the Active Isolated protocol used today was pioneered by kinesiologist Aaron L. Mattes and has become widely popular among clinicians, athletes, and the general public. **Active Isolated Stretching (AIS)** involves the use of the body's natural movements (flexion, extension, rotation, etc.) and physiology to achieve greater range of motion. It uses the principles of Sherrington's law (reciprocal innervation, see Chapter 2) as well as short, 2-second holds. To achieve a stretch, an agonist muscle contracts to move a body segment, and the antagonist muscle is lengthened, held in a short stretch, and then returned to the starting position. This is repeated in repetitions, with several sets, depending on muscle tightness (see Chapter 12, Table 12.1). This method theorizes that the short holds do not violate the stretch reflex and therefore minimize muscle-tissue injury. Additionally, AIS movements are performed with the body in an advantageous position. For example, to lengthen the hamstring group, the body is supine, with no isometric contraction holding the body up in gravity. This allows the hamstring group to be lengthened in a relaxed state, without the interference of another contraction.

THE IMPORTANCE OF "CLINICAL" FLEXIBILITY

Clinical flexibility is defined as stretching used in a clinical setting, and it is usually assisted by a therapist. A clinical setting is anywhere a health care provider works, whether an actual clinic, a hospital, or the client's home. Since physical therapists, athletic trainers, and massage therapists generally provide care for clients suffering from pain and injury issues, utilizing a safe stretching protocol helps prevent further injury and aids in recovery. There are many reasons that the AIS approach is best suited for the health care worker's toolbox:

1. The active component and client contribution increase blood flow, and muscle reeducation occurs with each repetition.
2. The method involves the use of natural joint movements and reciprocal innervation.
3. Short holds help avoid the myotatic reflex arc contraction. Less force is placed on injured areas.
4. AIS is easily taught to clients for self-care.
5. Specific isolation of muscle groups allows for dynamic stretching of dysfunctional areas.

The exercises presented later in this chapter consist of upper-extremity AIS, followed by strengthening for the same muscles that were stretched (antagonists). This makes understanding the functional actions of the agonist and antagonist easier. Table 4.2 shows the protocol for performing AIS. It should be noted that these AIS exercises are presented mainly for students to attempt so that they can better understand functional anatomy and movement. These exercises can be shown to clients only if the clinician is within the scope of his or her practice.

TABLE 4.2 Active Isolated Stretching Protocol

1. Use agonist muscles to stretch antagonists.
2. Perform 8 to 10 repetitions and 2 to 3 sets.
3. Return to the start position with each repetition.
4. Hold the stretch approximately 2 seconds.
5. Exhale on work phase; inhale on relaxation phase.
6. Position the body to perform the stretches comfortably, using core muscles to assist.

Individual Muscles of the Shoulder Girdle

OIAI MUSCLE CHART TRAPEZIUS (tra-pe´zi-us) Named for its shape—irregular four-sided figure

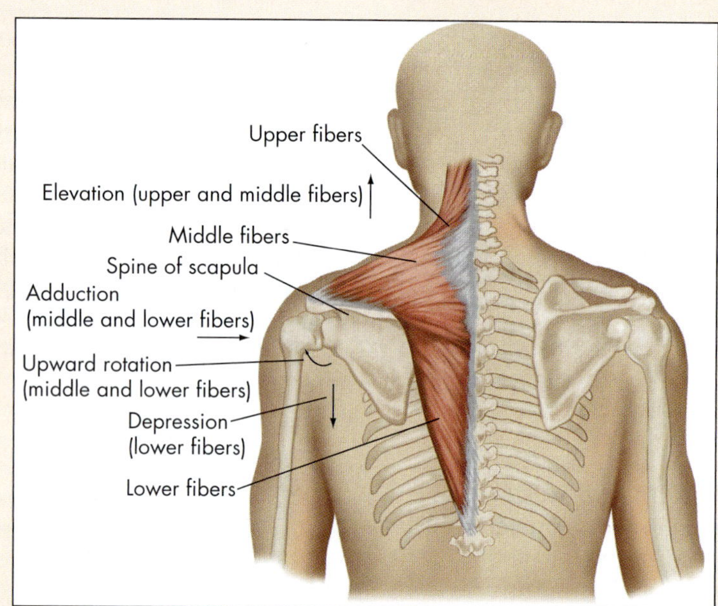

Name of Muscle	Origins	Insertion	Actions	Innervations
Trapezius	*Upper:* occiput, ligamentum nuchae	*Upper:* lateral clavicle	*Upper:* elevation, upward rotation of scapula	Accessory nerve (CN XI), branches of C3, C4
	Middle: spinous processes of C7, T1–T3	*Middle:* spine of scapula, acromion	*Middle:* adduction, elevation, upward rotation	
	Lower: spinous processes of T4–T12	*Lower:* root of spine of scapula	*Lower:* depression, upward rotation of scapula, adduction	
			bilateral extension of spine	

TRAPEZIUS MUSCLE

Palpation

Upper fibers: The upper fibers can be palpated halfway between occipital protuberance to C6 and laterally to acromion, particularly during elevation and extension of the head at the neck. Lift the shoulder, and then place a thumb under the upper trap inserting at the clavicle and an index finger on top, effectively making a pincer palpation of the upper trapezius.

Middle fibers: The middle fibers can be palpated from C7 to T3 and laterally to acromion process and scapula spine, particularly during adduction.

Lower fibers: The lower fibers can be palpated from T4 to T12 and medial aspect of scapula spine, particularly during depression and adduction.

See Chapter 5 for additional palpation techniques and the location of the upper, middle, and lower trapezius.

CLINICAL NOTES **Common Muscle Factors**

The sternocleidomastoid and trapezius share the same innervation of the spinal accessory nerve. This is noteworthy, as these two muscles oppose each other in flexion and extension of the head. As paired opposites, the muscles are caught in balancing the head on the neck. If the head is in a prolonged head-forward posture, the sternocleidomastoid shortens and the upper trapezius endeavors to hang on to the posterior head attachment with other posterior cervical muscles. Also, the accessory nerve can become entrapped by the sternocleidomastoid fibers and, in turn, make the trapezius weak. This means that the practitioner must treat both the sternocleidomastoid and the trapezius to unwind the chronic tension in the upper and middle trapezius. The trapezius is often involved in stiff neck, flexion and extension whiplash, repetitive actions, head-forward posture positions, and compensatory changes due to injury. Stretching of all the neck muscles is helpful for establishing better blood flow.

Muscle Specifics

Aptly named for its shape, the trapezius acts as its own all-in-one agonist and antagonist muscle. Thanks to its shape and attachments, the trapezius balances elevation with depression. Of the two actions, elevation is the stronger because it has to go against gravity and carry the extremities around as extra weight. The trapezius often has lengthened or stretched fibers, as the upper and middle trapezius may be kept in a constant state of elevation or shortening along with the levator scapulae. Unilaterally, one side of the trapezius may be shortened if one extremity is injured and in a sling. The active extremity will torque on the ipsilateral side of the entire trapezius and shoulder girdle muscles, while the injured contralateral side will be passively shortened.

The upper fibers are a thin and relatively weak part of the muscle; however, the muscle is thick and twisted where it attaches to the clavicle. The muscle must spirally attach in this way so that the head can fully rotate to the opposite side. The fibers assist the middle trapezius and levator scapulae in clavicle elevation, as well as elevation and upward rotation of the scapula.

Due to their origin on the base of the skull, the upper fibers assist in bilateral head extension and unilateral rotation. Ipsilaterally, the trapezius laterally flexes the head.

The middle fibers are stronger and thicker, and they provide strong elevation, upward rotation, and scapular adduction (retraction). The middle fibers are stronger because they position the shoulder for function and posture. As a result, the area is often a source of tenderness, discomfort, and chronic tension, usually caused by head-forward postures, repetitive shortening of the upper and middle fibers, rounded shoulders, or the weight of the upper extremities pulling on the shoulder.

The lower fibers assist in adduction (retraction), depression, and upward rotation of the scapula. The area is typically weak, and the fibers often are lengthened or stretched, particularly in individuals whose posture and activities demand a significant amount of scapular abduction.

When all the parts of the trapezius are working together, they tend to pull upward and adduct at the same time. Fixation of the scapula for deltoid action is a typical function of the trapezius muscle. For example, continuous upward rotation of the scapula permits one to raise the arms over the head; the muscle always prevents the glenoid fossa from being pulled down when the arms are lifting objects; and the muscle action enables one to hold an object overhead. Holding the arm at the side horizontally shows typical fixation of the scapula by the trapezius muscle, while the deltoid muscle holds the arm in that position. The muscle is used strenuously when lifting with the hands, as in picking up the handlebars of a heavy wheelbarrow. The trapezius must prevent the scapula from being pulled downward. Awkward repetitive actions that require frequent reaching in front of the body will shorten the upper and middle trapezius as the scapula abducts, effectively lengthening the lower trapezius. Dental hygienists, computer operators, truck drivers, and landscapers can all lay claim to shortened upper and middle trapezius, abducted scapulae, and lengthened lower trapezius.

Clinical Flexibility

In stretching the trapezius, it is important to remember its attachments and functional actions. The most vital areas to stretch are the upper and middle fibers because of their antigravity functions and history of inflicting chronic tension. The cervical region also is affected by these fibers because of the close proximity of attachments to the occipital bone. Because the middle fibers attach to the medial border of the acromion and upper border of the scapula, and the lower fibers attach to the base of the scapular spine, it is necessary to consider scapular action in stretching these fibers. To stretch these fibers, the scapula must be *protracted.* To achieve this, bring the extended arm across the front of the body (horizontal adduction) just under the chin. Using the other hand, assist by pushing just proximal to the elbow. Apply a gentle stretch for 2 seconds; repeat 8 to 10 times. A variation of this movement that will cause the scapula to protract with rotation, thus increasing the stretch to the trapezius and rhomboids, is to flex the elbow as it is brought across the body, reaching with the hand to the posterior contralateral shoulder; then apply the same gentle stretch. *Contraindications:* This exercise should be avoided with shoulder arthroplasty. Impingement, tendonitis, and other dysfunctions will benefit from this exercise, but movement must be slow and controlled.

Strengthening

Strengthening the upper and middle fibers can be accomplished through a *forward*-circle shoulder-shrugging exercise that consists of a forward, up, and back sequence to cause scapular retraction. This exercise also helps strengthen the rhomboids at the same time. The middle and lower fibers can be strengthened through bent-over rowing and shoulder-joint horizontal abduction exercises from a prone position. See Chapter 12 for more information. *Contraindications:* These exercises are safe with controlled movement.

OIAI MUSCLE CHART LEVATOR SCAPULAE (le-va´tor scap´u-lae) The lifter

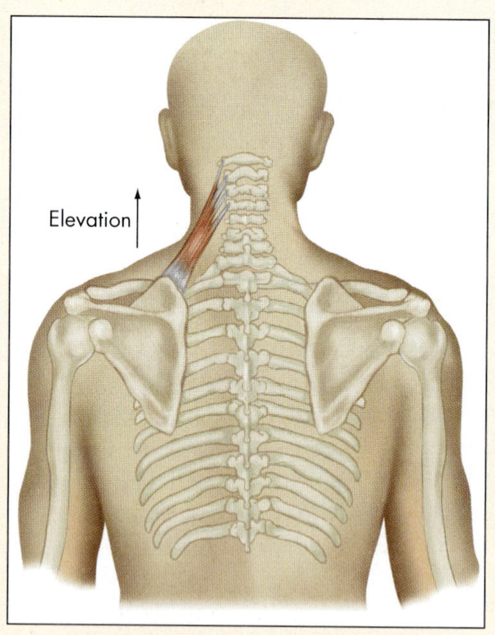

Name of Muscle	Origins	Insertion	Actions	Innervations
Levator scapulae	C1–C4 transverse processes	Vertebral border of scapula (medial) from superior angle to root of spine	Elevation of scapula	Dorsal scapular nerve (C5, C4, and C3)

LEVATOR SCAPULAE MUSCLE

Palpation

Deep to the trapezius, the levator scapulae is difficult to palpate posteriorly; it is best palpated at its insertion just medial to the superior angle of the scapula, particularly during slight elevation. Locate the insertion on the anterior scapula by approaching from under the middle and upper trapezius. For better access, passively shorten the upper and middle trapezius by lifting the inferior angle and elevating the scapula.

> **CLINICAL NOTES** — **Common Problems**
>
> In addition to the upper and middle trapezius, the levator scapulae is a common site for tightness, tenderness, discomfort, and chronic-tension (stiff-neck) conditions. Poor body mechanics such as head-forward posture, a nonergonomic computer station, and excessive lateral head tilt with a phone can contribute to dysfunction.

Muscle Specifics

The levator scapulae acts as a bilateral guy wire that runs from the upper four vertebrae to the scapula. If head movement is compromised or the muscle is shortened in any way, it upsets the balance with its connections to the transverse processes of C1, which it can easily rotate. It is important for therapists to remember this relationship when planning to release muscles prior to manipulation by another appropriate health care professional.

Clinical Flexibility

To stretch the levator scapulae, perform the same horizontal adduction stretch as that for the trapezius. Also, since the muscle has attachments along the cervical spine, the head can be moved contralaterally to facilitate a good stretch. Start with the head in the neutral position, eyes straight ahead. Leave one hand above the head to help assist in the stretch. Move the head in lateral flexion to the opposite shoulder, and apply a gentle stretch using the other hand. Return to the neutral position, and repeat 8 to 10 times. *Contraindications:* Use caution with cervical herniations.

Strengthening

Shrugging the shoulders involves the levator scapulae muscle, along with the upper and middle trapezius. Since fixation of the scapula by the pectoralis minor muscle allows the levator scapulae muscles on both sides to extend the neck or to flex it unilaterally, the levator scapulae should be strengthened the same way it is stretched—by flexion and extension of the neck. For the flexors, lie on one side, with head and arm off a therapy table or bed. Begin the movement with the lower ear toward the ground (lateral flexion). Lift the head into flexion to the opposite shoulder, and then gently return to the lower position. Extension can be performed in the prone position, lifting the head back into extension. Repeat 8 to 10 times. *Contraindications:* Use caution with disk herniations.

RHOMBOID MUSCLES: MAJOR AND MINOR

Palpation

Deep to the trapezius are the rhomboids. Though difficult, they may be palpated through the relaxed trapezius during adduction. This is best accomplished by placing the client's ipsilateral hand behind the back (glenohumeral medial rotation and scapula downward rotation), as this relaxes the trapezius and brings the rhomboid into action when the client lifts the hand away from the back. The rhomboid major makes a small triangle that is visible and superficial just medial to the inferior angle of the scapula. The lower trapezius slopes away from the scapula in its angle from the root of the spine to the spinous processes of the vertebrae.

> **CLINICAL NOTES** — **Postural Problems**
>
> Rounded shoulders may lead to a superficial ache in the rhomboids, particularly in the trigger points located around the medial border of the scapula. While the pectoralis minor and serratus anterior lock and hold the scapulae in abduction, the rhomboids in turn lengthen. Since the rhomboids are often weak, this muscle struggles to pull the scapulae back into an adducted position. This posture often leads to a head-forward position, causing torque and anterior wedging on the cervical and midthoracic vertebrae. Self-care could include using a tennis ball for ischemic compression, creating ergonomically correct computer stations, and maintaining postural awareness. A lumbar pillow can help support the upper body and maintain the curve in the lower back. The rhomboids should also be strengthened on a weekly basis, and the pectoralis minor and major should be stretched to facilitate scapular retraction.

Muscle Specifics

In the average person, the rhomboid muscles spend a disproportionate amount of time in lengthened (stretched) positions. The rounded-shoulder posture usually starts in elementary school, where heavy backpacks increase thoracic kyphosis. Because the rhomboids are antigravity muscles, and the opposite pectoralis major is developed and powerful, the

OIAI MUSCLE CHART RHOMBOIDS MAJOR AND MINOR (rom´boyd) Bilateral Christmas tree; means "diamond shaped"

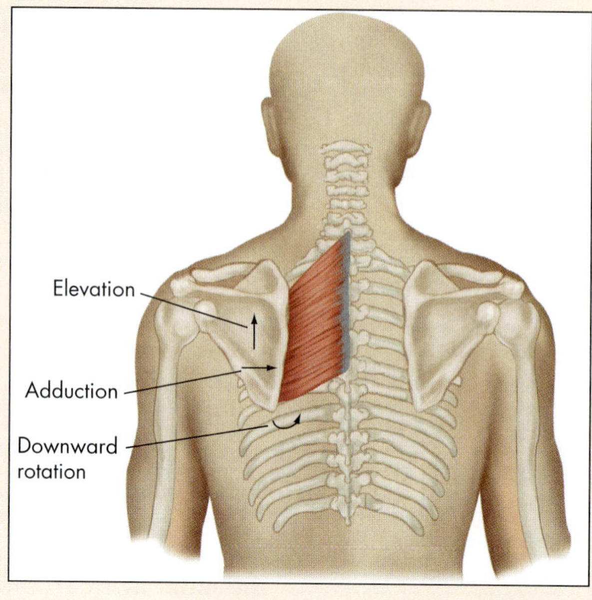

Name of Muscle	Origins	Insertion	Actions	Innervations
Rhomboid major	T2–T5 spinous processes	Vertebral border of scapula below root of spine	Adduction (retraction), elevation accompanying adduction, downward rotation of scapula	Dorsal scapular nerve (C5)
Rhomboid minor	C7, T1 spinous processes	Root of spine of scapula	Same	Same

rhomboids tend to become lengthened and atrophied. In a fitness program, they are one of the most overlooked muscles to strengthen because they lose favor over the "shapely" prime movers.

Clinical Flexibility

The rhomboids are extremely important muscles to stretch. Since their pain patterns are wide, often spreading into the occipital area or down the lower back, stretching can help restore blood flow and release trigger or energy points. The rhomboids are scapular retractors and therefore must be stretched with scapular *protraction.* The horizontal adduction stretches are excellent for this, as the rhomboids are stretched by passively moving the scapula into full protraction while maintaining depression. *Contraindications:* These stretches should be avoided with shoulder arthroplasty. Impingement, tendonitis, and other dysfunctions will benefit from this exercise, but movement must be slow and controlled.

Strengthening

The rhomboid muscles fix the scapula in adduction (retraction) when the shoulder joint muscles adduct or extend the arm. These muscles are used powerfully during chin-up exercises. As one hangs from the horizontal bar, suspended by the hands, the scapula pulls away from the top of the chest. When the chin-up movement begins, the rhomboid muscles rotate the medial border of the scapula down and back toward the spinal column. The rhomboid also works in a similar manner to prevent scapula winging. The trapezius and rhomboid muscles working together produce adduction with slight elevation of the scapula. The latissimus dorsi muscle opposes this action, as it adducts or extends the humerus.

OIAI MUSCLE CHART SERRATUS ANTERIOR (ser-a´tus an-tir´e-or) Named for shape and location—the saw in front

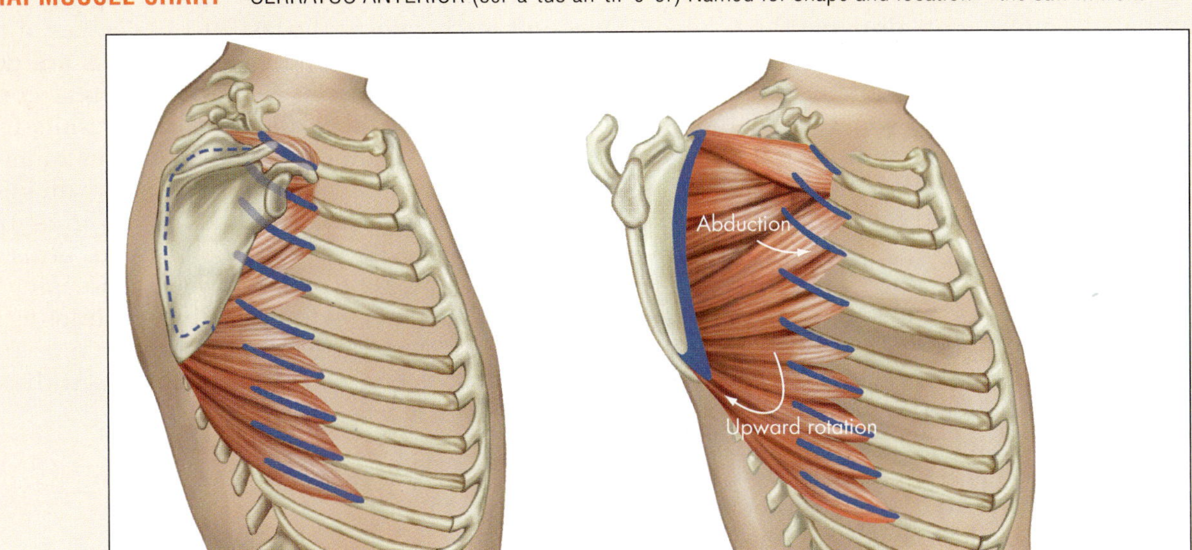

(a) Lateral view **(b) Lateral view with scapula reflected posteriorly to reveal anterior surface**

Name of Muscle	Origins	Insertion	Actions	Innervations
Serratus anterior	Surface of the upper nine ribs at the side of the chest	Anterior aspect of the whole length of the medial border of scapula	Abduction, upward rotation	Long thoracic nerve (C5–C7)

The rhomboids must be isolated in order to strengthen them. In the prone position on an exercise bench, with arms off the edge, hold dumbbells; then flex the elbows and wrist to form a "ball." With the head lowered completely so that there is no action in the upper trapezius, bring the elbows back as the scapula is retracted very tightly and hold for 2 seconds; then lower the weight to the starting position. Repeat 8 to 10 times. To see photos of this exercise, see Chapter 12. *Contraindications:* This exercise is generally safe with controlled movement.

SERRATUS ANTERIOR MUSCLE

Palpation

Palpate the serratus anterior on the front and lateral side of the chest below the 5th and 6th ribs just proximal to their origin during abduction, which is best accomplished from a supine position with the glenohumeral joint in 90 degrees of flexion. The upper fibers may be palpated in the same position between the lateral borders of the pectoralis major and latissimus dorsi in the axilla. See the side-lying techniques in Chapter 7 to locate and palpate the serratus anterior easily.

CLINICAL NOTES **Painful Actions of the Serratus Anterior**

Often forgotten as an accessory respiratory muscle, the serratus anterior comes from the upper nine ribs and thus interdigitates with the external oblique. Any actions that preclude abducted shoulder positions may shorten serratus anterior fibers. Running, scrubbing floors, and even repetitive massage techniques can lead to debilitating myofascial pain in the serratus anterior that could refer down the upper extremity. A point of tenderness is often found in the axilla region between the ribs. The serratus anterior is easily accessed in a side-lying position. See Chapter 7 for positions and techniques.

Muscle Specifics

Named for its shape, the serratus anterior muscle is used commonly in movements drawing the scapula forward with slight upward rotation, such as throwing a baseball, punching in boxing, shooting and guarding in basketball, and tackling in football. As a shoulder girdle anterior stabilizer, it helps prevent winging of the scapula. For this reason, it should not be overlooked in a strength and stretching program.

Clinical Flexibility

The serratus anterior can be stretched by reversing its action. Since it abducts the scapula, it can be stretched by causing the scapula to adduct. With arms at the sides in the fundamental position, lift one arm into abduction with the palms turned out, continuing into sideward elevation, with the arm passing just behind the head. Use the opposite hand to help stretch by pulling at the elbow for 2 seconds. Repeat 8 to 10 times. *Contraindications:* Impingement, tendonitis, and other dysfunctions will benefit from this exercise, but movement must be slow and controlled.

Strengthening

The serratus anterior muscle is used strongly in doing push-ups, especially in the last 5 to 10 degrees of motion. The bench press and overhead press are good exercises for this muscle. A winged scapular condition (lateral tilt of the scapula) usually results from weakness of the rhomboid or the serratus anterior. Serratus anterior weakness may result from an injury to the long thoracic nerve. Another way to strengthen this muscle is to lie on the floor supine, arms extended in front holding 5-pound weights. Keeping the arms extended, push up to the ceiling, protracting the scapula all the way. Repeat 8 to 10 times. *Contraindications:* These exercises are generally safe with controlled movement.

PECTORALIS MINOR MUSCLE

Palpation

The pectoralis minor is difficult to palpate, but it can be palpated under the pectoralis major muscle and just inferior to the coracoid process during resisted depression. This may be enhanced by placing the client's hand behind the back and having her actively lift the hand away, which brings the protractors into action.

OIAI MUSCLE CHART PECTORALIS MINOR (pek-to-ra´lis mi´nor) Brachial plexus entrapper—*pectus* means "chest"

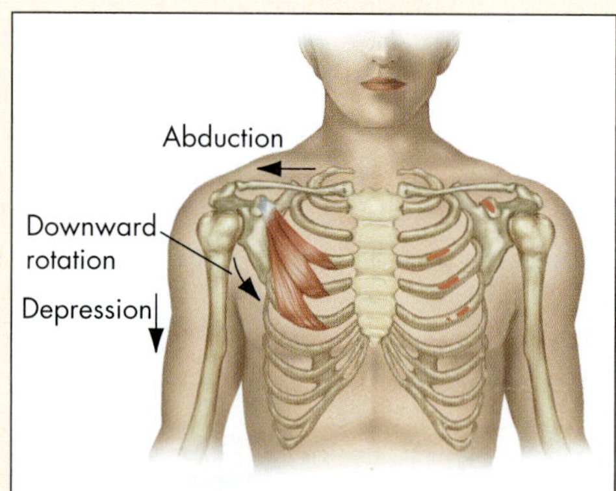

Name of Muscle	Origins	Insertion	Actions	Innervations
Pectoralis minor	Anterior surfaces of 3rd to 5th ribs	Coracoid process of scapula	Abduction, downward rotation as it abducts, depression from upward rotation	Medial pectoral nerve (C8–T1)

CLINICAL NOTES **Entrapment of the Brachial Plexus**

Sometimes people experience numbness or tingling in either parts of or the entire upper extremity if they sleep with the arm positioned over the head all night. The large nerve structure of the brachial plexus runs under the tendinous attachment of the pectoralis minor at the coracoid process. If the upper extremity is placed over the head, this position may be conducive to entrapping the brachial plexus, particularly the lateral cord that leads into the median nerve as well as the axillary artery, possibly diminishing a pulse at the wrist. In addition to sleeping in this position, incorrectly wearing an overly laden backpack compresses the pectoralis minor and can entrap the brachial plexus. Stretching the pectoralis minor and major can help "open" the thoracic space and is very helpful for thoracic outlet syndrome.

Muscle Specifics

The pectoralis minor muscle is used, along with the serratus anterior muscle, in true abduction (protraction) of the scapula without rotation, particularly in movements such as push-ups or rounding the shoulders. The serratus anterior draws the scapula forward with a tendency toward upward rotation, and the pectoralis minor pulls the scapula forward with a tendency toward downward rotation. The two pulling together give true abduction, which is necessary in many humeral flexed positions such as push-ups. These muscles work together in most movements that involve pushing with the hands.

Clinical Flexibility

The pectoralis minor is most used in depressing and rotating the scapula downward from an upwardly rotated position, as in pushing the body upward on dip bars. The pectoralis minor is often tight due to overuse in activities involving abduction, such as gardening or working at a desk. The result is often forward and rounded shoulders. It is also involved in thoracic kyphotic patterns and brachial plexus dysfunctions. To stretch the pectoralis minor, lift both arms up in flexion, palms facing each other, to about a 90-degree angle. Using the muscles on the posterior upper back, bring the arms back into horizontal abduction. The scapulae should retract in this movement. As you lift back, tighten the abdominals to prevent back hyperextension. Hold for 2 seconds, and repeat 8 to 10 times. *Contraindications:* Shoulder arthroplasty patients; client should move into only 70 degrees of horizontal abduction. Impingement, tendonitis, and other dysfunctions will benefit from this exercise, but movement must be slow and controlled.

Strengthening

The pectoralis minor can be strengthened by a standard chest fly, except the angle of the arms must be

OIAI MUSCLE CHART SUBCLAVIUS (sub-klá-ve-us) The stabilizer below the clavicle

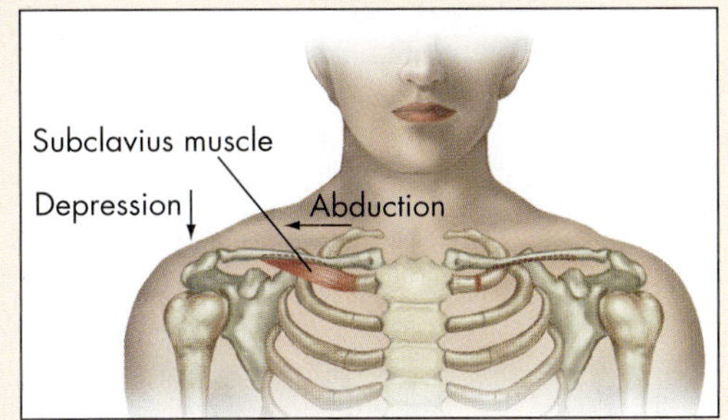

Name of Muscle	Origins	Insertion	Actions	Innervations
Subclavius	Superior aspect of 1st rib at its junction with its costal cartilage	Inferior groove in the midportion of clavicle	Stabilization of sternoclavicular joint, depression; draws clavicle down as shoulders abduct	Nerve fibers from C5 and C6

changed to better isolate the pectoralis minor. Lying supine on the floor or table with the arms flexed in front of the chest, bring the weight slowly out to the sides (horizontal abduction), keeping a 90-degree angle on the arms. Slowly return to the starting position. Repeat 8 to 10 times. *Contraindications:* This exercise is generally safe with controlled movement.

SUBCLAVIUS MUSCLE

Palpation

The subclavius is difficult to distinguish from the pectoralis major, but it may be palpated just inferior to the middle third of the clavicle with the client in the side-lying position. The clavicle is in an upward-rotated position, and the humerus is supported in a partially, passively flexed position. Slight active depression and abduction of the scapula may enhance palpation.

CLINICAL NOTES **Subclavius—the Stabilizer**

Although the subclavius is not a major prime mover, its stabilizing feature makes it a working muscle that almost never rests. If the scapulae are abducted and perpetuated in rounded shoulders, the subclavius fibers may shorten and develop trigger points with a painful referred pattern. This pattern might refer down the upper extremity distally toward the hand and wrist.

Muscle Specifics

The subclavius pulls the clavicle anteriorly and inferiorly toward the sternum. In addition to assisting in abduction and depression of the clavicle and the shoulder girdle, it has a significant role in protecting and stabilizing the sternoclavicular joint during upper-extremity movements.

Clinical Flexibility

The subclavius muscle can be stretched much like stretching the pectoralis minor, by starting with the arms flexed in front of the chest, palms facing each other. Using the muscles on the posterior shoulder, retract the scapula and bring the arms back into horizontal abduction. Hold 2 seconds, and repeat 8 to 10 times. This stretch also targets the pectoralis major. *Contraindications:* This exercise is generally safe with controlled movement.

Strengthening

The subclavius may be strengthened during activities in which there is active depression, such as dips, or active abduction, such as push-ups. A standard fly (explained earlier) is an effective way to strengthen this muscle. *Contraindications:* This exercise is generally safe with controlled movement.

CHAPTER *summary*

Introduction

✔ The shoulder girdle is a two-bone structure that surrounds the axial skeleton and provides dynamic stability for the shoulder joint.

Bones

✔ The two bones that make up the shoulder girdle are the clavicle and the scapula. Bony landmarks provide attachments for muscles to pull on and cause movement when contracting.

Joints

✔ The sternoclavicular joint is a gliding articulation that is formed by the sternum and the clavicle. The acromioclavicular joint is also a gliding joint, but with less motion than the sternoclavicular joint. The scapulothoracic joint is not a true synovial joint but moves over the rib cage with contractions of its muscles.

Movements

✔ The movements of the shoulder girdle include elevation, depression, abduction (protraction), adduction (retraction), upward rotation, and downward rotation. There are accessory tilt movements as well.

✔ The shoulder joint and shoulder girdle work together in performing upper-extremity activities. It is critical to understand that movement of the shoulder girdle is not dependent on the shoulder joint and its muscles.

Muscles

✔ The pectoralis minor, subclavius, and serratus anterior are located anteriorly, while the trapezius, rhomboids, and levator scapulae are located posteriorly.

Nerves

✔ The nerves for the shoulder girdle muscles stem primarily from the cervical plexus and brachial plexus.

Clinical Flexibility and Therapeutic Exercise

- ✔ The shoulder girdle muscles should be stretched and strengthened to help maintain their dynamic range of movement.
- ✔ Muscles should always be stretched before any resistance is applied.
- ✔ Strengthening the antigravity muscles of the shoulder is necessary to facilitate proper scapular movement.
- ✔ The synergistic movement in the shoulder joint between the glenohumeral joint and the scapulothoracic joint is known as the *scapulohumeral rhythm*.

Understanding Flexibility

- ✔ Flexibility is an important component in sports and general fitness, and it should not be overlooked in the study of kinesiology.
- ✔ Proper range of motion by increased flexibility has been shown to help poor posture, increase sports performance, and reduce wear and tear on joints.
- ✔ Flexibility is defined as the end motion of a segment, and it can occur by active contraction of the agonist (active range of motion) or by motion of an external force (passive range of motion).
- ✔ To protect a muscle from being overstretched, a primary afferent neuron initiates a stretch reflex (myotatic reflex arc, see Chapter 2), which causes a contraction of the muscle being stretched.
- ✔ This mechanism has been measured to fire after 1 to 2 seconds of a stretch hold, and its response is proportional to the amount of force placed on the stretch.
- ✔ Another important component of a stretched muscle is the Golgi tendon organ, or GTO (see Chapter 2).
- ✔ The GTO response occurs mostly in an active stretch, such as when the knee is extended and the hamstrings are being lengthened, and when pressure is applied to tendons.
- ✔ The GTO initiates an inverse stretch reflex, which relaxes the muscle being stretched.

Types of Flexibility

- ✔ There are many different types of stretching; these include ballistic, passive, static, proprioceptive neuromuscular facilitation (PNF), and Active Isolated Stretching (AIS).
- ✔ Active Isolated Stretching is used in this text as part of the *Clinical Flexibility and Therapeutic Exercise* modality.
- ✔ Active Isolated Stretching involves the use of the body's natural movements and physiology to achieve greater range of motion.
- ✔ AIS uses the principle of reciprocal innervation (Sherrington's law, see Chapter 3) as well as short, 2-second holds.
- ✔ To achieve a stretch in AIS, an agonist muscle contracts to move a body segment; then the antagonist muscle is lengthened, held in a 2-second stretch, and then returned to the start position.
- ✔ Clinical flexibility is defined as flexibility used in a clinical setting, and it is usually assisted by a therapist.
- ✔ A clinical setting can be anywhere a health care provider might work, whether it is a clinic, a hospital, or a client's home.
- ✔ Since physical therapists, athletic trainers, and massage therapists usually provide care for clients with pain and injury issues, utilizing a safe stretching protocol helps prevent further injury and aids in recovery.
- ✔ There are many reasons that the AIS approach is best suited for the clinic or the health care worker's toolbox.

Individual Muscles of the Shoulder Girdle

- ✔ *Trapezius* is a four-sided superficial posterior muscle that is divided into three sections: upper, middle, and lower. The trapezius lifts and depresses the clavicle and scapula and adducts and upwardly rotates the scapula. Bilaterally it extends the head, and unilaterally it can rotate and laterally flex the head to the ipsilateral side.
- ✔ *Levator scapulae* lifts the scapula. It lies underneath the trapezius and spans from the cervical vertebrae to the superior angle of the scapula.
- ✔ *Rhomboids,* major and minor, are deep to the trapezius. Shaped like a bilateral Christmas tree, the rhomboids connect the spinous processes of the thoracic spine to the vertebral edge of the scapula. Their major functions are adduction and downward rotation.
- ✔ *Serratus anterior* runs from the upper nine ribs and inserts into the anterior medial scapula. It abducts and upwardly rotates the scapula. Serratus anterior is also an accessory muscle of respiration.
- ✔ *Pectoralis minor* is an anterior muscle that originates on the ribs and inserts on the coracoid process of the scapula. It abducts and depresses the scapula. Pectoralis minor is an accessory respiratory muscle.
- ✔ *Subclavius* is a stabilizer and protects the sternoclavicular joint.

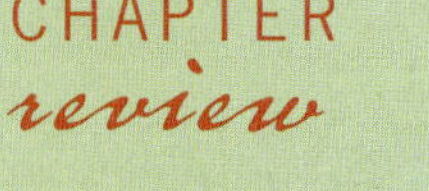

Worksheet Exercises

As an aid to learning, for in-class or out-of-class assignments, or for testing, tear-out worksheets are found at the end of the text, pages 519–522.

True or False

Write true *or* false *after each statement.*

1. The bones of the shoulder girdle include the tibia, clavicle, and humerus.
2. For the shoulder girdle bones to move, the muscles must insert on the ulna.
3. The pectoralis minor and serratus anterior are the primary abductors of the scapula for the shoulder girdle.
4. The trapezius acts as its own agonist and antagonist with the actions of elevation and depression.
5. The scapulothoracic joint is a true synovial joint.
6. The acromioclavicular joint is an arthrodial (gliding) joint.
7. The levator scapulae and the lower trapezius lift the scapula.
8. The rhomboids insert on the medial border of the scapula.
9. The serratus anterior originates on the upper nine ribs.
10. The subclavius is more of a stabilizer muscle for the shoulder girdle than a prime mover.
11. Strengthening the rhomboids will help correct rounded-shoulder posture.
12. By stretching the neck in lateral flexion, one can help stretch the levator scapulae.

Short Answers

Write your answers on the lines provided.

1. Name the muscles that adduct the scapula.

___
___
___

2. Name the gliding joint that connects the clavicle to the sternum.

___
___
___

3. What is the joint called that connects the clavicle to the scapula?

___
___
___

4. Why do you use the serratus anterior when you flex your upper extremity in front of the body?

___
___
___

5. Name the muscles that elevate the scapula.

___
___
___

6. Name the origin of the pectoralis minor.

___
___
___

7. What nerve structure might be entrapped by the pectoralis minor?

___
___
___

8. Name the insertion of the lower trapezius.

___
___
___

9. Name the origin of the levator scapulae.

___
___
___

10. What is the action of the lower trapezius that is the antagonist for the upper trapezius?

____

____

____

11. Name three muscles that affect posture on the posterior shoulder.

____

____

____

12. Describe the agonist and antagonist of horizontal flexion.

____

____

____

Multiple Choice

Circle the correct answers.

1. The muscle(s) that stabilizes the sternoclavicular joint, assists in depression, and draws the clavicle down as the shoulders abduct is the:
   a. pectoralis minor
   b. subclavius
   c. trapezius
   d. rhomboids
2. The muscle(s) that often lengthens with a rounded-shoulder posture is the:
   a. serratus anterior
   b. upper trapezius
   c. rhomboids
   d. pectoralis minor
3. Pectoralis minor inserts on the:
   a. coracoid process
   b. styloid process
   c. anterior ribs 3 to 5
   d. clavicle
4. The actions of the serratus anterior are:
   a. adduction and elevation
   b. elevation and depression
   c. abduction and upward rotation
   d. downward rotation and adduction

   Stiff neck muscles could be:
   e. the levator scapulae and upper trapezius
   f. the pectoralis minor and upper trapezius
   g. the levator scapulae and rhomboids
   h. none of the above
5. The origin of the rhomboid minor is the:
   a. transverse processes of C1–C4
   b. spinous processes of C7 and T1
   c. vertebral border of the scapula
   d. root of the spine of the scapula
6. The trapezius can contract bilaterally to cause:
   a. flexion of the neck
   b. abduction of the scapula
   c. extension of the neck
   d. none of the above
7. CFTE is a modality composed of:
   a. stretching and strengthening the muscles of the body
   b. just stretches
   c. just strengthening
   d. therapeutic massage techniques
8. Muscles that cause downward rotation of the scapula are the:
   a. pectoralis minor and serratus anterior
   b. pectoralis minor and rhomboids
   c. lower trapezius and serratus anterior
   d. subclavius and serratus anterior
9. An accessory movement of the scapula could be:
   a. downward rotation
   b. upward rotation
   c. lateral tilt
   d. abduction
10. The nerve that stimulates the trapezius is the:
    a. accessory nerve
    b. dorsal thoracic
    c. sciatic nerve
    d. brachial nerve
11. The stretch reflex is known as:
    a. the Golgi tendon organ
    b. the myotatic reflex arc
    c. GTO
    d. plyometrics

12. Sherrington's law exemplifies which neuromuscular principle?
    a. reciprocal innervation
    b. nerve conduction
    c. agonist contraction
    d. stretch reflex

13. Flexibility and strength for the entire body are important for:
    a. athletes only
    b. children in elementary school
    c. everyone regardless of sports involvement
    d. people over 50

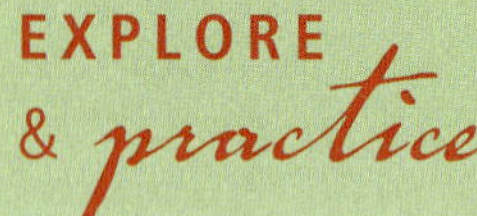

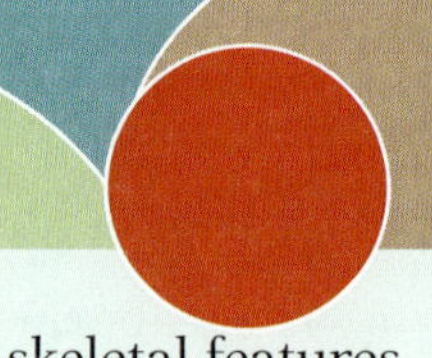

1. Locate the following prominent skeletal features on a human skeleton and on a subject:

   a. Scapula:
   1. Medial border
   2. Inferior angle
   3. Superior angle
   4. Coracoid process
   5. Spine of the scapula
   6. Glenoid cavity
   7. Acromion process
   8. Supraspinatus fossa
   9. Infraspinatus fossa

   b. Clavicle:
   1. Sternal end
   2. Acromial end

   c. Joints:
   1. Sternoclavicular joint
   2. Acromioclavicular joint

2. Palpate the following muscles on a human subject:
   a. Serratus anterior
   b. Trapezius
   c. Rhomboid major and minor
   d. Levator scapulae
   e. Pectoralis minor

3. Palpate the sternoclavicular and acromioclavicular joint movements and the muscles primarily involved while demonstrating the following shoulder girdle movements:
   a. Adduction
   b. Abduction
   c. Rotation upward
   d. Rotation downward
   e. Elevation
   f. Depression

4. Locate the origins and insertions of the muscles of the shoulder girdle on a skeleton and on a human subject.

5. *Muscle analysis chart:* Fill in the chart below by listing the muscles primarily involved in each movement.

Abduction	Adduction
Elevation	Depression
Upward rotation	Downward rotation

6. *Antagonistic muscle action chart:* Fill in the chart below by listing the muscle(s) or parts of muscles that are antagonists in their actions to the muscles in the left column.

Agonist	Antagonist
Serratus anterior	
Trapezius (upper fibers)	
Trapezius (middle fibers)	
Trapezius (lower fibers)	
Rhomboid	
Levator scapulae	
Pectoralis minor	

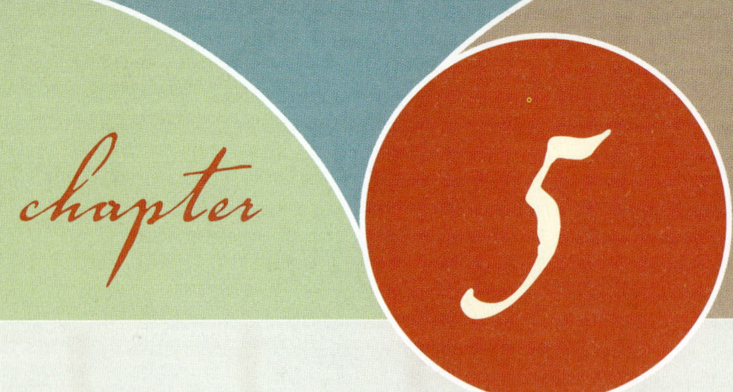

Dimensional Massage Techniques for the Shoulder Girdle Muscles

LEARNING OUTCOMES

After completing this chapter, you should be able to:

5-1 Define key terms.

5-2 List goals of individual techniques.

5-3 Describe deep-tissue therapy.

5-4 Give examples of some general principles of body mechanics.

5-5 Practice safe body mechanics.

5-6 Demonstrate specific techniques on shoulder girdle muscles.

5-7 Incorporate dimensional massage therapy techniques in a regular routine or use them when needed.

5-8 Identify two underlying principles for the theory of dimensional massage.

5-9 Determine safe treatment protocols and refer clients to other health professionals when necessary.

KEY TERMS

Body mechanics
Compression
Cross-fiber friction
Deep-tissue therapy
Deep transverse friction
Dimensional massage therapy
Elliptical movement
Functional unit
Ischemic compression
Jostling
Myofascial stretches
Parallel thumbs
Sequence
Splinting
Stripping
Technique goals
Treatment protocol
Trigger point release
Trigger points

Introduction

Although nothing can replace the kinesthetic quality of touch, it is important to learn about the body, its structure, and its functional foundation. The more knowledge a student retains about how the muscles work, where they are located, and how they are attached, the more she will be able to demonstrate critical thinking in a therapeutic setting. For the student, there are two very significant principles of motion:

- *Aggregate muscle action:* Muscles work in groups and in paired opposition.
- *Law of reaction:* For every action there is an opposite and equal reaction.

As discussed in Chapter 2, muscles perform specific roles in relation to the typical diarthrodial joint. Agonists and antagonists are both prime movers, but they oppose each other and are usually located on opposite sides of the joint; synergists assist; stabilizers protect the joint in movement and allow other muscles to function; and neutralizers resist actions or act as brakes to stop motion. All of these actors practice as the muscles pull on the bones to move the joints. Range of motion, or the joint's ability to function within its complete range, is dependent on the **functional unit:** muscles cooperating to work in groups and in paired opposition. A practitioner cannot ignore the work that the synergists perform or contribute to a joint's range of motion or to the stabilizers protecting the joint. When a muscle is injured, the remaining areas of the functional unit have to compensate for the less than normally functioning actor. It does not take long for the whole joint to debilitate. Treating the whole joint and all the muscles involved in the functional unit is a dimensional approach.

As the manual therapist works to unwind the soft tissue in an area of the body, she needs to be aware of which actions a client performed to overload the muscles, which joints are involved, and how the joints and muscles are dependent on each other for movement and stability. A practitioner always works on the muscles that operate together to provide the action and makes sure that the opposing muscles were not shortened or lengthened in the process of whatever repetitive action or injury took place. The shoulder girdle and shoulder joint are so dependent on one another that if a soft-tissue problem of the shoulder joint muscles exists, the shoulder girdle muscles are apt to be very tight, even splinting the problem in the shoulder joint. **Splinting** is a supportive action that a muscle or muscles may perform so that another joint and group of muscles can function appropriately. The splinting muscle may contract isometrically or dynamically. To treat all the offending soft-tissue structures, a therapist must explore the entire kinetic chain right up to the head, neck, and trunk.

Treatment Protocol

This book assumes that the student has learned how to perform an appropriate intake, including a medical history, client interview, and appropriate SOAP notes, and has had practice observing posture, gait, and the exploration of range of motion of joints. The **treatment protocol** below is a synopsis of an overall approach to a massage session.

Technique Goals and the Mystery of Deep-Tissue Therapy

Technique goals are the outcomes expected from choosing techniques for a particular purpose; because each person is unique, treatment goals should be based on the client's individual needs. A therapist's goals are to lengthen, separate, lift, and broaden fibers to release hypertonicities, increase range of motion, reduce pain and/or discomfort, increase circulation, and help relieve any joint restrictions. This book assumes that the student has practiced Swedish techniques (also called *classical Western*), such as effleurage, petrissage, friction, tapotement, vibration, and nerve strokes and that they require no further definition. Proficiency comes with practice; however, for a review of Swedish technique definitions, refer to the Glossary.

Deep-tissue therapy is simply a series of specific techniques designed to unwind the soft tissue in a particular pattern or sequence with an end result that includes meeting specific goals. *Deep* does not necessarily mean a lot of pressure; rather, it means more appropriate pressure that is determined by palpation and the

TREATMENT PROTOCOL

- Take the client's medical history, interview the client, and record SOAP notes.
- Observe postural assessment, gait, and the range of motion of joints.
- Perform palpation.
- Passively shorten muscles and/or position shoulders and scapula whenever possible.
- Work superficial to deep.
- Release hypertonic muscles.
- Use dual-hand distraction methods when possible.
- Work individual muscles, their attachments, synergists, stabilizers, and antagonists; study the functional unit.
- Do not overwork areas.
- Do trigger point work last on passively shortened muscles.
- Stretch tissue and joints as appropriate.
- Discuss additional massage sessions and suggested self-help measures.
- Refer to other health professionals when necessary.

client's need. Using deep-tissue techniques means that the practitioner is not randomly using a sequence but is, instead, critically thinking about a specific result. Compressive effleurage is an example of a valuable deep-tissue technique. Deep-tissue techniques do not have to be complicated; they are simply additional techniques that could be part of every practitioner's tool belt. Because each client is unique and has his own set of injuries, chronic and/or repetitive conditions, and specific structure, the same set of techniques is not likely to work on everyone. Practitioners need to practice with a wide variety of techniques and modalities in order to serve the tremendous variations they will inevitably find in their clients. The success of a practitioner's session depends on the critical use of her therapeutic skills.

Before beginning with the sequence itself, students are encouraged to read the following definitions, as well as "Sequence" later in the chapter, for more information on how to use the techniques in an orderly, intelligent fashion.

Dimensional massage therapy is a philosophical approach to therapy that is based on science, structure, and soft-tissue functions and that uses a variety of techniques for the client's benefit.

DEEP-TISSUE TECHNIQUES

Jostling rattles the fibers back and forth and is a form of vibration. Grasp the muscle loosely closest to the origin, apply a slight traction, and shake toward the insertion. For a better grasp of the tissues, do not use lubrication.

Compression efficiently speeds circulation to the area when executed correctly. This stroke can be combined with petrissage to make a dual-hand distraction technique. Press the muscle and soft tissue straight down against the bone, flattening and spreading tissues repeatedly with the palm and heel of the hand. Make sure that the surface is not slippery when applying compression.

Stripping is a deep-tissue technique that lengthens fibers and empties or pushes fluids. Place your thumb or forefinger of one or both hands at the distal end of the muscle and then slowly and deeply glide along the length of the muscle toward the origin. Use a minimal amount of lubrication. This technique should be used intelligently in the order of a sequence.

Deep transverse friction, or **cross-fiber friction,** is useful at tendinous attachments for releasing spasms and reducing adhesions; it can often be substituted with digital circular friction. Apply the technique against the fibers at a right angle with the fingers or thumb, using enough pressure to separate and flatten the fibers. Be careful, as the technique may be painful. Adjust pressure, and use the technique appropriately in the order of a sequence. (*Note to students:* This technique should be practiced only under the supervision of an instructor.)

Myofascial stretches are a series of techniques designed to stretch and warm up the tissues. The fascia is literally pulled off the structures in a rhythmic pace. As the fascia warms, it becomes more pliable, stretchy, and less "stuck" to the underlying soft tissue. Myofascial stretches are usually performed with little to no lubrication.

Elliptical movement is an alternating clockwise and counterclockwise distraction movement sometimes executed on joints such as the shoulder girdle and done most often while the therapist is engaged with muscles. The two alternating directions release any tension the client may be holding onto; this is because the client cannot focus on the direction of the movement and hold the tension at the same time. For a better grip, try to use this technique before applying lubrication.

Trigger points are irritated or hyperactive areas, often located in hypertonic tissue, that are either *active* (refer pain to a specific area) or *latent* (have a positive reaction to pain in the area of the trigger point). Sometimes trigger points form palpable nodules, but most often the therapist must rely on client feedback. *Satellite* trigger points are often located in functional units of synergistic muscles. **Ischemic compression,** or **trigger point release,** applies digital pressure, whereas a *pincer palpation* places the tissue between the thumb and the forefinger. The purpose of the digital pressure is to try to interrupt the pain pattern by robbing the tissue of oxygen for a short period of time. (*Note:* This book does not offer an exhaustive study on trigger points. Students seeking complete information about trigger points and treatment options for them should refer to books devoted to that topic. See Appendix A for suggested texts.)

Parallel thumbs is a deep-tissue technique executed by alternately applying pressure with the thumbs in a rolling-over motion. The thumbs face and are parallel to each other; they should be at a right angle to the muscle fibers.

Sequence

Sequence is a specific series of techniques chosen to accomplish a particular goal in a session. It is determined by the client's medical history, the structure, and the area of the body needing the work. Evaluation of pressure and technique may be determined by the stage of the condition: acute, subacute, or chronic. Therapists

A Few Words about Body Mechanics

How many treatments does a massage therapist complete in a day, week, month, or year? It would be easy to add them up, but the equation of repetitive action times the amount of clients sometimes equals injury instead of a successful practice. Fortunately, good **body mechanics** that utilize ergonomically safe methods and practices to execute techniques can prevent injury, support self-care, provide balanced energy, and promote a long career in the massage therapy industry.

Practicing *aikido,* a special form of martial arts, teaches balance, the location of one's center of energy, and effortless movement. Applied to massage therapy, aikido teaches the therapist how to utilize the body's momentum for strength by applying an Eastern philosophy to a Western style of bodywork so that, ultimately, the massage therapist sinks into the soft tissue rather than pressing into it. Achieving and practicing good body mechanics is actually quite easy. Lower the massage table to enable your fingertips to just brush the top of the table when you are standing by its side. Remember that adding a person to the table means you will actually be working higher. The larger the person, the lower the table has to be set. If a client requires a side-lying position, the table should be adjusted to an appropriate lower level.

Aikido teaches that when the body moves, it should be relaxed, and that strength is not in how much force one uses but is in how the body's momentum is utilized. It is a silent strength that comes from balance and movement from the center of one's energy. The "center" of energy in the abdominal area is a Japanese concept referred to as the *hara.* Shiatsu (the Japanese rendition of acupressure), aikido, and other modalities and martial arts utilize this philosophy. The energy itself is called *chi* (Chinese) or *ki* (Japanese). How a person directs her ki forms the basis of her body mechanics.

Here are some general principles of good body mechanics:

- Always keep your back as straight as possible. As soon as you find yourself bending at the waist, your body mechanics have been compromised.
- Always move with your technique, using the momentum of movement to assist in the action. Your ki will follow your momentum as long as you are in balance. For effleurage of the extremities, for example, keep your back straight and lunge with your lower extremities, using mostly the quadriceps for strength. Relax your hands, and use your body weight over your hands to sink into the soft tissues as your momentum carries you forward.
- Always maintain balance so that you do not fall over if you need to step back for a moment.
- When you are standing straight, bend your knees so that movement is easier and springier.
- Stay over your hands as much as possible. As soon as your hands are reaching out in front of your body (a position known as the "Superman complex"), you have lost the center of balance and have no body strength to support the technique.
- Relax your thumbs, hands, and arms between techniques. Bodyworkers tend to hurt themselves with the repetitive holding of tension in their hands and arms. Do not hold your fingers or thumbs in extension while you are executing techniques.
- Always place your feet in the direction you are headed so that your body can move in that direction efficiently and easily.
- Try not to press into soft-tissue structures. Lean or sink into the tissues with your body weight. Ki extends from the center of your body, allowing you to move into the tissues. You will be surprised at how much deeper the tissues will allow you to go when you do not force your way into their fibers. It is a myth that one must be Hercules to do bodywork! Too much pressure applied incorrectly will cause discomfort and invoke immediate instinctive tension in the client's tissues. If you do not have passive tissues to work with, it is very difficult to get an effective result.
- Never sacrifice yourself to a technique or to the client's structure.
- Breathe. Students often forget the importance of breathing. Breathing is rhythmic; it silently teaches grace, promotes relaxation, and makes centering easier.
- Center yourself often. Remember that the person on the table has engaged your services. Thus, you need to be "present" for that person.

If you have no experience with any martial arts, *tai chi* will add to your practice by helping you to understand energy, discipline, balance, and movement. Tai chi is meditation, grace, and dance. It is good for the soul. In *Care of the Soul,* Thomas Moore says, "Care of the soul requires craft—skill, attention, and art. To live with a high degree of artfulness means to attend to the small things that keep the soul engaged in whatever we are doing." Massage therapy is the art of touching other human beings; thus, therapists are engaged in a relationship of response. It is the therapists' ethical duty to prepare themselves well and practice self-care. Paying such attention to your craft will feed your soul.

Good body mechanics are the basis of your success with any type of bodywork. Having someone videotape you working will help you determine whether your body mechanics are still in good form. Are your shoulders elevated while you work? Are you bending over at the waist? More to the point, does your back hurt? Do your forearms or hands hurt anywhere? If the answer is yes to any of these questions, you need to revisit your body mechanics and take a critical look at how you are executing your techniques. Becoming a "wounded healer" makes it very difficult, if not impossible, to continue in your chosen profession.

If you are already injured, seek a diagnosis and appropriate care.

should never dive into the structure. Rather, they should use superficial strokes to experiment with various palpation skills and to prepare the involved joint or joints for further deep-tissue techniques. Unwinding an area involves patience, structural knowledge, and intelligent use of a sequence of techniques. Warm-up techniques include an efficient use of effleurage and myofascial stretches. Depending on the problem, therapists might begin with techniques that require no lubrication. If possible, they should place the body part and muscle in a passively shortened position.

Some of the techniques described below will be old friends from previous technique courses. Use them wisely, and combine them with newer techniques to add variety, flow, and skill to your repertoire. Remember that all parts of the body are connected entirely: When a technique is not working on a specific muscle group, the problem may not be the technique—it may be the opposing muscles that are causing restrictions and preventing complete relaxation, or it may be another area of the body. For example, many people have back and neck conditions from flat feet and gait issues.

The shoulder girdle surrounds the body and provides the mechanism for attachment that allows muscles to connect to the head and neck and gives the upper extremity free movement with the ball-and-socket joint. Sequentially it makes sense to start the client in a supine position to utilize the head to assist with passively shortening muscles efficiently.

The following sequence should give a solid basis for unwinding the shoulder girdle muscles and setting up a foundation for working on other areas of the body. Chapter 14 presents postural perspectives and additional techniques for the head and neck area.

Dimensional Massage Therapy for the Shoulder Girdle Muscles

SUPINE POSITION

Slide the client's shoulders superiorly to passively shorten the upper and middle trapezius. Test the trapezius for relaxation.

Effleurage around Shoulders

Use lubrication with this effleurage technique. Stand with one foot in front of the other at the head of the table. Place your hands just below the client's clavicle, facing your fingers of both hands toward the sternum. Follow the line of the clavicle, and stroke around the deltoids and up the back of the trapezius to the occipital ridge. Give a slight traction at the end of the stroke. Really feel the shape of the pectoralis major, and sink into the tissue there as you begin this stroke. Use your body weight. Lighten your pressure around

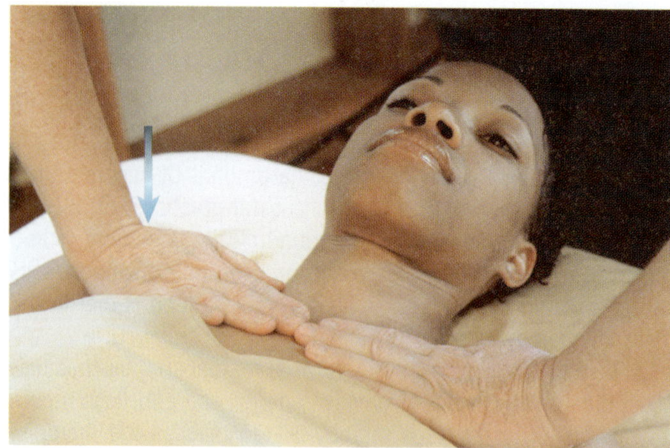

FIGURE 5.1 Effleurage around shoulders

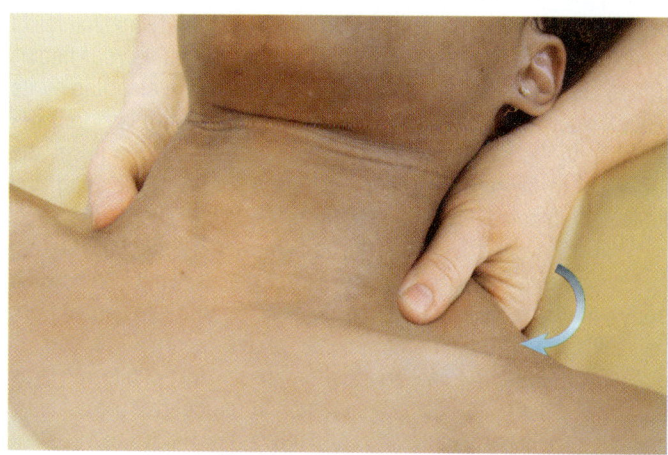

FIGURE 5.2 Petrissage of the trapezius

the shoulder joint, and use your backward momentum to help draw your hands to the back of the neck. Repeat several times. (See figure 5.1.)

Petrissage of the Trapezius

Petrissage the client's trapezius, alternately moving your whole body and keeping your forearms in alignment with your hands. While bracing the head with your other forearm, petrissage one side of the trapezius at a time. Repeat on the other side. Remember to relax your hands after the completion of each technique. (See figure 5.2.)

Closed-Palm Shaping

With the dorsal side of your hand, make a *relaxed*, loose fist, engage the client's trapezius, and stroke superiorly and inferiorly, posterior to sternocleidomastoid. Support the head on the opposite side with your forearm while you complete the stroke. Try to keep the head in a fairly neutral position, and use care, as always, to engage the tissues with an appropriate amount of pressure. Repeat on the opposite side. (See figure 5.3.)

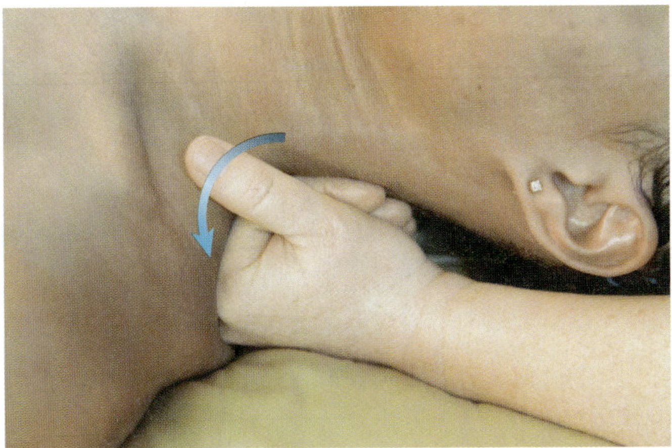

FIGURE 5.3 Closed-palm shaping of the trapezius

Alternating-Hands Neck Stretch

Start at the base of the neck (C7), and cup the cervical spine with one hand; the spine should be nestled between your thumb and index finger. As you stroke superiorly toward the C1 area, the other hand takes the place of the first hand, alternating and repeating the stretch stroke. The client's neck should arch in this technique, but the head should remain on the table. Again, the hands are in a straight line with the forearms. Do not compromise your wrists to complete the technique. (See figure 5.4.)

Cup-Stripping the Upper Trapezius

Place one hand under the client's head to give you access to the neck. Arch the neck, pointing the client's chin in the air. With your other hand, straddle the cervical spine with your index finger and thumb. Lift the head slightly, and glide down the upper trapezius to the 7th cervical. Repeat. This should be a fluid movement. (See figure 5.5.)

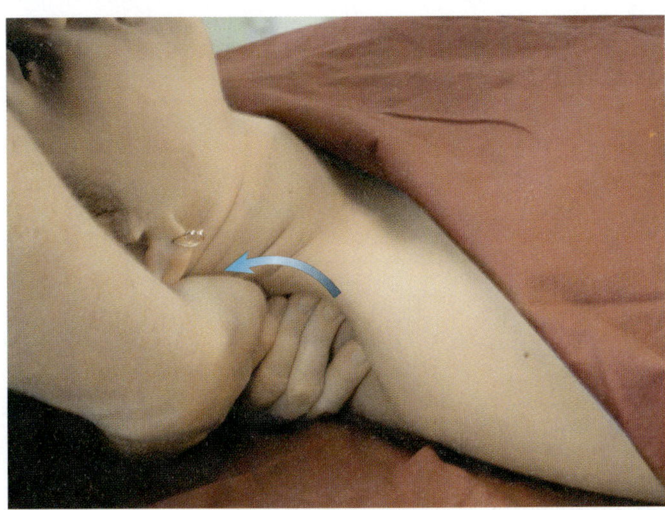

FIGURE 5.4 Alternating-hands neck stretch

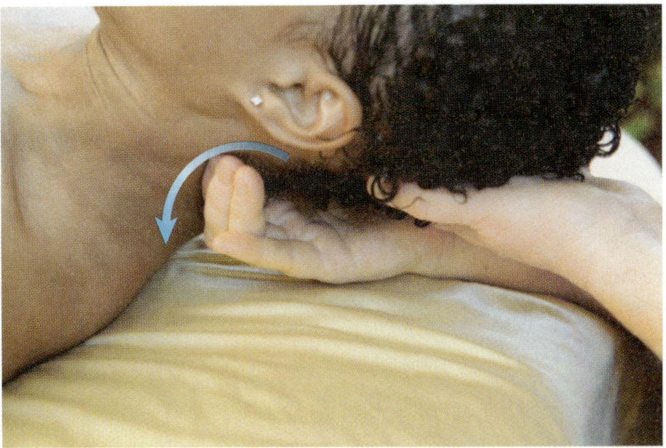

FIGURE 5.5 Cup-stripping the upper trapezius

Edging the Upper Trapezius

Stand at the head of the table behind your client, who is in a supine position. Bend the client's elbow to passively shorten the upper trapezius. For the left upper trapezius, place your right hand under the client's neck, and engage the edge of the upper trapezius at the occiput on the side you intend to stretch. Place your left thumb on the client's left upper trapezius close to the insertion at the clavicle, and draw your hands away from each other, stretching the trapezius in opposite directions. Be careful to use slight to no lubrication with this technique. Repeat with the other side, exchanging hand positions. (See figure 5.6.)

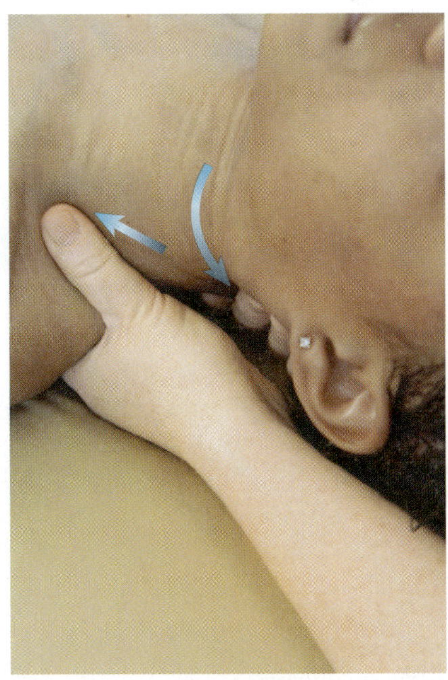

FIGURE 5.6 Edging the upper trapezius

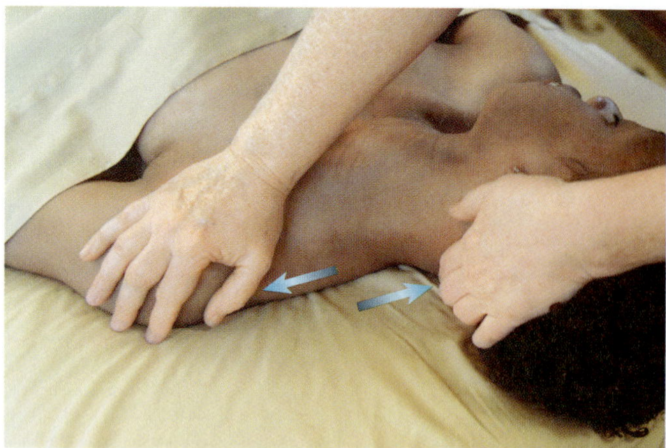

FIGURE 5.7 Neck stretch to side

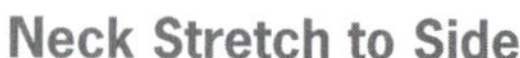

Neck Stretch to Side

Rotate the client's head to the side. Standing on the opposite side of the table (facing the client's face), place one hand on the shoulder and one hand on the back of the head. Glide the hand from the shoulder to the head. Take the other hand off the head, and place it on the shoulder. Stretch, glide, stretch. Do not bend the ear. (See figure 5.7.)

Opposite-Side Petrissage of the Trapezius—Comb the Trapezius

Standing to the side of the table, place your inferior hand under the client's head and grasp the opposite trapezius. Your fingers will comb and pull on the trapezius while your thumb completes a circular friction between the spine and the scapula. Your superior hand should brace the head while you complete the technique. (See figure 5.8.) Repeat the neck stretch and this technique on the opposite side.

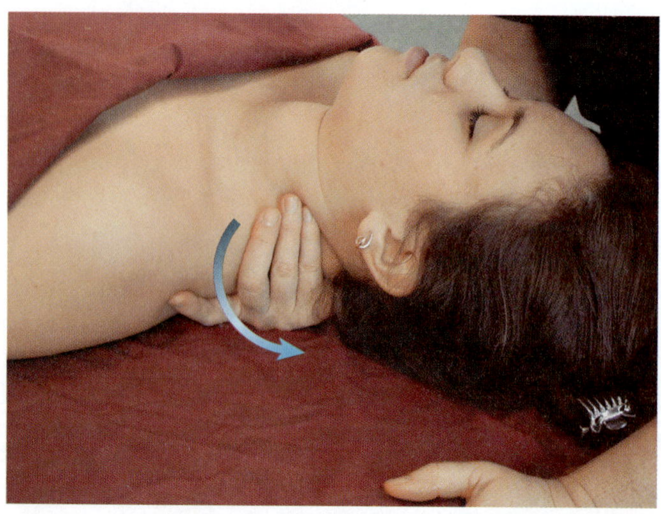

FIGURE 5.8 Opposite-side petrissage of the trapezius

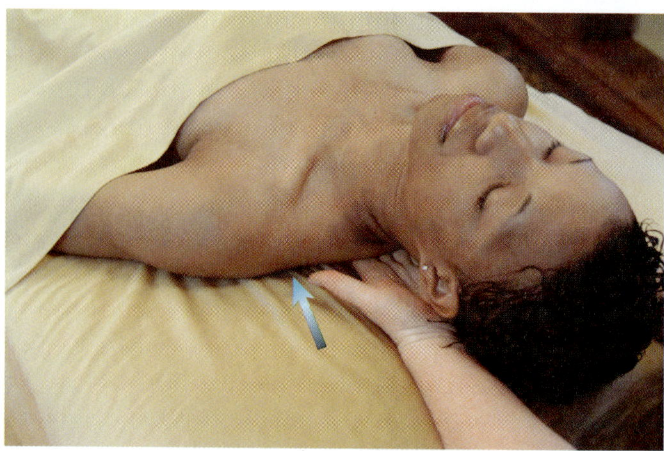

FIGURE 5.9 Hands under back

Hands under Back

This technique connects the lower trapezius with the upper trapezius and lengthens fibers of the erectors. Place your hands under the client's back, and push down on your forearms to slide down to the lower thoracic spine. Stroke superiorly in any combination of effleurage, vibration, or circular friction. End with a little traction on the occipital ridge. Keep your fingers stiff for extra pressure. Repeat several times. (See figure 5.9.)

Head Rock

With the client's head in the palms of your hands, slightly push on the head with your palms; the chin will lift. Retract the head with your fingertips by grasping the occipital ridge and bringing the chin back in. Repeat a few times slowly and with an even rhythm. (See figure 5.10.)

Head-Forward Stretch with Breath

Have the client inhale. On the exhale, lift the head forward in a slight passive flexion stretch, slowly and carefully. Ask the client to signal when she feels the

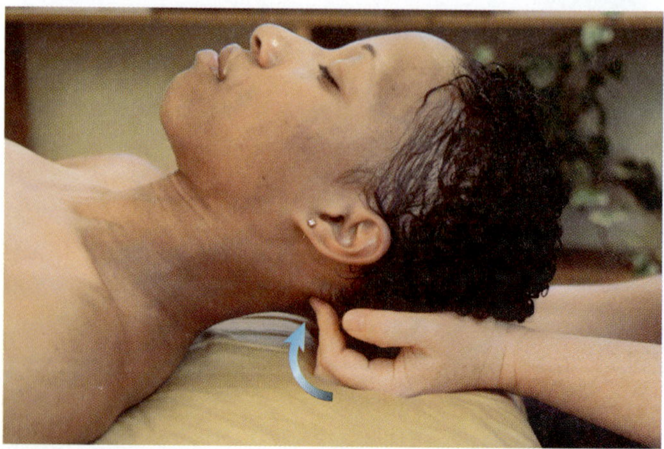

FIGURE 5.10 Head rock

stretch. Gently and slowly lower the head to the table. Finish with an effleurage around the shoulders and a slight traction to the occipital ridge.

PRONE

Myofascial Stretches and Techniques

Picking up the fascia and releasing it from underlying structures provides a unique opportunity for deep-tissue work. *Technique 1:* Push the fascia in a clockwise manner with one thumb into the opposite hand as it gathers the tissue between the thumb and the forefinger. All the fingers of the gathering hand should help with the momentum of the stroke. *Technique 2:* Pick up the tissue with the fingers of both hands in a slight half-moon, and draw it over the thumbs as the thumbs press forward toward the fingers. Both of these techniques are done repetitively over a region. (See figures 5.11 and 5.12.)

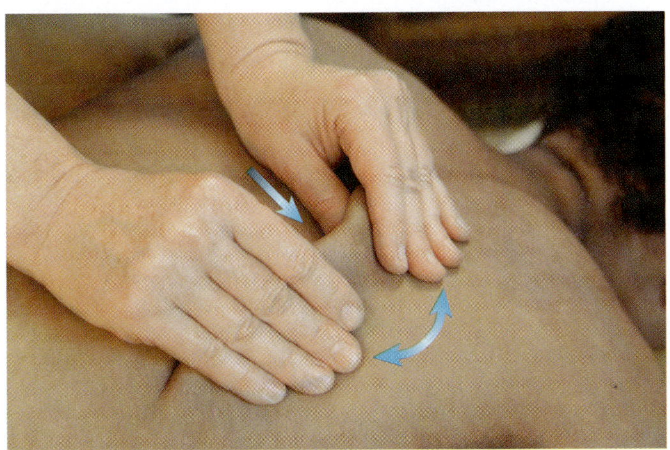

FIGURE 5.11 Myofascial warm-up half-moon

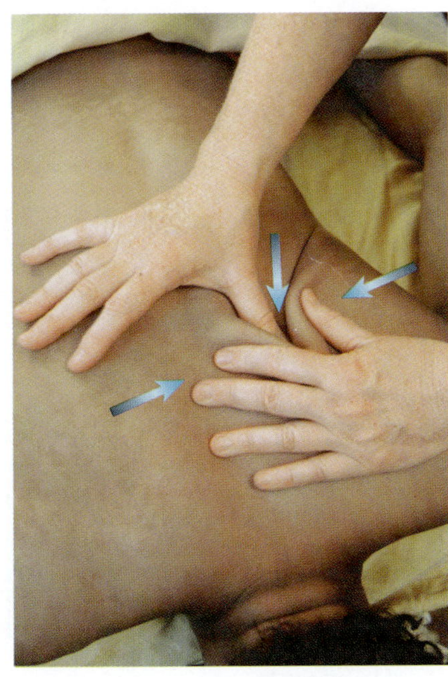

FIGURE 5.12 Myofascial warm-up technique

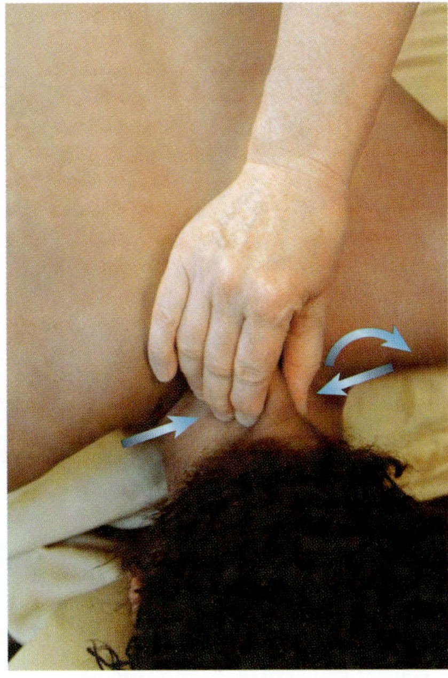

FIGURE 5.13 Myofascial pull on the upper trapezius

Myofascial Stretch on the Upper Trapezius

Stand facing the client's side. Straddle the client's neck with your thumbs parallel to each other on the closest side of the upper trapezius. Brace your thumbs on the closest side, and draw the tissue over your thumbs with the fingers from the opposite side of the upper trapezius. Repeat several times. (See figure 5.13.)

Myofascial Stretch on the Middle Trapezius

Stand facing the client's side. Grasp the opposite side of the middle trapezius, bracing your thumbs on the dorsal side. Draw the tissue over your thumbs with the fingers from the ventral side of the trapezius. Repeat several times. (See figure 5.14.)

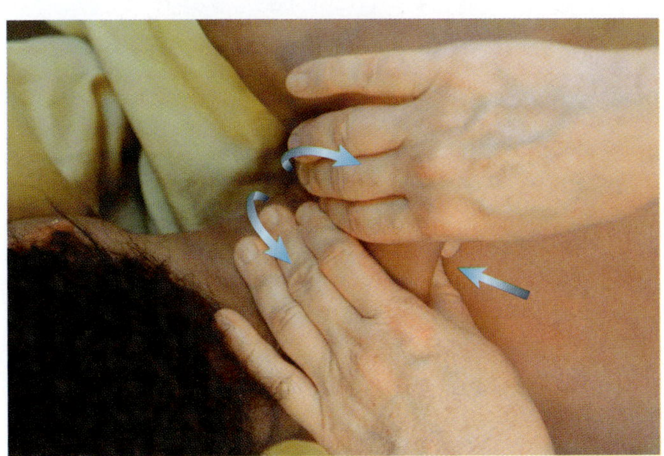

FIGURE 5.14 Myofascial pull on the middle trapezius

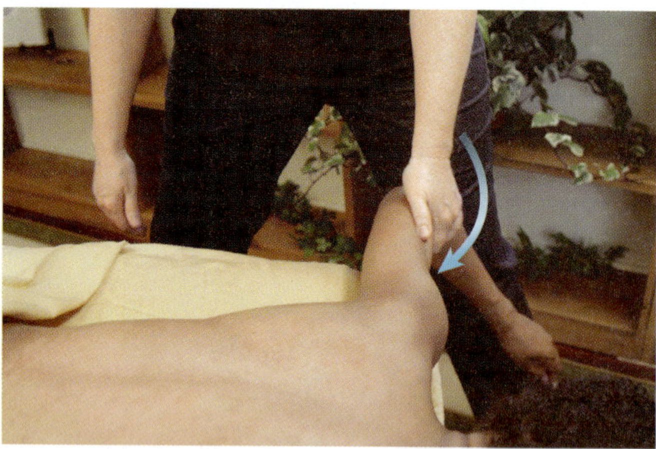

FIGURE 5.15 Movement 1

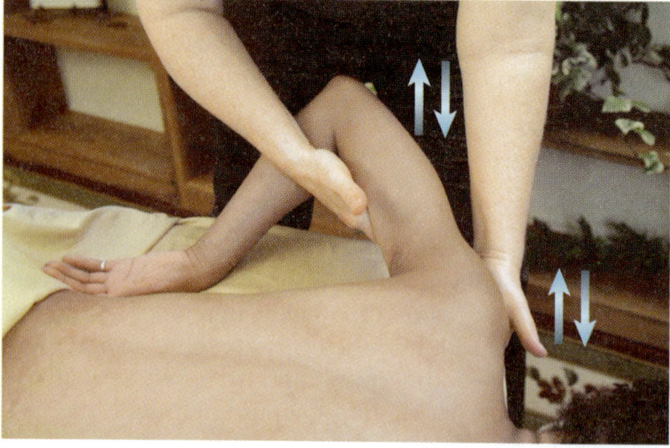

FIGURE 5.17 Movement 3

Range of Motion for the Shoulders

This is passive movement that will interact with the shoulder joint and shoulder girdle. Keep the movement easy, simple, and fluid. This is a simple technique that becomes a sequential automatic function. With the client prone, stand facing one upper extremity at the side of the table. Bend your knees slightly, and widen your leg stance. Keep your back straight. Pick up the client's arm just above the elbow with both of your hands. The forearm and hand will hang off the table.

1. Swing the arm passively in a back-and-forth motion (figure 5.15). Continue to hold and swing the arm, and with your hand that is closest to the client's feet, catch the client's ventral wrist.
2. Circulate the arm, first in one direction and then in the opposite direction, by leading with the elbow and guiding with the wrist. (See figure 5.16.)
3. Place the wrist on the table so that the elbow is bent out from the table. Place your hand that is closest to the client's feet on the inside of the arm grasping the biceps. Take your other hand and grasp the deltoid area. Alternate movement of the inside hand and deltoid hand in a one-two motion. (See figure 5.17.)
4. Draw the upper extremity down by the client's side. Place one hand underneath the shoulder and one on the dorsal side of the joint. Passively move the entire shoulder first ventrally in a circle and then dorsally in a circle. Repeat these motions until they blend quickly into each other and are done fluently and without effort. This takes a little practice. (See figure 5.18.)

Elliptical Movement of the Entire Scapula

Stand on the opposite side of the table. Place your superior hand on the middle trapezius above the

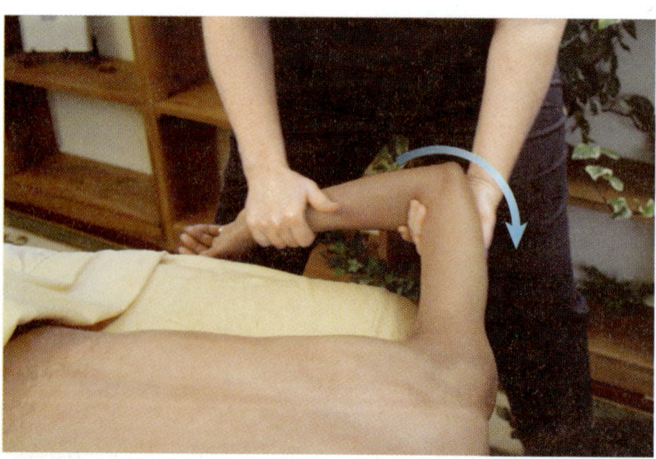

FIGURE 5.16 Movement 2

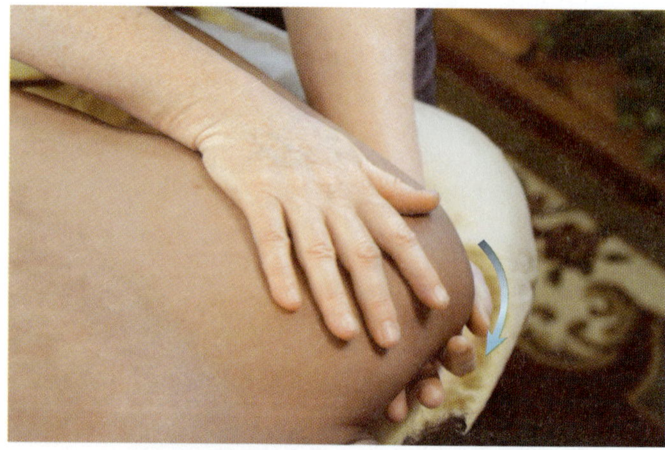

FIGURE 5.18 Movement 4

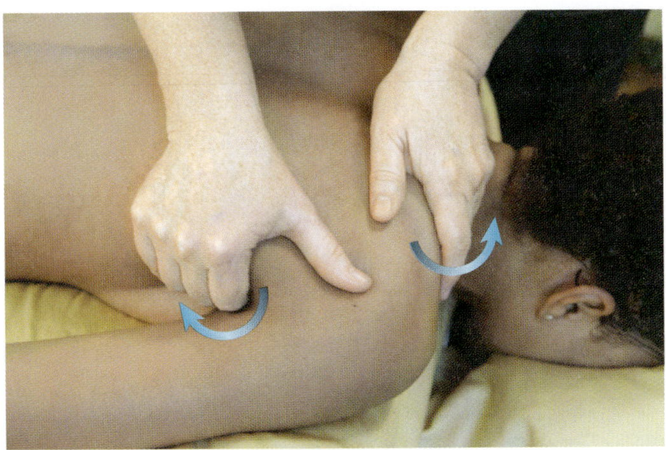

FIGURE 5.19 Elliptical movement of the entire scapula

spine of the scapula, with the thumb dorsal side up. Grasp the teres major–latissimus area with your inferior hand, with the thumb dorsal side up. Alternately rotate the shoulder by passively moving it first clockwise and then counterclockwise repetitively. Another option is to draw the vertebral side of the scapula over the thumbs in this position. *Variation—two-hand elliptical:* Anchor your hands on the back and engage the muscles in alternate directions. (See figure 5.19.)

Jostle and Stretch the Upper and Middle Trapezius

Facing the client at a right angle, grasp the upper and middle trapezius on the shoulder closest to its origin loosely with your thumb on the dorsal side and your fingers on the ventral side. Slightly traction the muscle, and shake with a drag toward its insertion. Repeat several times. (See figure 5.20.)

Compress the Rhomboids

Where you stand often depends on the size of the client. For this technique, position your hand so that your palm rests lightly on the rhomboid closest to you and your fingers rest lightly over the spine. Flatten the rhomboids with a pumping action of your wrist repeatedly, with the palm and heel of your hand. Be careful not to use the edge or bony part of your palm as doing so could potentially hurt the client. (See figure 5.21.)

Effleurage and Circular Friction

Apply regular Swedish techniques. Continue to deepen your effleurage to a compressive stroke. *Friction:* Using the entire ventral surface of your hands, broadly sweep in a circular motion; move one hand clockwise and move the other hand counterclockwise over the expanse of the back.

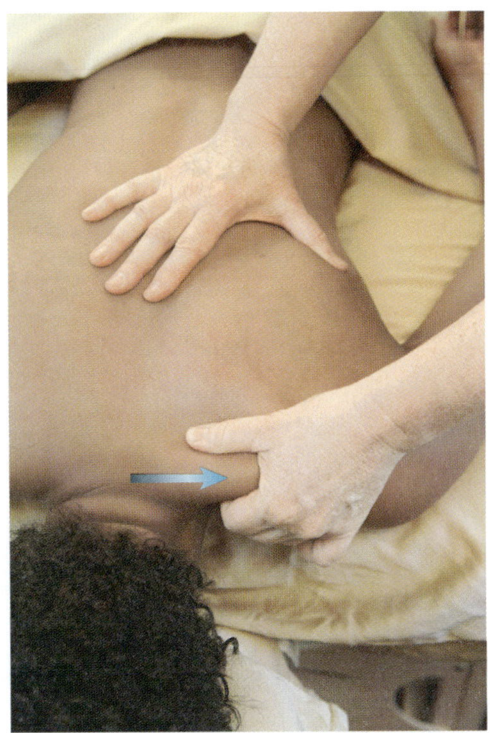

FIGURE 5.20 Jostling the middle trapezius

Alternating Petrissage of the Upper and Middle Trapezius and Compression of the Rhomboids

This is a dual-hand maneuver. Depending on the size of your client, stand on the same side or opposite side of the table. Place the hand closest to the head on the trapezius and the other hand over the rhomboids. Alternately petrissage the trapezius and compress the rhomboids. (See figure 5.22.)

Claw-Strip the Rhomboids

Place your curled fingers at the origin of the muscles at the spinous processes on one side of the client's

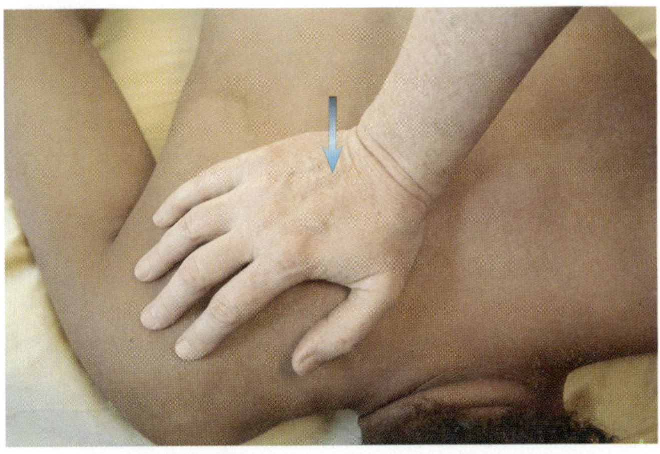

FIGURE 5.21 Compression of the rhomboids

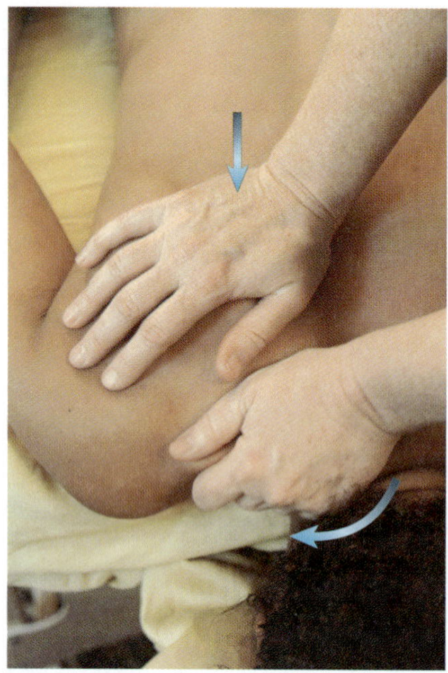

FIGURE 5.22 Alternating petrissage of the upper and middle trapezius and compression of the rhomboids

body. Apply pressure with your other hand by placing it on top of the hand that is already in position on the rhomboid. Draw both hands toward the insertion of the muscles on the vertebral side of the scapula. You are essentially stripping the fibers, so keep a steady, even pressure as you draw your fingers toward the insertion of the muscles. (See figure 5.23.)

Deep Transverse Friction of the Interspinales between the Spinous Processes

Place your thumbs between the spinous processes of thoracic 12 (T12) and thoracic 11 (T11). Make a half-circular motion with your alternating thumbs as you travel in a superior direction up the spine. Keep the stroke fluid and continuous. (See figure 5.24.)

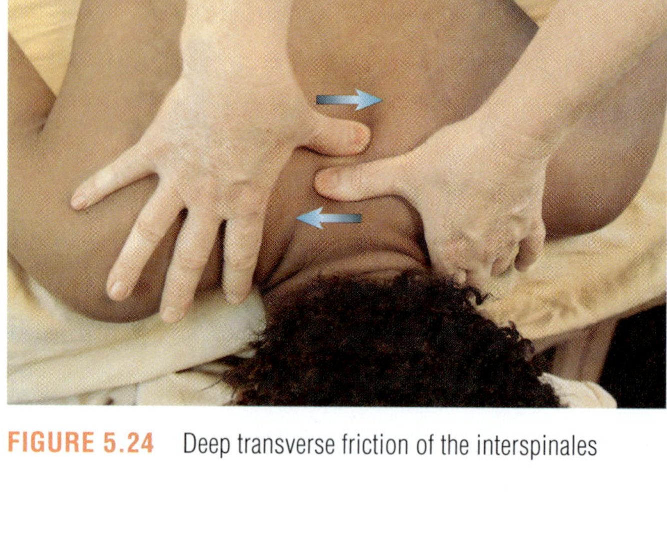

FIGURE 5.24 Deep transverse friction of the interspinales

Straddle the Spine and Claw Down the Spine with Support over the Fingers

Start at about C7 if possible, and straddle the spine with the fingers of one hand. Place your other hand at a right angle over the hand in position on the spine. Slowly drag your fingers down the spine to the lumbar region. Effleurage superiorly up the back and repeat. (See figure 5.25.)

Strip the Levator

Stand to the side of the table, and place your closest hand on the top of the shoulder, depressing it slightly. Place your thumb of your opposite hand on the insertion of the levator. Strip toward the origins of the muscle with a little bit of lubrication. Repeat four times going toward each origin (C1–C4 transverse

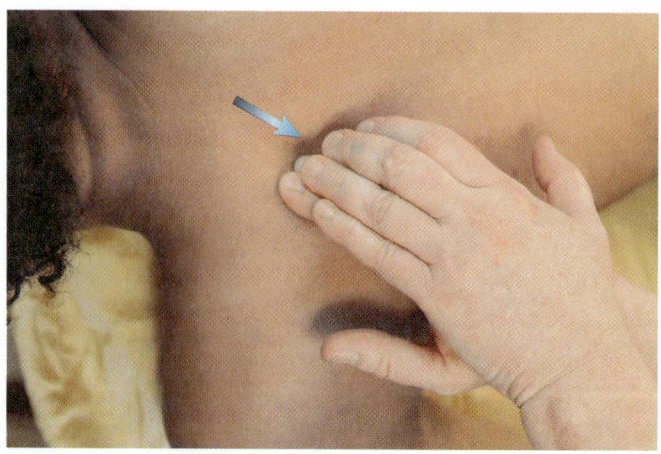

FIGURE 5.23 Claw-strip of the rhomboids

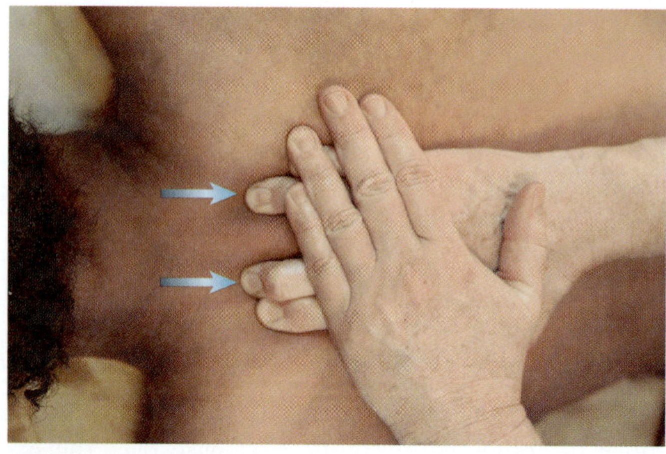

FIGURE 5.25 Straddling the spine and clawing down

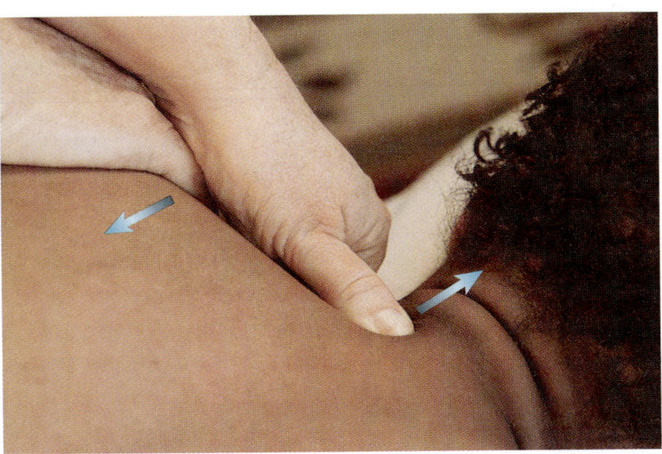

FIGURE 5.26 Stripping the levator scapulae

processes). Be careful not to press hard on C1, as it moves easily. (See figure 5.26.)

Anchor and Stretch the Upper and Middle Trapezius

Stand to the client's side, facing the head. Place your inside hand with your thumb on the upper trapezius at the base of the skull. Grasp the middle trapezius with your other hand, and stretch the two hands away from each other, stretching the trapezius. (See figure 5.27.)

Deep Transverse Friction of the Rhomboid Insertion

Open the shoulder region as you normally would to apply pressure on the muscles in the medial vertebral region of this bone. As you brace the ventral side of the shoulder with one hand, apply steady pressure with the thumb of your other hand to the vertebral border of the scapula. Start inferiorly and move superiorly. (See figure 5.28.)

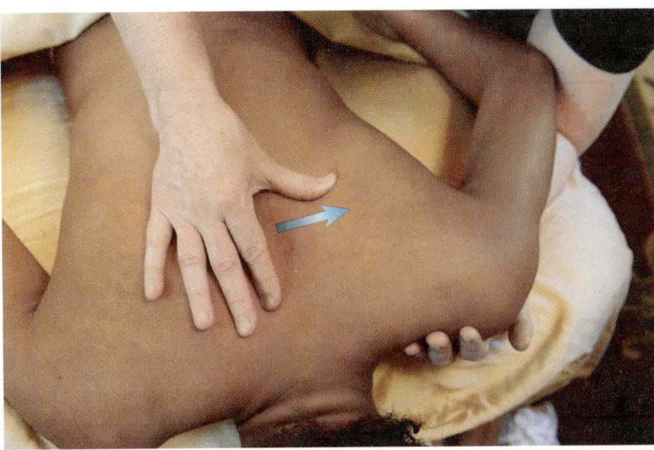

FIGURE 5.28 Deep transverse friction of the rhomboid insertion

Parallel Thumbs on the Lower Trapezius

Locate the lower trapezius closest to the lowest thoracic attachment. Place your thumbs facing and parallel to each other and proceed to apply pressure alternately, first with one thumb and then the other, as one thumb replaces the other in the thumb-over-thumb movement. Move toward the vertebral border and the root of the spine of the scapula. (See figure 5.29.)

Locate Trigger Points

Passively shorten the muscle, if possible. Determine whether the trigger points are active or latent. Determine pressure tolerance. Apply tolerable pressure until either there is a release or you have spent enough time on the area. Remember to use the client's breathing

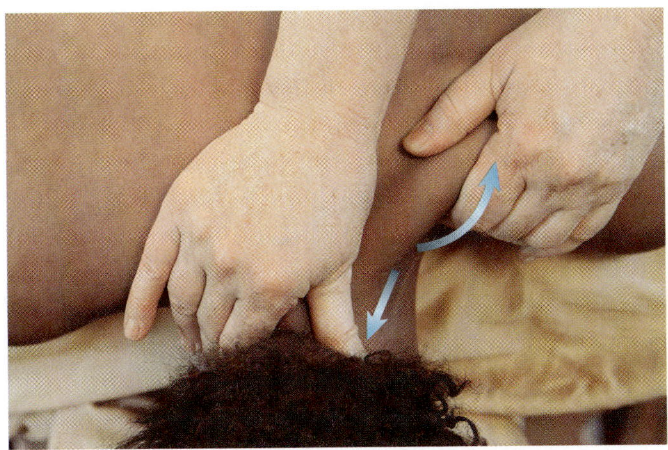

FIGURE 5.27 Anchoring and stretching the upper and middle trapezius

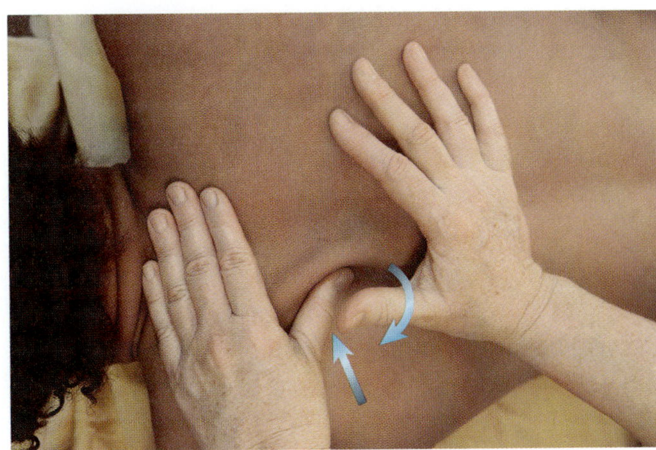

FIGURE 5.29 Parallel thumbs on the lower trapezius

with the application of pressure. Stretch the tissue after applying pressure.

Serratus Anterior Trigger Point

Locate the trigger point in the axilla region between the ribs; apply tolerable pressure to this point as the client exhales. Stretch the tissue. See Chapter 7 for technique directions for the serratus anterior in the side-lying position.

Claw-Strip the Serratus Anterior and Intercostals between the Ribs

Stand on the opposite side of the table, and separate your fingers (with one hand on top of the other) between the ribs. Draw them toward your body from ventral to dorsal. Repeat several times.

Vibration and Friction

These techniques should be interwoven within the above routine. For example, one can vibrate down the spine instead of gliding. Intersperse vibration after deep work to add variety to applied techniques. Make a habit of locating attachments, and apply deep transverse friction or digital circular friction to them.

Techniques for the pectoral region and serratus anterior are included in Chapter 7. Chapter 14 has additional techniques for the soft tissue of the head and neck.

CHAPTER *summary*

Introduction

- ✔ Dimensional massage therapy is a philosophical approach to therapy that is based on science, structure, and soft-tissue functions and that uses a variety of techniques for the client's benefit. Two underlying principles of motion are important to remember with dimensional massage therapy: (1) *aggregate muscle action:* Muscles work in groups and in paired opposition; and (2) *the law of reaction:* For every action there is an opposite and equal reaction.
- ✔ Muscles *perform* roles in the functional unit. Agonists, antagonists, synergists, stabilizers, and neutralizers make up a functional unit.

Treatment Protocol

- ✔ A treatment protocol is a synopsis of an overall approach to a massage session.
- ✔ It must be based on a medical history, interview and SOAP notes, structure of the client, observation skills, palpation, and a dimensional approach to treatment.

Technique Goals and the Mystery of Deep-Tissue Therapy

- ✔ Each technique that is chosen for use in a sequence has a purpose. Practitioners should be familiar with the use and purpose of each technique to obtain a particular goal or outcome.
- ✔ Deep-tissue therapy is a series of techniques executed on soft tissue for a specific outcome.
- ✔ Deep-tissue techniques include, but are not limited to, jostling, compression, stripping, deep transverse friction, circular friction, myofascial stretches, elliptical movement, ischemic pressure and pincer palpations for trigger point therapy, parallel thumbs, and dual-hand distraction combinations.
- ✔ The therapist must practice safe body mechanics when performing a sequence of techniques.
- ✔ To avoid injury, the therapist must use the correct positioning to apply the techniques, adjust the table to the correct height, stay in balance during the session, and use body weight and momentum to execute the techniques.
- ✔ Practitioners must always practice safe body mechanics, or they risk sustaining an injury. Wounded healers are clients, not practitioners.

Sequence

- ✔ Always use treatment protocols to determine the sequence of a therapeutic session.
- ✔ Use warm-up techniques first, and determine pressure intelligently.
- ✔ Follow a dimensional approach, and critically think about the involved joints and kinetic chain.

Dimensional Massage Therapy for the Shoulder Girdle Muscles

- ✔ Try the supine position first to efficiently prepare the neck and shoulder muscles for further work.
- ✔ Prone techniques assist with further unwinding of the shoulder girdle muscles.

CHAPTER *review*

True or False

Write true *or* false *after each statement.*

1. Synergists assist only antagonists.
2. Myofascial techniques can help to warm up and loosen soft tissue.
3. Jostling is a form of ischemic pressure.
4. Compression should be accomplished with a soft hand flattening out the tissue in a pumping action of the wrist.
5. Medical history, interview, and SOAP notes are all part of the treatment protocol.
6. Deep-tissue therapy is only trigger point therapy.
7. It is a good idea to use a lot of pressure on the rhomboids because the soft tissue is so thick.
8. It is necessary to passively shorten muscles for more immediate results with techniques.
9. For good body mechanics, practitioners should set the table higher than their waist.
10. Deep transverse friction strokes are in the direction of the fibers.

Short Answers

Write your answers on the lines provided.

1. List two principles that assist in critical thinking for practicing a dimensional approach to massage therapy.

____

____

____

2. Give examples of agonists, antagonists, synergists, and stabilizers of the shoulder girdle.

____

____

____

3. List some components on which treatment protocols of a session should be based.

____

____

____

4. Define *jostling, compression, stripping, deep transverse friction, myofascial stretches, elliptical movement, trigger points, ischemic pressure, pincer palpation,* and *parallel thumbs.*

____

____

____

____

____

____

____

____

____

____

5. How does a practitioner determine an appropriate sequence for a massage session?

____

____

____

Multiple Choice

Circle the correct answers.

1. It makes sense to unwind the ____ trapezius first.
   a. upper
   b. lower
   c. middle
   d. none of the above
2. Muscles work in groups and in ____ opposition.
   a. singular
   b. paired
   c. no
   d. none of the above
3. Sequence is:
   a. a specific series of techniques chosen to accomplish a particular goal in a session
   b. a haphazard approach to massage

c. not necessary
d. determined by guesswork

4. A medical history is:
   a. never necessary
   b. a part of treatment protocol
   c. a ridiculous idea
   d. only necessary if the client is seeing a physician
5. Stripping:
   a. is a technique that shortens fibers
   b. is never necessary
   c. is a deep-tissue technique that lengthens fibers
   d. can always be used first
6. Claw-stripping can be easily used on the:
   a. levator scapulae
   b. rhomboids
   c. biceps
   d. pectineus
7. Body mechanics:
   a. that utilize ergonomically safe methods to execute techniques can prevent injury, support self-care, provide balanced energy, and promote a long career in the massage therapy industry
   b. decribe how to fix a car
   c. are never useful
   d. do not help therapists stay in the field
8. The coracoid process is palpable on the ____ side of the body.
   a. posterior
   b. lateral
   c. medial
   d. anterior
9. The upper and lower trapezius act as agonist and:
   a. antagonist
   b. stabilizer
   c. synergist
   d. none of the above
10. People often carry their tension in the ____ trapezius.
    a. lower
    b. middle
    c. upper and middle
    d. upper

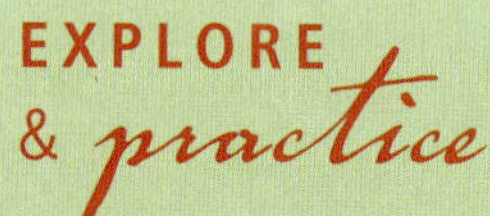

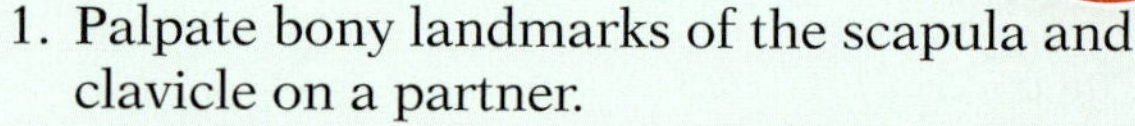

1. Palpate bony landmarks of the scapula and clavicle on a partner.
2. Palpate the origin and insertions of the shoulder girdle muscles on a partner.
3. Demonstrate how to passively shorten the upper and middle trapezius.
4. Demonstrate some principles of safe body mechanics while you perform massage techniques.
5. Demonstrate warm-up techniques without lubrication.
6. Practice deep-tissue techniques individually and in a sequence on a willing participant.

chapter 6

The Shoulder Joint

LEARNING OUTCOMES

After completing this chapter, you should be able to:

6-1 Define key terms.

6-2 Identify on a human skeleton or human subject selected bony structures of the shoulder joint.

6-3 Label on a skeletal chart selected bony landmarks of the shoulder joint.

6-4 Draw on a skeletal chart the muscles of the shoulder joint and indicate, using arrows, shoulder joint movements.

6-5 Demonstrate with a partner all the movements of the shoulder joints.

6-6 Describe how movements of the scapula accompany movements of the humerus in achieving movement of the entire shoulder complex.

6-7 Explore the origins and insertions of the muscles of the shoulder joint on a partner.

6-8 Organize and list the muscles that produce the movements of the shoulder girdle and the shoulder joint.

6-9 Practice flexibility and strengthening exercises for each muscle group.

KEY TERMS

Adhesive capsulitis
Aponeurosis
Coracobrachialis
Deltoid
Frozen shoulder
Glenohumeral
Glenoid labrum
Humerus
Infraspinatus
Latissimus dorsi
Pectoralis major
Rotator cuff group
Subscapularis
Supraspinatus
Tendonitis
Tendonosis
Teres major
Teres minor

Introduction

The shoulder joint enables the upper extremity to perform all manner of repetitive actions using the hands. The shoulder joint has a wide range of motion in so many different planes, but it also has a significant amount of laxity, which can often result in pathologic conditions and injuries. Common injury sites are the rotator cuff, capsule, ligaments, bursa, and glenohumeral joint. The price of mobility is reduced stability. While it's generally true that the more mobile a joint is, the less stable it is, this is particularly the case with the shoulder joint.

The only attachment of the shoulder joint to the axial skeleton is via the scapula at the glenoid fossa and its attachment through the clavicle at the sternoclavicular joint. Shoulder joint movements are many and varied. It is unusual, if not impossible, to have complete movement of the humerus without scapula movement. When the humerus is flexed above shoulder level, the scapula

TABLE 6.1 Pairing of Shoulder Girdle and Shoulder Joint Movements

Shoulder joint actions	Shoulder joint agonists	Shoulder girdle actions	Shoulder girdle agonists
Abduction	Supraspinatus, deltoid, upper pectoralis major	Upward rotation/elevation	Serratus anterior, middle and lower trapezius, levator scapulae, rhomboids
Adduction	Latissimus dorsi, teres major, lower pectoralis major	Downward rotation	Pectoralis minor, rhomboids
Flexion	Anterior deltoid, upper pectoralis major	Elevation/upward rotation	Levator scapulae, serratus anterior, upper and middle trapezius, rhomboids
Extension	Latissimus dorsi, teres major, lower pectoralis major, posterior deltoid	Depression/downward rotation	Pectoralis minor, lower trapezius
Internal rotation	Latissimus dorsi, teres major, pectoralis major, subscapularis	Abduction (protraction)	Serratus anterior, pectoralis minor
External rotation	Infraspinatus, teres minor	Adduction (retraction)	Middle and lower trapezius, rhomboids
Horizontal abduction	Middle and posterior deltoid, infraspinatus, teres minor	Adduction (retraction)	Middle and lower trapezius, rhomboids
Horizontal adduction	Pectoralis major, anterior deltoid, coracobrachialis	Abduction (protraction)	Serratus anterior, pectoralis minor
Diagonal abduction (overhand activities)	Posterior deltoid, infraspinatus, teres minor	Adduction (retraction)/ upward rotation/elevation	Trapezius, rhomboids, serratus anterior, levator scapulae
Diagonal adduction (overhand activities)	Pectoralis major, anterior deltoid, coracobrachialis	Abduction (protraction)/ depression/downward rotation	Serratus anterior, pectoralis minor

is elevated, rotated upward, and abducted. With glenohumeral abduction above shoulder level, the scapula is rotated upward and elevated. Adduction of the humerus results in rotation downward and depression, whereas extension of the humerus results in depression, rotation downward, and adduction of the scapula. The scapula abducts with humeral internal rotation and horizontal adduction. Scapula adduction accompanies external rotation and horizontal abduction of the humerus. For a summary of these movements and the muscles primarily responsible for them, see table 6.1. When the muscles of the shoulder joint (second column) perform the actions (in the first column) through any substantial range of motion, the muscles of the shoulder girdle (fourth column) work in concert by performing the actions (in the third column).

Bones

The scapula, clavicle, and **humerus** serve as attachments for most of the shoulder joint muscles. Locating the specific bony landmarks is critical to learning the functions of the shoulder girdle–joint complex. Important scapular landmarks are the supraspinous fossa, infraspinous fossa, subscapular fossa, spine of the scapula, glenoid cavity, coracoid process, acromion process, and inferior angle. Humeral landmarks are the head, greater tubercle, lesser tubercle, bicipital groove, and deltoid tuberosity. (Review figures 4.1 and 4.2 on pages 77 and 78, and see figures 6.1, 6.2, and 6.3.)

Joint

The shoulder joint, specifically known as the **glenohumeral** joint, is a multiaxial ball-and-socket joint classified as enarthrodial (figure 6.1). As such, it moves in all planes and is the most movable joint in the body. Its stability is enhanced slightly by the **glenoid labrum,** a cartilaginous ring that surrounds the

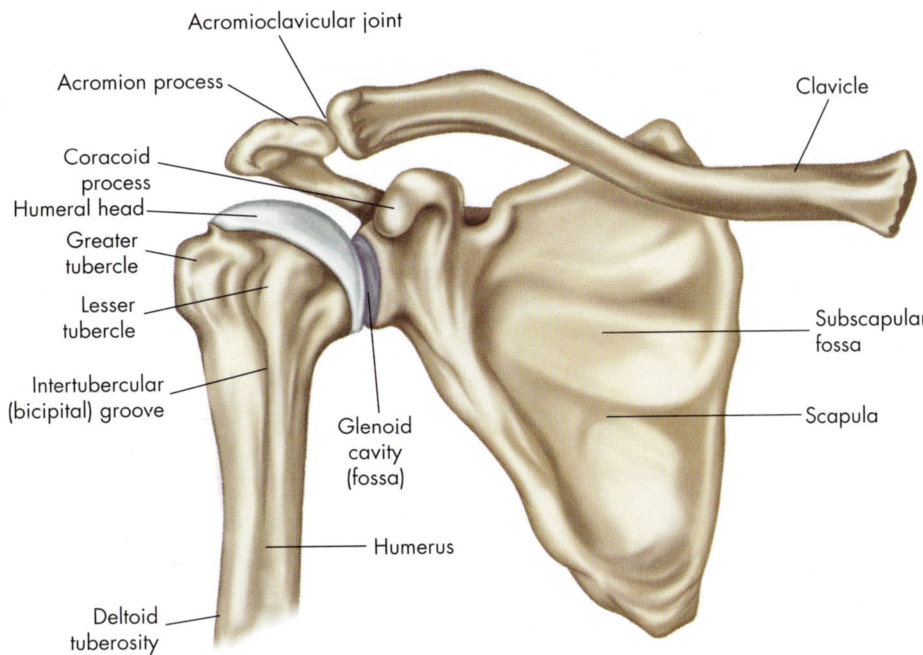

FIGURE 6.1 Glenohumeral joint

glenoid fossa just inside its periphery. The joint is further structurally supported by the glenohumeral ligaments, especially anteriorly and inferiorly. The anterior glenohumeral ligaments become taut as external rotation, extension, abduction, and horizontal abduction occur, whereas the very thin posterior capsular ligaments become taut in internal rotation, flexion, and horizontal adduction. In recent years, the importance of the inferior glenohumeral ligament in providing both anterior and posterior support has come to light (figures 6.2 and 6.3). However, due to the wide range of motion involved in the glenohumeral joint, the ligaments are quite lax until the extreme ranges of motion are reached; stability is sacrificed to gain mobility.

Movement of the humerus from the side position is common in throwing, tackling, and striking activities. Shoulder joint flexion and extension are performed frequently when supporting body weight in a hanging position or in movement from a prone position on the ground.

Determining the exact range of each movement for the glenohumeral joint is difficult because of the accompanying shoulder girdle movement; however, if the shoulder girdle is prevented from moving, the glenohumeral joint movements are generally thought to be in the following ranges: 90 to 95 degrees abduction, 0 degrees adduction (prevented by the trunk) or 75 degrees anterior to the trunk, 40 to 60 degrees of

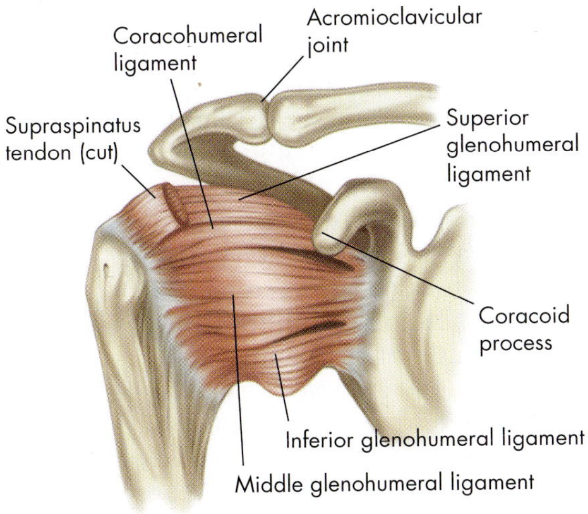

Coracohumeral ligament
Acromioclavicular joint
Supraspinatus tendon (cut)
Superior glenohumeral ligament
Coracoid process
Inferior glenohumeral ligament
Middle glenohumeral ligament

FIGURE 6.2 Glenohumeral ligaments

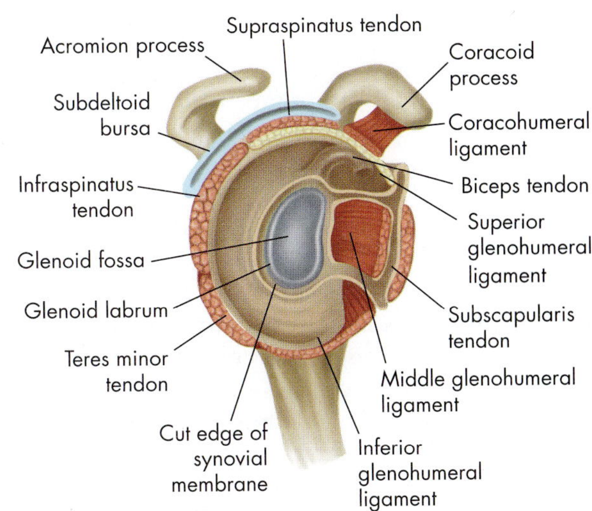

FIGURE 6.3 Glenohumeral joint with humerus removed

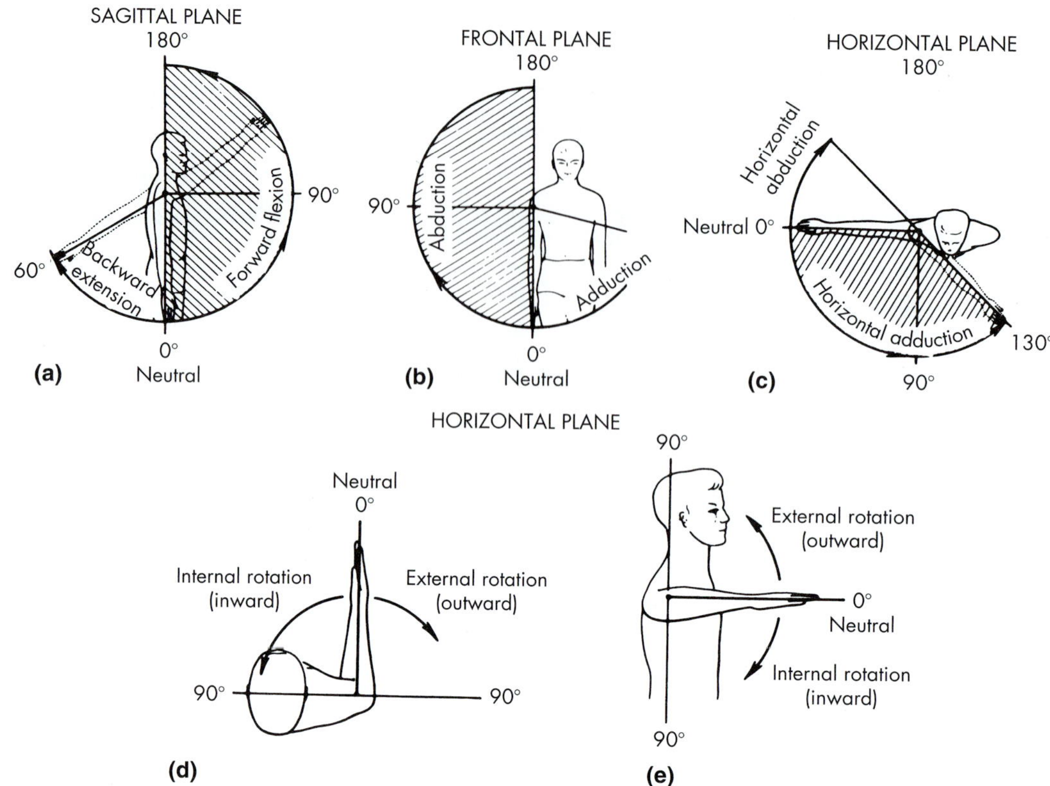

FIGURE 6.4 Range of motion of the shoulder

extension, 90 to 100 degrees of flexion, 70 to 90 degrees of internal and external rotation, 45 degrees of horizontal abduction, and 135 degrees of horizontal adduction. If the shoulder girdle is free to move, the total range of the combined joints is 170 to 180 degrees of abduction and 170 to 180 degrees of flexion (see figure 6.4).

The shoulder joint is frequently injured because of its anatomical design. A number of factors contribute to its injury rate, including the shallowness of the glenoid fossa, the laxity of the ligamentous structures necessary to accommodate its wide range of motion, and the lack of strength and endurance in the muscles, which are essential in providing dynamic stability to the joint. Additionally, the shape of the acromion varies from person to person, and it can be categorized as one of three distinct types. A type 1 acromion is considered a "normal" or flat bone. Type 2 is more curved and dips downward. Type 3 is hooked and dips downward and, as a result, is more likely to abrade the supraspinatus tendon. Types 2 and 3 have been shown to increase the incidence in rotator cuff tears. Anterior or anteroinferior glenohumeral subluxations and dislocations are quite common with physical collision activities such as football. Although posterior dislocations are fairly rare, problems about the shoulder due to posterior instability are somewhat commonplace.

The rotator cuff also experiences frequent injuries, and its small muscles are often weak and may lack an appropriate amount of endurance. The supraspinatus, infraspinatus, teres minor, and subscapularis muscles make up the rotator cuff. The tendons of these muscles cross the top, rear, and front of the head of the humerus to attach on the greater and lesser tubercles, respectively. All of these muscles and tendons must fit under the acromion, and when they become inflamed, impingement results. Their point of insertion enables them to rotate the humerus, an essential movement in this freely movable joint. Most important, however, is the vital role as stabilizers that the rotator cuff muscles play in maintaining the humeral head; without them, there would be no stability in the glenohumeral joint. Biomechanical principles also figure in the injury equation. If the body is too far away from the source of its activity, the result can be injury. For example, a person attempting to hang a heavy wooden door will extend his arms to prevent the door from falling, should it suddenly slip. The result can be a torn or ruptured biceps muscle or rotator muscle. The shoulder joint is simply too small and too mobile to complete repetitive actions such as handling a power tool at chest level, using hedge clippers, or carrying water buckets without fatiguing shoulder joint muscles or putting the rotator cuff at risk. To enable the body to perform these movements without injury, the shoulder must be strengthened and maintain optimal flexibility.

Movements

Flexion (Forward Elevation)

Flexion is movement of the humerus straight anteriorly from any point in the sagittal plane.

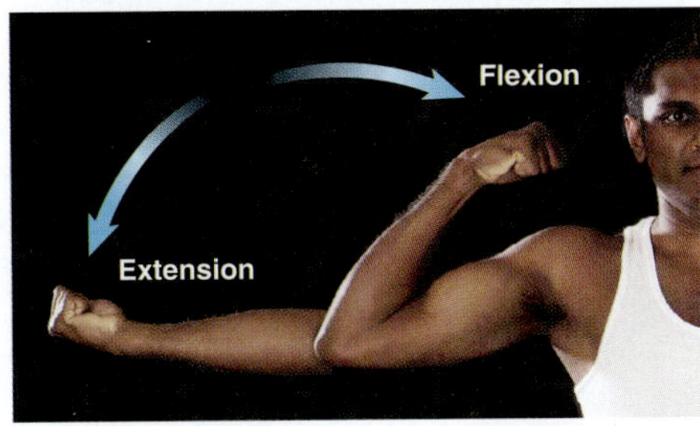

Extension (Hyperextension)

Extension involves movement of the humerus straight posteriorly from any point in the sagittal plane; it is sometimes referred to as *hyperextension*.

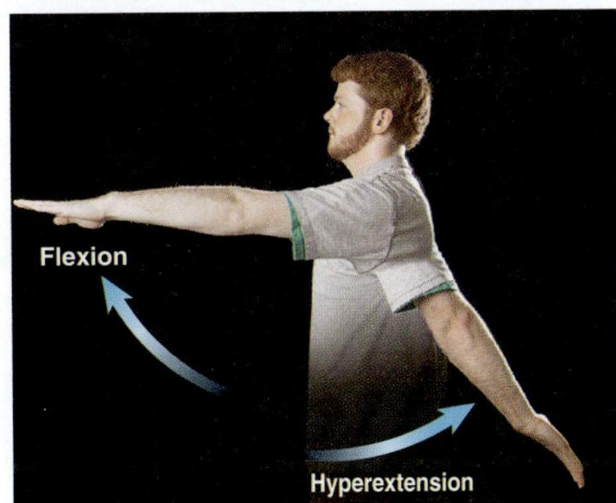

Abduction

Abduction is upward lateral movement of the humerus in the frontal plane out to the side, away from the body.

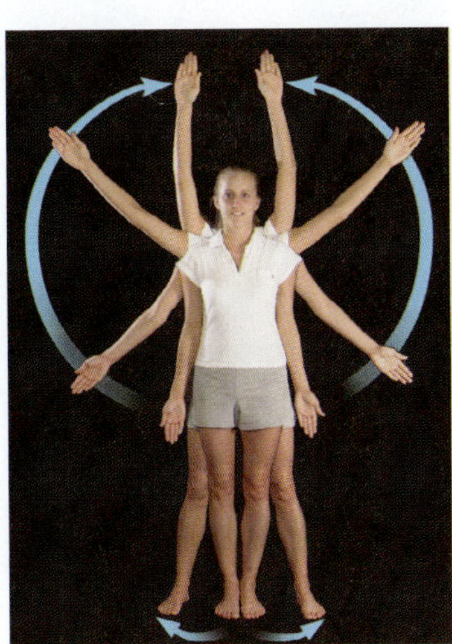

Adduction

Adduction is downward movement of the humerus in the frontal plane medially toward the body from abduction.

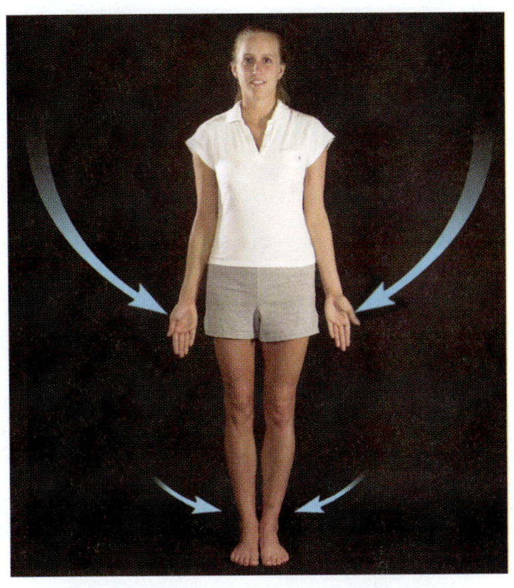

Lateral Rotation

Lateral rotation is movement of the humerus laterally in the transverse plane around its long axis away from the midline.

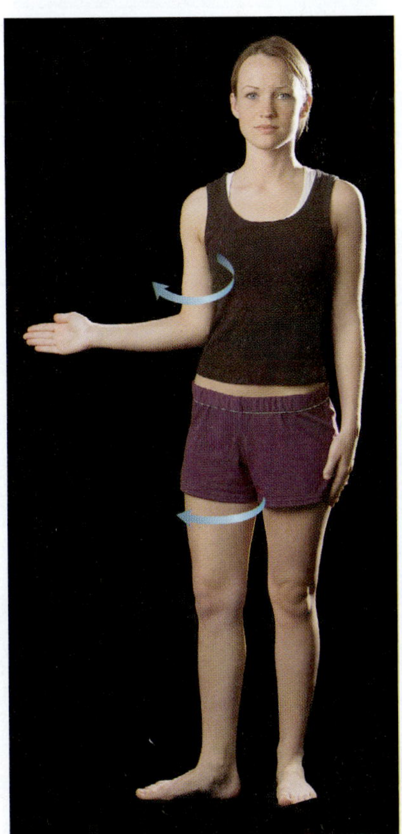

Medial Rotation

Medial rotation is movement of the humerus in the transverse plane medially around its long axis toward the midline.

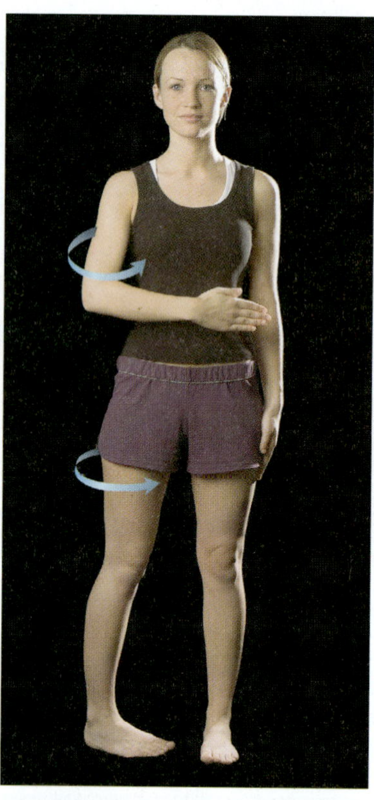

Horizontal Adduction (Flexion)

Horizontal adduction is movement of the humerus in a horizontal or transverse plane toward and across the chest.

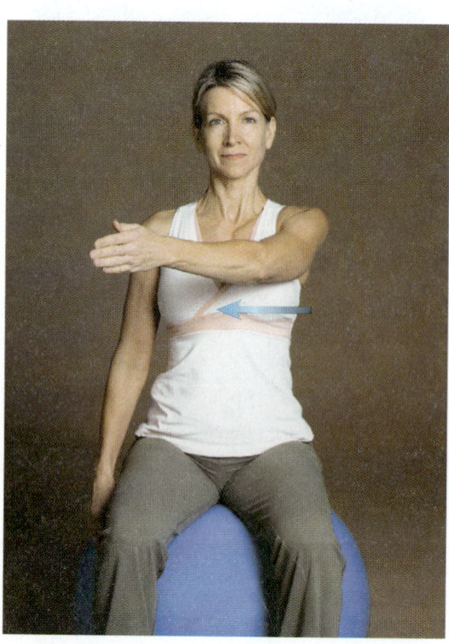

Horizontal Abduction (Extension)

Horizontal abduction is movement of the humerus in a horizontal or transverse plane away from the chest.

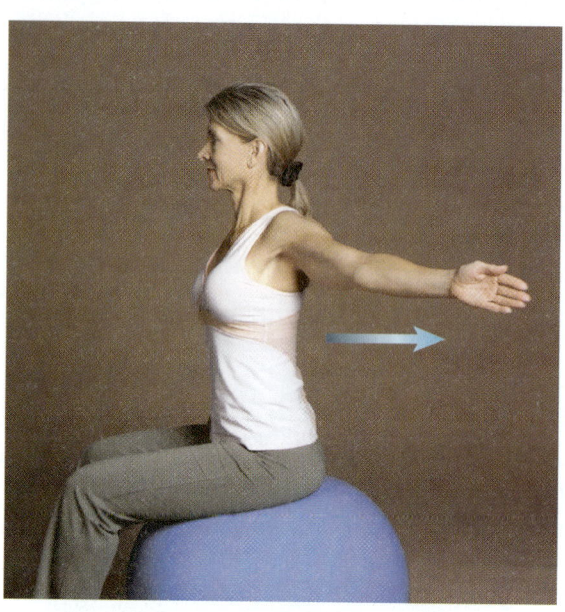

Diagonal Abduction

Diagonal abduction is movement of the humerus in a diagonal plane away from the midline of the body. If the humerus continues toward the midline in abduction, the movement is called *sideward elevation*.

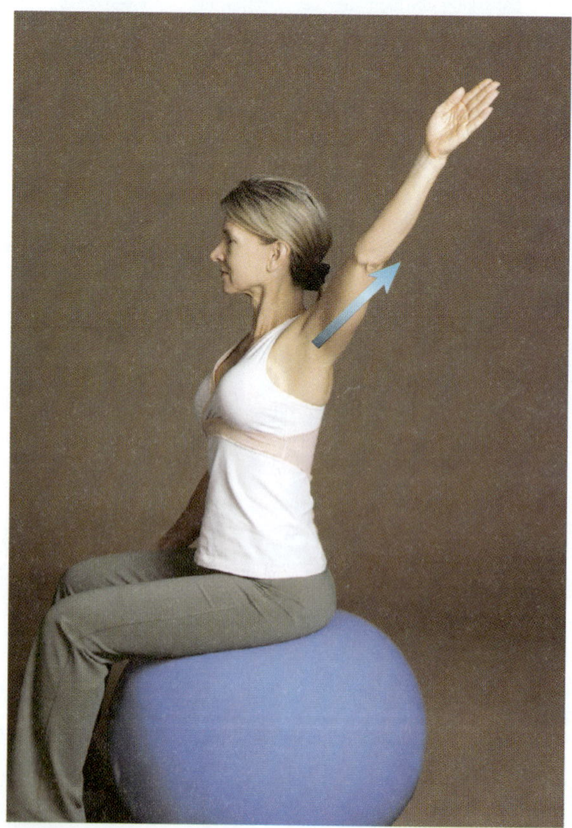

Diagonal Adduction

Diagonal adduction is movement of the humerus in a diagonal plane toward the midline of the body.

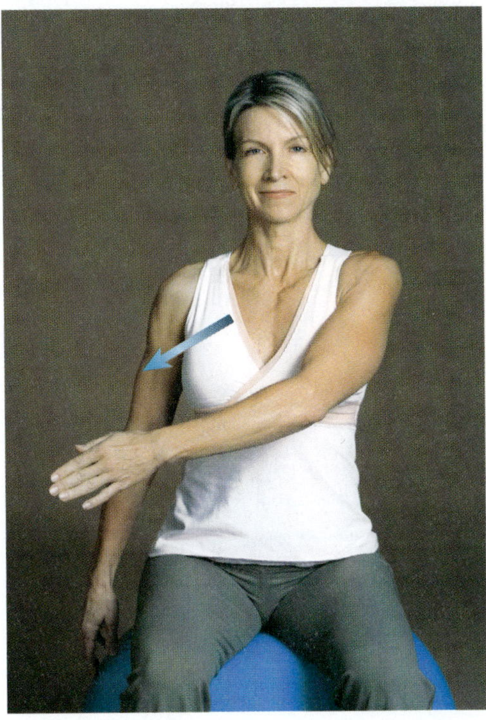

Muscles

When studying the muscles of the glenohumeral joint, it can be helpful to group them according to their location and function. Muscles that originate on the scapula and clavicle and insert on the humerus may be thought of as muscles *intrinsic* to the glenohumeral joint, whereas muscles originating on the trunk and inserting on the humerus are considered *extrinsic* to the joint. The intrinsic muscles include the **deltoid,** the **coracobrachialis,** the **teres major,** and the **rotator cuff group,** which is composed of the **supraspinatus, infraspinatus, teres minor,** and **subscapularis.** Extrinsic glenohumeral muscles are the **latissimus dorsi** and the **pectoralis major,** even though it has a clavicular attachment. It can also be helpful to organize the muscles according to their general location. The pectoralis major, coracobrachialis, and subscapularis are anterior muscles. Located superiorly are the deltoid and supraspinatus. The latissimus dorsi, teres major, infraspinatus, and teres minor are located posteriorly.

MUSCLE IDENTIFICATION

Figure 6.5 identifies the anterior and posterior muscles of the shoulder joint and shoulder girdle. Refer to table 6.2 for a detailed breakdown of the agonist muscles for the glenohumeral joint.

The biceps brachii and triceps brachii (long head) are also involved in glenohumeral movements as agonists and antagonists. Primarily, the biceps brachii assists in flexing and horizontally adducting the shoulder, whereas the long head of the triceps brachii assists in extension and horizontal abduction. See Chapter 8 on the elbow and radioulnar joints for further discussion of these muscles.

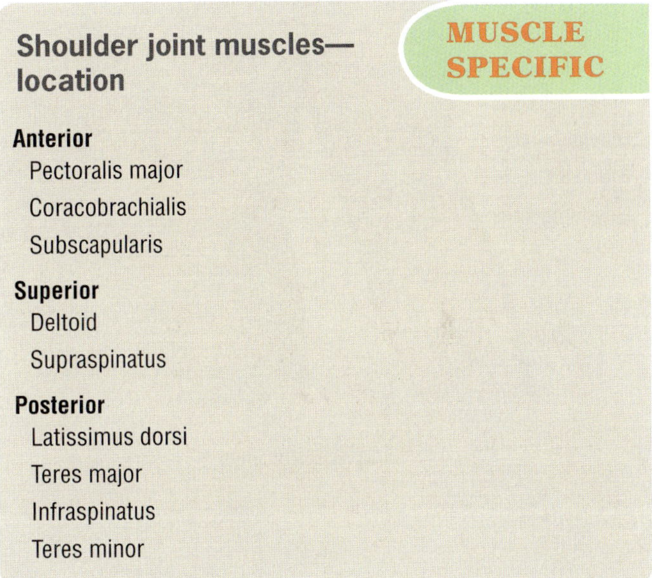

Shoulder joint muscles—location

MUSCLE SPECIFIC

Anterior

Pectoralis major
Coracobrachialis
Subscapularis

Superior

Deltoid
Supraspinatus

Posterior

Latissimus dorsi
Teres major
Infraspinatus
Teres minor

Nerves

The shoulder joint muscles are all innervated from the nerves of the brachial plexus (figure 6.6). The pectoralis major is innervated by the pectoral nerves. Specifically, the lateral pectoral nerve arising from C5, C6, and C7 innervates the clavicular head, while the medial pectoral nerve arising from C8 and T1 innervates the sternal head. The thoracodorsal nerve, arising from C6, C7, and C8, supplies the latissimus dorsi. The axillary nerve, branching from C5 and C6, innervates the deltoid and teres minor. The axillary nerve supplies sensation to a lateral patch of skin over the deltoid region of the arm. Both the upper and lower subscapular nerves arising from C5 and C6 innervate the subscapularis, while only the lower subscapular nerve supplies the teres major. The supraspinatus and infraspinatus are innervated by the suprascapular nerve, which originates from C5 and C6. The musculocutaneous nerve, as seen in figure 6.6, branches from C5, C6, and C7 and innervates the coracobrachialis. It supplies sensation to the radial aspect of the forearm.

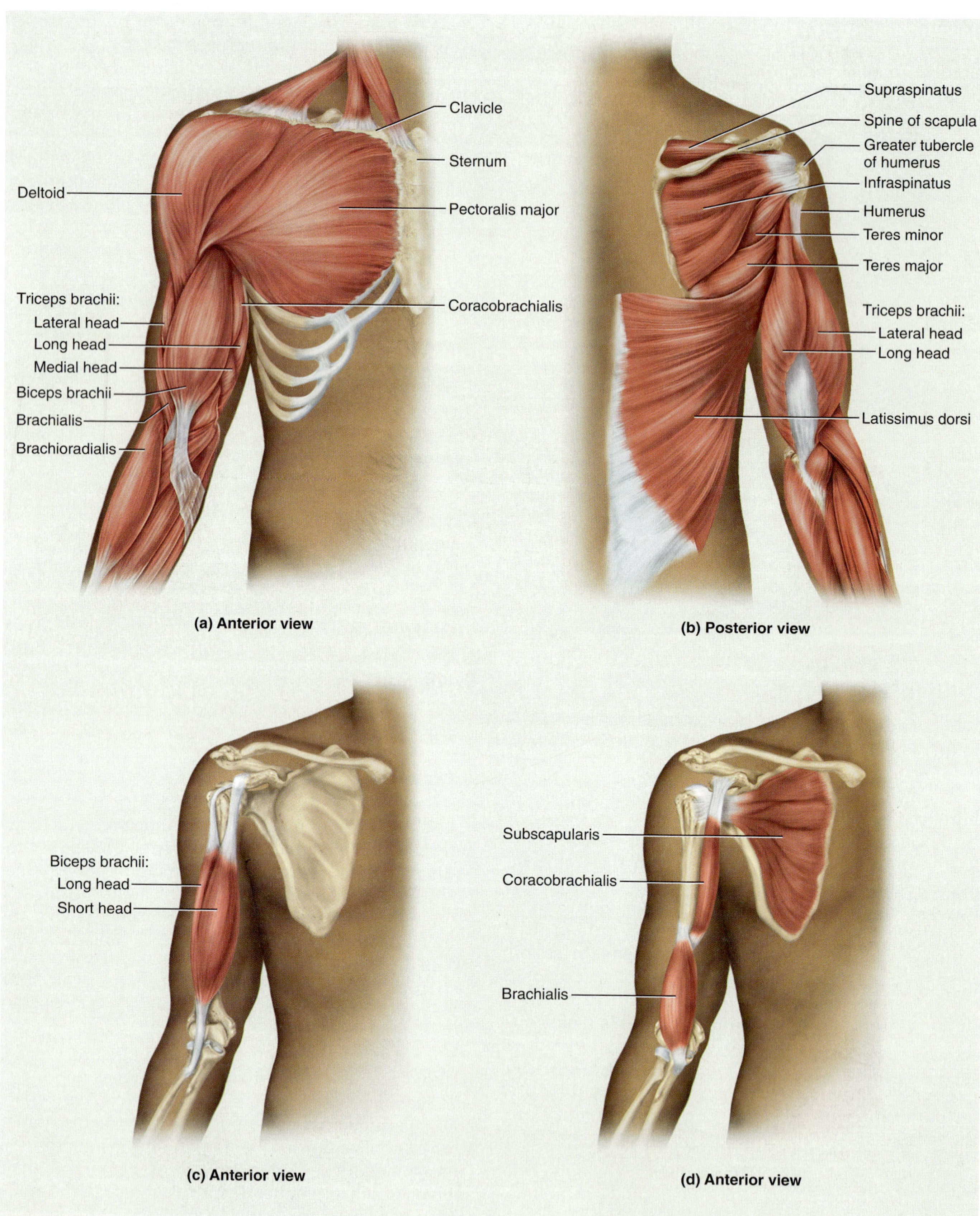

FIGURE 6.5 Pectoral and brachial muscles

TABLE 6.2 Agonist Muscles of the Glenohumeral Joint

Name of Muscle	Origins	Insertion	Actions	Innervations
Deltoids	*Anterior:* lateral 1/3 of clavicle	Deltoid tuberosity of humerus	*Anterior:* abduction, flexion, horizontal adduction, medial rotation of humerus	Axillary nerve (C5, C6)
	Middle: lateral acromion	Same	*Middle:* abduction of humerus to 90 degrees	
	Posterior: spine of scapula	Same	*Posterior:* abduction, extension, horizontal abduction, lateral rotation of humerus	
Rotator cuff:				
Supraspinatus	Supraspinous fossa of scapula	Superior facet, greater tubercle of humerus	Weak abduction, stabilization of head of humerus to initiate abduction	Suprascapular nerve (C5)
Infraspinatus	Infraspinous fossa of scapula	Greater tubercle of humerus, middle facet	Lateral rotation, extension of humerus, horizontal abduction	Suprascapular nerve (C5, C6)
Teres minor	Upper axillary border of scapula	Greater tubercle of humerus, inferior facet	Lateral rotation, extension, horizontal abduction	Axillary nerve (C5, C6)
Subscapularis	Subscapular fossa of scapula	Lesser tubercle of humerus	Medial rotation of humerus, adduction of arm, extension	Upper and lower subscapular nerve (C5, C6)
Latissimus dorsi	Thoracolumbar aponeurosis from T7 to iliac crest, lower three or four ribs, inferior angle of scapula	Floor of bicipital groove of humerus	Extension, medial rotation, horizontal abduction, adduction	Thoracodorsal nerve (C6–C8)
Teres major	Posterior inferior angle of scapula	Medial lip of bicipital groove of humerus	Extension, medial rotation, adduction	Lower subscapular nerve (C5, C6)
Pectoralis major	*Clavicular head:* medial 1/2 of clavicle	Lateral lip of bicipital groove of humerus	*Clavicular head:* medial rotation, horizontal adduction, flexion, abduction (once the arm is abducted 90 degrees, the upper fibers assist in further abduction), adduction (with the arm below 90 degrees of abduction)	*Clavicular head:* lateral pectoral nerve (C5–C7)
	Sternal head: sternum, cartilage of upper six ribs		*Sternal head:* medial rotation, horizontal adduction, extension, adduction	*Sternal head:* medial pectoral nerve (C8, T1)
Coracobrachialis	Coracoid process of scapula	Middle of medial border of humeral shaft	Flexion, adduction, horizontal adduction	Musculocutaneous nerve (C5–C7)

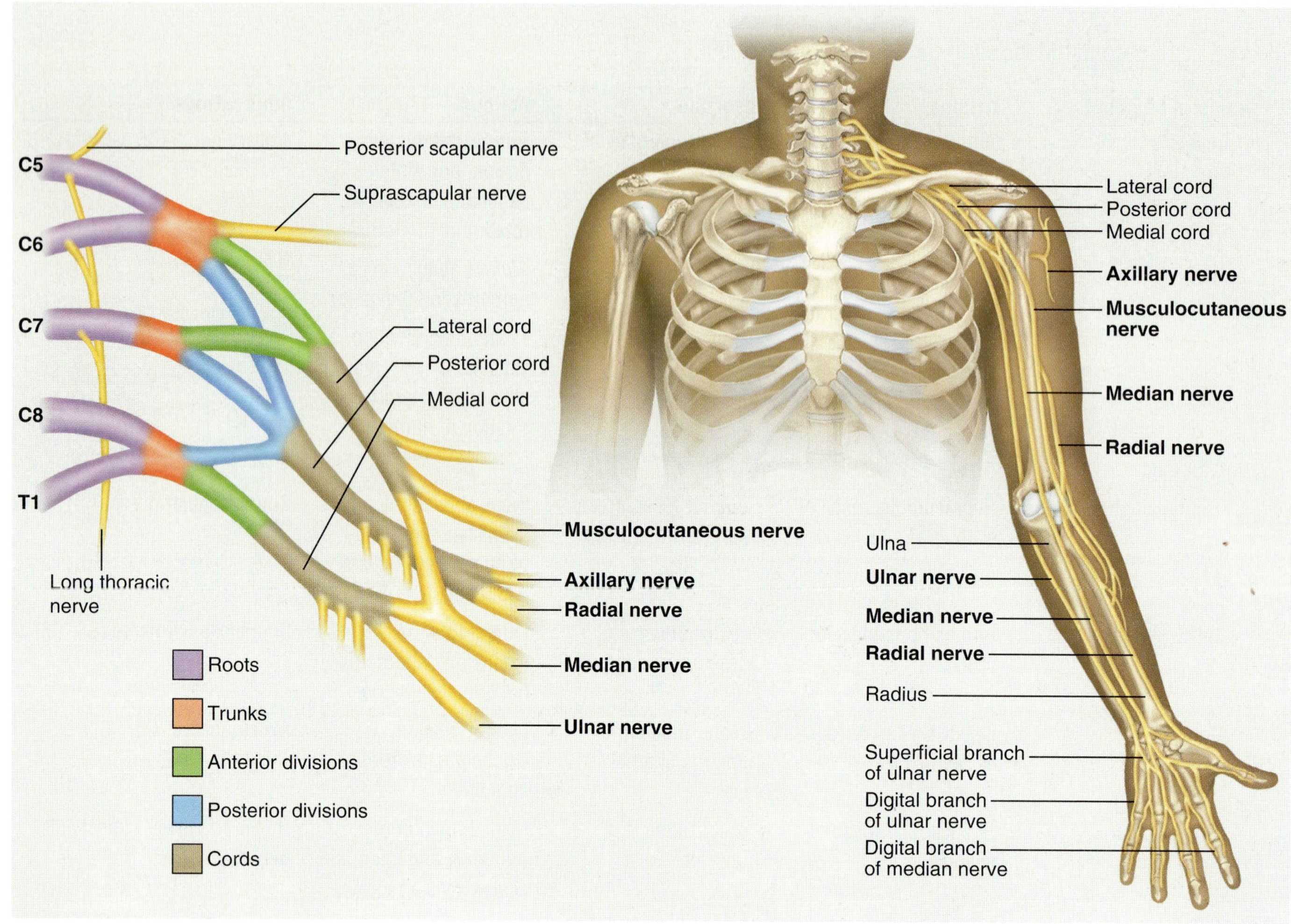

FIGURE 6.6 The brachial plexus

Individual Muscles of the Shoulder Joint

DELTOID MUSCLE

Palpation

Passively shorten by flexing the humerus superior to the client's head. Cradle the arm in your hands. In this position, all three sections of the deltoid can be palpated easily. See Chapter 7 for deltoid techniques.

Anterior fibers: Palpate the anterior fibers from the clavicle toward the anterior humerus during resisted flexion or horizontal adduction.

Middle fibers: Palpate the middle fibers from the lateral border of the acromion down toward the deltoid tuberosity during resisted abduction.

Posterior fibers: Palpate the posterior fibers from the lower lip of the spine of the scapula toward the posterior humerus during resisted extension or horizontal abduction.

CLINICAL NOTES — **Cautionary Note**

Actions that preclude flexion of the upper extremity and rounded shoulders will shorten fibers of the anterior deltoid while lengthening the posterior deltoid. Stretching and releasing the anterior deltoid while encouraging strengthening of the posterior deltoid will help balance the deltoid muscles and support better posture. Practitioners should also note that the subdeltoid bursa is located just below the anterior deltoid. Therapists must use caution and avoid using compressive techniques that can irritate the subdeltoid bursa. Specific stretching, however, is extremely beneficial in healing inflamed bursae.

OIAI MUSCLE CHART DELTOID (del-toyd´) Multifaceted superficial muscle

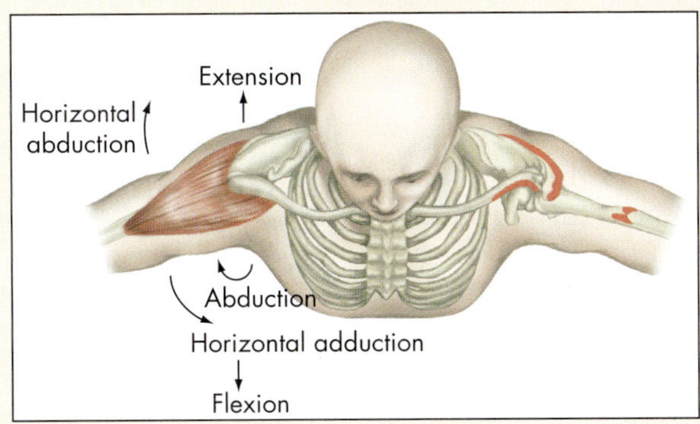

Name of Muscle	Origins	Insertion	Actions	Innervations
Deltoid	*Anterior:* lateral 1/3 of clavicle	Deltoid tuberosity of humerus	*Anterior:* abduction, flexion, horizontal adduction, medial rotation of humerus	Axillary nerve (C5, C6)
	Middle: lateral acromion	Same	*Middle:* abduction of humerus to 90 degrees	
	Posterior: spine of scapula	Same	*Posterior:* abduction, extension, horizontal abduction, lateral rotation of humerus	

Muscle Specifics

The deltoid muscle is used commonly in activities such as driving a car, poling in cross-country skiing, and doing any lifting movement. The trapezius muscle stabilizes the scapula as the deltoid pulls on the humerus. The anterior fibers of the deltoid muscle flex and internally rotate the humerus and oppose the posterior fibers that extend and externally rotate the humerus. The anterior fibers also horizontally adduct the humerus, while the posterior fibers horizontally abduct it. The deltoid muscle is used in all lifting movements. Any movement of the humerus on the scapula will involve part or all of the deltoid muscle.

Clinical Flexibility

Stretching the deltoid requires varying positions, depending on the fibers to be stretched. To stretch the anterior deltoid, take the humerus into extreme hyperextension. Start with arms at the sides and, using the posterior shoulder muscles, lift the arm back into hyperextension. Hold 2 seconds and repeat. This movement also stretches the biceps brachii. To further isolate the anterior deltoid, while the arms are in hyperextension, squeeze the arms together in horizontal abduction. To stretch the middle and posterior deltoid, take the humerus into horizontal adduction. Begin with arms at the sides. Lift one arm up into flexion in front, elbow extended, and bring it across the chest just under the chin (horizontal adduction). Use the other hand to assist by pulling above the elbow toward the chest. Hold 2 seconds and then repeat, bringing the arm down to the side of the body each time. *Contraindications:* Avoid horizontal adduction with shoulder arthroplasty clients; they can, however, perform the extension movement.

Strengthening

Lifting the humerus from the side to the position of abduction is a typical action of the deltoid. Side-arm dumbbell raises are excellent for strengthening the deltoid, especially the middle fibers. The anterior deltoid fibers can be emphasized by abducting the humerus in a slightly horizontally adducted (30-degree) position. The posterior fibers can be strengthened better by hyperextending the arm with a weight, lifting it as high as possible. The eccentric (down phase) movement is extremely important, so the dumbbell in these strength exercises should be returned slowly to the start position each time. *Contraindications:* These exercises are generally safe with controlled movement.

ROTATOR CUFF MUSCLES

Muscle Specifics

The figure in the chart illustrates the rotator cuff muscle group, which, as previously mentioned, is most important in maintaining the humeral head in its proper location within the glenoid cavity. The acronym *SITS* may be used in learning the names *supraspinatus, infraspinatus, teres minor,* and *subscapularis*. These muscles, which are not very large in comparison with the deltoid and pectoralis major, must possess not only adequate strength but also a

OIAI MUSCLE CHART ROTATOR CUFF Stabilizers for the head of the humerus

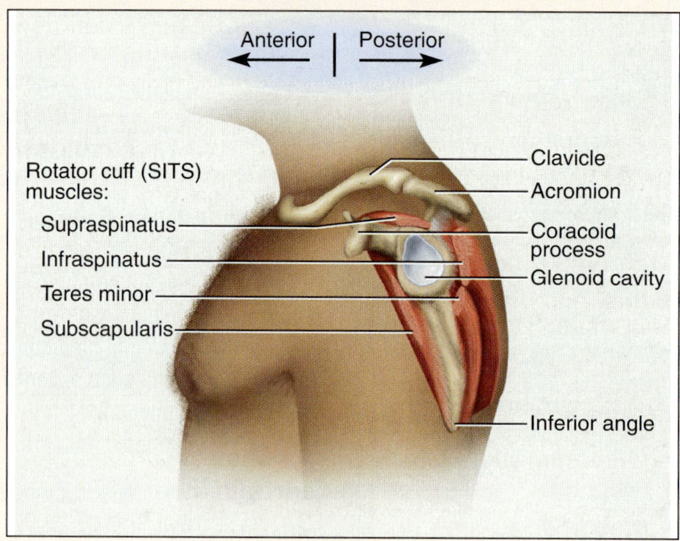

Name of Muscle	Origins	Insertion	Actions	Innervations
Supraspinatus	Supraspinous fossa of scapula	Superior facet, greater tubercle of humerus	Weak abduction, stabilization of head of humerus to initiate abduction	Suprascapular nerve (C5)
Infraspinatus	Infraspinous fossa of scapula	Greater tubercle of humerus, middle facet	Lateral rotation, extension of humerus, horizontal abduction	Suprascapular nerve (C5, C6)
Teres minor	Upper axillary border of scapula	Greater tubercle of humerus, inferior facet	Lateral rotation, extension, horizontal abduction	Axillary nerve (C5, C6)
Subscapularis	Subscapular fossa of scapula	Lesser tubercle of humerus	Medial rotation of humerus, adduction of arm, extension	Upper and lower subscapular nerve (C5, C6)

significant amount of muscular endurance to ensure their proper functioning, particularly in repetitious overhead activities such as throwing, swimming, and pitching. When these and similar activities are repetitive actions or are carried out using poor technique, or when the muscles are fatigued or have not been adequately warmed up or conditioned, the rotator cuff muscle group, particularly the supraspinatus, fails to dynamically stabilize the humeral head in the glenoid cavity, leading to further rotator cuff problems such as tendonosis, tendonitis, or rotator cuff impingement within the subacromial space. **Tendonosis** is a breakdown of collagen fibers within the tendon, while **tendonitis** is an inflammation of a tendon. See Chapter 9 for different types of tendonitis.

SUPRASPINATUS MUSCLE

Palpation

Palpate the supraspinatus anterior and superior to the spine of the scapula in the supraspinatus fossa during initial abduction in the scapular plane. The tendon also may be palpated just off the acromion on the greater tubercle with the arm placed behind the back.

CLINICAL NOTES **Weak Abductor**

Supraspinatus is often called the "briefcase" or "suitcase" muscle. The repetitive action of carrying something slightly away from the body in weak abduction is enough to apply strain to this often-weak muscle. It is a much better stabilizer than it is an abductor. The development of supraspinatus tendonitis or tendonosis is common for this weak link of the rotator cuff, and it is likely to become impinged under the acromion when its tendon is inflamed.

Muscle Specifics

The supraspinatus muscle holds the head of the humerus in the glenoid fossa. When the body is engaged in a throwing movement, the supraspinatus provides important dynamic stability by maintaining the proper relationship between the humeral head and the glenoid fossa. In the cocking phase of throwing, the humeral head has a tendency to subluxate anteriorly. In the follow-through phase, the humeral head tends to move posteriorly.

OIAI MUSCLE CHART SUPRASPINATUS (su´pra-spi-na´tus) Above the spine of the scapula

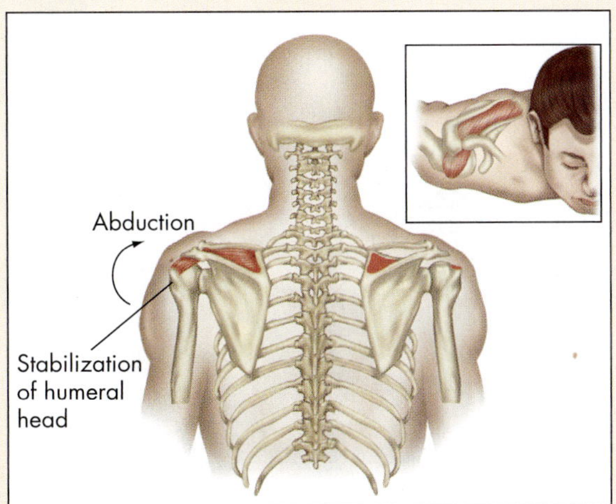

Name of Muscle	Origins	Insertion	Actions	Innervations
Supraspinatus	Supraspinous fossa of scapula	Superior facet, greater tubercle of humerus	Weak abduction, stabilization of head of humerus to initiate abduction	Suprascapular nerve (C5)

The supraspinatus, along with the other rotator cuff muscles, must have excellent strength and endurance to prevent abnormal and excessive movement of the humeral head in the fossa.

The supraspinatus is the most often injured rotator cuff muscle. Acute and severe injuries may occur with trauma to the shoulder. However, mild to moderate strains or tears often occur with athletic activity, particularly if the activity involves repetitious overhead movements, such as throwing or swimming.

Injury or weakness in the supraspinatus may be detected when the athlete attempts to substitute the scapula elevators and upward rotators to obtain humeral abduction. An inability to smoothly abduct the arm against resistance with the thumb turned down is indicative of possible rotator cuff injury.

Clinical Flexibility

To stretch the supraspinatus, the humerus must rotate internally to isolate the muscle attachments. With the arm in abduction and the elbow flexed 90 degrees, palms open facing anterior, rotate the humerus down and stretch for 2 seconds. Repeat 8 to 10 times. Rotate the arm back to the starting position each time; during the stretch, the scapula area should remain as relaxed as possible. *Contraindications:* It may be difficult to hold the arm in abduction if bursitis or tendonitis issues exist.

Strengthening

The supraspinatus muscle may be called into action whenever the middle fibers of the deltoid muscle are used. An "empty-can" exercise may be used to isolate supraspinatus action. To perform, internally rotate the humerus and abduct the arm to 90 degrees in a 30- to 45-degree horizontally adducted position, as if one were emptying a can. A dumbbell is then lifted from the midline, up into abduction, with the pinky finger leading and the thumb turned down. A person with an injury to the supraspinatus will have difficulty performing this movement. *Contraindications:* It may be difficult to lift the arm into abduction if bursitis or tendonitis issues exist. In these cases, a modification of the empty-can exercise may be done in exactly the same position except with the thumb turned up for a "full-can" exercise.

OIAI MUSCLE CHART INFRASPINATUS (in´fra-spi-na´tus) Under the spine of the scapula

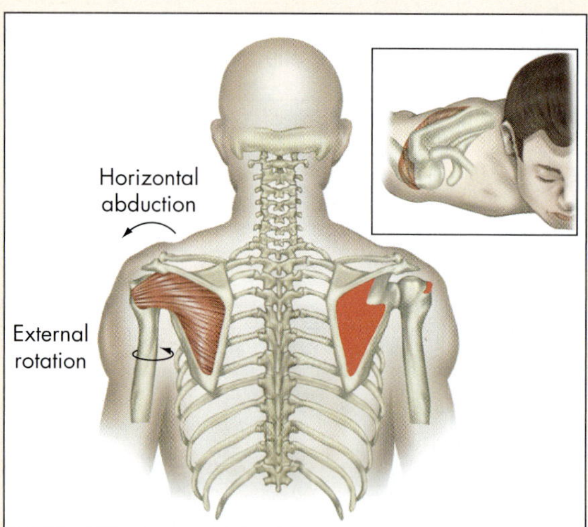

Name of Muscle	Origins	Insertion	Actions	Innervations
Infraspinatus	Infraspinous fossa of scapula	Greater tubercle of humerus, middle facet	Lateral rotation, extension of humerus, horizontal abduction Stabilization of humeral head in glenoid fossa	Suprascapular nerve (C5, C6)

INFRASPINATUS MUSCLE

Palpation

Palpate the infraspinatus superficially just below the spine of the scapula, passing upward and laterally to the humerus during resisted external rotation.

> **CLINICAL NOTES** **Extension Tendonitis**
>
> Consider infraspinatus involvement if the client has difficulty fastening a seat belt or placing an arm through a sleeve. Sports injury or other trauma, such as hauling a wheeled suitcase or excessive poling with cross-country skis, could also contribute to infraspinatus tendonitis or tendonosis. The infraspinatus tendon is often tender at the attachment site of the humerus.

Muscle Specifics

The infraspinatus and teres minor muscles are effective when the rhomboid muscles stabilize the scapula. When the humerus is laterally rotated, the rhomboid muscles flatten the scapula to the back and fixate it so that the humerus may be rotated. Agonists to the infraspinatus include the teres minor as well as the posterior deltoid.

Clinical Flexibility

Stretching the infraspinatus is accomplished with medial rotation and extreme horizontal adduction. Start with the shoulder flexed in front, elbow extended, palms facing the midline. Using the anterior shoulder muscles, move the arm across the chest (horizontal adduction), just under the chin. Use the other hand to assist in a gentle 2-second stretch at the end movement. This exercise protracts the scapula, stretching the infraspinatus as a horizontal abductor. To stretch these fibers as rotators, use the same medial rotator stretch for the supraspinatus. *Contraindications:* Use caution with shoulder arthroplasty clients with this movement or avoid altogether.

Strengthening

An appropriate amount of strength and endurance is critical in both the infraspinatus and teres minor, as they are called on eccentrically to slow the arm down from high-velocity medial rotation activities, such as pitching a baseball and serving a tennis ball. The

OIAI MUSCLE CHART TERES MINOR (te´rez mi´nor) Small round muscle

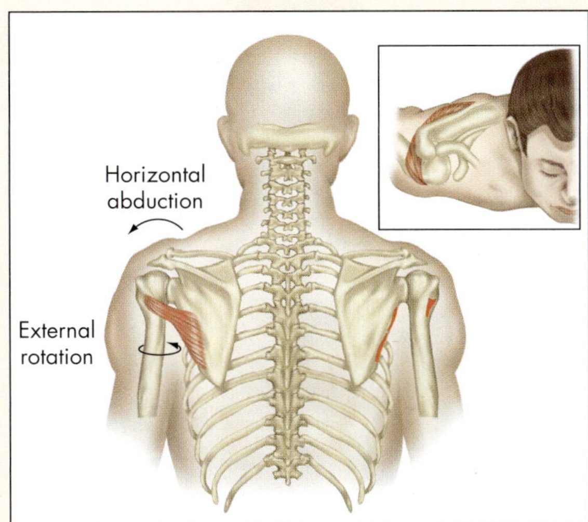

Name of Muscle	Origins	Insertion	Actions	Innervations
Teres minor	Upper axillary border of scapula	Greater tubercle of humerus, inferior facet	Lateral rotation, extension, horizontal abduction Stabilization of humeral head in glenoid fossa	Axillary nerve (C5, C6)

infraspinatus is vital to maintaining the posterior stability of the glenohumeral joint. It is the most powerful of the lateral rotators and is the second most commonly injured rotator cuff muscle.

Both the infraspinatus and the teres minor can best be strengthened by laterally rotating the arm against resistance in the 15- to 20-degree abducted position and the 90-degree abducted position. Begin on your side, elbow bent at 90 degrees, and fixed at the hip. Using a dumbbell, start at the navel and lift the weight up into external rotation. Return to the starting position, slowly lowering the weight. *Contraindications:* This exercise is generally safe with controlled movement.

TERES MINOR MUSCLE

Palpation

Palpate the teres minor just above the teres major on the posterior scapula surfacc, moving diagonally upward and laterally from the inferior angle of the scapula during resisted lateral rotation.

CLINICAL NOTES **Satellite Pain**

Since the teres minor has the same actions as the infraspinatus, it usually does not develop problems until the infraspinatus is weakened. That said, the teres minor can be included in rotator cuff tendonosis or tendonitis simply because of its close proximity to the infraspinatus and therefore should not be overlooked in treatment.

Muscle Specifics

The teres minor functions similarly to the infraspinatus in providing dynamic posterior stability to the glenohumeral joint. Both of these muscles perform the same actions together.

Clinical Flexibility

The teres minor is stretched similarly to the infraspinatus by moving into extreme horizontal adduction and

OIAI MUSCLE CHART SUBSCAPULARIS (sub-skap-u-la´ris) Below the scapula

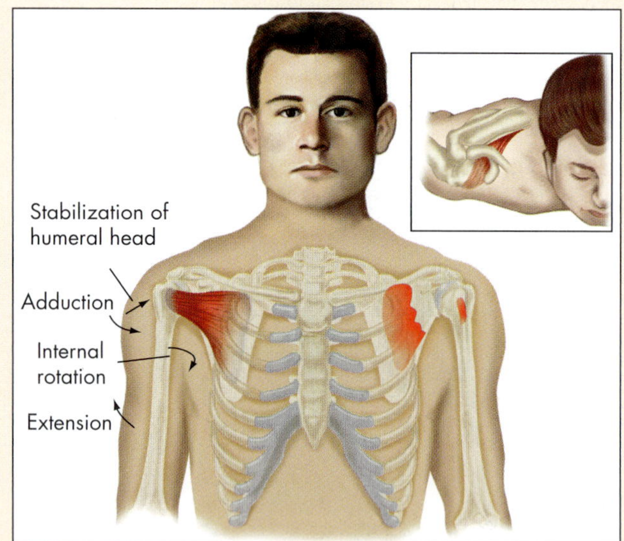

Name of Muscle	Origins	Insertion	Actions	Innervations
Subscapularis	Subscapular fossa of scapula	Lesser tubercle of humerus	Medial rotation of humerus, adduction of arm, extension Stabilization of the humeral head in the glenoid fossa	Upper and lower subscapular nerve (C5, C6)

medially rotating the shoulder. Use the same stretches for the teres minor that are used for the infraspinatus.

Strengthening

The teres minor is strengthened with the same exercises that are used in strengthening the infraspinatus. Any exercise with resistance that forces lateral rotation is appropriate.

SUBSCAPULARIS MUSCLE

Palpation

The subscapularis, in conjunction with the latissimus dorsi and teres major, forms the posterior axillary fold. Most of the subscapularis is inaccessible on the anterior scapula behind the rib cage. The lateral portion may be palpated with the client supine and the arm in slight flexion and adduction so that the elbow is lying across the abdomen. Use one hand posteriorly to grasp the medial border and pull it laterally while palpating between the scapula and rib cage with the other hand. To assist the palpation, the client presses the forearm against the chest, further protracting the scapula. The thick tendon of subscapularis can be palpated between the coracoid process and the lesser tubercle of the humerus.

CLINICAL NOTES **Painful Shoulder**

The subscapularis becomes subject to trigger points and pain patterns when there is little to no scapular range of motion. **Adhesive capsulitis,** often called **frozen shoulder,** is a progressive, painful condition that starts with limited motion of the shoulder joint and progresses to a frozen stage. Small adhesions form in the joint capsule, creating an extremely debilitating condition. With lack of movement, the subscapularis becomes weak and atrophies; as a result, it adds to the restriction of normal range of motion.

Muscle Specifics

The subscapularis muscle, another rotator cuff muscle, holds the head of the humerus in the glenoid fossa from an anterior position. It acts with the latissimus dorsi and teres major muscles in its typical movement; however, it is less powerful in its action because of its proximity to the joint. The muscle also requires the help of the rhomboids in stabilizing the scapula to make it effective in the movements described. The subscapularis is relatively hidden behind the rib cage in its location on the anterior aspect of the scapula in the subscapular fossa.

OIAI MUSCLE CHART LATISSIMUS DORSI (lat-is´i-mus dor´si) Broad flat back

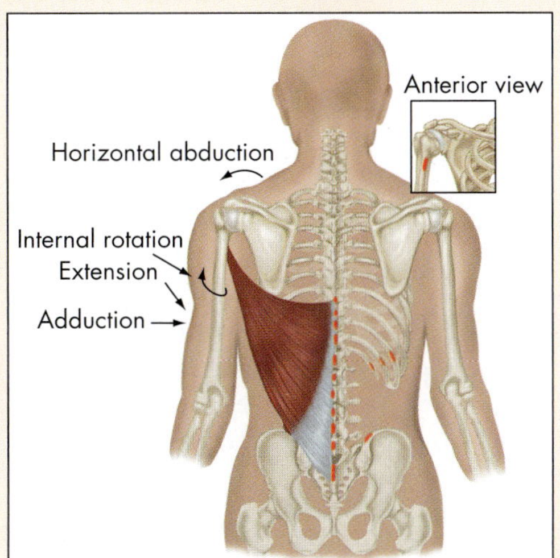

Name of Muscle	Origins	Insertion	Actions	Innervations
Latissimus dorsi	Thoracolumbar aponeurosis from T7 to iliac crest, lower three or four ribs, inferior angle of scapula	Floor of bicipital groove of humerus	Extension, medial rotation, horizontal abduction, adduction	Thoracodorsal nerve (C6–C8)

Clinical Flexibility

Lateral rotation of the humerus stretches the subscapularis. With the shoulder flexed at 90 degrees and abducted in the same manner as in the supraspinatus stretch, rotate the humerus laterally to gently stretch for 2 seconds. This targets the rotary action of this muscle. Since it also adducts the shoulder, the subscapularis should be stretched in horizontal abduction. Begin with arms flexed in front, palms facing each other. Using the muscles on the back of the shoulder, bring the arms back into horizontal abduction. Stretch for 2 seconds. This stretch also targets the pectoralis major. *Contraindications:* These movements are generally safe, although it may be difficult to hold the arm in abduction if shoulder dysfunctions exist.

Strengthening

The subscapularis can be strengthened with exercises similar to those used for the latissimus dorsi and teres major (see below), such as rope climbing and latissimus pulls. It should, however, be strengthened by challenging it during every action. A specific exercise for its development is done by medially rotating the arm against resistance in the beside-the-body position at 0 degrees of glenohumeral abduction. This is accomplished with the client in the side-lying position, with the bottom arm tucked under the body and bent at 90 degrees. Start at the floor and internally rotate the arm to bring the weight up. *Contraindications:* This movement may be difficult if bursitis or tendonitis issues exist.

LATISSIMUS DORSI MUSCLE

Palpation

The latissimus dorsi tendon may be palpated as it passes under the teres major at the posterior wall of the axilla, particularly during resisted extension and medial rotation. The muscle can be palpated in the upper-lumbar–lower-thoracic area during extension from a flexed position. The muscle may be palpated throughout most of its length during resisted adduction from a slightly abducted position.

CLINICAL NOTES **Thin Tissue**

Often injured because of its very large plastic wrap–like tissue, the **aponeurosis,** the latissimus dorsi is not designed to pick up weights in a flexed trunk position. It is more suited for powerful movements such as rowing and pulling. This fascia connects the thoracic vertebrae from T6 or T7 to all the spinous processes of the lumbar vertebrae and sacrum to the iliac crest. Muscle fibers at the ribs interdigitate with the external oblique, which sometimes makes it hard to take a deep breath when torn tissues are present.

Muscle Specifics

The latissimus dorsi, along with the teres major, forms the posterior axillary fold. The latissimus twists around the teres major, and the two are partially intertwined before they insert in their respective positions on the medial lip of the bicipital groove. This of course provides a strong insertion into the humerus and supports the shoulder joint in actions such as adduction, extension, and medial rotation. Due to the upward rotation of the scapula that accompanies glenohumeral abduction, the latissimus effectively downwardly rotates the scapula by way of its action in pulling the entire shoulder girdle downward in active glenohumeral adduction. It is one of the most important extensor muscles of the humerus, and it contracts powerfully in performing chin-ups. The teres major assists the latissimus in all of its actions. The latissimus dorsi is sometimes referred to as the "swimmer's muscle" because of its function in pulling the body forward in the water during medial rotation, adduction, and extension.

Clinical Flexibility

The latissimus dorsi is stretched with the teres major when the shoulder is laterally rotated in a 90-degree abducted position. It can be stretched using the same movements as those for the pectoralis major and subscapularis and using lateral side bends with the arm in sideward elevation. Lift one arm up into sideward elevation, and laterally bend the torso to the opposite side. *Contraindications:* This stretch is generally safe. Impingement clients may feel some discomfort when the arm is in sideward elevation.

Strengthening

Exercises in which the arms are pulled down bring the latissimus dorsi muscle into powerful contraction; examples are chin-ups, rope climbing, and dips on parallel bars. In barbell exercises, the basic rowing and pullover exercises are good for developing the "lats." Pulling the bar of an overhead pulley system down toward the shoulders, known as a "lat pull," is a common exercise for this muscle. *Contraindications:* These exercises are generally safe with controlled movement.

TERES MAJOR MUSCLE

Palpation

Palpate the teres major just above the latissimus dorsi and below the teres minor on the posterior scapula surface, moving diagonally upward and laterally from the inferior angle of the scapula during resisted medial rotation.

Muscle Specifics

The teres major muscle is effective only when the rhomboid muscles stabilize the scapula or move the scapula

OIAI MUSCLE CHART TERES MAJOR (te´rez ma´jor) Large round muscle

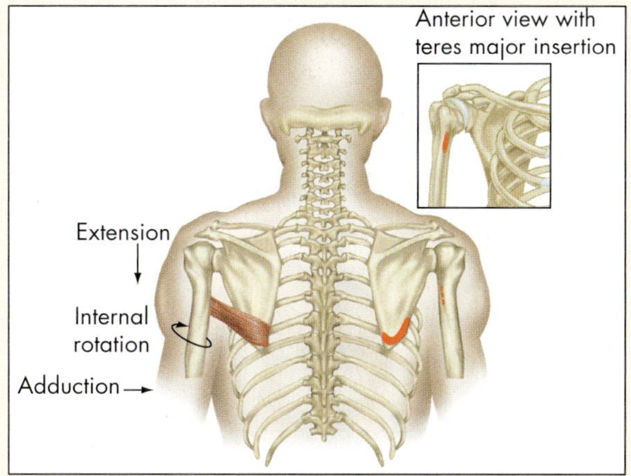

Name of Muscle	Origins	Insertion	Actions	Innervations
Teres major	Posterior inferior angle of scapula	Medial lip of bicipital groove of humerus	Extension, medial rotation, adduction	Lower subscapular nerve (C5, C6)

CLINICAL NOTES **Friend to the Latissimus Dorsi**

The teres major is easily accessible for soft-tissue work, especially in a side-lying position. It is less likely to be injured than the latissimus dorsi, as it is not as spread out with as many attachments. The teres major does get fatigued with use; thus it is beneficial to massage the entire scapula region, as the teres major will compensate for the latissimus dorsi. See Chapter 7 for side-lying techniques.

in downward rotation. Otherwise, the scapula would move forward to meet the arm. The teres major completes extension of the glenohumeral joint, particularly from the flexed position to the posteriorly extended position, as well as adduction of the glenohumeral joint, particularly from the abducted position down to the side and toward the midline of the body.

This muscle works effectively with the latissimus dorsi and also assists the pectoralis major and subscapularis in adducting, medially rotating, and extending the humerus. It is said to be the latissimus dorsi's "little helper" and, as such, can be labeled as a synergist.

Clinical Flexibility

Laterally rotating the shoulder in a 90-degree abducted position stretches the teres major. The stretches described for the latissimus are also effective for the teres major.

Strengthening

Like the latissimus, the teres major may be strengthened by lat pulls, rope climbing, and medial rotation exercises against resistance.

PECTORALIS MAJOR MUSCLE

Palpation

Upper fibers: Palpate the upper fibers of the pectoralis major from the medial end of the clavicle to the bicipital groove of the humerus, during flexion and adduction from the anatomical position.

Lower fibers: Palpate the lower fibers of the pectoralis major from the ribs and sternum to the bicipital groove of the humerus, during resisted extension from a flexed position and resisted adduction from the anatomical position.

CLINICAL NOTES **Breast Supporters**

Although it seems natural to work on the more developed pectoralis major on men, this muscle is often forgotten for women. Breast tissue adds to the weight of the front of the shoulders and sits on top of the pectoralis major in women. This large muscle is often contracted, forming rounded shoulders exacerbated by breast weight. It is therefore important to release contracted tissue and stretch the pectoralis major to help with

OIAI MUSCLE CHART PECTORALIS MAJOR (pek-to-ra´lis ma´jor) Large chest muscle

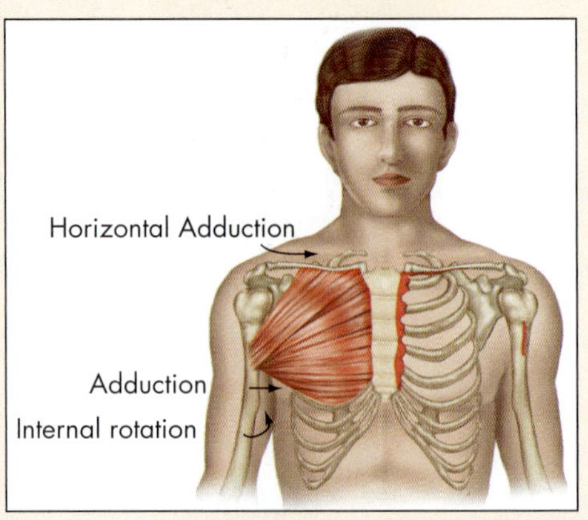

Name of Muscle	Origins	Insertion	Actions	Innervations
Pectoralis major	*Clavicular head:* medial 1/2 of clavicle	Lateral lip of bicipital groove of humerus	*Clavicular head:* medial rotation, horizontal adduction, flexion, abduction (once the arm is abducted 90 degrees, the upper fibers assist in further abduction), adduction (with the arm below 90 degrees of abduction)	*Clavicular head:* lateral pectoral nerve (C5–C7)
	Sternal head: sternum, cartilage of upper six ribs		*Sternal head:* medial rotation, horizontal adduction, extension, adduction	*Sternal head: medial* pectoral nerve (C8, T1)

postural problems and support back muscles. The rhomboids should be strengthened to help assist in scapular retraction. Compression, myofascial stretches, elliptical movements, and jostling are all great techniques for unwinding this powerful muscle. See Chapter 7 for techniques for the pectoralis major.

Muscle Specifics

The anterior axillary fold is formed primarily by the pectoralis major. It has a fanlike structure that completely twists at the insertion on the lateral lip of the bicipital groove. The insertion is superficial to the latissimus dorsi and teres major. The pectoralis major aids the serratus anterior muscle in drawing the scapula forward as it moves the humerus in flexion and medial rotation. Even though the pectoralis major is not attached to the scapula, it is effective in scapula protraction because of its anterior pull on the humerus, which joins to the scapula at the glenohumeral joint. A typical action is throwing a baseball. As the glenohumeral joint is flexed, the humerus is medially rotated and the scapula is drawn forward with upward rotation. The pectoralis major also works as a helper of the latissimus dorsi muscle when extending and adducting the humerus from a raised position.

Clinical Flexibility

Due to the popularity of bench pressing and other weight-lifting exercises that emphasize the pectoralis major, as well as this muscle's use in most sporting activities, the pectoralis major is often overdeveloped in comparison to its antagonists. Bodybuilders will stand with rounded, medially rotated shoulders and the palms facing posterior. As a result, stretching is often needed and can be done by active lateral rotation. The muscle is also stretched when the shoulder is horizontally abducted. Begin with arms flexed in front, palms facing each other. Using the muscles on the back of the shoulder, bring the arms back into horizontal abduction. Stretch for 2 seconds. You can also perform this movement in a doorway, reaching with one arm into abduction as the torso twists. *Contraindications:* This stretch is generally safe with controlled movement.

Strengthening

The pectoralis major and the anterior deltoid work closely together. The pectoralis major is used powerfully in push-ups, pull-ups, throwing, and tennis serves. With the client in the supine position on a bench and holding a barbell with the arms at the side, move the arms to a horizontally adducted position. This exercise, known as bench pressing, is widely used for pectoralis major development. *Contraindications:* Bench pressing is generally safe with controlled movement. Use caution with heavy weight, and avoid hyperextension of the humerus.

CORACOBRACHIALIS MUSCLE

Palpation

The belly of the coracobrachialis may be palpated high up on the medial arm just posterior to the short head of the biceps brachii and toward the coracoid process, particularly with resisted adduction.

CLINICAL NOTES **Compensatory Pain**

The coracobrachialis can develop a painful referred pattern that traverses down the extremity to the hand in a pulsing fashion. This is usually a compensating factor to adhesive capsulitis or to an injury that limits movement of the shoulder joint. When the coracobrachialis is shortened, the client will not be able to place the hand behind the back, as the movement will be too painful.

OIAI MUSCLE CHART CORACOBRACHIALIS (kor-a-ko-bra´ki-a´lis) Named for its attachments

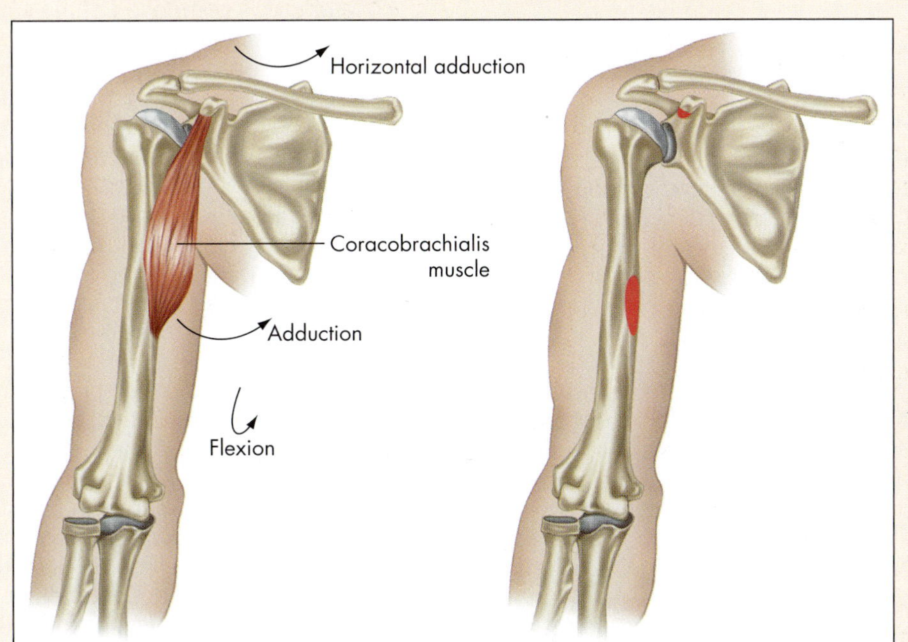

Name of Muscle	Origins	Insertion	Actions	Innervations
Coracobrachialis	Coracoid process of scapula	Middle of medial border of humeral shaft	Flexion, adduction, horizontal adduction	Musculocutaneous nerve (C5–C7)

Muscle Specifics

The coracobrachialis is not a powerful muscle, but it does assist in flexion and adduction and is most functional in moving the arm horizontally toward and across the chest. It is mostly buried under the pectoralis major and has a long tendon that runs side by side with the biceps short-head tendon. The practitioner needs to be cautious with locating the coracobrachialis, as the brachial plexus enters the upper extremity in close quarters to the muscle.

Clinical Flexibility

The coracobrachialis can be stretched in extreme horizontal abduction and in extreme extension, the same way the pectoralis major is stretched.

Strengthening

Like the pectoralis major, the coracobrachialis is best strengthened by horizontally adducting the arm against resistance, as in bench pressing or flys. Review the pectoralis major exercises for details.

CHAPTER *summary*

Introduction

- ✔ The mobile shoulder joint enables multiple movements, but it can sustain many injuries due to its lack of stability.

Bones

- ✔ The three bones that make up the shoulder joint are the clavicle, scapula, and humerus. Bony landmarks provide muscular attachment to make movement possible.

Joint

- ✔ The glenohumeral joint is a multiaxial, enarthrodial ball-and-socket joint.

Movements

- ✔ The glenohumeral joint enjoys complete range as a ball-and-socket joint. Shoulder joint actions include flexion, extension, abduction, adduction, and medial and lateral rotation. Other movements of this diarthrodial joint include horizontal adduction and abduction and diagonal plane movements.

Muscles

- ✔ The pectoralis major and coracobrachialis are located anteriorly, whereas the deltoid is located laterally. The rotator cuff includes supraspinatus, infraspinatus, teres minor, and subscapularis. Supraspinatus is located superior to the spine of the scapula, and infraspinatus is located posteriorly below the spine of the scapula. Teres minor is located laterally and posteriorly on the scapula, whereas the subscapularis has an anterior location on the scapula. Teres major is located inferiorly on the posterior scapula; latissimus dorsi is located posteriorly on the trunk.

Nerves

- ✔ The nerves for the shoulder joint muscles stem primarily from the brachial plexus.

Individual Muscles of the Shoulder Joint

- ✔ *Deltoid* is a superficial lateral muscle that is divided into three sections: anterior, middle, and posterior. The deltoid originates on the clavicle and scapula and inserts on the humerus. It is a major abductor of the humerus and is its own agonist and antagonist, as the anterior deltoid and posterior deltoid perform opposite actions. The anterior deltoid performs flexion, medial rotation, and horizontal adduction, whereas the posterior deltoid performs extension, lateral rotation, and horizontal abduction. The middle deltoid has very strong abduction to 90 degrees.
- ✔ *Rotator cuff* is composed of the supraspinatus, infraspinatus, teres minor, and subscapularis (SITS). These stabilize the head of the humerus. The supraspinatus originates on the supraspinous fossa, and its insertion lines up next to the infraspinatus and teres minor on the greater tubercle of the humerus. Infraspinatus originates on the infraspinous fossa; the teres minor attaches to the superior axillary border of the scapula. Supraspinatus performs weak abduction; infraspinatus and teres minor perform extension, lateral rotation, and horizontal abduction. Subscapularis originates on the subscapular fossa and inserts on the lesser tubercle. It adducts, extends, and medially rotates the humerus.
- ✔ *Latissimus dorsi* means "broad flat back." It spans superficially over most of the posterior trunk and inserts on the bicipital groove of the humerus. Its functions are adduction and extension, medial rotation, and horizontal abduction of the humerus. It is easily injured when used to pick up too much weight in an unbalanced position.
- ✔ *Teres major* is a posterior muscle that originates on the inferior angle of the scapula and inserts on the bicipital groove of the humerus. It forms the back aspect of the axilla region with the latissimus dorsi. It is a strong extensor and adductor and medially rotates the humerus.
- ✔ *Pectoralis major* has attachments on the clavicle, sternum, and costal ribs of the anterior trunk. Because of its fanlike structure coming from different directions on the trunk, it performs all shoulder joint movements with the exception of lateral rotation and horizontal abduction.
- ✔ *Coracobrachialis* is named for its attachments on the coracoid process of the scapula and the humerus. It flexes and horizontally adducts the humerus.

CHAPTER *review*

Worksheet Exercises

As an aid to learning, for in-class or out-of-class assignments, or for testing, tear-out worksheets are found at the end of the text, pages 523–526.

True or False

Write true *or* false *after each statement.*

1. The bones of the shoulder joint include the humerus, scapula, clavicle, and ulna.
2. Pectoralis major is a strong horizontal adductor.
3. The deltoid is an intrinsic muscle and inserts on the deltoid tuberosity.
4. The latissimus dorsi is often easily injured partially because of the very thin tissue attachments at its origin.
5. The rotator cuff includes supraspinatus, infraspinatus, teres major, and subscapularis.
6. Part of the job of the rotator cuff is to stabilize the head of the humerus.
7. The capsule of the head of the humerus is vulnerable to adhesive capsulitis.
8. The origin of the supraspinatus is the spine of the scapula.
9. The latissimus dorsi and the subscapularis both claim internal rotation as an action.
10. The anterior deltoid does extension, whereas the posterior deltoid does flexion.
11. One way to stretch the pectoralis major is to move the arms into horizontal abduction.

Short Answers

Write your answers on the lines provided.

1. Why is it essential that both anterior and posterior muscles of the shoulder joint be properly developed?

2. Bench presses or flys will help strengthen what muscles of the shoulder joint?

3. List the rotator cuff muscles. What action or job do they all share?

4. How does the pectoralis major contribute to a round shoulder posture?

5. What major nerve plexus innervates the shoulder joint muscles?

6. What happens to the scapula when the humerus is in an abducted position?

7. What muscle's name means "broad flat back"?

8. What is the name of the valley between the lesser and greater tubercles?

9. On what facets does the rotator cuff line up on the greater tubercle?

10. Explain how the subscapularis can be a synergist to the latissimus dorsi and teres major.

____

____

____

11. Explain how the pectoralis major can do flexion and extension.

____

____

____

Multiple Choice

Circle the correct answers.

1. The muscle that works with the latissimus dorsi is the:
   a. supraspinatus
   b. teres major
   c. teres minor
   d. coracobrachialis
2. The supraspinatus does weak ________as an action.
   a. abduction
   b. adduction
   c. flexion
   d. extension
3. When the latissimus dorsi causes medial rotation, the scapula will abduct with the help of the:
   a. trapezius and levator scapulae
   b. teres major
   c. serratus anterior and pectoralis minor
   d. pectoralis major
4. Adhesive capsulitis is often called frozen shoulder because:
   a. the condition progresses to a stage where there is little, if any, range of motion of the upper extremity and scapula
   b. it is easier to call it that
   c. the shoulder really gets cold
   d. none of the above
5. If the coracobrachialis is shortened, the individual will not be able to put the arms:
   a. in extension
   b. behind the back
   c. in front of the body
   d. across the body
6. The pectoralis major is able to generate many different actions because of:
   a. its insertion
   b. its location on the front of the body
   c. its shape and multiple origins
   d. none of the above
7. Teres major originates on the:
   a. posterior inferior angle of the scapula
   b. upper axillary border
   c. superior facet of the greater tubercle
   d. inferior facet of the greater tubercle
8. Rowing is a good exercise to develop the:
   a. trapezius
   b. supraspinatus
   c. pectoralis minor
   d. latissimus dorsi
9. The anterior and posterior deltoids do opposite actions because:
   a. of their location and opposite origins
   b. they are located on the humerus
   c. they both attach on the humerus
   d. none of the above
10. The bicipital groove divides the:
    a. coracoid process and acromion
    b. greater trochanter and lesser trochanter
    c. greater tubercle and lesser tubercle
    d. supraspinous fossa and infraspinous fossa

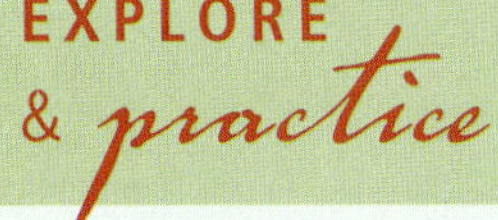

1. Locate the following parts of the humerus and scapula on a human skeleton and on a subject:
   a. Greater tubercle
   b. Lesser tubercle
   c. Neck
   d. Shaft
   e. Bicipital groove
   f. Medial epicondyle
   g. Lateral epicondyle
   h. Trochlea
   i. Capitulum
   j. Supraspinous fossa
   k. Infraspinous fossa
   l. Spine of the scapula

2. How and where can the following muscles be palpated on a human subject?
   a. Deltoid
   b. Teres major
   c. Infraspinatus
   d. Teres minor
   e. Latissimus dorsi
   f. Pectoralis major (upper and lower)

   Note: Using the pectoralis major muscle, indicate how various actions allow muscle palpation.

3. Demonstrate and locate on a partner the muscles that are primarily used in the following shoulder joint movements:
   a. Abduction
   b. Adduction
   c. Flexion
   d. Extension
   e. Horizontal adduction
   f. Horizontal abduction
   g. Lateral rotation
   h. Medial rotation

4. Using an articulated skeleton, compare the relationship of the greater tubercle to the undersurface of the acromion in each of the following situations:
   a. Flexion with the humerus medially rotated versus laterally rotated.
   b. Abduction with the humerus medially versus laterally rotated.
   c. Horizontal adduction with the humerus medially versus laterally rotated.

5. Pair up with a partner with his or her back exposed. Use your hand to grasp your partner's right scapula along the lateral border to prevent scapula movement. Have your partner slowly abduct the glenohumeral joint as much as possible. Note the difference in total abduction possible when conditions are normal as opposed to when you restrict movement of the scapula. Repeat the same exercise, except this time hold the inferior angle of the scapula tightly against the chest wall while your partner medially rotates the humerus. Note the difference in total medial rotation possible when conditions are normal as opposed to when you restrict movement of the scapula.

6. The movements of the scapula in relation to the humerus can be explained by discussing the movement of the shoulder complex in its entirety. How does the position of the scapula affect shoulder joint abduction? How does the position of the scapula affect shoulder joint flexion?

7. Describe the bony articulations and movements specific to shoulder joint rotation during the acceleration phase of the throwing motion, and explain how an athlete can work toward increasing the velocity of the throw. What factors affect the velocity of the throw?

8. Using the information from this chapter and other resources, how would you strengthen the four different rotator cuff muscles? Give several examples of how they are used in everyday activities.

9. *Antagonistic muscle action chart:* Fill in the chart below by listing the muscle(s) or parts of muscles that are antagonistic in their actions to the muscles in the left column.

Agonist	Antagonist
Deltoid (anterior fibers)	
Deltoid (middle fibers)	
Deltoid (posterior fibers)	
Supraspinatus	
Subscapularis	
Teres major	
Infraspinatus/Teres minor	
Latissimus dorsi	
Pectoralis major (upper fibers)	
Pectoralis major (lower fibers)	
Coracobrachialis	

10. *Muscle analysis chart:* Fill in the chart below by listing the muscles primarily involved in each joint movement.

Shoulder Girdle		Shoulder Joint	
Upward rotation		Abduction	
Downward rotation		Adduction	
Depression		Extension	
Elevation		Flexion	
Abduction		Horizontal adduction	
		Internal rotation	
Adduction		Horizontal abduction	
		External rotation	

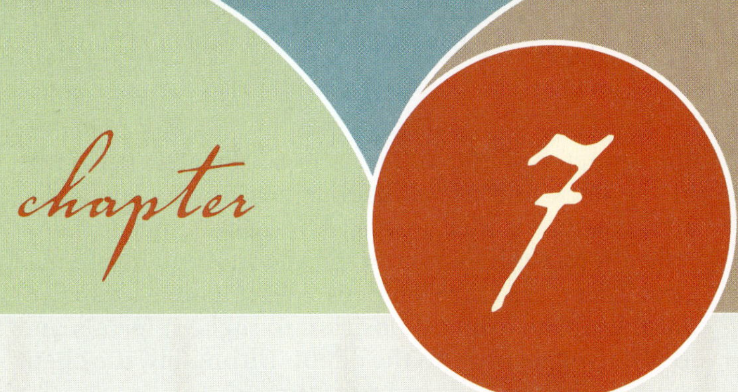

Deep-Tissue Techniques for the Shoulder Joint Muscles

LEARNING OUTCOMES

After completing this chapter, you should be able to:

7-1 Define key terms.

7-2 Name three stages of the inflammatory response.

7-3 List five signs and symptoms of the acute stage of the inflammatory response.

7-4 Demonstrate with a partner the active and passive movements of the muscles of the shoulder joint.

7-5 Identify the locations of the subdeltoid and subacromial bursae.

7-6 Describe and practice safe body mechanics.

7-7 Practice specific techniques on shoulder joint muscles.

7-8 Demonstrate appropriate supportive structures for side-lying positions.

7-9 Incorporate dimensional massage therapy techniques in a regular routine or use them when needed.

7-10 Determine safe treatment protocols and refer clients to other health professionals when necessary.

KEY TERMS

Active movement
Acute
Arc of pain
Bursae
Chronic
Crepitus
Passive movement
RICE
Somatic pain
Subacute

Introduction

There are so many muscles involved in the variety of shoulder movements that it is often difficult to see which muscle groups are most compromised in each soft-tissue problem. Occupational repetition, traumatic injury, and pathologic conditions add to this complex issue. For clients who do not have a diagnosis, it is best to follow the treatment protocol outlined in Chapter 5, starting with the client's medical history. This helps determine whether contraindications exist and enables the practitioner to have all the information necessary to create treatment goals. If any red flags arise, it is the practitioner's professional responsibility to refer the client to the appropriate health care provider because the client's welfare and benefit are the practitioner's top priorities.

Active and Passive Ranges of Movement

Aside from providing data for the medical history, clients have the ability to reveal a wealth of information about their condition; unfortunately, most do not. It is up to the practitioner to use critical thinking and to draw information out of the client by asking appropriate questions. Employing active and passive range-of-motion activities is useful to help determine more information about the client's soft-tissue problems.

The shoulder joint is the perfect location to explore how much active and passive movement the client is able to perform without pain or restriction. **Active movement** shortens muscles, as it contracts and pulls on the engaged bone. To determine active range of motion, the practitioner must first demonstrate the action for the client. The shoulder joint is complicated, as it is able to perform multiple actions. Thus, the practitioner should start with flexion of a nonpainful joint and then demonstrate the action and have the client replicate the movement. It is important to ask if the client feels any pain or restriction in the action and to take written notes if the client is compensating in the action by lifting the shoulder to complete the movement. Some useful information to document includes which muscles work together to complete flexion, as well as their antagonists. (See Chapter 6.) The practitioner should move through all the actions of the shoulder joint until he forms a clear evaluation of the client's range of motion. A soft-tissue problem could exist if pain or soreness is present during active movement.

Eliciting pain in passive motion is another issue altogether. **Passive movement** is action that does not shorten the soft tissues; there is no contraction and, therefore, no shortening. If pain is present during passive movement, probably some other structure around or within the joint is causing the complaint. Other involved structures include, but are not limited to, **bursae** (synovial sacs of fluid needed to lubricate joints), ligaments, joint capsules, cartilage, and nerves. If a client complains of pain during passive movement and has not been diagnosed, it is probably best to refer the client to another health care provider. That said, the soft tissue around a joint could benefit from the additional circulation of massage treatment, even if the problem is inside the joint. For the client's benefit, a holistic approach to the problem should involve more than one health care professional. For example, a client diagnosed with adhesive capsulitis could benefit from an orthopedic physician for diagnosis and clinical treatment, a physical therapist for determing degrees of motion and exercises, and a massage therapist to keep the involved soft tissue of the joint passively moving and circulated. A chiropractor might relieve the subluxated vertebrae in the neck and upper back, since movement in the area causes so much pain. An acupuncturist and/or reflexologist might encourage the movement of energies. There are many choices, and massage and manual therapists are in a position to make referrals and to offer suggestions to the client. Ultimately, the client must decide on a course of action.

To determine passive range of movement, the practitioner must move the joint into its range, starting with flexion and moving through all the actions of the joint. The practitioner should always demonstrate the passive movement first and, if possible, apply the passive movement to the shoulder joint that has no pain or problem. The client should then be asked if there is any pain during the movement. The practitioner may be able to feel restrictions, clicking, or crepitus in the joint. **Crepitus** is any grinding, grating, or popping elicited during the movement of the joint. Examples include the grinding of the head of the humerus if it hits the acromion in abduction and the movement of the scapula if it makes noises rubbing on the ribs. The practitioner should never force passive range and should move only within the comfort level of the client's range, taking note of the results of each passive movement.

Arc of Pain

An **arc of pain** is a pain response during a portion of active or passive movement. One example of an arc of pain occurs when a client abducts the humerus and does not feel pain until the arm is about 90 degrees abducted and then the pain subsides as the arm continues to move in abduction. In this example, the cause could be the acromion and the humerus interacting a bit too closely. Remember, the rotator cuff lines up on the greater tubercle of the humerus. If there is not enough room for the humerus to slide under the acromion in abduction, it might impinge the parts of the rotator cuff muscles. Additionally, there is a subacromion bursa that could be irritated by the close proximity of the humerus. Arcs of pain are noteworthy no matter what position the humerus is in.

Pain

Pain is a warning sign: It keeps clients awake at night; it keeps muscles in a constant state of tension, splinting joints that hurt when moved; and it provides a reason why so much money is spent on analgesics and narcotics. Pain is not necessarily reliable. Just because pain is felt in one area does not mean the root cause of the problem is in the same area. For example, nerves could be compressed by arthritis in the neck and cause a spiraling, lightninglike pain down the upper extremity.

The pronator teres could entrap the median nerve and cause carpal tunnel symptoms in the hand. Myofascial pain refers often to remote areas and may not be located at all in the vicinity of the problem. However, all pain should be noted, and questions must be asked to draw out complete information about its severity. Clients should be questioned about the *quality* of the pain, which may be described as:

- Shooting or burning
- Numbness or tingling
- A dull ache
- Superficial or deep
- Deep in the joint
- Radiating
- Hurting in one spot

There is a difference between compressed nerve pain and somatic pain. Pain from muscles, skin, and joints is called **somatic pain**. *Compressed nerve pain* is often of the shooting, radiating, or burning variety, whereas somatic pain can range from dull ache to deep joint pain. Some pain or discomfort may not be expressed until the therapist finds a sore area or attachment. The therapist must take care and use caution when palpating areas of concern to prevent irritating painful attachments, tendons, or soft tissue. Undiagnosed pain in and of itself is enough to constitute the need for a referral.

Acute, Subacute, and Chronic

There are three stages of the inflammatory response, which are commonly referred to as **acute, subacute,** and **chronic.** The acute stage has all the signs and symptoms of inflammation: redness, heat, swelling, pain, and loss of function. The acute stage is the most common arena of contraindications. A person who sprains her ankle experiences immediate swelling, pain, and lack of motion. Additionally, bruising and heat are readily apparent. When this occurs, the client needs to apply the rescue recipe of **RICE:** rest, ice, compression, and elevation. Massage would be contraindicated for the ankle until it is in a chronic stage.

The subacute stage has the same signs and symptoms as those of the acute stage with the exception that none of the signs or symptoms are worsening. Swelling has reached a peak; it may not have diminished, but it is not getting worse. The client may still have to use ice on the ankle to lessen the existing swelling and to help reduce discomfort. The bruising is very obvious, and putting weight on the foot may not be an option.

The chronic stage of pain might also have signs of the inflammatory process, but the symptoms have significantly decreased to manageable levels. Swelling subsides; pain is reasonable, if not gone; and the ankle and foot may be able to manage some weight bearing. The massage therapist sees most clients in the chronic stage of injury. Some of these clients have been in chronic pain for months or years.

It is important for the massage therapist to think about the stages of inflammation when clients present with injuries, especially if the client appears to be hopping or otherwise incapacitated. Levels of pain must be examined for possible referrals. Shoulder joint and capsule injuries, rotator cuff conditions, bursa pathologies, and tendonitis and/or tendonosis all share stages of the inflammatory process. Therapists must take careful medical histories and proceed with caution, even keeping a pathology text nearby for reference when necessary.

More Synergy

The close relationship between the shoulder girdle and shoulder joint reflects a dependency that needs to be examined to develop an effective and reasonable treatment goal. Chapter 5 introduced techniques for the shoulder girdle muscles. It is important to start with the shoulder girdle because the muscles that act on the clavicle and scapula are foundational to the shoulder joint. Chapters 4 and 6 determined that there exists a certain synergy between the shoulder girdle and the shoulder joint. The humerus hangs off the scapula perilously and must depend on the muscles and ligaments to prevent force, momentum, and direction from dislocating the joint. The muscles have to oppose each other to stop the action, add another action, and stabilize the joint all at the same time. The shoulder girdle muscles provide stability for the shoulder joint and therefore often share the pain and soreness of the soft-tissue problem. Therapists could compare the soft tissue to unwinding a ball of twine. Generally, a person would not start in the center of the ball to unravel the twine. Instead, he would start at the easiest location and work inward, unwinding as the ball got smaller. This is also a good approach for soft-tissue work—palpating first and then progressively unwinding. Therapists should start on the foundational shoulder girdle muscles and work out to the shoulder joint, working opposing muscles to create balance as the process continues. Additionally, the muscles will respond better if the joint is treated as a whole instead of in pieces. It is important to remember that massage is a conservative approach to health care and benefits the client in a natural process. Although the tissues might soften or release, the process of circulation will continue after the area has been worked. This is the body's natural response.

The side-lying shoulder posture is useful in a variety of circumstances, especially if the client cannot lay supine or prone on the table. Pregnancy after the first trimester prohibits the prone position; thus side-lying is the obvious alternative. Shoulder injuries, specifically adhesive capsulitis, benefit from the passive movement of the side-lying position. Therapists should practice using this position frequently so that they will feel comfortable providing support to the client with pillows and draping. Shoulder techniques discussed in this chapter utilize the side-lying position.

Dimensional Massage Therapy for the Shoulder Joint Muscles

SIDE-LYING SHOULDER POSITION AND SEQUENCE

Working with an individual in a side-lying position provides a unique opportunity to access muscles and areas denied by the usual supine and prone positions. Passive movement of the shoulder region is accessible in this position. Adjusting table height for side-lying techniques may be necessary; the table may need to be slightly lower, as a person on her side will be higher on the table than she would be in the supine position. Therapists should not sacrifice proper body mechanics in regard to table height or the side-lying position.

Make sure the client is comfortable, with enough support to make the side-lying position worth the extra effort. Support the head with a small pillow or rolled towel, and place a pillow or bolster under the superior knee and thigh to maintain a flexed-knee position. Straighten the inferior lower extremity. Try to keep the client's neck and spine fairly straight on the table and not collapsed forward in the trunk region. The head and neck need to be in alignment with the spine. Prop a pillow under the superior extremity to help prevent the client from moving into a fetal position and out of a side-lying posture.

Draping can often be a challenge in the side-lying position. Use a twin sheet and a few extra towels if necessary. The pillow under the superior upper extremity often helps with draping, especially on a female client.

The following techniques can be used entirely as a sequence and, when used wisely, also can be incorporated into other treatment sequences. Remember to:

- Always use treatment protocols to determine the sequence of a therapeutic session.
- Palpate soft tissue.
- Use warm-up techniques first, and determine the appropriate pressure.
- Passively shorten the muscles whenever possible.
- Follow a dimensional approach, and critically think about the involved joints and kinetic chain.
- Work on healthy soft tissue and joints first; work on painful areas or those with restricted motion last.

Elliptical Movement of the Shoulder

Assist the client with the side-lying position, and stand facing the client at the shoulder region. Lift the superior upper extremity, and drape it over your forearm closest to the client's feet. Place your inferior hand on the client's teres major–latissimus area. Take your other hand and position it on the supraspinatus–upper trapezius region. Slowly, passively move the whole shoulder in an alternating clockwise and then counterclockwise motion. (See figure 7.1.)

Middle Trapezius Petrissage

With the client in the same side-lying position and using the same support for the client's arm, grasp the middle trapezius with the fingers of your superior hand moving between the scapula and the spine and your thumb on the ventral side of the trapezius. Using your inferior hand, push the shoulder superiorly to further access the middle trapezius. Petrissage the middle trapezius. (See figure 7.2.)

Upper Trapezius Petrissage

Using the same position as above, grasp the upper trapezius with your superior hand and petrissage the muscle. Bring the whole shoulder toward the head to passively shorten the upper trapezius a bit more while you are massaging the muscle. (See figure 7.3.)

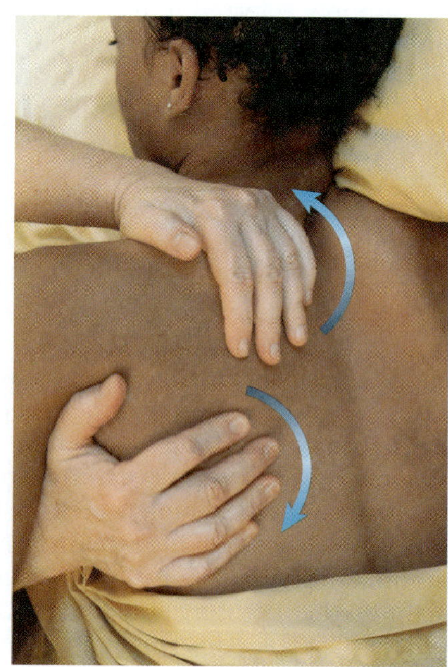

FIGURE 7.1 Elliptical movement of the shoulder

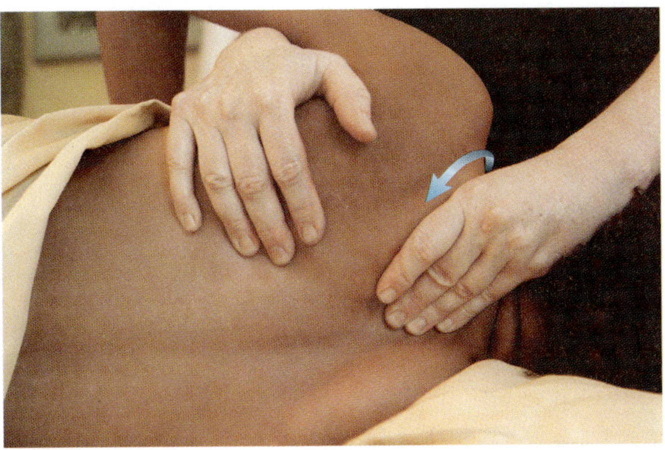

FIGURE 7.2 Middle trapezius petrissage

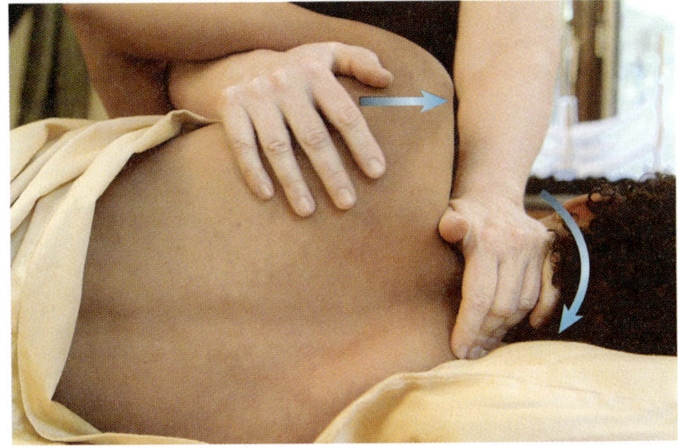

FIGURE 7.3 Upper trapezius petrissage

Upper and Middle Trapezius Myofascial Stretch

Using the same position as above, position your superior hand on the upper trapezius; straddle the spine by bracing your thumb on one side and your fingers on the other side. While bracing your thumb, gently draw the tissues over the spine toward you. Start as close to the occiput as possible, and move inferiorly toward C7. (See figure 7.4.) Apply the same procedure to the middle trapezius. (See figure 7.5.)

Open the Scapula

Using the same position as above, mobilize the scapula so that you can curl your fingers around the vertebral border. Jiggle and move the shoulder so that you can have better access to the area. (See figure 7.6.)

Locate the Supraspinatus Trigger Point

Locate the acromioclavicular joint. With your superior hand, place your thumb on the supraspinatus closest to the AC joint. Bring the shoulder superior

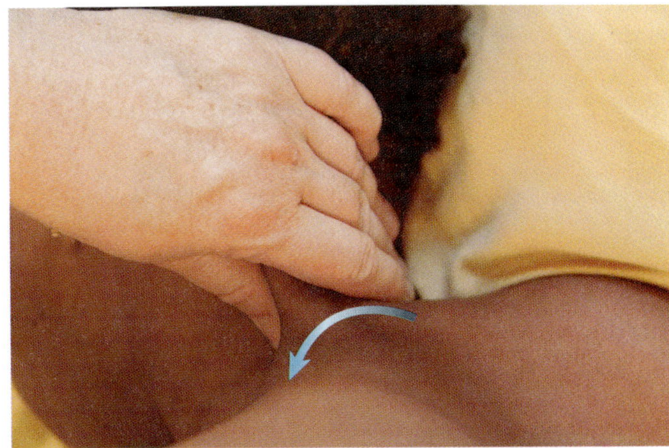

FIGURE 7.4 Upper trapezius myofascial stretch

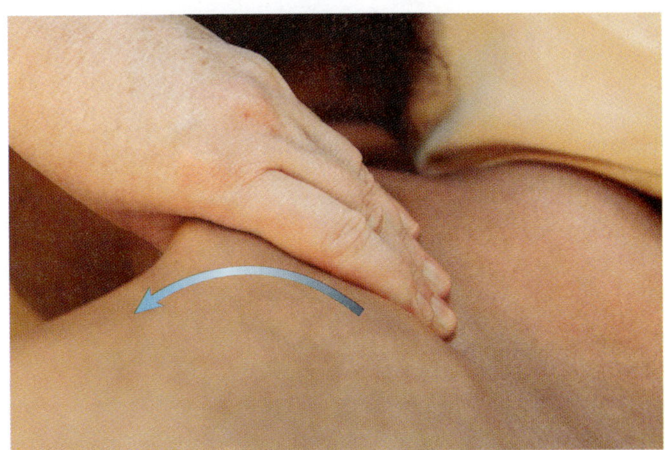

FIGURE 7.5 Middle trapezius myofascial stretch

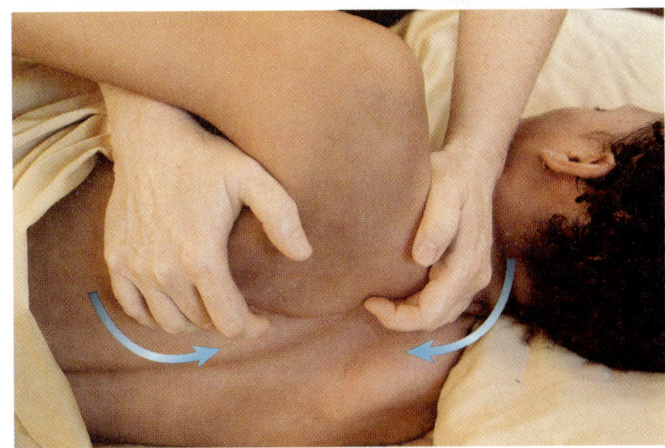

FIGURE 7.6 Opening the scapula

with your other supportive forearm-hand combination. Apply ischemic pressure, and check with the client for feedback about discomfort levels. Only apply pressure for 7 to 10 seconds. Stretch the surrounding tissue after release. (See figure 7.7.)

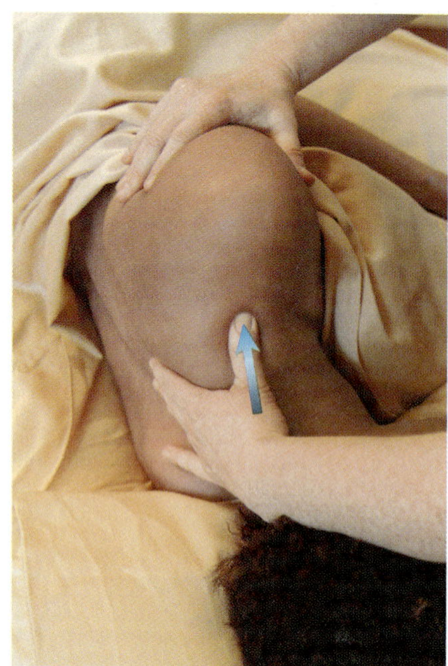

FIGURE 7.7 Supraspinatus trigger point

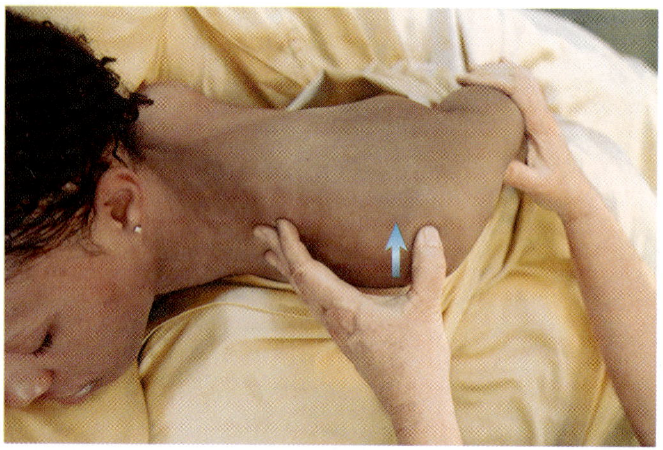

FIGURE 7.8 Supraspinatus tendon

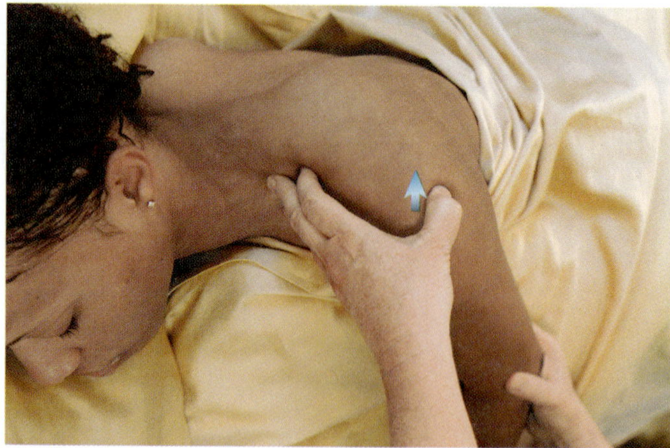

FIGURE 7.9 Infraspinatus tendon

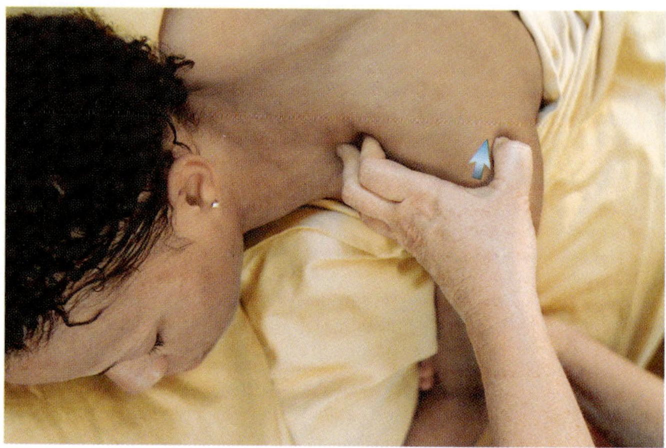

FIGURE 7.10 Teres minor tendon

Deep Transverse Friction of the Rotator Cuff Tendons

Remember that you will be palpating through the deltoid when you are locating the rotator cuff tendons. Position the client's arm behind the back to locate the supraspinatus tendon on the superior facet of the greater tubercle; the head of the humerus rolls out from under the acromion in this position. Locate the tendon and apply deep transverse friction or circular friction to it. (See figure 7.8.) To locate the infraspinatus tendon, drop the arm down in front of the client. Locate the middle facet of the greater tubercle and the infraspinatus tendon. Apply deep transverse friction or circular friction to it. (See figure 7.9.) For teres minor, draw the arm a bit more forward, and locate the tendon on the inferior facet of the greater tubercle; apply deep transverse friction or circular friction. (See figure 7.10.) The subscapularis is located on the lesser tubercle anteriorly. Position the client's arm behind the back, and locate the coracoid process. The subscapularis tendon will be between the coracoid process and the lesser tubercle. Apply deep transverse friction or circular friction to the tendon. (See figure 7.11.)

Compression of the Teres Major

Face the table and hold the client's arm with your superior hand as you compress with the inferior hand. Angle your hand to compress the muscle into the axillary border of the scapula. There will be a slight one-two motion as you compress the muscle and slightly pull on the arm at the same time. Repeat several times. (See figure 7.12.)

Compression and Myofascial Pull of the Latissimus Dorsi

Repeat as above with compression on the latissimus. Place your thumb under the lip of the latissimus just below the axillary region. With your fingers, pull the teres major and latissimus over your thumb. (See figure 7.12.)

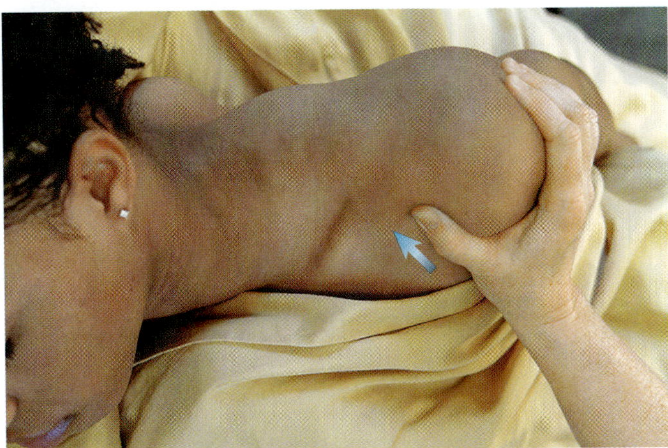

FIGURE 7.11 Subscapularis tendon

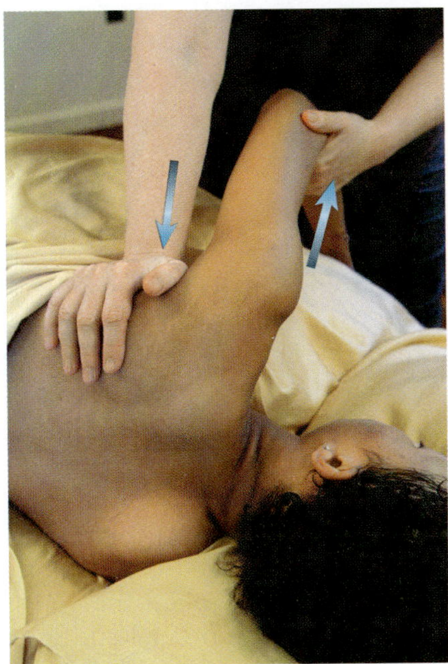

FIGURE 7.12 Compression of the teres major

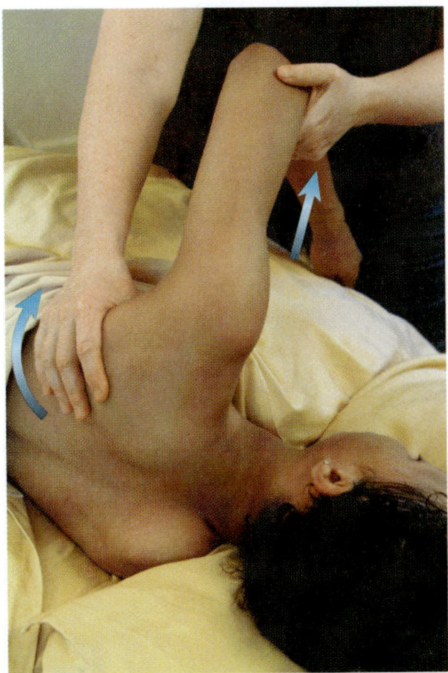

FIGURE 7.13 Serratus anterior access

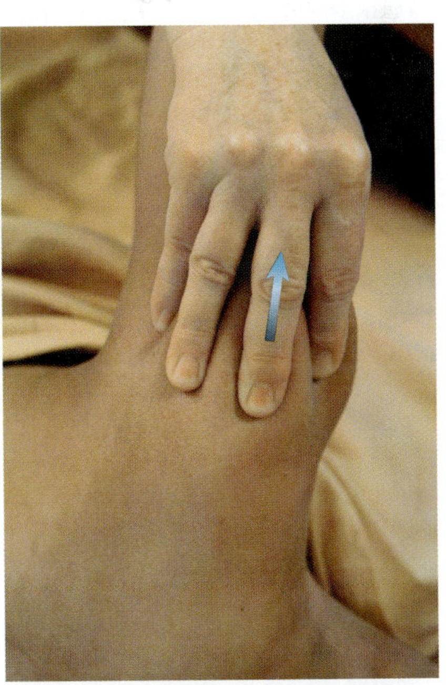

FIGURE 7.14 Jostling the deltoids

Serratus Anterior Access

Hold the client's arm at the elbow joint with your superior hand as you face the table. Slide your thumb anterior to the scapula in the axillary region. Access the serratus anterior fibers on the ribs. Pin the fibers and gently pull the arm toward you. This process will give you access to apply ischemic pressure to the fibers of the serratus anterior. Ask the client for feedback, as this area may be very tender. Adjust your pressure. Hold for a short period of time, and then try to move to a different place on the fibers. (See figure 7.13.)

Jostle the Deltoids

Assist the client with the side-lying position, flex the arm, and hold the arm at the elbow joint. With your other hand, grasp the deltoid (anterior, posterior, and middle), stretch slightly, and jostle it from origin to insertion. Repeat several times. (See figure 7.14.)

Side-Lying Stretch of the Upper Extremity

In the over-the-head position, stretch the upper extremity and place one hand on the ribs while pulling with the elbow joint. This will effectively stretch the serratus anterior, external oblique, and posterior deltoid. (See figure 7.15.)

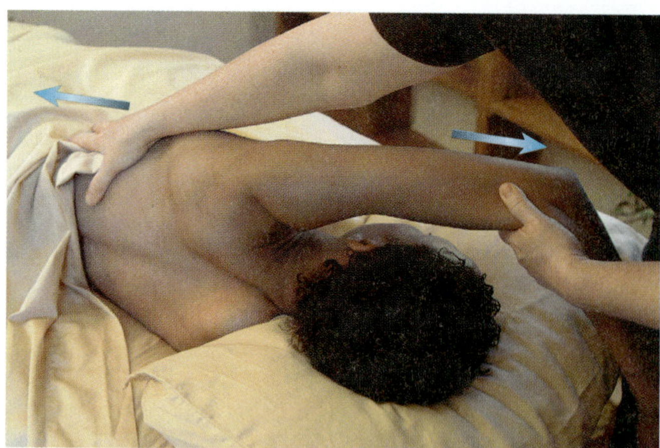

FIGURE 7.15 Side-lying stretch of the upper extremity

SUPINE POSITION

Pectoralis Major Compression

Standing next to the client at the side of the table, place your hand closest to the client on the pectoralis major. Your fingers should drape over the anterior deltoid without pressure. Hold the client's arm at about 90 degrees from his body. Compress the pectoralis major while you pull the arm at the wrist away from the body. To prevent irritating the subdeltoid bursa, be careful not to compress the anterior deltoid. (See figure 7.16.)

Pectoralis Major Jostling and Stretch

Place your hand on the pectoralis major with your fingers on the ventral side of the muscle and your thumb in the axillary region. Slightly stretch and jostle the muscle. (See figure 7.17.) For a myofascial stretch, position your hand in the same manner as above. Instead of jostling, pull the tissues from the clavicle toward the axillary region. Two hands can also be used on a larger pectoralis major.

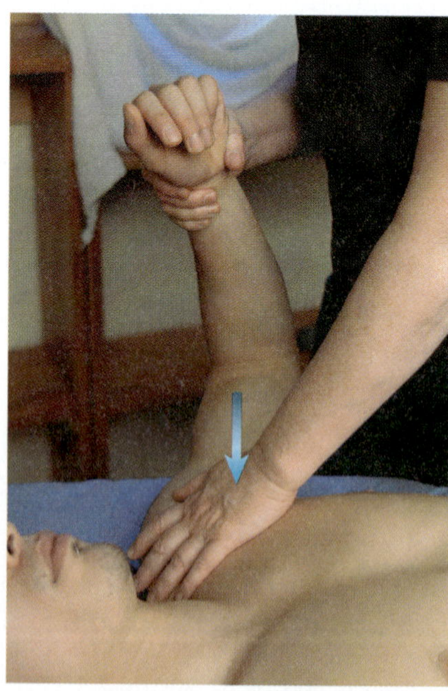

FIGURE 7.16 Pectoralis major compression

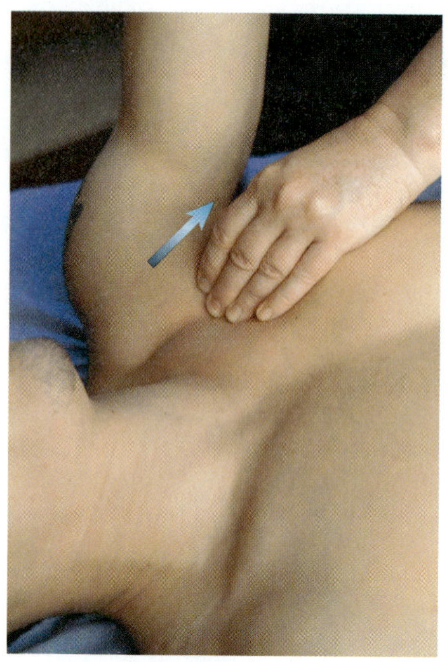

FIGURE 7.17 Jostling and stretching the pectoralis major

Elliptical Movement of the Pectoralis Major

Lift the upper extremity with your outside hand at the wrist. Place the fingers of your inside hand on the pectoralis major and your thumb in the axillary region. Now that you have gentle access, place the upper extremity on the table and join your other hand in a like position. Gently grasp the muscle and alternately move the pectoralis major in a clockwise and then counterclockwise movement. (See figure 7.18.) Stretching from the clavicle can follow this technique as well.

Deep Transverse Friction and Circular Friction for Pectoralis Major Attachments

Locate the clavicular head of the pectoralis major. Apply deep transverse friction and/or circular friction just below the clavicle at the attachments. (See figure 7.19.) Repeat to the sternal attachments. (See figure 7.20.) For a female client, you may need to work over a towel on sternal attachments.

Unwind the Twine

Stand at a right angle to the table, facing the client's head. Pick up the client's wrist with your outside hand, and lift the upper extremity into flexion. Grasp the strings of the humeral attachment of the pectoralis major with your

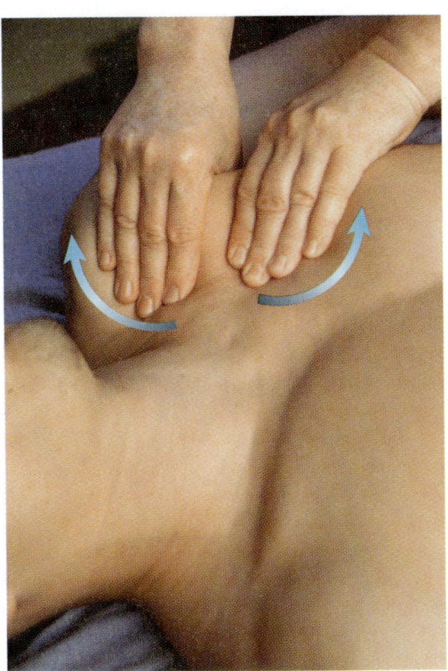

FIGURE 7.18 Elliptical movement of the pectoralis major

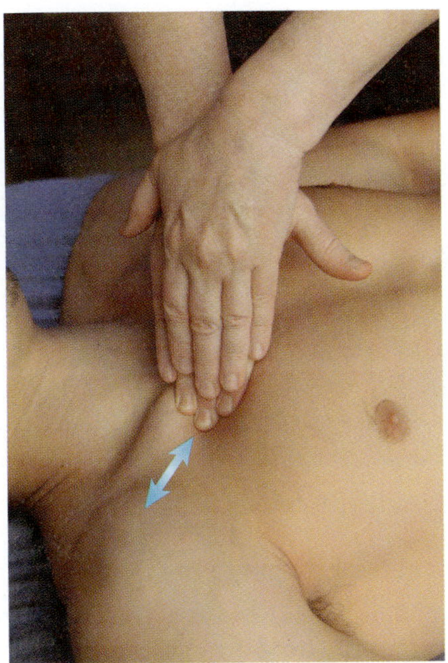

FIGURE 7.19 Clavicular attachments

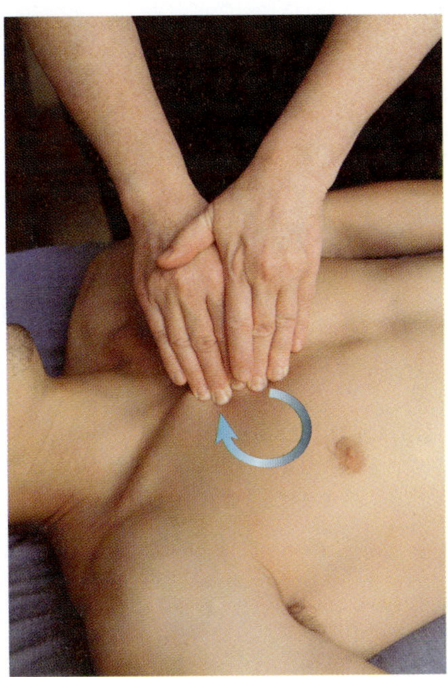

FIGURE 7.20 Sternal attachments

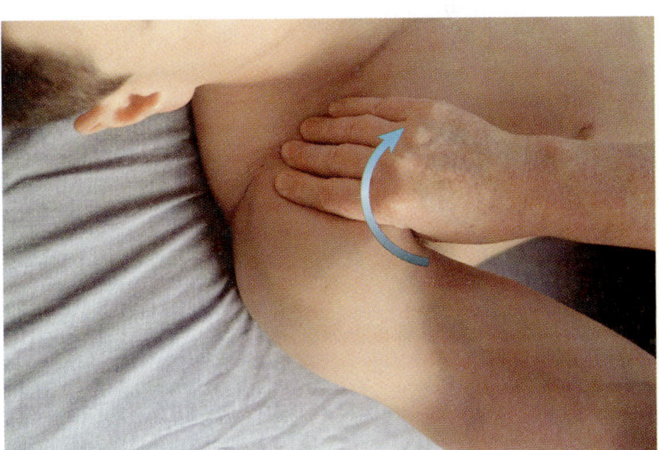

FIGURE 7.21 Unwinding the twine

thumb, and place your forefingers on the anterior muscle mass. Draw your grasping fingers and thumb from distal to proximal along the fibers of the attachments while moving the arm in a horizontal abduction movement, passively stretching the fibers. (See figure 7.21.)

Strip the Coracobrachialis

Pick up the client's arm at the elbow, and hold it over the trunk at a right angle (horizontal adduction). Locate the coracoid process with your hand that is closest to the body. Palpate the coracobrachialis from the coracoid process to the humeral attachment. Locate the coracobrachialis underneath the pectoralis major and anterior deltoid. Slightly strip as much of the muscle as possible. It will be tender. Be careful of the brachial plexus, and work in cooperation with your client. (See figure 7.22.)

Subscapularis

Locate the sore points, and apply circular friction to the fibers. Standing next to the supine client, grasp the client's arm above the elbow with your superior hand. Bring the arm out to about 90 degrees laterally in an abducted position. Place your inferior fingers under the scapula and your thumb in the axillary region. The client's forearm will rest over the forearm of the hand that is in position to work

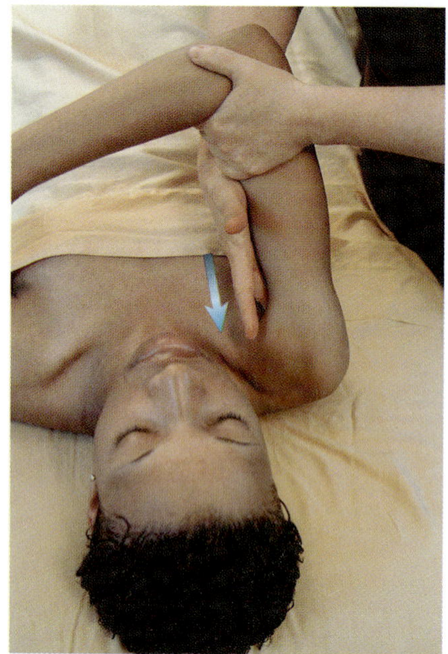

FIGURE 7.22 Stripping the coracobrachialis

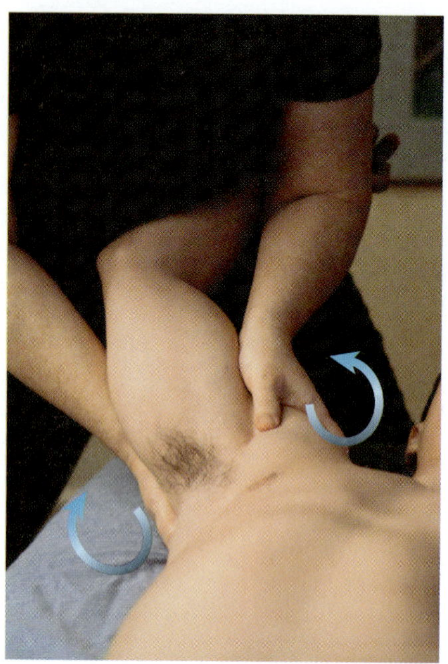

FIGURE 7.24 Elliptical movement of the deltoids

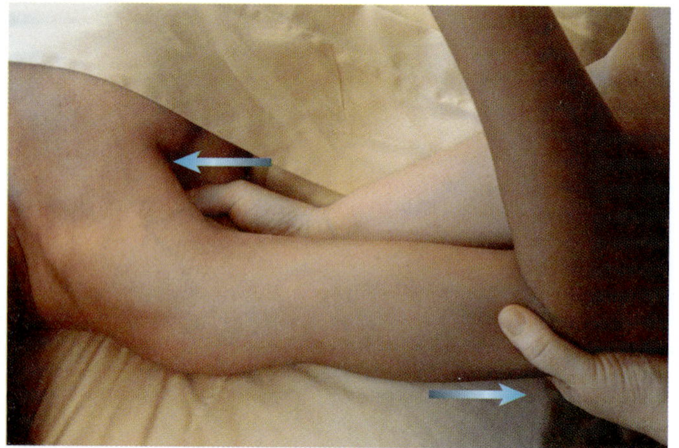

FIGURE 7.23 Subscapularis

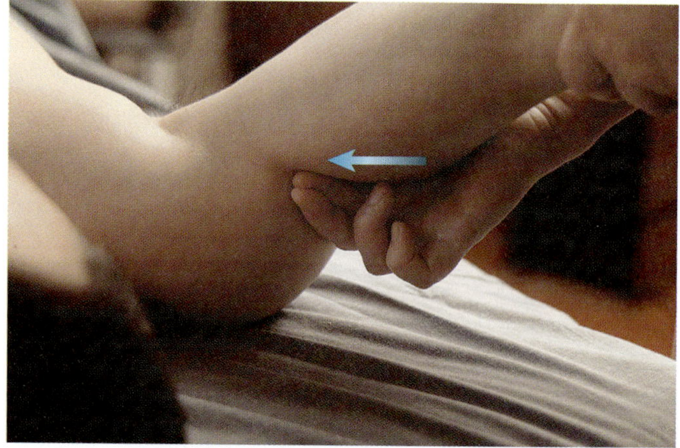

FIGURE 7.25 Deep transverse friction to the deltoid tuberosity

the subscapularis. Locate the anterior scapula with your thumb. Apply pressure on sore points and fibers. Be aware that this area may be very tender, so make sure to work with the client and elicit feedback. (See figure 7.23.)

Elliptical Movement of the Deltoids

Perform an over-the-head stretch. Standing next to the client, facing her head, place your inside hand on the shoulder, and pick up the wrist with your outside hand. Take a step and pivot at the end of the table. Switch hands so that you are now holding the arm with both hands on either side of the shoulder joint. The elbow can be tucked in at your waist. In this position, grasp the deltoid on both sides of the muscle. Gently but firmly alternate moving the muscle in a clockwise and counterclockwise motion. (See figure 7.24.)

Deep Transverse Friction to the Deltoid Tuberosity

Locate the deltoid tuberosity, the insertion of the deltoids, and apply deep transverse friction to the attachment. (See figure 7.25.) Apply circular friction to the origins on the clavicle, acromion, and spine of the scapula.

Rock and Roll the Deltoids

Roll the deltoids around the humerus, and petrissage the muscles alternately. (See figure 7.26.)

Stretch the Deltoids

Cradle the client's arm over the top of the head in hyperflexion for the humeral tease stretch. Hold one hand under the shoulder joint and one hand on the client's flexed elbow joint. Instead of just stretching, alternate

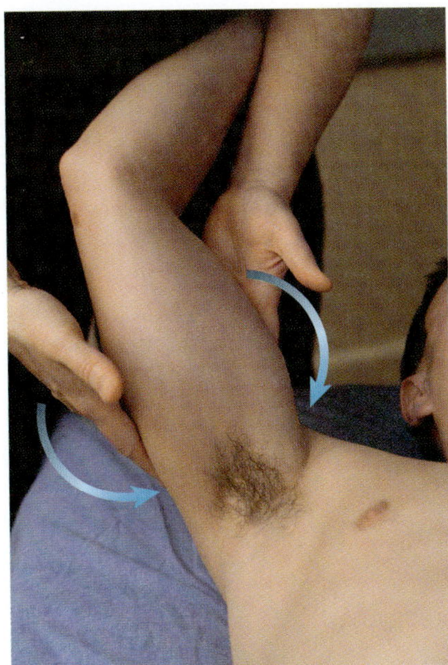

FIGURE 7.26 Rocking and rolling the deltoids

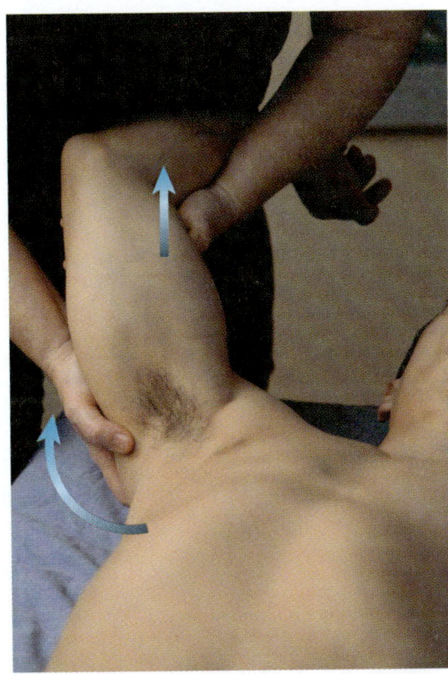

FIGURE 7.27 Humeral tease stretch

stretching and relaxing the shoulder joint in hyperflexion in a bit of an arc. Move the entire joint. (See figure 7.27.) Place your inferior hand under the scapula. Hold the client's upper extremity at the elbow joint, and draw the arm across the body. (See figure 7.28a.) Circle the head with the upper extremity, and place your forearm on the table. Brace the client's arm next to your forearm; pull laterally using the hand underneath the scapula and the hand holding the elbow joint. (See figure 7.28b.) Your hand will slide out from underneath the scapula; slide down the upper extremity distally with your other hand. (See figure 7.28c.)

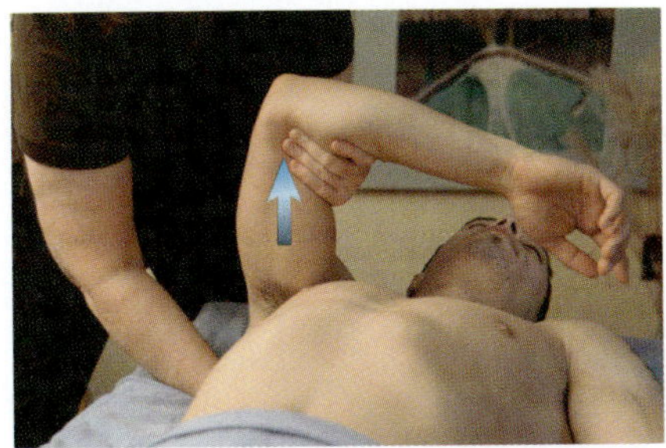

FIGURE 7.28a Stretching to the side, step 1

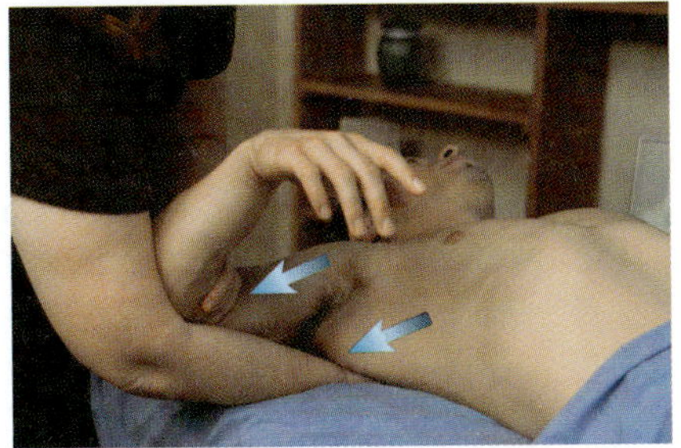

FIGURE 7.28b Stretching to the side, step 2

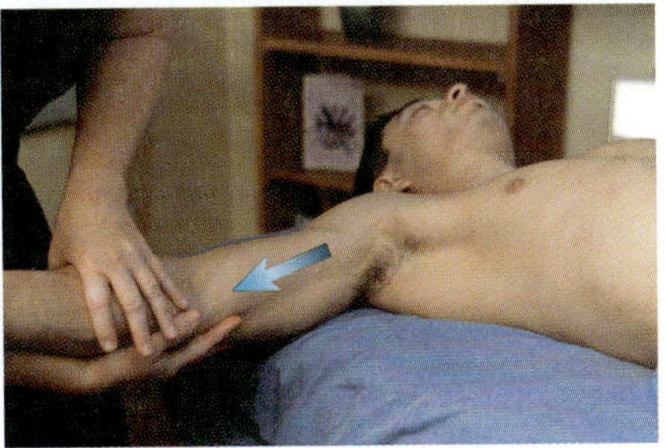

FIGURE 7.28c Stretching to the side, finish

PRONE

Latissimus Dorsi

Always work the "good" side first as a means of comparison and for the client's psychological preparation. Generally, stretch the fibers of the latissimus toward its humeral attachment. Finishing strokes can be done bilaterally, but most detail work is done unilaterally. Perform deep effleurage from the lower back to the axillary region. Apply circular friction on the aponeurosis attachments. Petrissage the muscle. Use elliptical motion with the muscle and myofascial stretches. Remember the interdigitation of the external oblique and the latissimus dorsi and the close proximity of serratus anterior. Locate potential short areas at these attachments, and stretch the tissues. Drag your fingers through the lower ribs for the attachments. Vibration along the spinal attachments addresses taut fibers.

Pictures and additional descriptions for back muscle techniques are included in Chapter 16, "Deep Tissue of the Low Back and Posterior Pelvis."

CHAPTER summary

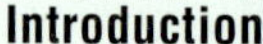

Introduction

- ✔ For clients who do not have a diagnosis, it is best to follow the treatment protocol, starting with the client's medical history. This helps determine whether contraindications exist and enables the practitioner to have all the information necessary to create treatment goals.

Active and Passive Ranges of Movement

- ✔ Active movement is the range of motion of a particular joint that is performed by the client.
- ✔ Passive movement is the range of motion of a particular joint that the practitioner administers to the client, who does not participate in the action.
- ✔ The therapist should demonstrate the action, whether active or passive, on an unrestricted pain-free side first. Then she should complete the activity and get feedback from the client.
- ✔ Pain or restriction in active movements often can be soft-tissue dysfunction.
- ✔ Pain or restriction in passive movements can involve structures that are not soft tissue. They include, but are not limited to, joint capsules, nerves, ligaments, bursae, and cartilage.
- ✔ Undiagnosed clients with pain and/or restriction in passive movement should be referred to the appropriate health care professional.
- ✔ Restrictions in the joint sometimes make noise called crepitus.

Arc of Pain

- ✔ An arc of pain is a pain response that is positive in a portion of the range of motion.
- ✔ Any positive pain response should be noted in the medical history and SOAP notes.

Pain

- ✔ Somatic pain is pain from muscles, skin, and joints.
- ✔ Nerve pain may come from bony compression or soft-tissue entrapment.
- ✔ The severity of pain can be described by the client on the basis of how it feels, including burning, radiating, dull, achy, superficial, deep, numbness, or tingling.
- ✔ All pain must be noted and is a reason for referral.

Acute, Subacute, and Chronic

- ✔ There are three stages of the inflammation response: acute, subacute, and chronic.
- ✔ Acute has all the signs and symptoms of inflammation: redness, heat, pain, swelling, and loss of function.
- ✔ Subacute also may have all the signs and symptoms of inflammation, but the swelling has reached a zenith and is not increasing.
- ✔ Chronic may still have signs of inflammation but does not have the intensity of acute or subacute. Signs and symptoms diminish in chronic. The chronic stage may last months or years in some cases.

More Synergy

- ✔ The shoulder joint relies on the shoulder girdle for support, attachment, and muscular cooperation.
- ✔ It is important to treat the shoulder girdle muscles first.

Dimensional Massage Therapy for the Shoulder Joint Muscles

- ✔ Always use treatment protocols to determine the sequence of a therapeutic session.
- ✔ Use warm-up techniques first, and determine pressure intelligently.
- ✔ Follow a dimensional approach, and critically think about the involved joints and kinetic chain.
- ✔ Try the supine position first to efficiently prepare neck and shoulder muscles for further work.
- ✔ The side-lying posture works well for accessing the shoulder joint.
- ✔ Prone techniques assist with further unwinding of the shoulder girdle and shoulder joint muscles.

CHAPTER review

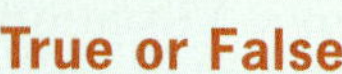

True or False

Write true *or* false *after each statement.*

1. *Bursa* is another name for *ligament*.
2. An arc of pain begins and ends with the same constant pain.
3. Somatic pain is nerve pain.
4. Nerve pain can be suspected if the client is complaining of radiating, burning pain.
5. Medical history, interview, and SOAP notes help determine whether there are any contraindications.

6. It is always safe to massage someone with an acute condition.
7. The joint capsule is a structure that could cause pain in passive movement.
8. Compression of the pectoralis major should be done carefully to avoid irritating the subdeltoid bursa.
9. For side-lying techniques, the therapist should raise the table to maintain good body mechanics.
10. Elliptical movement of the shoulder is a passive movement.

Short Answers

Write your answers on the lines provided.

1. List the muscles of the shoulder joint.

____

____

____

2. Why would there be pain in active movements and not in passive movements?

____

____

____

3. What structures might cause pain in passive movement?

____

____

____

4. Why would a therapist refer a client experiencing pain during passive movement to an appropriate health care provider?

____

____

____

5. What is crepitus?

____

____

____

6. What function does a bursa perform?

____

____

____

7. List the signs and symptoms of the inflammatory process.

____

____

____

8. What are the three stages of the inflammatory process?

____

____

____

9. What should a therapist do if a client literally hopped into the office and claimed that he had just sprained his ankle? Should the therapist give the client a massage?

____

____

____

10. What is the difference between somatic pain and compressed nerve pain?

____

____

____

Multiple Choice

Circle the correct answers.

1. The first step in conducting an active range-of-motion test is:
   a. to demonstrate the action
   b. to tell the client to flex the muscle
   c. to lift the joint without the help of the client
   d. none of the above
2. Pain is:
   a. to be ignored in the client
   b. overrated
   c. a warning sign
   d. always a contraindication

3. An arc of pain:
   a. is a pain response that is positive in a portion of the range of motion
   b. hurts during the entire range of motion
   c. goes away as soon as there is range of motion
   d. none of the above
4. The signs and symptoms of the acute stage of the inflammatory process include:
   a. only swelling
   b. only pain
   c. heat, pain, swelling, loss of function, and redness
   d. only loss of function
5. In an acute sprained shoulder, the signs and symptoms would include:
   a. heat, redness, and pain
   b. heat, redness, pain, swelling, and loss of function
   c. heat, redness, and swelling
   d. no heat or redness, just swelling
6. A client who cannot lie in the supine or prone position can be positioned:
   a. upright
   b. side-lying
   c. comfortably in the supine only
   d. none of the above
7. The practitioner may often have to __________ the table for side-lying clients.
   a. raise
   b. do nothing to
   c. lower
   d. bolster
8. Chronic pain can last for:
   a. 48 hours only
   b. 72 hours only
   c. years
   d. 24 hours only
9. The only difference between acute and subacute is:
   a. 24 hours
   b. pain is no longer present
   c. no difference
   d. the swelling is no longer increasing but has leveled off
10. The quality of pain could be described as:
    a. burning
    b. radiating, numbness, or tingling
    c. dull, achy, superficial, deep
    d. all of the above
11. The practitioner should investigate the state of the muscles of the __________ before working on the shoulder joint.
    a. shoulder girdle
    b. abdomen
    c. lower back
    d. lower extremities

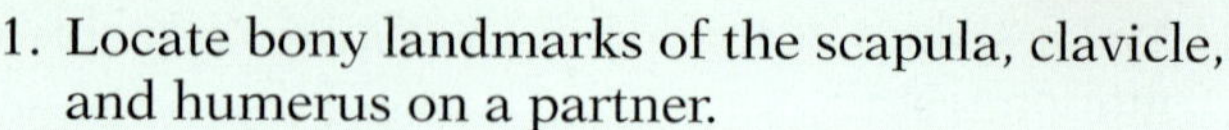

EXPLORE & *practice*

1. Locate bony landmarks of the scapula, clavicle, and humerus on a partner.
2. Locate the origin and insertions of the shoulder joint muscles on a partner.
3. Locate the rotator cuff on a partner.
4. Demonstrate how to passively shorten muscles of the shoulder joint in the side-lying position.
5. Demonstrate some principles of safe body mechanics while performing massage techniques.
6. Demonstrate active and passive movements of the shoulder joint with a partner.
7. Practice supine-position deep-tissue techniques individually and in a sequence on a willing participant.
8. Demonstrate placing a partner in a side-lying position on a table with the correct table height and support for the individual.
9. Demonstrate appropriate draping techniques for the side-lying position. Please refer to pictures in the text depicting appropriate draping techniques.

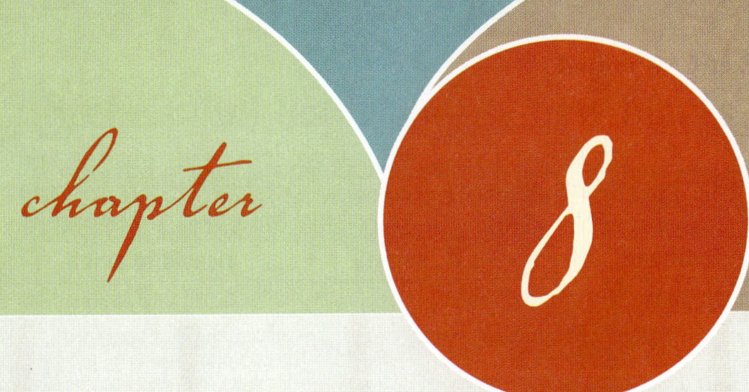

The Elbow and Radioulnar Joints

LEARNING OUTCOMES

After completing this chapter, you should be able to:

8-1 Define key terms.

8-2 Locate on a human skeleton all bony landmarks of the elbow and radioulnar joints.

8-3 Label on a skeletal chart all bony landmarks of the elbow and radioulnar joints.

8-4 Draw and identify the muscles of the elbow and radioulnar joints on a skeletal chart.

8-5 Palpate the muscles of the elbow and radioulnar joints on a partner.

8-6 Explore the origins and insertions of the muscles of the elbow and radioulnar joints on a partner.

8-7 Organize and list the agonists, antagonists, and synergists of the elbow and radioulnar joints.

8-8 Demonstrate with a fellow student all the active and passive movements of the elbow and radioulnar joints.

8-9 Practice basic stretching and strengthening appropriate for the elbow and radioulnar joints.

KEY TERMS

Anconeus
Biceps brachii
Brachialis
Brachioradialis
Elbow joint
Median nerve
Musculocutaneous nerve
Pronator quadratus
Pronator teres
Radial nerve
Radioulnar joint
Radius
Supinator
Triceps brachii
Ulna

Introduction

Almost every upper-extremity movement involves the elbow and radioulnar joints. Repetitive action could be said to originate in the elbow joint region, as most muscles that control the hand and wrist have attachments there. Using a screwdriver, turning a doorknob, or dragging products over a supermarket scanner require the unique mechanism of supination and pronation made possible by the radioulnar pivot joint. Coupled with its ability to flex the forearms, the upper extremity has a dynamic range of motion available to perform many complex movements.

This text has grouped the elbow and radioulnar joints together because of their close anatomical relationship. The **elbow joint** is formed by the ulna articulating with the humerus; the radius pivots with the ulna to form the **radioulnar joint.** Under close inspection, elbow joint movements are clearly distinguishable as flexion and extension. Radioulnar joint actions include supination and pronation, also known as *radioulnar internal rotation* and *external rotation,* respectively. These movements are quite different from those of the hand and wrist. The wrist is a condyloid joint that is capable of flexion, extension, abduction, and adduction. There is no rotary movement that takes place at the wrist. Students can avoid confusing these joint functions by isolating the movements and studying them one at a time.

Bones

The **ulna** is much larger proximally than the **radius,** but distally the radius is much larger than the ulna (figure 8.1). The scapula and humerus serve as the proximal attachments for the muscles that flex and extend the elbow. The ulna and radius serve as the distal attachments for the same muscles. The scapula, humerus, and ulna serve as proximal attachments for the muscles that pronate and supinate the radioulnar joints. The distal attachments of the radioulnar joint muscles are located on the radius.

The medial condyloid ridge, olecranon process, coronoid process, and radial tuberosity are important bony landmarks for these muscles. Additionally, the medial epicondyle, lateral epicondyle, and lateral supracondylar ridge are key bony landmarks for the wrist and hand muscles, which are discussed in Chapter 10.

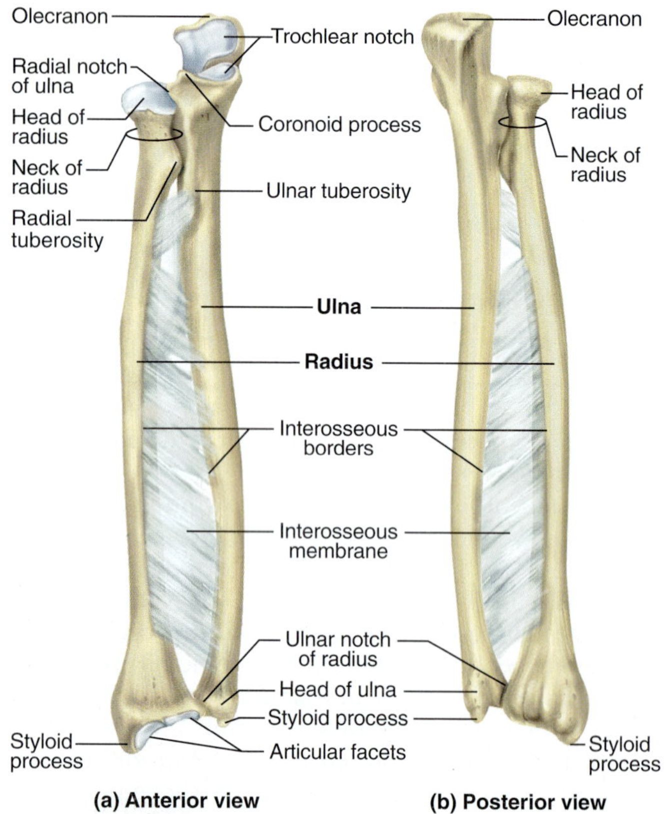

FIGURE 8.1 Radius and ulna

Joints

The elbow joint is classified as a *ginglymus* or *hinge-type* joint that allows only flexion and extension. The elbow may actually be thought of as two interrelated joints: the humeroulnar and the radiohumeral joints (figures 8.2 and 8.3). Elbow motions primarily involve movement between the articular surfaces of the humerus and the ulna—specifically, the humeral trochlea fitting into the trochlear notch of the ulna. The head of the radius has a relatively small amount of contact with the capitulum of the humerus. As the elbow reaches full extension, the olecranon process of the ulna is received by the olecranon fossa of the humerus. This arrangement provides increased joint stability when the elbow is fully extended.

As the elbow flexes approximately 20 degrees or more, its bony stability is somewhat unlocked, allowing for more side-to-side laxity. The stability of the elbow in flexion is more dependent on the collateral ligaments, such as the lateral or radial collateral ligament and especially the medial or ulnar collateral ligament (figure 8.3). The ulnar collateral ligament is critical to providing medial support to prevent the elbow from abducting (not a normal movement of the elbow) when stressed in physical activity. Many contact sports, particularly sports that involve throwing activities, place stress on the medial aspect of the joint, and this could result in injury. The radial collateral ligament on the opposite side provides lateral stability and is rarely injured. Additionally, the annular ligament is located laterally, providing a sling effect around the radial head to secure its stability.

The elbow is capable of moving from 0 degrees of extension to approximately 145 to 150 degrees of flexion, as detailed in figure 8.4.

The radioulnar joint is classified as a *trochoid* or *pivot-type* joint. The radial head rotates in its location at the proximal ulna. This rotary movement is accompanied by the distal radius rotating around the distal ulna. The radial head is maintained in its joint by the annular ligament. The radioulnar joint can supinate approximately 80 to 90 degrees from the neutral position. Pronation varies from 70 to 90 degrees (figure 8.5).

Because the radius and ulna are held tightly together between the proximal and distal articulations by an interosseous membrane, the joint between the shafts

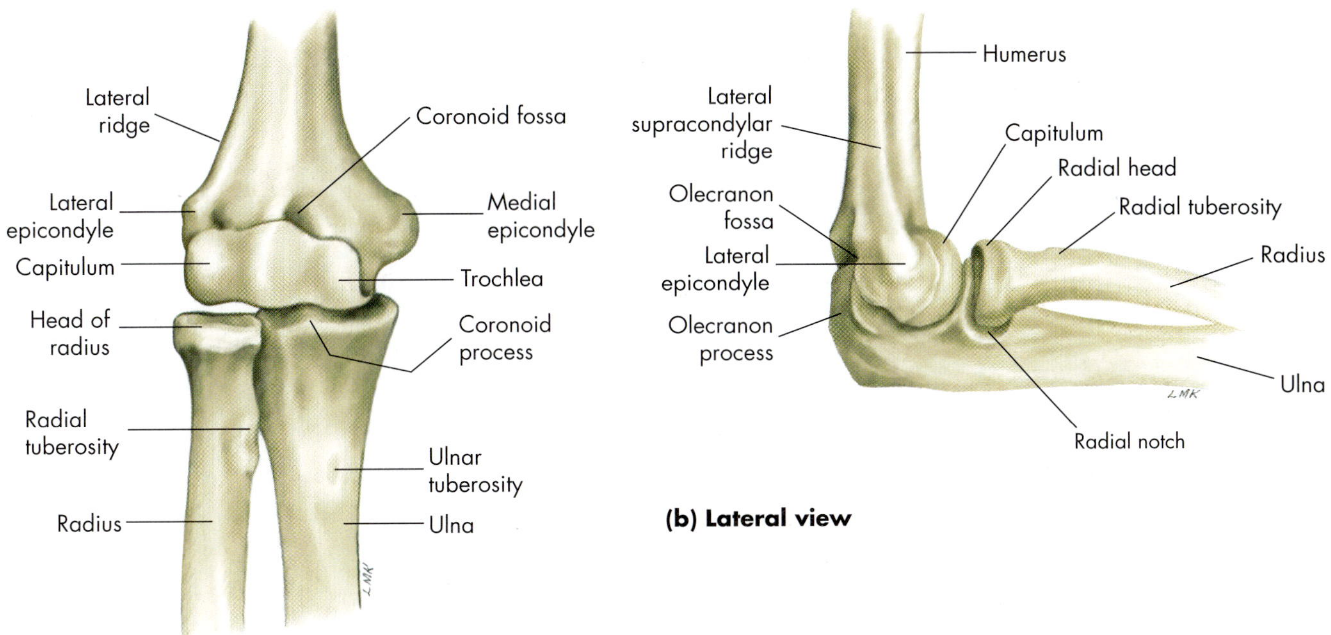

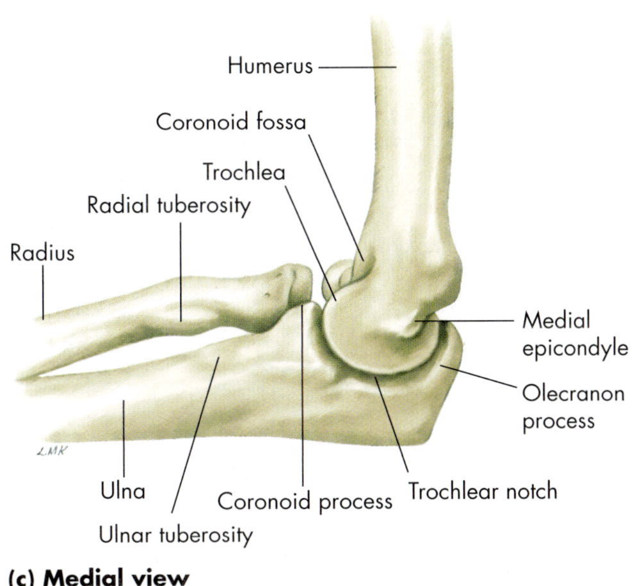

FIGURE 8.2 Right elbow joint

of these bones is often referred to as a *syndesmosis* type of joint. There is substantial rotary motion between the bones despite this classification.

Although the elbow and radioulnar joints can and do function independently of each other, the muscles controlling each work together in synergy to perform actions at both that benefit total upper-extremity function. For this reason, dysfunction at one joint may affect normal function at the other.

SYNERGY BETWEEN THE GLENOHUMERAL, ELBOW, AND RADIOULNAR JOINT MUSCLES

Just as there is synergy between the shoulder girdle and the shoulder joint in accomplishing upper-extremity activities, there is also synergy between the glenohumeral joint and the elbow and radioulnar joints.

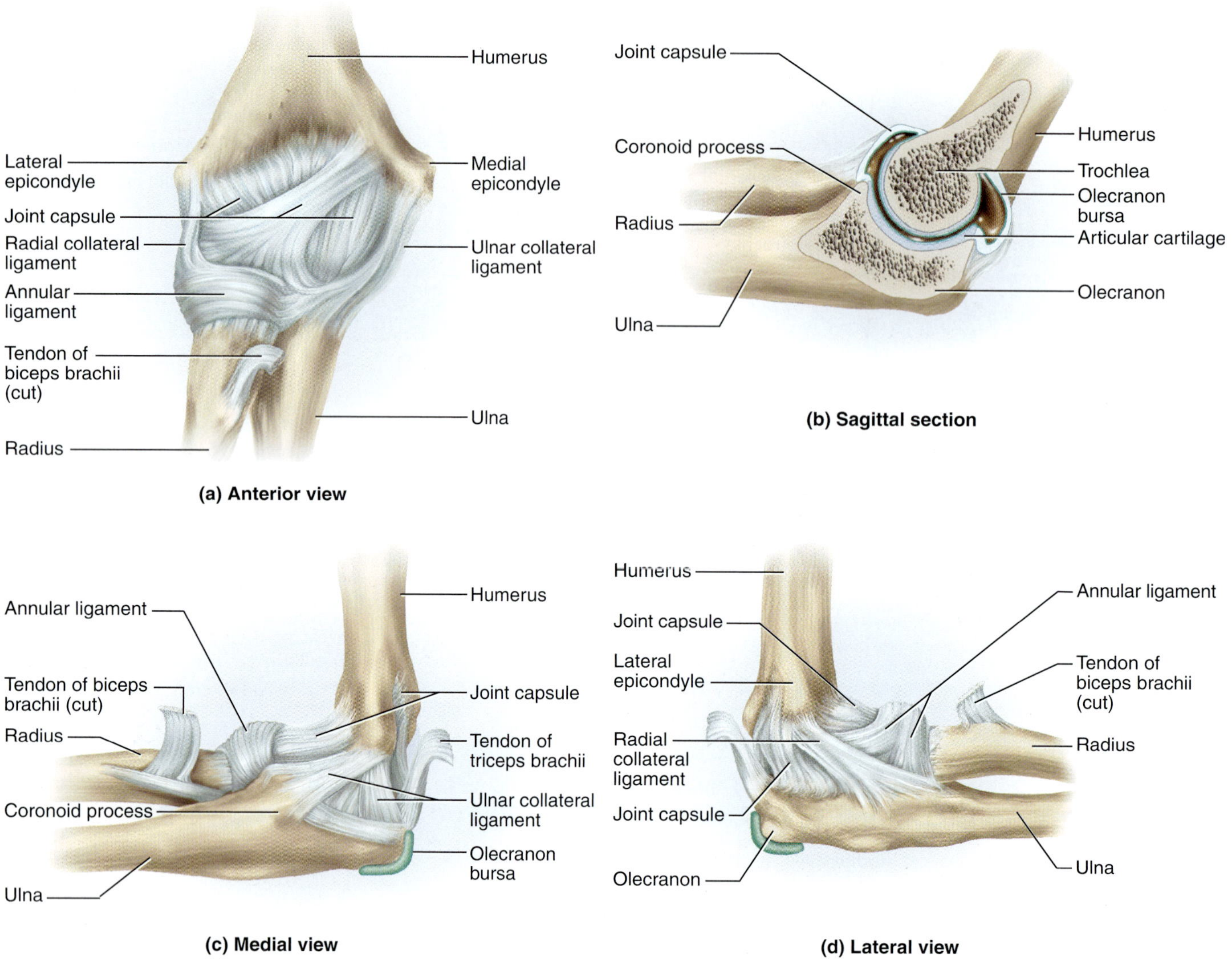

(a) Anterior view

(b) Sagittal section

(c) Medial view

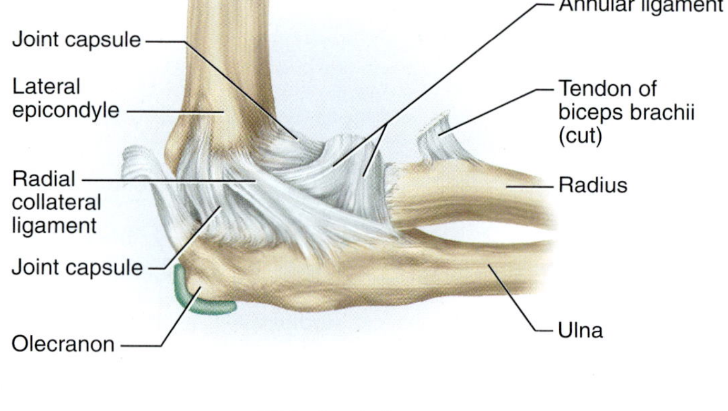

(d) Lateral view

FIGURE 8.3 Right elbow joint

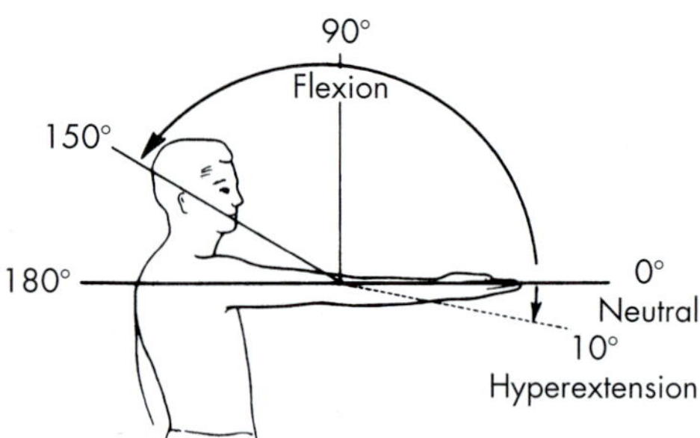

FIGURE 8.4 ROM of the elbow

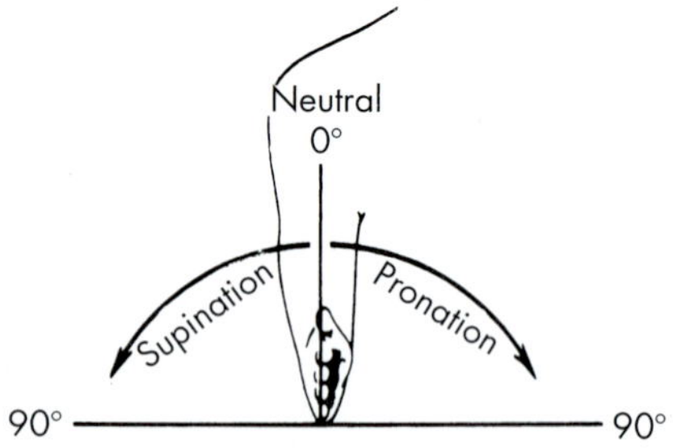

FIGURE 8.5 ROM of the forearm: supination and pronation

As the radioulnar joint goes through its ranges of motion, the glenohumeral and elbow muscles contract to stabilize or assist in the effectiveness of movement at the radioulnar joint. For example, when one holds a screwdriver in the right hand and attempts to fully tighten a screw, the movement consists of radioulnar supination, which usually involves laterally rotating and flexing the glenohumeral and elbow joints, respectively. Conversely, when one attempts to loosen a tight screw, the movement consists of pronation, which usually involves medially rotating and extending the elbow and glenohumeral joints, respectively. In either case, the body depends on both the agonists and the antagonists in the surrounding joints to assist in an appropriate amount of stabilization with the required task. This information is important to remember when analyzing actions and determining which muscles may be involved in injuries or engage in compensatory actions. Clearly, all movement is connected up the kinetic chain of the upper extremity to the shoulder girdle and neck.

Movements

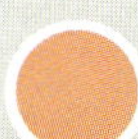

FLEXIBILITY & STRENGTH

Movements of the Humerus

See figures 8.6 and 8.7.

Elbow Movements

FLEXION

Movement of the forearm to the shoulder by bending the elbow to decrease its angle.

EXTENSION

Movement of the forearm away from the shoulder by straightening the elbow to increase its angle.

Radioulnar Joint Movements

PRONATION (RADIAL ROTATION)

Medial rotary movement of the radius on the ulna that results in the hand moving from the palm-up to the palm-down position.

SUPINATION (ULNAR ROTATION)

Lateral rotary movement of the radius on the ulna that results in the hand moving from the palm-down to the palm-up position.

Muscles

The muscles of the elbow and radioulnar joints are located in synergistic groups and are separated by function. The elbow flexors, located anteriorly (figure 8.8), are the **biceps brachii,** the **brachialis,** and the **brachioradialis,** with some weak assistance from the **pronator teres.**

The **triceps brachii,** located posteriorly, is the primary elbow extensor, with assistance provided by the **anconeus** (figure 8.9). The pronator group, located anteriorly, consists of the pronator teres, the **pronator quadratus,** and the brachioradialis. The **supinator** and biceps brachii perform supination assisted by the neutrally positioned brachioradialis. The supinator muscle is located posteriorly.

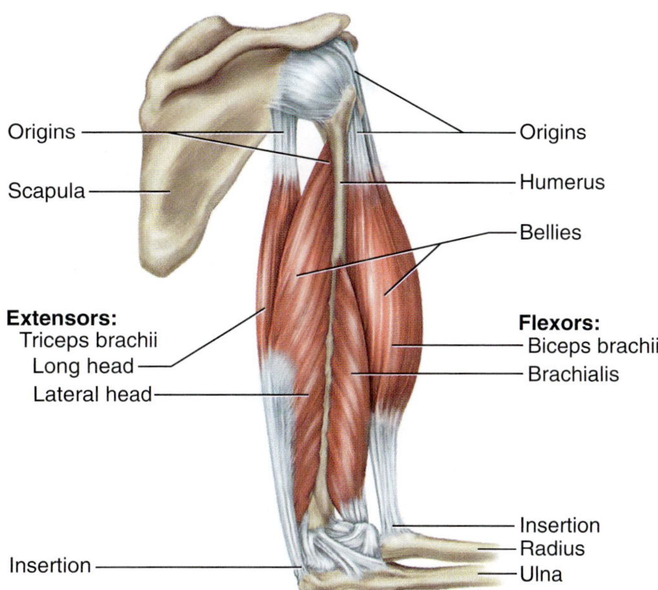

FIGURE 8.6 Flexion, extension, pronation, supination movement

CLINICAL NOTES — Tennis Elbow

A common problem associated with the elbow muscles is "tennis elbow," which involves the extensor digitorum muscle near its origin on the lateral epicondyle, brachioradialis, supinator, extensor carpi radialis, biceps, triceps, anconeus, and brachialis. (*Note:* Although the biceps and brachialis may not be directly related to lateral epicondylitis, they are included for a dimensional massage approach.) This condition, known technically as *lateral epicondylitis,* or tendonitis, is frequently associated with gripping and lifting activities, as well as many repetitive actions of the hand and wrist. *Medial epicondylitis,* or "golfer's elbow," a somewhat less common problem, is associated with the wrist flexors and pronator group near their origin on the medial epicondyle. Both of these conditions involve muscles that cross the elbow, arm, and shoulder but act primarily on the wrist and hand. Because of the association with the wrist and finger muscles, rehabilitation of epicondyle dysfunction should include exercises that target wrist and finger flexion and extension. Ulnar and radial rotation (supination and pronation) with resistance is also important.

The forearm muscles and different types of tendonitis are discussed in Chapter 10. See Chapter 9 for elbow muscle and radioulnar joint techniques and Chapter 11 for hand and wrist muscle techniques. See Table 8.1 for a summary of the agonist muscles of the elbow and radioulnar joints.

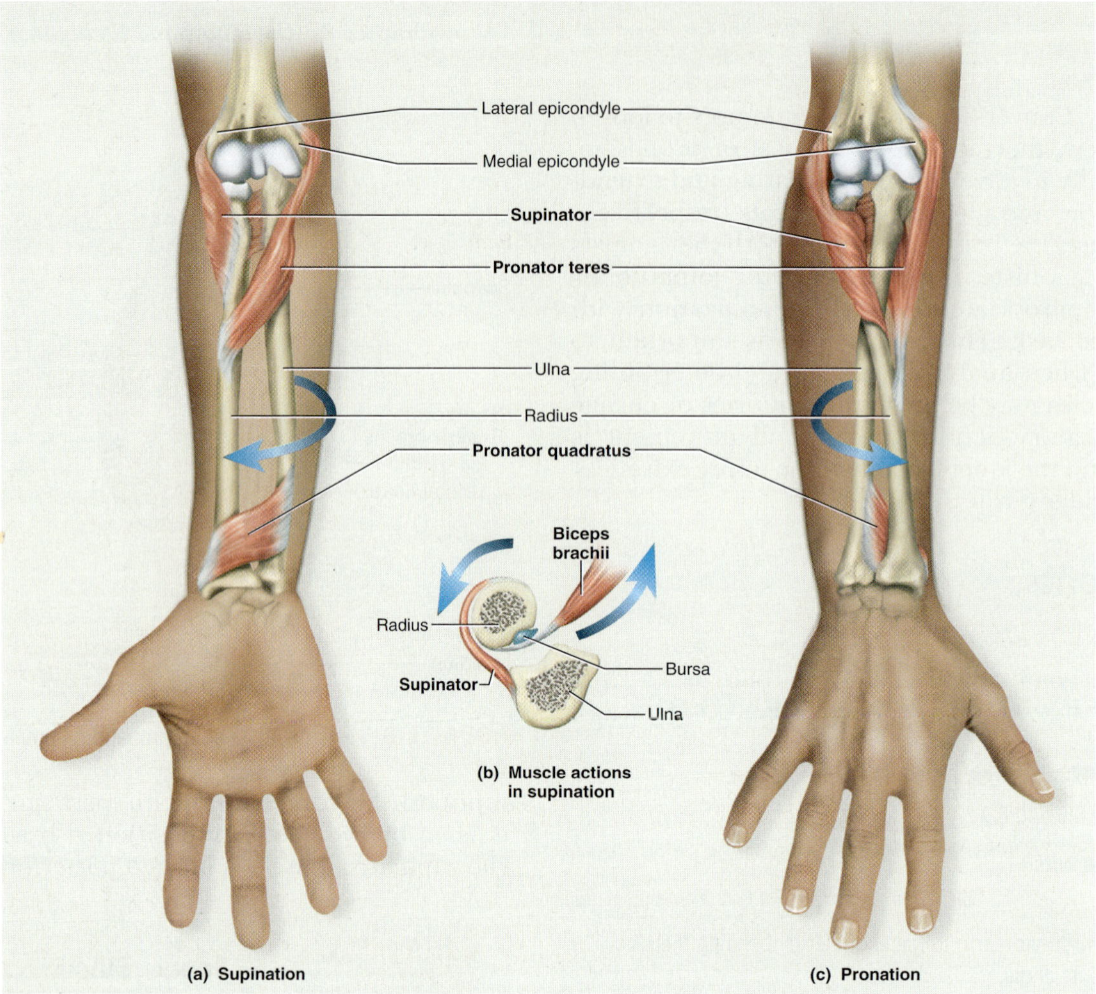

FIGURE 8.7 Supination and pronation

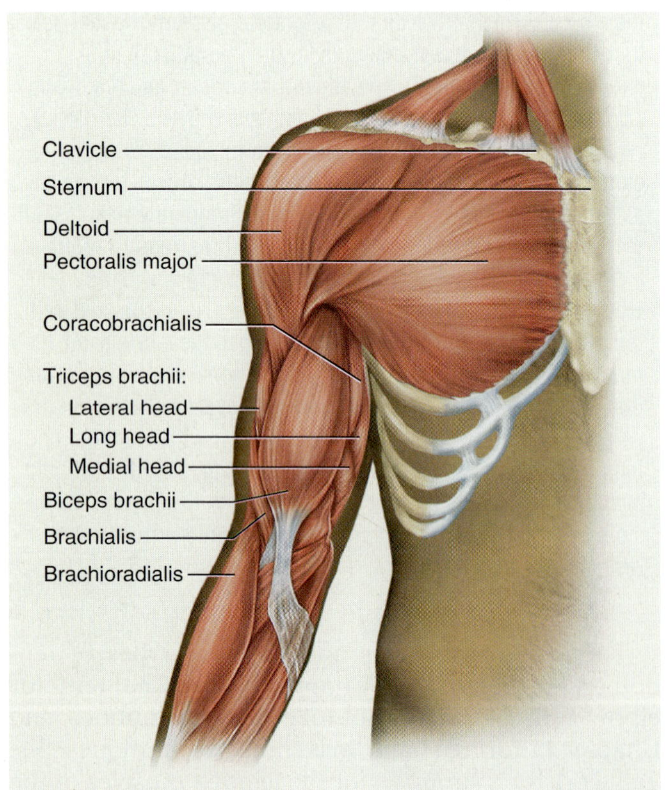

FIGURE 8.8 Elbow flexors, anterior view

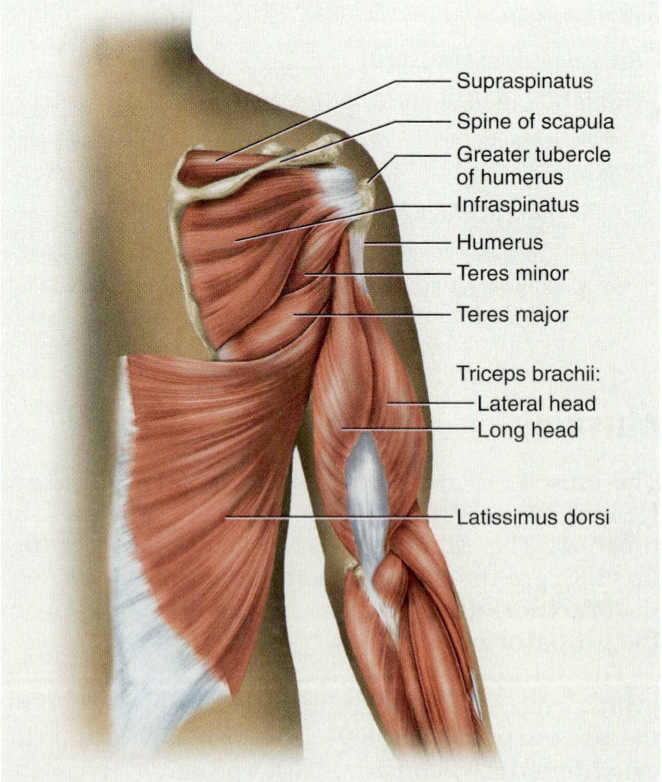

FIGURE 8.9 Elbow extensors, posterior view

TABLE 8.1 Agonist Muscles of the Elbow and Radioulnar Joints

Name of Muscle	Origins	Insertion	Actions	Innervations
Biceps brachii	*Short head:* coracoid process of scapula *Long head:* supraglenoid tubercle of scapula	Tuberosity of the radius and bicipital aponeurosis (Lacertus fibrosis)	Flexion of elbow, supination of forearm, weak flexion of shoulder joint	Musculocutaneous nerve (C5, C6)
Brachialis	Lower-half anterior shaft of humerus	Coronoid process of ulna	True flexion of elbow	Musculocutaneous nerve and sometimes branches from radial and median nerves (C5, C6)
Brachioradialis	Lateral supracondylar ridge of humerus	Styloid process of radius	Flexion of elbow in neutral position, pronation from supinated position, supination from pronated position	Radial nerve (C5, C6)
Triceps brachii	*Long head:* infraglenoid tubercle of scapula *Lateral head:* posterior humerus above spiral groove *Medial head:* posterior humerus below spiral groove	Olecranon process of ulna	Extension of elbow, long head: extension of humerus, adduction and horizontal abduction of shoulder joint	Radial nerve (C7, C8)
Anconeus	Posterior surface of lateral condyle of humerus	Posterior surface of olecranon process of ulna and dorsal surface of ulna	Extension of elbow, contracts with triceps	Radial nerve (C7, C8)
Pronator teres	Distal part of medial condyloid ridge of humerus and medial side of ulna	Middle third of lateral surface of radius	Pronation of forearm, weak flexion of elbow	Median nerve (C6, C7)
Pronator quadratus	Distal fourth of anterior side of ulna	Distal fourth of anterior side of radius	Pronation of forearm	Median nerve (palmar interosseous branch) (C6, C7)
Supinator	Lateral epicondyle ridge of humerus, dorsal surface of ulna	Lateral surface of upper third of radius	Supination of forearm	Radial nerve (C6)

MUSCLE SPECIFIC

Elbow and Radioulnar Joint Muscles—Location

Anterior	Posterior
Biceps brachii	Triceps brachii
Brachialis	Anconeus
Brachioradialis	Supinator
Pronator teres	
Pronator quadratus	

Nerves

The muscles of the elbow and radioulnar joints are all innervated from the **median nerve, musculocutaneous nerve,** and **radial nerve** of the brachial plexus. The radial nerve, originating from C5, C6, C7, and C8, provides innervation for the triceps brachii, brachioradialis, supinator, and anconeus (figure 8.10). More specifically, the posterior interosseous nerve, derived from the radial nerve, supplies the supinator. The radial nerve also provides

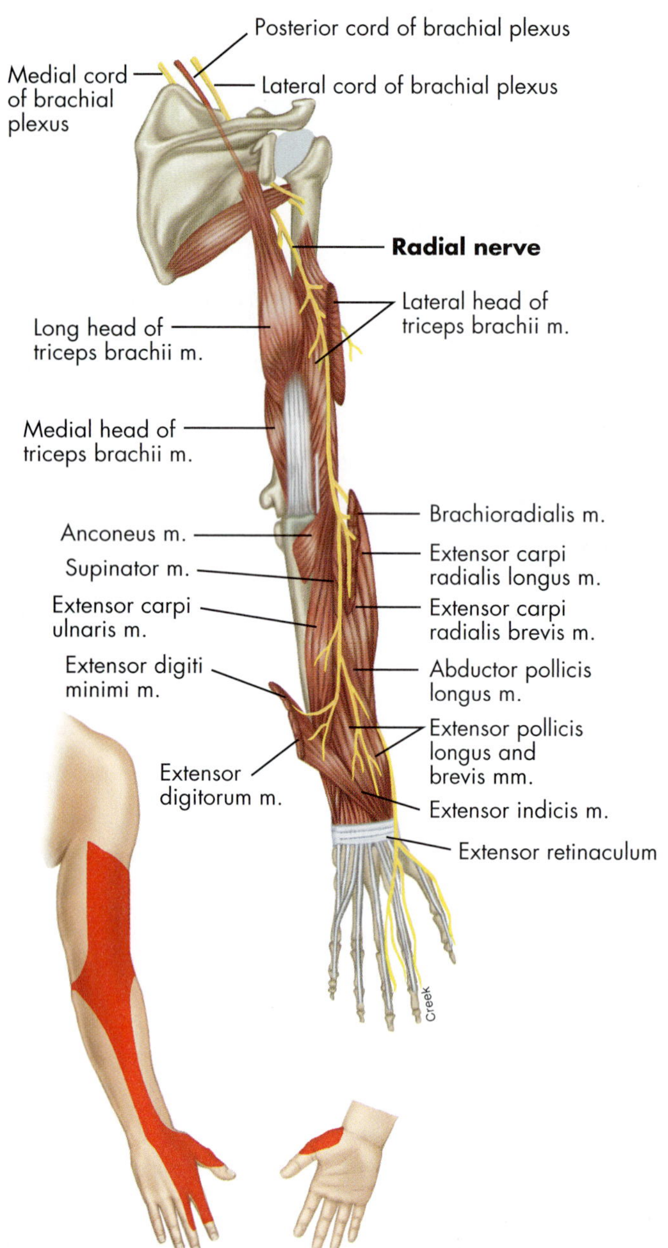

FIGURE 8.10 Radial nerve

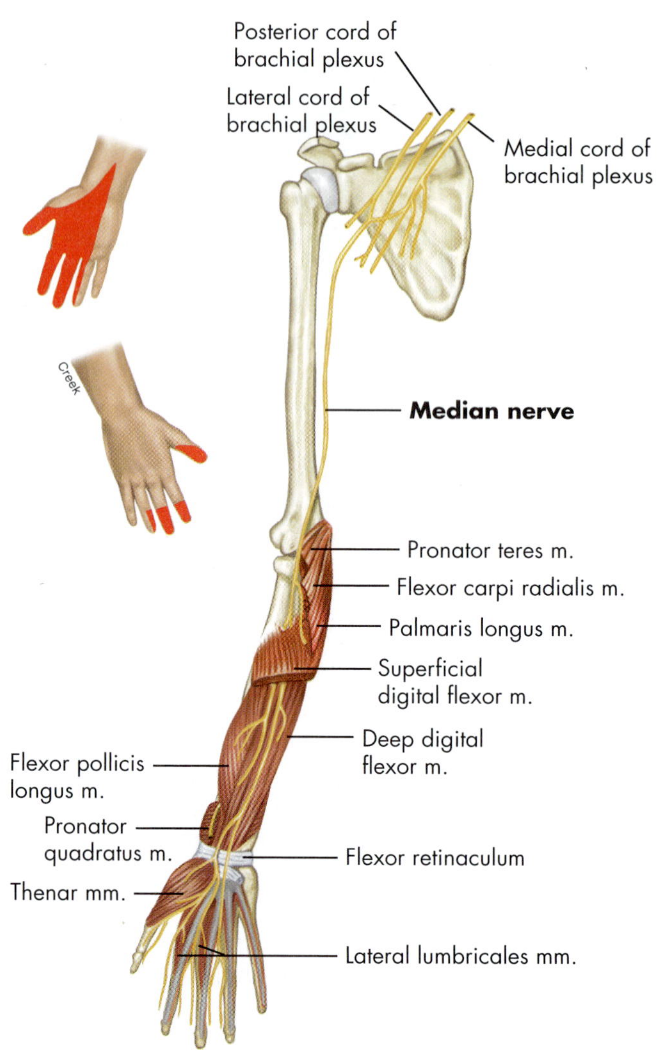

FIGURE 8.11 Median nerve

sensation to the posterolateral arm, forearm, and hand. The median nerve, illustrated in figure 8.11, innervates the pronator teres and further branches to become the anterior interosseous nerve, which supplies the pronator quadratus. The median nerve's most important related derivations are from C6 and C7. It provides sensation to the palmar aspect of the hand and the first three phalanges. It also supplies sensation to the palmar aspect of the radial side of the fourth finger, along with the dorsal aspect of the index and long fingers. The musculocutaneous nerve (shown in Chapter 6, figure 6.5, page 122) branches from C5 and C6 and supplies the biceps brachii and brachialis.

Individual Muscles of the Elbow and Radioulnar Joints

BICEPS BRACHII MUSCLE

Palpation

The biceps brachii is easily palpated on the anterior humerus. The long-head tendon may be palpated in the bicipital groove, and the short-head tendon may be palpated just inferior to the coracoid process. Distally, the biceps tendon is palpated just anteromedial to the elbow joint during supination and flexion.

OIAI MUSCLE CHART BICEPS BRACHII (bi´seps bra´ki-i) Two-headed arm muscle

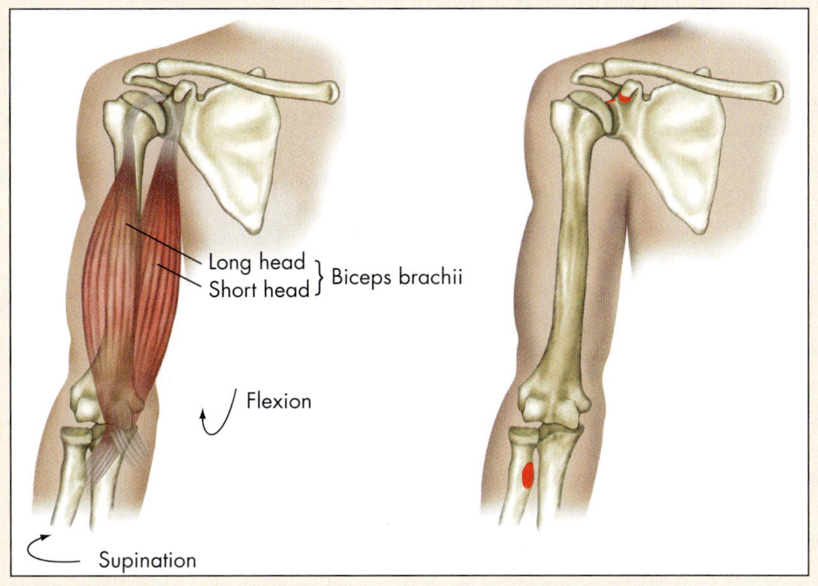

Name of Muscle	Origins	Insertion	Actions	Innervations
Biceps brachii	*Short head:* coracoid process of scapula *Long head:* supraglenoid tubercle of scapula	Tuberosity of the radius and bicipital aponeurosis (Lacertus fibrosis)	Flexion of elbow, supination of forearm, weak flexion of shoulder joint	Musculocutaneous nerve (C5, C6)

CLINICAL NOTES **Frequently Used Muscle**

The biceps brachii is used so frequently for common activities that almost everyone has experienced fatigued anterior arm muscles at one time or another. Shoveling snow, performing a hard tennis serve, playing the violin, engaging in heavy lifting—all stress the biceps brachii repetitively. Usually the resultant ache prevails superficially and is not deep into the shoulder joint; pain can refer down the arm or laterally. The long head of the biceps is much like a rope stretched over a pulley (the humerus). Wear and tear on the long-head tendon causes attachment tenderness at the origin. Injury to the long-head tendon can cause bicipital tendonitis, which may involve slipping from its position in the bicipital groove. When this occurs, the constant movement across the groove can irritate the tendon. A tell-tale snap may indicate rubbing over the lesser tubercle. Movement from humeral hyperextension to the midline with resistance can help stabilize the groove slippage.

Muscle Specifics

The biceps is actually considered a three-joint (multiarticular) muscle—shoulder, elbow, and radioulnar. It is weak in shoulder joint actions, although it does assist in providing dynamic anterior stability to maintain the humeral head in the glenoid fossa. It is more powerful in flexing the elbow when the radioulnar joint is supinated. It is also a strong supinator, particularly if the elbow is flexed. Palms away from the face (pronation) decrease the effectiveness of the biceps, partly as a result of the disadvantageous pull of the muscle as the radius rotates. The biceps brachii works with the brachialis and brachioradialis to flex the elbow joint. The biceps brachii abducts the arm at the shoulder joint, though weakly, when it is laterally rotated with the middle deltoid and supraspinatus, and it assists the coracobrachialis and the clavicular head of pectoralis major in horizontal adduction. The triceps brachii is the main antagonist.

Clinical Flexibility

Due to the multiarticular orientation of the biceps brachii, all three joints must be positioned appropriately to achieve optimal stretching. To stretch the long head, begin with the arms at the sides, palms facing midline. Lift back into hyperextension with the triceps, keeping the elbow extended. The anterior capsule, including the biceps, is stretched at the end movement. Hold 2 seconds and repeat. To stretch the short head, clasp your hands behind your back and turn the palms posterior. This pronates the forearm. Lift the arms up into hyperextension, stretching gently. Another way to dynamically stretch the anterior capsule and biceps is with assistance. After reaching back into hyperextension on the first movement, the arms are moved into horizontal abduction by a partner and a stretch is applied to the anterior shoulder. *Contraindications:* Caution should be used if preexisting anterior-capsule issues are present. Arthroplasty patients should avoid the partner-assisted stretch with both arms. Instead, one arm may be stretched at a time.

Strengthening

Flexion of the forearm with a barbell in the hands, known as *curling,* is an excellent exercise for developing the belly of the biceps brachii. Since developing the belly makes for nice tone, using a dumbbell is usually the preferred method of strengthening this muscle, particularly in gyms. This movement can be performed one arm at a time with dumbbells or both arms simultaneously with a barbell. A more important movement, and one that strengthens the proximal portion of the biceps at the shoulder, is shoulder flexion with resistance. Holding a dumbbell thumbs up, bring the shoulder into flexion, hold for 3 seconds at the highest point, and return slowly to the start position. This exercise helps keep the long-head tendon stable in the bicipital groove. *Contraindications:* These exercises are safe with controlled movement.

BRACHIALIS MUSCLE

Palpation

Palpate the brachialis muscle deep on either side of the biceps tendon during flexion/extension with the forearm in partial pronation. The lateral margin of the brachialis may be palpated between the muscles of the biceps brachii; the triceps brachii and the belly may be palpated through the biceps brachii when the forearm is in pronation during light flexion.

OIAI MUSCLE CHART BRACHIALIS (bra´ki-a´lis) True flexor of the forearm

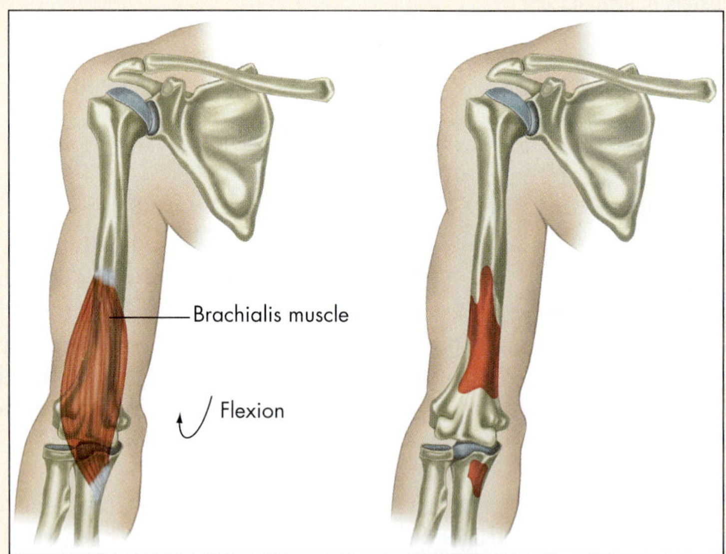

Name of Muscle	Origins	Insertion	Actions	Innervations
Brachialis	Lower-half anterior shaft of humerus	Coronoid process of ulna	True flexion of elbow	Musculocutaneous nerve and sometimes branches from radial and median nerves (C5, C6)

CLINICAL NOTES **Heavy Lifting**

Heavy lifting, as occurs in shoveling snow, can lead to discomfort in the brachialis muscle. This muscle is easily strained during elbow flexion with heavy resistance, especially if the biceps brachii is weak. When injured, the brachialis is extremely painful. Massage, along with wet heat, usually relieves muscle soreness. Passively shorten the brachialis by sleeping with a pillow in the flexed elbow. Stretching this muscle by gentle extension of the elbow can help restore blood flow (see below).

Muscle Specifics

The brachialis muscle is used along with other flexor muscles, regardless of pronation or supination. It pulls on the ulna, which does not rotate, thus making this muscle the only true flexor of the elbow. Synergists include the biceps brachii and the brachioradialis.

Clinical Flexibility

Since the brachialis is a true flexor of the elbow, it can be stretched maximally only by extending the elbow. Forearm positioning should not affect the stretch on the brachialis unless the forearm musculature itself limits elbow extension, in which case the forearm is probably best positioned in neutral. To stretch, flex one arm up in front of the body, elbow flexed, thumb up. Place the other hand under the elbow to brace it. Extend the elbow, using the other hand to stabilize, and when the elbow is fully extended, ulnar flex the wrist. Stretch for 2 seconds. Repeat. *Contraindications:* This stretch is safe with controlled movement.

Strengthening

The brachialis muscle is called into action whenever the elbow flexes. It is exercised along with elbow curling exercises, as described for the biceps brachii, pronator teres, and brachioradialis muscles. Elbow flexion activities that occur with the forearm pronated isolate the brachialis to some extent by reducing the effectiveness of the biceps brachii. *Contraindications:* Strengthening is safe with controlled movement.

OIAI MUSCLE CHART BRACHIORADIALIS (bra´ki-o-ra´di-a´lis) The neutral muscle

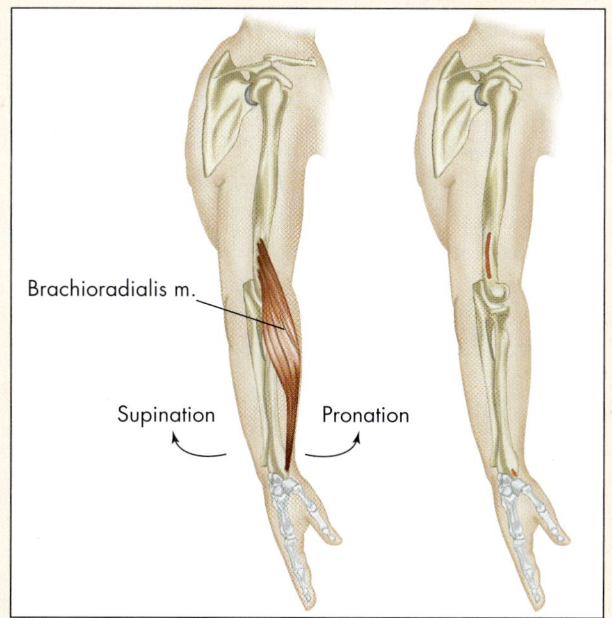

Name of Muscle	Origins	Insertion	Actions	Innervations
Brachioradialis	Lateral supracondylar ridge of humerus	Styloid process of radius	Flexion of elbow in neutral position, pronation from supinated position, supination from pronated position	Radial nerve (C5, C6)

BRACHIORADIALIS MUSCLE

Palpation

Palpate the brachioradialis muscle anterolaterally on the proximal forearm during resisted elbow flexion with the radioulnar joint positioned in neutral.

> **CLINICAL NOTES** **Neutral Worker**
>
> Since the brachioradialis is used a great deal in the neutral position, carpenters, roofers, and grocery cashiers all experience muscle exhaustion. Palpation reveals tenderness at the supracondylar ridge of the humerus and a much contracted muscle body. Fortunately, massage and stretching techniques can easily unwind this important forearm muscle. The brachioradialis may be involved in tendonitis or tendonosis of the lateral epicondyle region because of its close proximity to the overused extensors of the forearm that serve the hand and wrist. For this reason, it is important to release the brachioradialis first before working on the smaller muscles in the forearm. See Chapter 9 for techniques specific to the brachioradialis.

Muscle Specifics

The brachioradialis is one of three muscles on the lateral forearm sometimes known as the "mobile wad of three." The other two muscles are the extensor carpi radialis brevis and extensor carpi radialis longus, to which the brachioradialis lies directly anterior. The brachioradialis muscle acts best as a flexor in a midposition or neutral position between pronation and supination. In a supinated forearm position, it tends to pronate as it flexes. In a pronated position, it supinates as it flexes. This muscle is favored in its action of flexion when the neutral position between pronation and supination is assumed, as previously suggested. Its insertion at the styloid process at the distal end of the radius makes it a strong elbow flexor. Its ability as a supinator decreases as the radioulnar joint moves toward neutral. Similarly, its ability to pronate decreases as the forearm reaches neutral. Because of its action of rotating the forearm to a neutral thumb-up position, it is referred to as the "hitchhiker muscle," although it has no action at the thumb. As you will see in Chapter 10, nearly all the muscles originating off the lateral epicondyle have some action as weak elbow extensors. This is not the case with the brachioradialis because its line of pull is anterior to the elbow's axis of rotation.

Clinical Flexibility

The brachioradialis is stretched by maximally extending the elbow with the shoulder in flexion and with the forearm in either maximal pronation or maximal supination. The stretch for brachialis, described above, can be performed for this muscle. *Contraindications:* These stretches are safe with controlled movement.

Strengthening

The brachioradialis may be strengthened by performing elbow curls against resistance, particularly with the radioulnar joint in the neutral position, often called the "hammer curl," in which the thumb is up. In addition, the brachioradialis may be developed by performing pronation and supination movements through the full range of motion against resistance. Lying on your side on a massage table, flex the elbow at 90 degrees and tuck it under your body. The wrist should be off the table at the crease, so move to the edge if necessary. Clasp a 12-inch dumbbell sleeve at the top, thumbs up, and slowly supinate, lifting the end of it. Return to the start position. Switch to thumb down and clasp the sleeve again. This time, pronate the sleeve up. This is an excellent exercise for epicondylitis dysfunctions. *Contraindications:* Strengthening is safe with controlled movement.

TRICEPS BRACHII MUSCLE

Palpation

Palpate the triceps brachii on the posterior arm during resisted extension from a flexed position and distally just proximal to its insertion on the olecranon process.

Long head: proximally as a tendon on the posteromedial arm to underneath the posterior deltoid during resisted shoulder extension/adduction.

Lateral head: easily palpated on the proximal two-thirds of the posterior humerus.

Medial head (deep head): medially and laterally just proximal to the medial and lateral epicondyles.

> **CLINICAL NOTES** **Forceful Extension**
>
> The golf and tennis swing would be impossible without the use of the triceps brachii. Because one of its main actions is forceful extension of the forearm, fatigue can develop in overuse activities. The long head of the triceps will often have tenderness at the origin on the scapula. Stretching the long head of the triceps is necessary to maintain forward elevation movement of the shoulder. Passively shorten the triceps by working on the muscle in an overhead position. Roll and elliptically move the triceps and biceps around the humerus for efficient release. See more techniques in Chapter 9.

OIAI MUSCLE CHART TRICEPS BRACHII (tri´seps bra´ki-i) Three-headed muscle

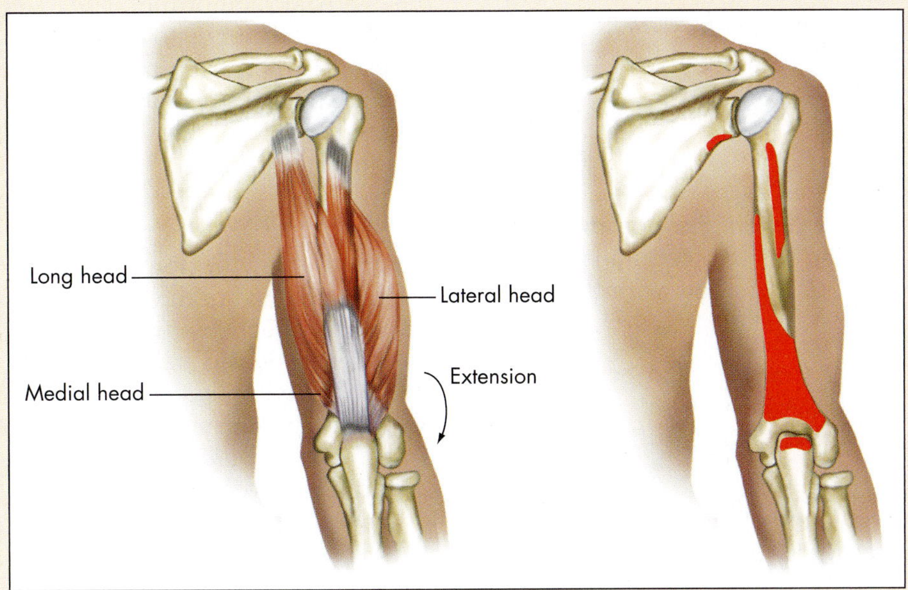

Name of Muscle	Origins	Insertion	Actions	Innervations
Triceps brachii	*Long head:* infraglenoid tubercle of scapula *Lateral head:* posterior humerus above spiral groove *Medial head:* posterior humerus below spiral groove	Olecranon process of ulna	Extension of elbow, long head: extension of humerus, adduction and horizontal abduction of shoulder joint	Radial nerve (C7, C8)

Muscle Specifics

Typical action of the triceps brachii is shown in push-ups when there is powerful extension of the elbow. This muscle is used in hand balancing and in any pushing movement involving the upper extremity. The long head is an important extensor of the shoulder joint. Two muscles extend the elbow: the triceps brachii and the anconeus.

Clinical Flexibility

The triceps brachii should be stretched with both the shoulder and the elbow in maximal flexion. To achieve this, stand with arms at the sides. Lift one arm up into flexion, elbow extended. At the top, flex the elbow, touching the palm to the posterior shoulder. Use the other hand to help assist a gentle 2-second stretch. Repeat. *Contraindications:* This stretch is safe with controlled movement.

Strengthening

Push-ups demand strenuous contraction of the triceps brachii. Dips on the parallel bars are even more difficult to perform. Bench pressing a barbell or a dumbbell is an excellent exercise. Overhead presses and triceps curls (elbow extensions from an overhead position) emphasize the triceps. Yet, as with the biceps brachii, the long head of the triceps at the shoulder is often overlooked. This proximal end should be strengthened to help maintain shoulder stability. To strengthen, use a dumbbell to perform shoulder extensions from a standing or forward-leaning, but supported, position. Start with your arms at your sides, thumbs forward, and lift the weight into shoulder hyperextension. Hold 3 seconds and slowly lower the weight. It is helpful to bend the knees during this movement, and the torso may flex forward slightly. *Contraindications:* Strengthening is safe with controlled movement.

ANCONEUS MUSCLE

Palpation

Palpate the anconeus muscle on the posterolateral aspect of the proximal ulna to the olecranon process during resisted extension of the elbow with the wrist in flexion.

CLINICAL NOTES **An Assistant Role**

When anconeus is fatigued, it tends to have attachment tenderness at the lateral epicondyle area. This muscle works with the triceps brachii and extends only the forearm, but, perhaps because of its size and attachment to the lateral condyle, it also can be involved in tennis elbow syndrome.

Muscle Specifics

The chief function of the anconeus muscle is to pull the synovial membrane of the elbow joint out of the way of the advancing olecranon process during extension of the elbow. It contracts along with the triceps brachii and is more of a stabilizer for the elbow. Some clinicians believe that the anconeus may be a continuation of the triceps.

Clinical Flexibility

Maximal elbow flexion stretches the anconeus, so it can be stretched in the same way as the triceps. Since its action affects elbow extension only, focus during the stretch should be full flexion of the elbow. The elbow is maximally flexed as the humerus moves into flexion during the stretch, thus isolating the anconeus fibers. *Contraindications:* This stretch is safe with controlled movement.

Strengthening

The anconeus is strengthened with any elbow extension exercise against resistance, in the same manner as the triceps. *Contraindications:* Strengthening is safe with controlled movement.

OIAI MUSCLE CHART ANCONEUS (an-ko´ne-us) Little elbow extensor

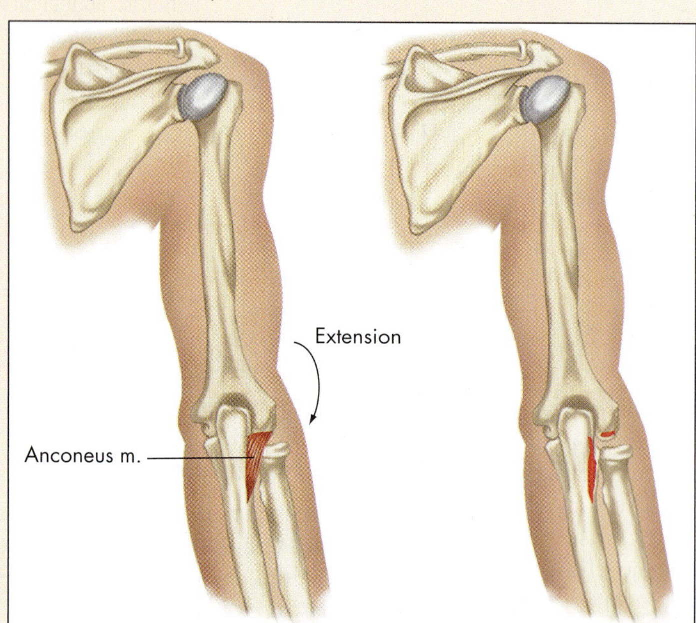

Name of Muscle	Origins	Insertion	Actions	Innervations
Anconeus	Posterior surface of lateral condyle of humerus	Posterior surface of olecranon process and dorsal surface of ulna	Extension of elbow, contracts with the triceps	Radial nerve (C7, C8)

PRONATOR TERES MUSCLE

Palpation

Palpate the pronator teres muscle on the anteromedial surface of the proximal forearm during resisted midpronation to full pronation.

CLINICAL NOTES **Median Nerve Entrapper**

It is helpful to remember that the median nerve travels through the pronator teres. Continual repetitive pronation can fatigue this muscle enough to annoy the median nerve. Symptoms may reflect carpal tunnel syndrome. Although carpal tunnel syndrome must be diagnosed by a physician, the massage therapist can take a conservative approach to releasing muscles that may entrap the median nerve. Appropriate diagnosis, rest from repetitive action, physical therapy, and massage therapy combined can promote recovery.

Muscle Specifics

Typical movement of the pronator teres muscle occurs with the forearm pronating as the elbow flexes. Movement is weaker in flexion with supination. The use of the pronator teres alone in movement tends to bring the back of the hand to the face as it contracts. Repetitive actions in the supine to prone position tend to promote stress on pronator teres and fatigue to the forearm muscles.

Clinical Flexibility

The elbow must be fully extended while taking the forearm into full supination to stretch the pronator teres. It can be stretched by holding a dumbbell sleeve or hammer handle. With the arm extended, pull on the end of the sleeve into supination, and stretch gently for 2 seconds. Repeat. *Contraindications:* This stretch is safe with controlled movement.

OIAI MUSCLE CHART PRONATOR TERES (pro-na´tor te´rez) Round pronator

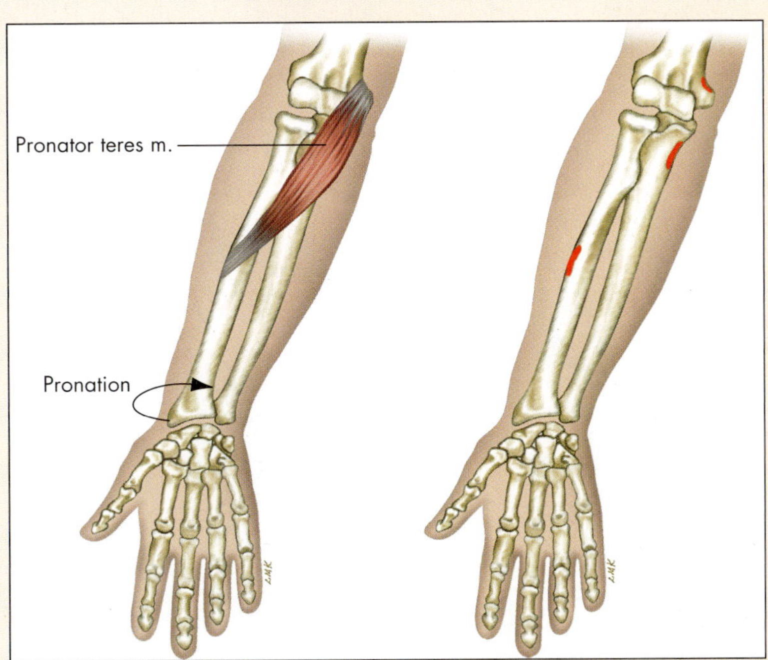

Name of Muscle	Origins	Insertion	Actions	Innervations
Pronator teres	Distal part of medial condyloid ridge of humerus and medial side of ulna	Middle third of lateral surface of radius	Pronation of forearm, weak flexion of elbow	Median nerve (C6, C7)

Strengthening

Pronation of the forearm with a dumbbell sleeve in the hand localizes action and develops the pronator teres muscle. Using the same exercise as that for the brachioradialis can help strengthen pronator teres. Lying on your side on a massage table, flex the elbow at 90 degrees and tuck it under your body. The wrist should be off the table at the crease, so move to the edge if necessary. Clasp a 12-inch dumbbell sleeve at the top, thumbs down. Pronate the sleeve up; then slowly return to the start position. *Contraindications:* This exercise is safe with controlled movement.

PRONATOR QUADRATUS MUSCLE

Palpation

The pronator quadratus is very deep and difficult to palpate, but with the forearm in supination, palpate the pronator quadratus muscle immediately on either side of the radial pulse with resisted pronation.

CLINICAL NOTES **Deep Location**

Because of the deep location of the pronator quadratus, specific therapeutic techniques are difficult, if not impossible, to complete. It can, however, be stretched and strengthened along with the other pronator muscles. All the flexor tendons to the hand and wrist pass over this muscle. Techniques for the hand and wrist can be found in Chapter 11.

Muscle Specifics

The pronator quadratus muscle works in pronating the forearm in combination with the triceps in extending the elbow. It is commonly used in turning a screwdriver or in movements requiring extension and pronation. It is also used in throwing a curve ball, which requires elbow extension and pronation.

OIAI MUSCLE CHART PRONATOR QUADRATUS (pro-na´tor kwad-ra´tus) Named for its action and shape

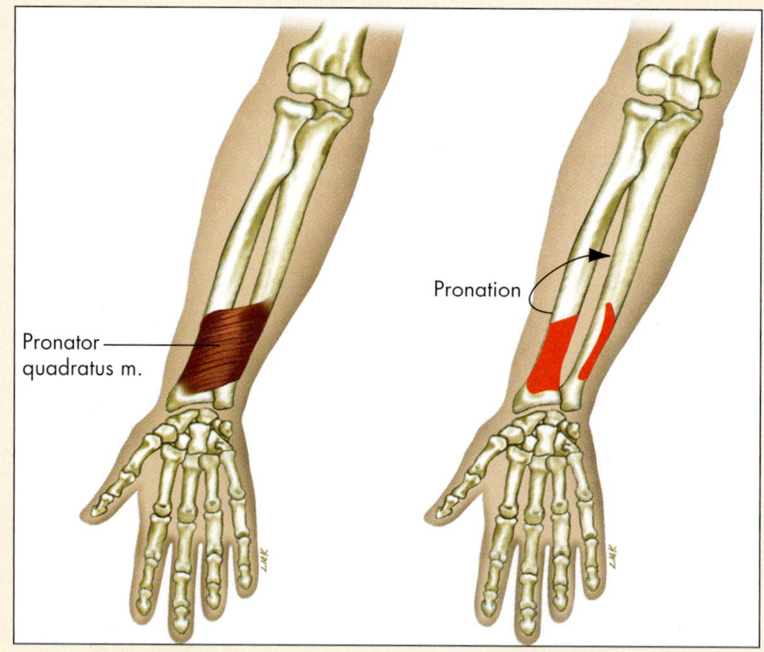

Name of Muscle	Origins	Insertion	Actions	Innervations
Pronator quadratus	Distal fourth of anterior side of ulna	Distal fourth of anterior side of radius	Pronation of forearm	Median nerve (palmar interosseous branch) (C6, C7)

Clinical Flexibility

Because the pronator quadratus is a small muscle and its attachments are within inches of each other, stretching it is difficult. Using the dumbbell sleeve again and moving it into extreme supination will help stretch this muscle (see the previous stretch). *Contraindications:* This stretch is safe with controlled movement.

Strengthening

The pronator quadratus may be developed with pronation exercises against resistance, as described for the pronator teres. *Contraindications:* These exercises are safe with controlled movement.

SUPINATOR MUSCLE

Palpation

Position the elbow and forearm in relaxed flexion and pronation, respectively, and palpate the supinator muscle deep to the brachioradialis, extensor carpi radialis longus, and extensor carpi radialis brevis on the lateral aspect of the proximal radius with slight resistance to supination.

CLINICAL NOTES **Radial Nerve Entrapper**

The radial nerve travels through the supinator in the arcade of Frohse. Should the radial nerve become entrapped, the clinical approach would be to surgically release the tissue to free up the radial nerve. Diagnostic tests determine the radial nerve entrapment. Otherwise, the supinator stabilizes pronation and may be part of the tendonitis or tendonosis that can develop at the lateral epicondyle area. A dimensional approach to tennis elbow symptoms should include icing attachments, treatment protocols of isolated stretching and strengthening, and massage. See Chapter 9 for elbow and radioulnar muscle techniques.

OIAI MUSCLE CHART SUPINATOR MUSCLE (su´pi-na´tor) Named for its action

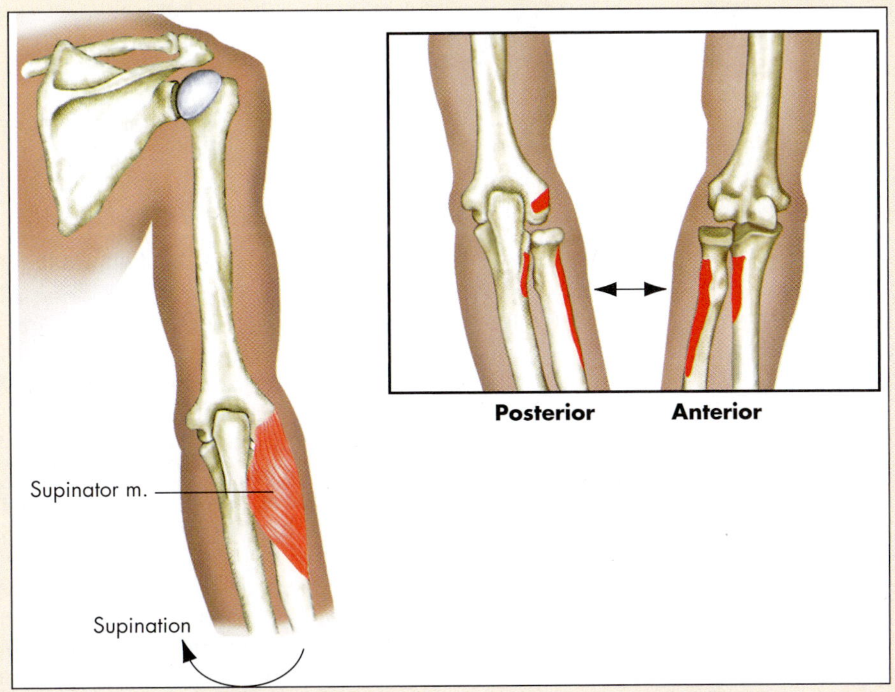

Name of Muscle	Origins	Insertion	Actions	Innervations
Supinator	Lateral epicondyle ridge of humerus, dorsal surface of ulna	Lateral surface of upper third of radius	Supination of forearm	Radial nerve (C6)

Muscle Specifics

The supinator muscle performs supination when movements of extension are required, as in turning a screwdriver or throwing a curve ball. The supinator acts as the elbow is extended just before ball release. It is most isolated in activities that require supination with elbow extension because the biceps brachii assists with supination most when the elbow is flexed. It can, however, be strengthened along with biceps brachii with the elbow flexed.

Clinical Flexibility

The supinator is stretched when the forearm is maximally pronated, so taking the weight sleeve into pronation with a gentle 2-second stretch will help stretch it. The elbow should be extended when pronating to better isolate this muscle. *Contraindications:* This stretch is safe with controlled movement.

Strengthening

The dumbbell sleeve exercise used for the pronator teres muscle may be modified to develop the supinator. With the thumb up clasping the sleeve, the forearm is supinated to the thumb-down position to strengthen this muscle. *Contraindications:* This exercise is safe with controlled movement.

CHAPTER *summary*

Introduction

✔ Almost every upper-extremity movement involves the elbow and radioulnar joints. Supination and pronation come from both the proximal and distal radioulnar joints. These movements are also known as radial and ulnar rotation.

Bones

✔ The two bones that make up the elbow joint are the humerus and the ulna. The radius and the ulna articulate and are the two bones of the radioulnar joint. The medial and lateral epicondyles of the humerus on the distal end are important landmarks for muscles that control the hand and wrist. Other bony landmarks provide muscular attachment to make movement possible for the elbow and radioulnar joints.

Joints

✔ The elbow joint is a hinge, or ginglymus, joint, while the radioulnar joint is a pivot, or trochoid, joint.

Movements

✔ Elbow joint actions include flexion and extension of the forearm.

✔ Radioulnar joint actions are supination and pronation.

Muscles

✔ The biceps brachii and brachialis are located anteriorly, while the triceps brachii and anconeus are located posteriorly on the humerus.

✔ The brachioradialis is considered to be the neutral muscle that spans from the lateral humerus to the thumb side of the hand at the styloid process of the radius.

✔ Muscles that act on the radius insert on the radius. The biceps brachii is a strong supinator and inserts on the tuberosity of the radius.

✔ The supinator is located posteriorly and laterally. It originates from the lateral epicondyle and ulna, and it inserts on the radius.

✔ The pronator teres originates from the medial epicondyle and ulna and inserts on the radius. It is located anteriorly and medially on the forearm.

✔ The pronator quadratus is at the distal end of the forearm anteriorly and spans from the ulna to insert on the radius.

Nerves

✔ The nerves that innervate the elbow joint and radioulnar joint muscles stem primarily from the brachial plexus. They include the median nerve, the radial nerve, and the musculocutaneous nerve.

Individual Muscles of the Elbow and Radioulnar Joints

✔ *Biceps brachii* is a two-headed muscle that originates on the supraglenoid tubercle and coracoid process of the scapula and inserts on the tuberosity of the radius. The scapula attachments enable this muscle to flex the shoulder joint, as well as flex and supinate the radius. In this way, the biceps brachii acts on the elbow and radioulnar joints.

✔ *Brachialis* is considered the true flexor of the elbow joint as it does not originate on the shoulder girdle but, instead, begins on the humerus. It inserts on the ulna, which gives a true line of pull for flexion of the elbow joint.

✔ *Triceps brachii* is a three-headed muscle that has one attachment for the long head on the infraglenoid tubercle of the scapula. Its attachment to the scapula enables the muscle to perform weak extension of the humerus. The lateral head and medial head begin on the humerus. All three heads insert on the olecranon process of the ulna and together extend the forearm.

✔ *Anconeus* is a small triangular-shaped muscle that attaches at the lateral epicondyle of the humerus and inserts on the olecranon process of the ulna. It works with the triceps in extension of the forearm.

✔ *Brachioradialis* is named for its locations on the humerus and on the styloid process of the radius. It governs the neutral position of the forearm and flexes the elbow joint. The brachioradialis enables movement from supination to pronation and back.

- ✔ *Supinator* begins on the humerus and ulna and inserts on the radius. Supination is its only true action.
- ✔ *Pronator teres* is located on the opposite side of the forearm from the supinator. It originates on the medial epicondyle of the humerus and ulna, and it inserts on the radius. The pronater teres pronates the forearm and assists in flexing the forearm.
- ✔ *Pronator quadratus* is located anteriorly, distally, and deeply close to the wrist. It assists in pronation of the forearm.

Worksheet Exercises

As an aid to learning, for in-class and out-of-class assignments, or for testing, tear-out worksheets are found at the end of the text, pages 527–530.

True or False

Write true *or* false *after each statement.*

1. The elbow joint is composed of the humerus and the radius.
2. The humerus has two important medial and lateral epicondyles on the distal part of the bone near the elbow area.
3. The biceps brachii is easy to palpate, whereas the brachialis is somewhat more difficult to palpate due to its location.
4. The biceps brachii has two heads and originates on the head of the humerus.
5. The insertion of the biceps brachii is on the ulna, and this is why it is able to rotate.
6. The triceps brachii muscle inserts on the olecranon process.
7. The brachioradialis can be exercised and strengthened by the hammer curl.
8. The median nerve goes through the pronator quadratus.
9. The radial nerve innervates the supinator.
10. The supinator, biceps brachii, pronator teres, and pronator quadratus all insert on the radius and have action on the radius.
11. An effective way to help strengthen the forearm in supination and pronation is through resistance in ulnar and radial rotation.

Short Answers

Write your answers on the lines provided.

1. Why is the brachialis considered a true flexor?

___

___

___

2. What muscle controls the neutral position of the forearm?

___

___

___

3. How can the long head of the triceps be involved in shoulder joint extension?

___

___

___

4. What nerve runs through pronator teres?

___

___

___

5. What nerve runs through the triceps?

___

___

___

6. How is it possible for the biceps to be involved with supination?

___

___

___

7. What are the two bones that articulate in the act of supination and pronation?

___

___

___

8. What action does the anconeus perform, and what muscle or muscles does it assist?

____

____

____

9. Where is the coronoid process, and what flexor of the elbow attaches to it?

____

____

____

10. Name all the muscles that are antagonists of the supinator.

____

____

____

11. If a client developed tennis elbow, what other areas would you recommend strengthening besides the forearm muscles?

____

____

____

12. For shoulder stability, what area of the biceps brachii is most important to strengthen?

____

____

____

Multiple Choice

Circle the correct answers.

1. The biceps brachii inserts on the:
   a. greater tubercle
   b. coronoid process of the ulna
   c. tuberosity of the radius
   d. coracoid process of the scapula
2. The pronator quadratus inserts on the:
   a. distal radius
   b. proximal radius
   c. tuberosity of the radius
   d. distal ulna
3. The largest muscle in the forearm is the:
   a. biceps brachii
   b. triceps brachii
   c. brachioradialis
   d. supinator
4. The supinator and pronator teres are perfectly designed to oppose each other because:
   a. their origins are located on the lateral and medial epicondyles of the humerus
   b. they originate on the radius
   c. they insert on the radius
   d. they do not originate on the humerus
5. The biceps brachii is able to flex the forearm in what position?
   a. extended position
   b. supinated position
   c. pronated position only
   d. none of the above
6. The elbow joint is classified as a:
   a. ball-and-socket joint
   b. hinge or ginglymus joint
   c. pivot
   d. condyloid
7. The pivot action of the radioulnar joint happens at:
   a. the wrist
   b. the shoulder joint
   c. the proximal and distal ends between the radius and the ulna
   d. none of the above
8. If you were turning a doorknob, you would be actively operating the:
   a. biceps brachii
   b. triceps brachii
   c. pronator teres only
   d. brachioradialis
9. The brachioradialis inserts on the:
   a. coronoid process of the ulna
   b. styloid process of the radius
   c. tuberosity of the radius
   d. medial epicondyle of the radius
10. As the baseball comes into contact with the bat, the baseball player is actively using the:
    a. brachioradialis
    b. supinator
    c. triceps brachii
    d. biceps brachii only

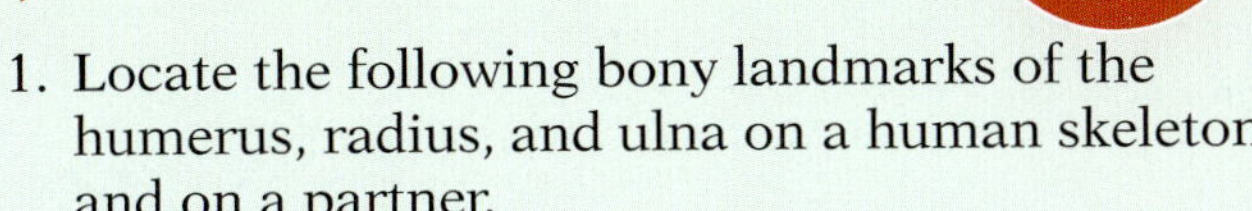

1. Locate the following bony landmarks of the humerus, radius, and ulna on a human skeleton and on a partner.

   a. Skeleton:

   1. Medial epicondyle
   2. Lateral epicondyle
   3. Lateral supracondylar ridge
   4. Trochlea
   5. Capitulum
   6. Olecranon fossa
   7. Olecranon process
   8. Coronoid process
   9. Coronoid fossa
   10. Tuberosity of the radius
   11. Ulnar tuberosity

   b. Subject:

   1. Medial epicondyle
   2. Lateral epicondyle
   3. Lateral supracondylar ridge
   4. Proximal radioulnar joint
   5. Olecranon process
   6. Olecranon fossa
   7. Styloid process

2. Palpate the following muscles and their origins and insertions on a partner:
   a. Biceps brachii
   b. Brachioradialis
   c. Brachialis
   d. Pronator teres
   e. Supinator
   f. Triceps brachii
   g. Anconeus

3. Palpate and list the muscles primarily responsible for the following movements as you demonstrate each:
   a. Flexion
   b. Extension
   c. Pronation
   d. Supination

4. Discuss the difference between flexing the forearm in a prone position and flexing it in a supine position. Describe the synergists used in the actions, and explain what muscles are stronger with the actions.

5. Analyze and list the differences in elbow and radioulnar joint muscle activity between turning a doorknob clockwise and pushing the door open and turning the knob counterclockwise and pulling the door open.

6. *Antagonistic muscle action chart:* Fill in the chart by listing the muscle(s) or parts of muscles that are antagonistic in their actions to the muscles in the left column.

Agonist	Antagonist
Biceps brachii	
Brachioradialis	
Brachialis	
Pronator teres	
Supinator	
Triceps brachii	
Anconeus	

7. *Muscle analysis chart:* Fill in the chart by listing the muscles primarily involved in each movement.

Flexion	Extension
Pronation	Supination

8. The elbow joint is the insertion of what biarticular muscle? Describe what motions it is involved in at the elbow and at the superior joint of its muscular origin.

9. Lifting a television set as you help your roommate move in requires appropriate lifting techniques and an effective angle of pull. Describe the angle of pull chosen at the elbow joint, and explain why it is chosen as opposed to other angles.

chapter 9

The Radioulnar Riddle: Techniques for Repetitive Action

LEARNING OUTCOMES

After completing this chapter, you should be able to:

9-1 Define key terms.

9-2 List several median nerve disorders.

9-3 Locate the medial and lateral epicondyles of the humerus to palpate muscles above and below the elbow and radioulnar joints.

9-4 Discuss symptoms of a subacute flare-up.

9-5 Practice safe body mechanics.

9-6 Demonstrate specific techniques on the muscles of the elbow and radioulnar joints.

9-7 Incorporate dimensional massage therapy techniques in a regular routine or use them when needed.

9-8 Determine safe treatment protocols and refer clients to other health professionals when necessary.

KEY TERMS

Bursitis
Carpal tunnel syndrome
Double-crush syndrome
Golfer's elbow
Hypertonic
Lateral epicondylitis
Medial epicondylitis
Median nerve disorders
Pronator teres syndrome
Radial nerve entrapment
Subacute flare-up
Tennis elbow
Ulnar nerve compression

Introduction

Picking up a cup of coffee and lifting it to take a drink involves a number of movements. Not including specific movements of the hand and the stabilized wrist, the actions involved include flexion of the shoulder joint, flexion of the elbow joint, and a neutral position of the forearm with a little pronation from the radioulnar joint. Activities like drinking from a cup are easy to take for granted because these repetitive actions are a part of daily life. The elbow and radioulnar joints are strategically located between the shoulder and the hand and wrist. The shoulder joint allows for movement that enables the elbow joint and the radioulnar joint to work synergistically together. The elbow and radioulnar joints further enable the distal hand and wrist to perform intricate detail work, including grasping, and individual digital actions in specific forearm positions.

The muscles involved in the actions of the elbow and radioulnar joints span from parts of the scapula to the wrist. This expansion of attachments protects the midway-spaced joints with integrity. It also connects the kinetic chain of the upper extremity and spreads the discomfort levels from repetitive actions. Flexion and extension are straightforward. Any muscle inserting on the ulna has something to do with flexion or extension. The radioulnar joint adds complexity to the forearm activities with supination and pronation. Muscles that insert on the radius have the additional ability to be involved in supination and/or pronation. Many of the muscles that contribute to the functions of the hand and wrist originate on or near the medial and lateral epicondyles of the humerus. The added soft-tissue links complicate this area and produce a lot of torque, force, and pull on muscles and tendons and at attachments. Thus, the muscles and soft tissue of the elbow joint region are a frequent source of tenderness and overactivity.

Injuries and Overuse Syndromes

FRACTURES AND DISLOCATIONS

There are a variety of soft-tissue problems and bony injuries that can occur in the elbow region. Like any joint in the body, the elbow and radioulnar joints are susceptible to dislocation and fracture from trauma. The journey to recovery from a fracture to the head of the radius as it articulates with the ulna can be difficult. Because the radius rotates against the ulna, the mobility necessitates no casting. A cast would immobilize the joint and likely "fuse" or severely limit motion as the joint heals. Massage would be contraindicated, as the condition heals very slowly and has to retain movement. Additional circulation in the limited area could inflame and irritate the joint.

Dislocated elbow joints are painful and warrant a trip to the emergency room. The elbow joint is a confined area with nerves and vessels traversing distally to the hand and wrist. A dislocated elbow joint could constrict circulation or nerve function locally as well as distally. Ligaments are often torn in the process, and tendons—if not torn—could be strained in the injury. Even after the dislocation has been safely reduced, massage should be avoided on the affected area until bruising is minimal or gone, swelling is significantly reduced, circulation is normal, and it is safe to apply pressure to the soft tissue. Whenever an isolated joint in the body suffers trauma, the rest of the body compensates for the injury. Massage therapy is beneficial and supports the individual emotionally and physically during the recovery process.

BURSITIS AND TENDONITIS

Bursitis is a condition that produces painful movement in the elbow area. Often coupled with medial epicondylitis, **bursitis** is simply an inflammation of a bursa. The swelling of a bursa in this area can get bigger than a golf ball. The bursa is often treated medically and drained. **Medial epicondylitis,** or **golfer's elbow** as it is commonly called, is simply tendonitis, an overuse condition that is not simple in nature or healing.

On the lateral side of the elbow joint around the lateral epicondyle is a highly torqued area that is the site of **lateral epicondylitis,** or **tennis elbow.** Commonly caused by overuse, this tendonitis produces painful movement and discomfort in the hand and wrist. Other overuse conditions are tendonosis and tenosynovitis. See Chapter 11 for a closer look at tendonitis, tendonosis, and tenosynovitis.

Soft-Tissue Issues

Chronic, painful repetitive injuries often have spells of **subacute flare-ups.** A subacute flare-up is a response to a chronic injury that is not allowed to rest. The site is not a new injury but, instead, is a badly abused area that generally evokes more vociferous complaints of pain from its sufferers. It may have all the symptoms of the acute stage. Overuse has made the area worse and pushed it from a chronic stage to a subacute stage. It is not necessary for an injury to be new to appear in its symptoms as acute. An ice bag or ice massage is a good initial step for the subacute flare-up to reduce the inflammation, swelling, and pain.

Using the forearm and arm muscles repeatedly can cause sore and often **hypertonic** muscles. Muscles go through an involved process every time they contract, and they need oxygen, which is obtained through circulation, in order to perform. After continuous activity, the muscle begins to fatigue and can no longer function to its optimum capacity without producing pain and discomfort. Massage therapy can provide relief for hypertonic muscles. Manual movement of tissues assists in circulation and relieves congestion in the muscle fibers by promoting oxygen supply and eliminating waste, such as lactic acid.

The origins and insertions of tendons are often tender at the attachment sites. If a rope was secured to a tree and a person pulled on the rope continuously, it would be only a matter of time before the rope would start to fray. Many tendons have tenuous attachments. Some are even ropelike, which adds more strength to the connection of soft tissue to bone. Like a rope, however, given enough pull and torque, the tendon can start to tear. This can be the beginning of tendonitis or tendonosis, but it is most certainly the beginning of tenderness at the attachment site.

Nerve Complaints

The cubital tunnel is an area between the medial epicondyle and the olecranon process. The ulnar nerve resides in the cubital tunnel. **Ulnar nerve compression** occurs when the ulnar nerve does not have enough room in the tunnel, usually from the placement of the elbow joint. One clinical solution is to surgically move the ulnar nerve so that it is no longer in jeopardy of compression.

The radial nerve runs through a variety of arm and forearm muscles before it ends distally in the hand. Entrapment of the radial nerve can occur in the triceps as well as the supinator. Surgery to the supinator can release **radial nerve entrapment** if all conservative measures fail.

Median nerve disorders include carpal tunnel syndrome, pronator teres syndrome, and double-crush syndrome. Median nerve disorders are all vulnerable to median nerve entrapment from the brachial plexus to the wrist. As discussed in Chapter 4, the pectoralis minor controls abduction of the scapula and can entrap the brachial plexus. The median nerve travels through the fibers of the pronator teres that can entrap the nerve and cause **pronator teres syndrome.** Repetitive action of pronation with the upper extremity in front of the body and the scapula abducted can set up an entrapment environment by the pectoralis minor and pronator teres known as the **double-crush syndrome.** The carpal tunnel has very little room, and the median nerve sits on top of the tendons just below the flexor retinaculum. Median nerve inflammation in the carpal tunnel is called **carpal tunnel syndrome,** and surgery is a common solution for this condition. See Chapters 10 and 11 for more on carpal tunnel syndrome.

Unraveling the Riddle

Addressing an area of the body that sees constant repetitive action requires treating the entire extremity, generally starting with the shoulder girdle muscles. It is important for the client to be suitably relaxed before the practitioner begins working on a painful area. As discussed in Chapters 4 and 6 on the shoulder girdle and shoulder joint, respectively, the upper extremity is attached to the scapula, and the soft tissue contains a massive communication network. The upper trapezius and levator often will shorten to elevate the scapula while the rest of the upper extremity tries to protect the injury site. Although there may be nothing wrong with the shoulder joint, pain in the elbow joint can subconsciously prevent a person from trying to move the entire limb. Relaxing the shoulder girdle muscles that have been compensating for tension creates a positive response pattern.

It is beneficial for the manual therapist to work first on the upper extremity that has fewer or no clinical problems. This gives the practitioner valuable information about the client's healthy soft tissue and its density. The client benefits from the psychological support, as there is no discomfort in those tissues, and subsequently experiences less anxiety.

Start on the joint above the troubled area first; then work on the arm muscles for the elbow area. Using no lubrication to start, apply techniques that are not painful or area-specific. Rolling, elliptical movement, myofascial techniques, jostling, and compression are useful methods to begin massaging a limb. Begin with the hyperflexed position for passive shortening of the deltoids and easy access to the biceps and triceps; then use dual-hand distraction techniques to unwind tight tendons and joints. Next, intersperse regular Swedish techniques, and remember to work on the attachment sites. The attachments are tender for a reason. Circular friction will increase circulation and increase activity inside the fibers. It is sometimes useful to ice the attachments that are painful before working on them, especially if there is a subacute flare-up.

With the client still in a supine position, move from the arm muscles to the brachioradialis. It is the largest of the forearm muscles and carries a big workload. The brachioradialis performs flexion of the elbow and also supports supination and pronation. Approach the area in the manner suggested above for the arm muscles, using no lubrication at first and following the treatment techniques described below. Be careful around the lateral epicondyle area, and unwind the whole area before performing any deep-tissue techniques that may be painful. Although you should sequentially treat painful attachments last, never end with a technique that elicits a painful memory. One good technique for closing the session includes effleurage to the entire extremity.

To review, remember to:

- Always use treatment protocols to determine the sequence of a therapeutic session.
- Palpate tissues.
- Apply techniques to the uninvolved upper extremity first.
- Use warm-up techniques first, and determine pressure intelligently.
- Follow a dimensional approach, and critically think about the involved joints and kinetic chain.
- Passively shorten the muscles whenever possible.

- Work on the shoulder girdle muscles first.
- Move onto the arm muscles and their attachments.
- Approach the forearm methodically, superficial to deep.

The group of techniques described below can be used as a complete sequence or be incorporated into other treatment sequences. These techniques support your purpose of reducing hypertonicities, lengthening fibers, separating tissues, reducing soreness and pain levels, increasing flexibility, and increasing movement to restricted action.

Dimensional Massage Therapy for the Muscles of the Radioulnar and Elbow Joints

Before beginning with technique application, do not forget to palpate the tissues and use touch to determine where tension exists in the tissue and if hypertonicity is present. Then assess the client's response to your touch.

SUPINE—FLEXED-ARM POSITION

Stand at the head of the table in a balanced position. Bring your body down to the client's level so that the client's arm remains at a comfortable angle. Make sure you are able to move with the application of the techniques and do not stay in a stagnant position.

Rock and Roll

With the client's arm flexed over his head and with his forearm cradled at your waist, lightly grasp the triceps and biceps with your hands and roll the muscles around the humerus. (See figure 9.1.)

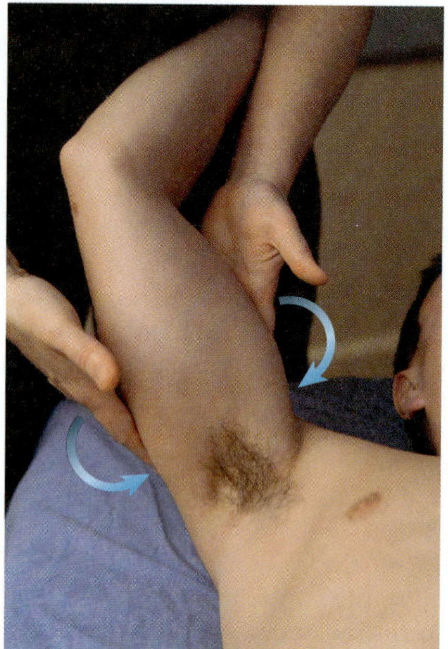

FIGURE 9.1 Rock and roll of the biceps and triceps

Elliptical Movement of the Deltoids, Biceps, and Triceps

Using the same arm position as above, elliptically move the deltoids, biceps, and triceps. (See figure 9.2.)

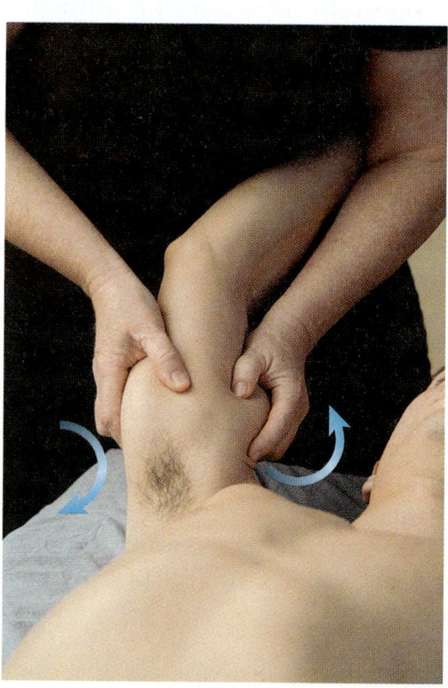

FIGURE 9.2 Elliptical movement of the biceps and triceps

Humeral Joint Tease

Using the same flexed-arm position as described above, grasp the deltoids close to the shoulder joint as you are cradling the arm with your other hand. Move the shoulder in a circular movement, effectively bringing the joint together and separating the bones.

Jostle the Deltoids, Biceps, and Triceps

Hold the client's arm at the elbow joint with one hand. With the other hand, jostle the anterior, middle, and posterior deltoids while the arm is in the flexed position. In the same over-the-head position, grasp the biceps with a loose grip, slightly stretch the tissue, and jostle from origin to insertion. Repeat several times. Switch hands holding the client's arm, and repeat the procedure with the triceps. (See figure 9.4 for the hand position.)

Deep Transverse Friction to the Deltoid Tuberosity

While the client's upper extremity is in the flexed position, locate the deltoid tuberosity and apply deep transverse friction to the insertion with your thumb.

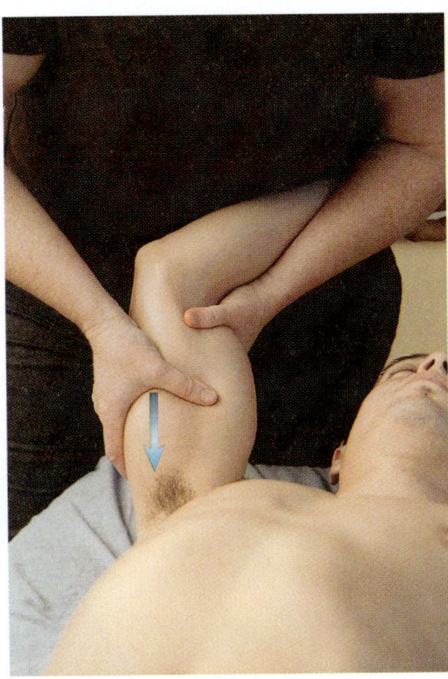

FIGURE 9.3 Alternating compressive effleurage for the triceps and biceps

Alternate Compressive Effleurage

With the client's arm in the flexed position, stroke the triceps and biceps toward the shoulder first with one hand and then the other. Use deep, fluid strokes and some lubrication. (See figure 9.3.)

Alternate Petrissage on the Triceps and Biceps

Pick up tissues and alternate applying petrissage to the biceps and triceps while you pin the client's arm in the flexed position to your waist. (See figure 9.4.)

Petrissage the Elbow Joint with Distraction

With the client's upper extremity in the flexed position, lightly grasp the distal end of the triceps with one hand and grasp the brachioradialis with the other hand. Petrissage the triceps and the forearm muscles as you slightly flex and extend the elbow repeatedly. This stretches the soft tissues at the elbow joint as you massage the muscles. (See figure 9.5.)

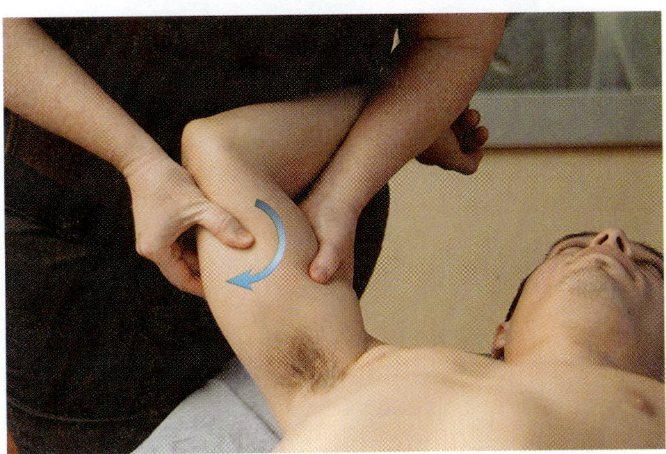

FIGURE 9.4 Alternating petrissage on the triceps and biceps

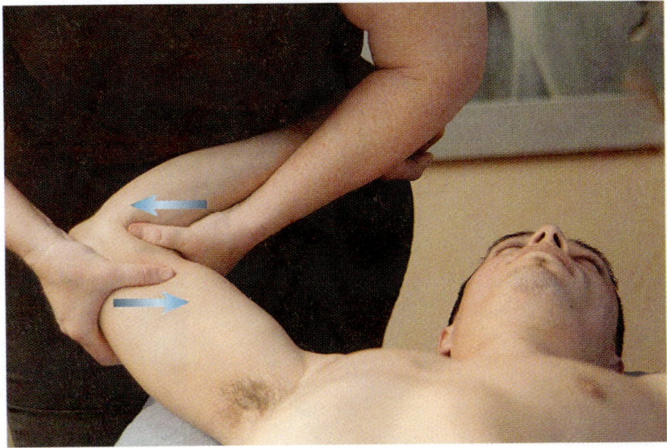

FIGURE 9.5 Petrissage of the elbow joint with distraction

Locate the Origin of the Long Head of the Triceps

With the client's upper extremity in the flexed position over her head, locate the infraglenoid tubercle on the scapula. Use circular friction on the origin of the long head of the triceps. Use caution with your pressure; this attachment could be unexpectedly sore. (See figure 9.6.)

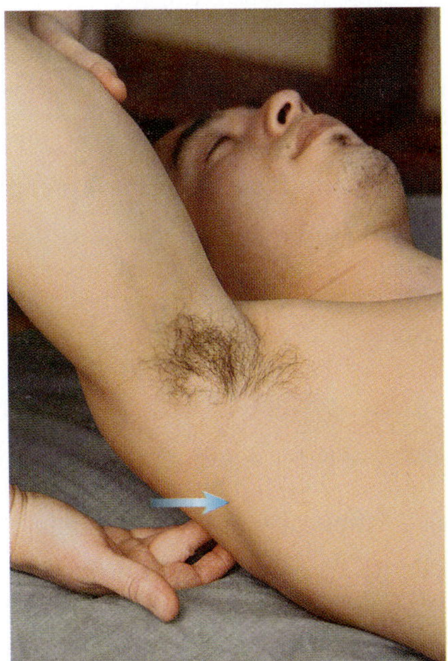

FIGURE 9.6 Locating the long head of the triceps

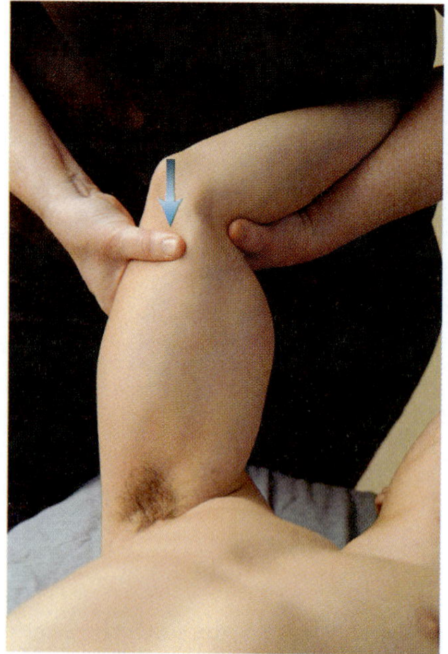

FIGURE 9.7 Broad stripping the triceps tendon

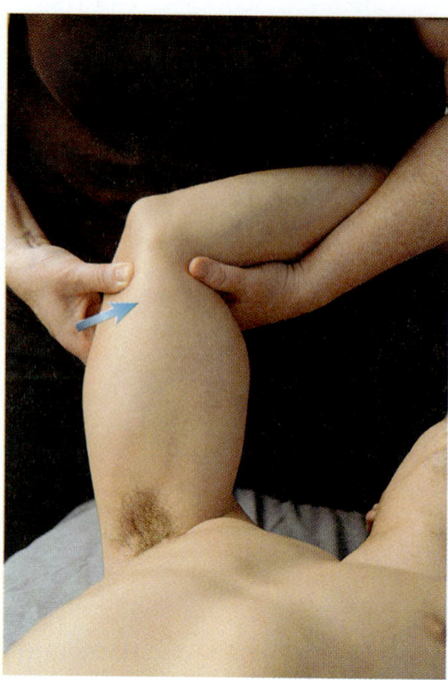

FIGURE 9.8 Deep transverse friction of the triceps insertion

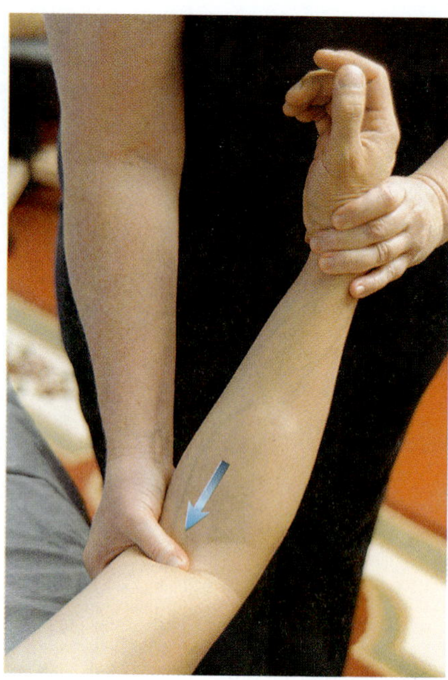

FIGURE 9.9 Stripping the radial insertion of the biceps

Broad Strip the Triceps Tendon

Using the same position for the upper extremity as described above, locate the triceps insertion, and broad strip it with one thumb or with alternating thumbs. Slide from the olecranon process into the bulk of the muscle. (See figure 9.7.)

Deep Transverse Friction of the Triceps Insertion

In the same flexed position, locate the olecranon process and apply deep transverse friction to the triceps insertion broadly with your thumb in one direction or with two thumbs in opposing directions. (See figure 9.8.)

Locate and Strip the Biceps Radial Attachment

Place the client's forearm in a supine position, and locate the insertion of the biceps tendon at the radial tuberosity. Flex and extend the elbow joint as you strip the insertion. (See figure 9.9.)

SUPINE

Use ice if necessary for acute tendon conditions.

Compressive Effleurage of the Brachialis

With the client's forearm in a supine position, apply compressive effleurage with relaxed soft hands to the lateral side of the arm. Use your body weight and momentum to sink into the tissues.

Compression to the Forearm and Brachioradialis

Use the palm of one hand to compress the belly of brachioradialis. Passively shorten the brachioradialis by flexing the client's elbow joint or laying the forearm flat on the table. (See figure 9.10.)

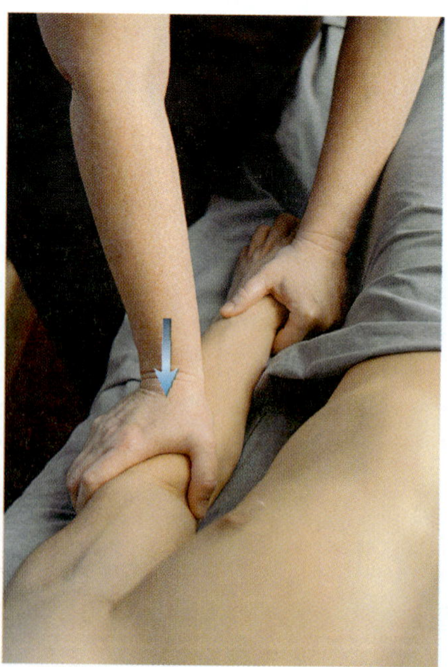

FIGURE 9.10 Compression of the brachioradialis

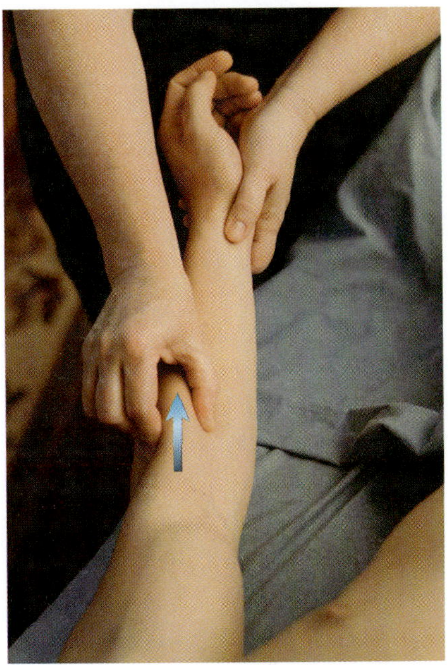

FIGURE 9.11 Jostling the brachioradialis

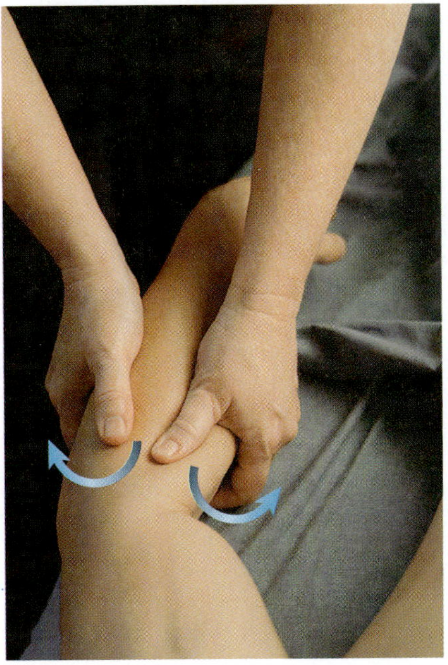

FIGURE 9.12 Elliptically moving the forearm muscles

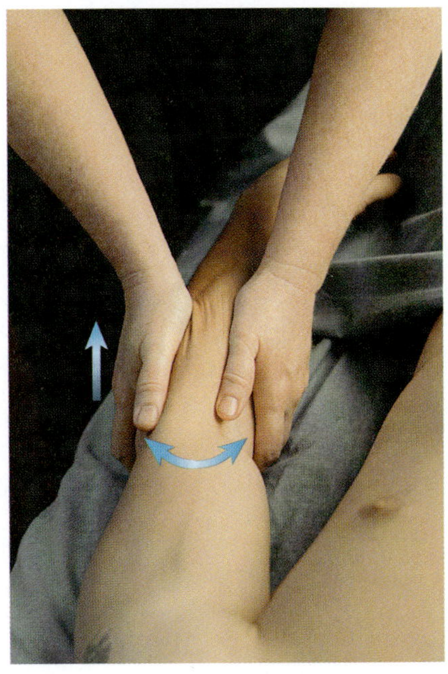

FIGURE 9.13 Broadening the brachioradialis

Jostle the Brachioradialis

Pick up the bulk of the muscle close to the client's elbow joint, apply a bit of a stretch, and jostle the brachioradialis toward the wrist. Repeat several times. (See figure 9.11.)

Elliptically Move the Forearm Muscles

Pick up the client's forearm (palm down), and grasp the muscles on both sides with your thumbs top-side-up and fingers positioned on the other side of the forearm. Elliptically move the forearm muscles. Notice how the radius shows movement. Move your hands in a variety of positions from proximal to distal. (See figure 9.12.)

Friction, Broadening, and Vibration of the Brachioradialis

Use any or all of these strokes to the brachioradialis to isolate it and loosen it from other sticky tendons. For broadening, place the client's forearm in a neutral position. Place your hands proximal to the elbow joint, and begin lifting and spreading the brachioradialis with your thumbs and the thenar side of your palm; then move distally toward the wrist and repeat the process. (See figure 9.13 for broadening.)

Myofascial Stretch for the Brachioradialis

At a right angle to the forearm, pick up the belly of the muscle and draw the tissue over your thumbs. Start close to the client's elbow joint, and work toward the wrist. Repeat. (See figure 9.14.)

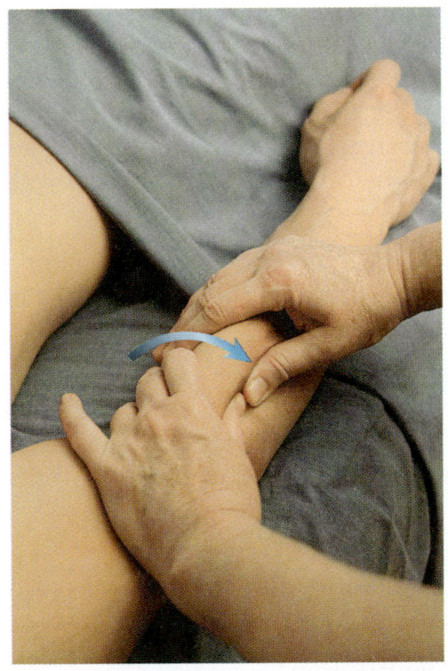

FIGURE 9.14 Myofascial stretch for the brachioradialis

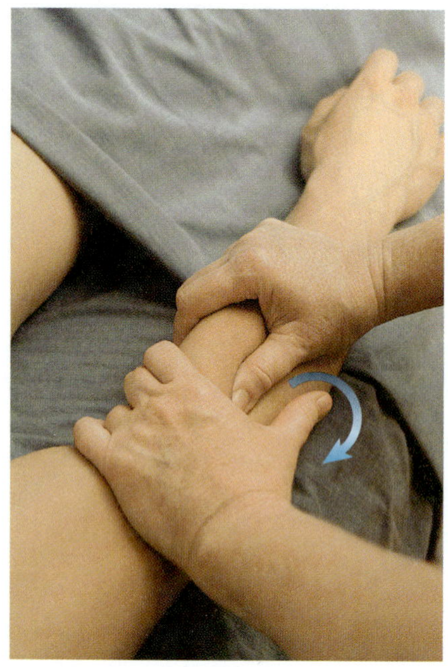

FIGURE 9.15 Parallel thumbs on the brachioradialis

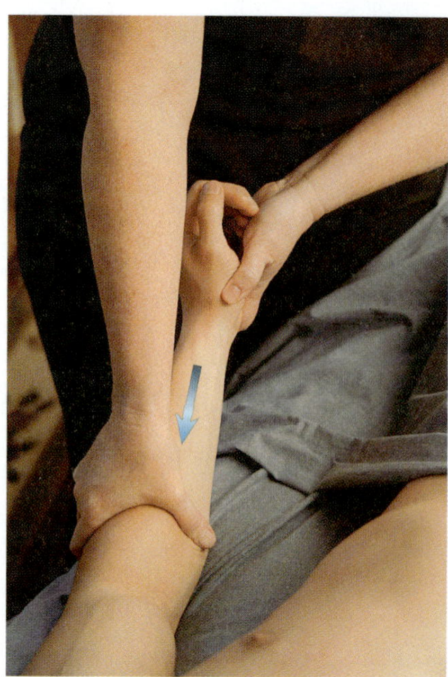

FIGURE 9.16 Compressive effleurage of the brachioradialis

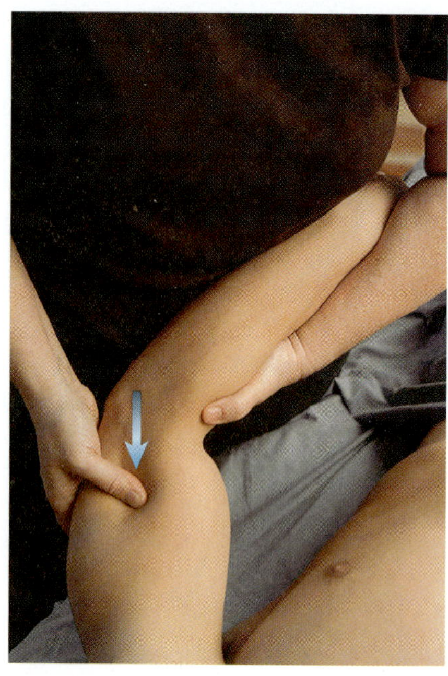

FIGURE 9.17 Stripping the origin of the brachioradialis

Parallel Thumbs on the Brachioradialis

At a right angle to the client's forearm, pick up the tissue with an alternating thumb-over-thumb technique, moving from the elbow to the wrist. (See figure 9.15.)

Compressive Effleurage of the Brachioradialis

Hold the ulnar side of the client's hand. With your other hand, straddle the brachioradialis muscle in neutral. Using your body weight and momentum, stroke from the distal end toward the elbow with a soft, compressive hand instead of hard hand pressure. Repeat several times. (See figure 9.16.)

Deep Transverse Friction, Circular Friction, or Stripping of the Origin of the Brachioradialis

Locate the supracondylar ridge, and apply deep transverse friction, stripping, or circular friction to the origin of the muscle. Locate the radial attachment, and apply deep transverse friction to the tendinous attachment. (See figure 9.17 for the origin and figure 9.19 for the insertion.)

Deep Transverse Friction or Circular Friction of the Anconeus

In the supine position, locate and apply deep transverse friction and/or use circular friction on attachments of the anconeus between the lateral epicondyle of the humerus and the olecranon process of the ulna. (See figure 9.18.)

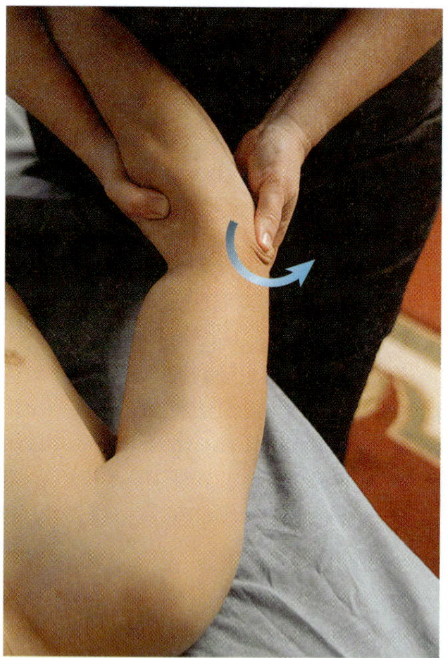

FIGURE 9.18 Circular friction of the anconeus

Strip the Radial Attachment of the Brachioradialis with Movement

Hold the client's wrist and hand in neutral with one hand. Locate the radial attachment at the wrist, and

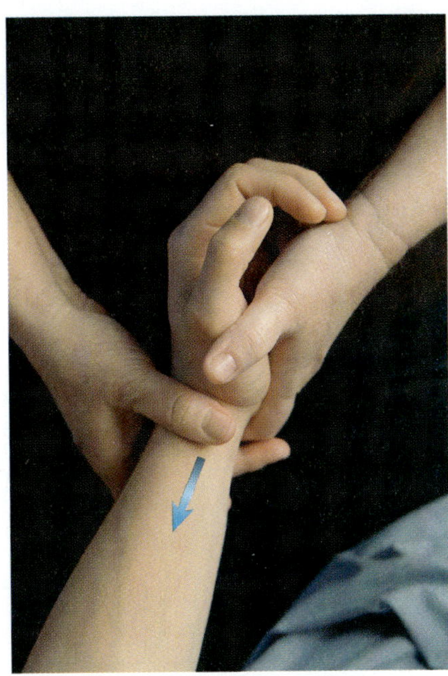

FIGURE 9.19 Stripping the radial attachment of the brachioradialis

as you move the wrist in an alternating sideways direction (radial flexion and ulnar flexion), strip the tendon with the thumb of your opposite hand. (See figure 9.19.)

Alternating Petrissage of the Brachioradialis

At a right angle to the muscle, alternate your hands in a petrissage technique.

Compressive Effleurage to the Entire Extremity

Note: The supinator as well as other forearm muscles will be worked with elliptical movement of the forearm. The pronator teres has been included in the flexors of the hand and wrist in Chapter 11, and there are additional techniques listed in Chapter 11 that will complete work on the forearm.

CHAPTER *summary*

Introduction

- ✔ Repetitive actions are a part of one's daily activities.
- ✔ The elbow joint and radioulnar joint are strategically located between the shoulder joint and the hand and wrist.
- ✔ The location of the joints provides more action for the hand and wrist, but often at the expense of overuse.

Injuries and Overuse Syndromes

- ✔ Dislocations and fractures are not uncommon to the elbow region.
- ✔ Bursitis often accompanies medial epicondylitis, or golfer's elbow.
- ✔ Lateral epicondylitis is a tendonitis located on the lateral side of the elbow joint.

Soft-Tissue Issues

- ✔ A subacute flare-up is a response to a chronic injury that has not been allowed to rest.
- ✔ Hypertonicity is a condition of soft tissue that is in a state of fatigue with too much congestion in the muscle.
- ✔ Attachment sites often have tenderness.

Nerve Complaints

- ✔ Ulnar nerve compression takes place when the ulnar nerve does not have enough room in the cubital tunnel.
- ✔ The triceps and supinator can entrap the radial nerve.
- ✔ Median nerve disorders include carpal tunnel syndrome, pronator teres syndrome, and the double-crush syndrome.

Unraveling the Riddle

- ✔ Shoulder girdle muscles contribute to compensatory discomforts.
- ✔ Work on the uninvolved upper extremity first.
- ✔ Follow a dimensional approach, and critically think about the involved joints and kinetic chain.
- ✔ Always use treatment protocols to determine the sequence of a therapeutic session.

Dimensional Massage Therapy for the Muscles of the Radioulnar and Elbow Joints

- ✔ The purpose of massage therapy is to reduce hypertonicities, lengthen fibers, separate tissues, reduce soreness and pain levels, increase flexibility, and increase restricted movements.
- ✔ Palpate the tissues and use touch to determine where tension exists in the tissue and whether hypertonicity is present; then assess the client's response to your touch.
- ✔ Begin with the client in a supine position.
- ✔ Approach techniques methodically, unwinding soft tissue superficially to deep.

CHAPTER *review*

True or False

Write true *or* false *after each statement.*

1. Muscles that insert on the ulna can perform extension only.
2. Massage can immediately be applied to the elbow area after a radial head fracture.
3. Hypertonic soft tissue can benefit from massage therapy.
4. The radial nerve goes through the carpal tunnel.
5. Active and passive range of motion can help determine whether to refer a client to another health professional.
6. The ulnar nerve lies in the cubital tunnel.
7. There are no areas of tenderness around the medial or lateral epicondyles.
8. The brachioradialis is used for hammering a nail or twisting a doorknob.
9. Ischemic pressure or deep transverse friction can be applied immediately on painful tendon attachments without any warm-up anywhere else.
10. A subacute flare-up of a chronic injury may require ice treatments.

Short Answers

Write your answers on the lines provided.

1. List the muscles of the elbow region through which the radial nerve can travel.

2. Give examples of agonists, antagonists, synergists, and stabilizers of the elbow joint and radioulnar joint.

3. What nerve can be entrapped by the pronator teres?

4. What muscles are involved in the double-crush syndrome?

5. How does a practitioner determine an appropriate sequence for a massage session that includes problems of the elbow region?

6. What is the significance of the biceps brachii inserting on the radius?

7. What forearm technique can the therapist use that will not be painful but will mobilize the soft tissue and deeply move the radius and ulna?

8. An undiagnosed client presenting with burning, radiating pain down the upper extremity to the hand in a particular pattern should be:

9. What concerns are involved when a client diagnosed with carpal tunnel syndrome makes an appointment for a massage?

10. Why is it important to work on the brachioradialis substantially in the forearm?

____

____

____

Multiple Choice

Circle the correct answers.

1. Median nerve disorders include:
   a. double-crush syndrome
   b. pronator teres syndrome
   c. carpal tunnel syndrome
   d. all of the above
2. Shoulder girdle muscles:
   a. contribute to compensatory discomforts
   b. have nothing to do with the elbow region
   c. attach to the humerus
   d. none of the above
3. A subacute flare-up is:
   a. something the practitioner will never have to deal with
   b. a response to a chronic injury that has not been allowed to rest
   c. an issue following acute
   d none of the above
4. A therapist's purpose is to:
   a. reduce hypertonicities and lengthen fibers
   b. separate tissues and reduce soreness and pain levels
   c. increase flexibility and increase restricted movements
   d. all of the above
5. A physician may not cast a fracture to the head of the radius because:
   a. the head of the radius is part of the elbow joint
   b. the radius must continue to move, and immobilizing it might ultimately affect the joint's complete range of motion
   c. it is not important
   d. none of the above
6. Bursitis often accompanies:
   a. fractures
   b. sore muscles
   c. golfer's elbow
   d. none of the above
7. Another name for golfer's elbow is:
   a. lateral epicondylitis
   b. medial epicondylitis
   c. bursitis
   d. tendonosis
8. Hypertonicity is:
   a. a tendonitis
   b. bursitis
   c. a condition of soft tissue that is in a state of fatigue with too much congestion in the muscle
   d. none of the above
9. Techniques used initially with no lubrication to the arm might include:
   a. effleurage, deep transverse friction, and tapotement
   b. rolling, elliptical movement, and jostling
   c. digital circular friction, deep transverse friction, and stripping
   d. friction, effleurage, and nerve strokes
10. When the client has a clinical soft-tissue problem in one extremity and not the other, it is important to:
    a. work on the uninvolved side first
    b. work on the soft-tissue problem first
    c. do deep transverse friction and stripping on the soft-tissue problem first
    d. not work on either extremity

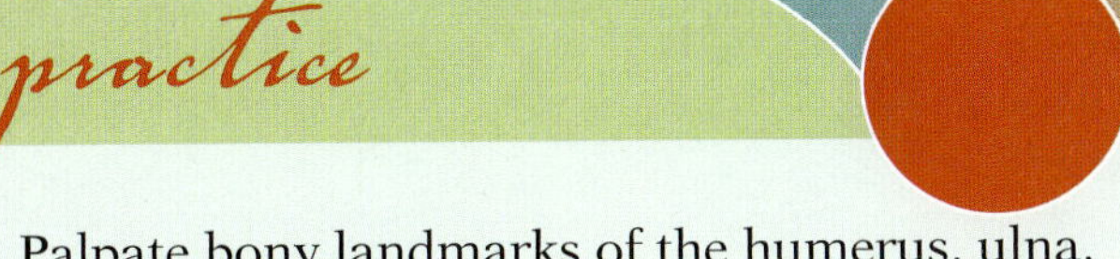

1. Palpate bony landmarks of the humerus, ulna, and radius on a partner.
2. Locate the origin and insertions of the elbow joint and radioulnar joint muscles on a partner.
3. Demonstrate how to passively shorten the biceps, triceps, and brachioradialis.
4. Demonstrate passive range of motion of the elbow joint with a partner.

5. Demonstrate active range of motion of the elbow joint with a partner.
6. Demonstrate passive range of motion of the radioulnar joint with a partner.
7. Demonstrate active range of motion of the radioulnar joint with a partner.
8. Demonstrate some principles of safe body mechanics while performing massage techniques.
9. Demonstrate warm-up techniques without lubrication.
10. Practice deep-tissue techniques individually and in a sequence on a willing participant.

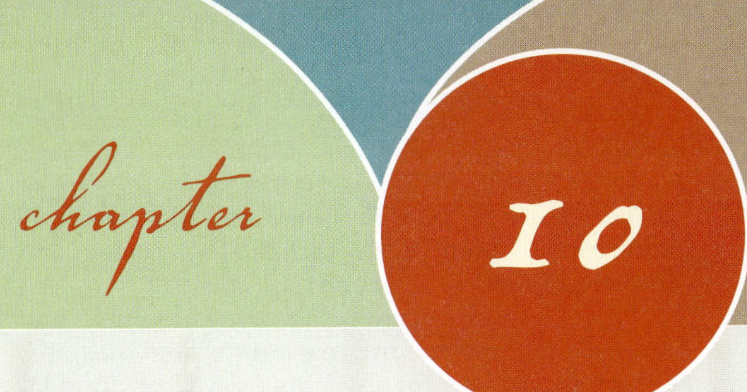

The Wrist and Hand Joints

LEARNING OUTCOMES

After completing this chapter, you should be able to:

10-1 Define key terms.

10-2 Locate on a human skeleton selected bony structures of the arm, forearm, wrist, hand, and fingers.

10-3 Label selected bony landmarks of the wrist and hand on a skeletal chart.

10-4 Name the bones of the hand.

10-5 Draw and identify the muscles involved in the hand and wrist on a skeletal chart.

10-6 Palpate the bony structures and the muscles of the forearm, hand, and wrist on a partner.

10-7 Explore the origins and insertions of the muscles of the forearm, hand, and wrist on a partner.

10-8 Demonstrate with a partner all the active and passive movements of the hand and wrist joints.

10-9 Organize and list the muscles that produce the primary movements of the wrist, hand, and fingers.

10-10 List the antagonists and synergists of the muscles of the wrist and hand.

10-11 Determine the names of the muscles and nerve that travel through the carpal tunnel.

10-12 Practice flexibility and strengthening exercises for each muscle group.

KEY TERMS

Abductor pollicis longus
Capitate
Carpals
Carpometacarpal (CMC)
Distal interphalangeal (DIP)
Extensor carpi radialis brevis
Extensor carpi radialis longus
Extensor carpi ulnaris
Extensor digiti minimi
Extensor digitorum
Extensor indicis
Extensor pollicis brevis
Extensor pollicis longus
Flexor carpi radialis
Flexor carpi ulnaris
Flexor digitorum profundus
Flexor digitorum superficialis
Flexor pollicis longus
Hamate
Lunate
Metacarpophalangeal (MCP)
Palmaris longus
Pisiform
Proximal interphalangeal (PIP)
Saddle-type joint
Scaphoid
Trapezium
Trapezoid
Triquetrum
Ulnar nerves

Introduction

Repetitive hand and wrist actions occur daily. Indeed, writing, pointing, drawing, typing, and numerous other everyday activities would be impossible to perform without the normal functioning of the hand and wrist joints and muscles; moreover, overuse of these multifaceted tools often leads to tenderness, strains, sprains, tendonitis, and other soft-tissue conditions.

The numerous muscles, bones, and ligaments in the hand and wrist illustrate the complex functional anatomy in this relatively small package; however, grouping the muscles into the major action categories can help simplify the learning process. Muscles work in groups and in paired opposition, and this is especially true in the hand and wrist. Primary hand and wrist actions include flexion, extension, abduction, and adduction, and they employ the use of several muscles. Anatomically and structurally, the hand and wrist have highly developed, complex mechanisms capable of a variety of movements thanks to the arrangement of the 29 bones; more than 25 joints; and more than 30 muscles, of which 18 are intrinsic (both origin and insertion found in the hand) muscles.

This chapter reviews the bones, joints, and movements involved in gross motor activities; discusses the nerves involved; and provides foundational information on the forearm muscles and the primary extrinsic muscles of the hand, wrist, and fingers. Each prime mover is discussed in detail to show how the muscles work together and in paired opposition. For ease of comprehension, the flexors are presented first as a group, superficial to deep, followed by the extensors, arranged in the same pattern. Clinical Notes boxes offer snapshots of conditions and problems associated with many of these muscles. The chapter also provides specific exercises to help stretch and strengthen the hand, wrist, and fingers, and it addresses why the small muscles of the hand and wrist should be included in a prescribed exercise program for forearm injuries. The end of the chapter reviews the intrinsic muscles to a limited degree. References in Appendix A provide additional resources.

Bones

The wrist and hand contain 29 bones, including the radius and ulna (figure 10.1). Eight **carpal** bones in two rows of four bones form the wrist. The proximal row consists of, from the radial (thumb) side to the ulnar (little-finger) side, the **scaphoid** (boat-shaped), or navicular as it is commonly known; the **lunate** (moon-shaped); the **triquetrum** (three-cornered); and the **pisiform** (pea-shaped) bones. The distal row, from the radial side to the ulnar side, consists of the **trapezium** (greater multangular), the **trapezoid** (lesser multangular), the **capitate** (head-shaped), and the **hamate** (hooked) bones. The trapezium, the trapezoid, the capitate, and the hamate form a three-sided arch that is either oval or square on the palmar side. This bony arch, from the hook of the hamate to the tubercle of the trapezium, is spanned by the transverse carpal (flexor retinaculum) and volar carpal ligaments to create the carpal tunnel, which is frequently a source of problems and conditions known as *carpal tunnel syndrome* (See figure 10.1). One of the many conditions that can contribute to carpal tunnel syndrome is a depressed capitate. The capitate sits on the roof of the carpal tunnel and can shrink the size of the tunnel if it is in a depressed position, thereby contributing to compression of the median nerve.

Of these carpal bones, the scaphoid is by far the one most commonly fractured, usually due to severe wrist hyperextension from falling on the outstretched hand. Unfortunately, this particular fracture is often dismissed as a sprain after the initial injury; however, it can cause significant problems in the long term if not properly treated. While treatment often requires precise immobilization for periods longer than needed with many other fractures, beginning range-of-motion exercises for the fingers and wrist can help prevent prolonged stiffness.

Five metacarpal bones, numbered 1 to 5 from the radial side to the ulnar side, join the wrist bones. There are 14 phalanxes (digits), 3 for each phalange except the thumb, which has only 2. The phalanxes are indicated as proximal, middle, and distal from the metacarpals. Additionally, the thumb has a sesamoid bone within its flexor tendon, and other sesamoids may be present in the fingers.

The medial epicondyle, medial condyloid ridge, and coronoid process serve as a point of origin for many of the wrist and finger flexors, whereas the lateral epicondyle and lateral supracondylar ridge serve as the point of origin for many extensors of the wrist and fingers. (Refer to figure 8.1 on page 156.) Distally, the key bony landmarks for the muscles involved in wrist motion are the base of the 2nd, 3rd, and 5th metacarpals and the pisiform and hamate. The finger muscles, which also are involved in wrist motion, insert on the base of the proximal, middle, and distal phalanxes. The base of the 1st metacarpal

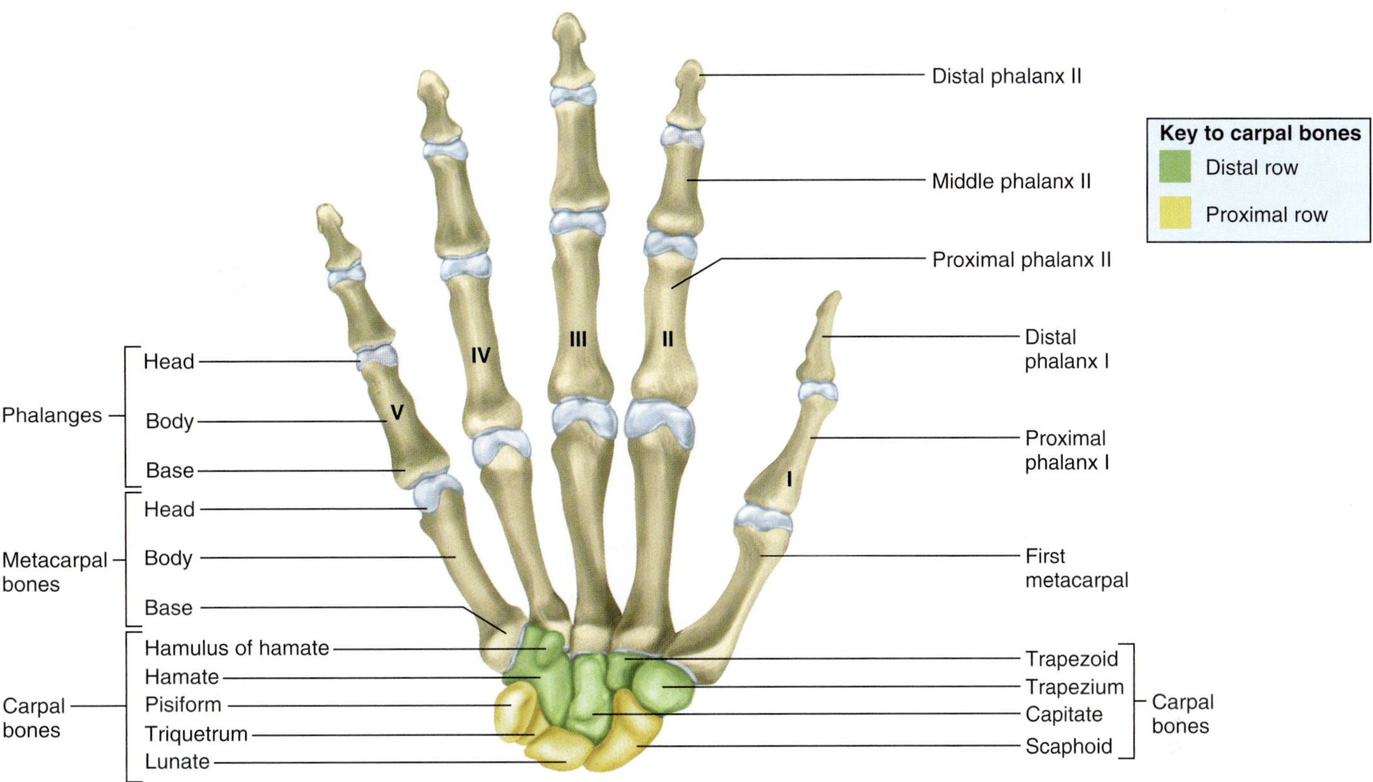

FIGURE 10.1 Bones of the wrist and hand

and the proximal and distal phalanxes of the thumb serve as key insertion points for the muscles involved in thumb motion.

Joints

The wrist joint is classified as a *condyloid*-type joint, which enables movement in two planes, allowing flexion, extension, abduction (radial flexion or deviation), and adduction (ulnar flexion or deviation). (See figure 10.2.) Wrist motion occurs primarily between the distal radius and the proximal carpal row, consisting of the scaphoid, lunate, and triquetrum. The joint allows 70 to 90 degrees of flexion and 65 to 85 degrees of extension. The wrist can abduct 15 to 25 degrees and adduct 25 to 40 degrees. (See figure 10.3.)

Each finger has three joints. The **metacarpophalangeal (MCP)** joint is classified as condyloid and is commonly called *knuckle*. In this joint, 0 to 40 degrees of extension and 85 to 100 degrees of flexion are possible. The next joint of the phalange is called the **proximal interphalangeal (PIP)** joint, classified as *ginglymus,* and it can move from full extension to approximately 90 to 120 degrees of flexion. At the end of the finger is the **distal interphalangeal (DIP)** joint, also classified as ginglymus; it can flex 80 to 90 degrees from full extension. (See figure 10.5.)

The interphalangeal and metacarpophalangeal joints of the thumb are classified as ginglymus. The metacarpophalangeal joint moves from full extension into 40 to 90 degrees of flexion. The interphalangeal (IP) joint can flex 80 to 90 degrees. The **carpometacarpal (CMC)** joint of the thumb is a unique **saddle-type joint,** which has 50 to 70 degrees of abduction. It can flex approximately 15 to 45 degrees and extend 0 to 20 degrees (figure 10.6). The ability of the thumb to touch each finger is called opposition; this movement is unique to humans.

Ligaments, too numerous to mention in this discussion, support and provide static stability to the many joints of the wrist and hand. Some of the finger ligaments are detailed in figure 10.4. Ligaments are often injured in stubbing the fingers in basketball and other sports, as well as in slip-and-fall injuries.

Movements of the Wrist and Hand

The common actions of the wrist are flexion, extension, abduction (radial flexion or deviation), and adduction (ulnar flexion or deviation). The fingers can only flex and extend, except at the metacarpophalangeal joints, where abduction and adduction are controlled by the intrinsic hand muscles. (See figure 10.7.) In the hand, the middle phalange is regarded as the reference point by which to differentiate abduction and adduction. Abduction of the index and middle fingers occurs when they move laterally toward the radial side of the forearm. Abduction of the ring and

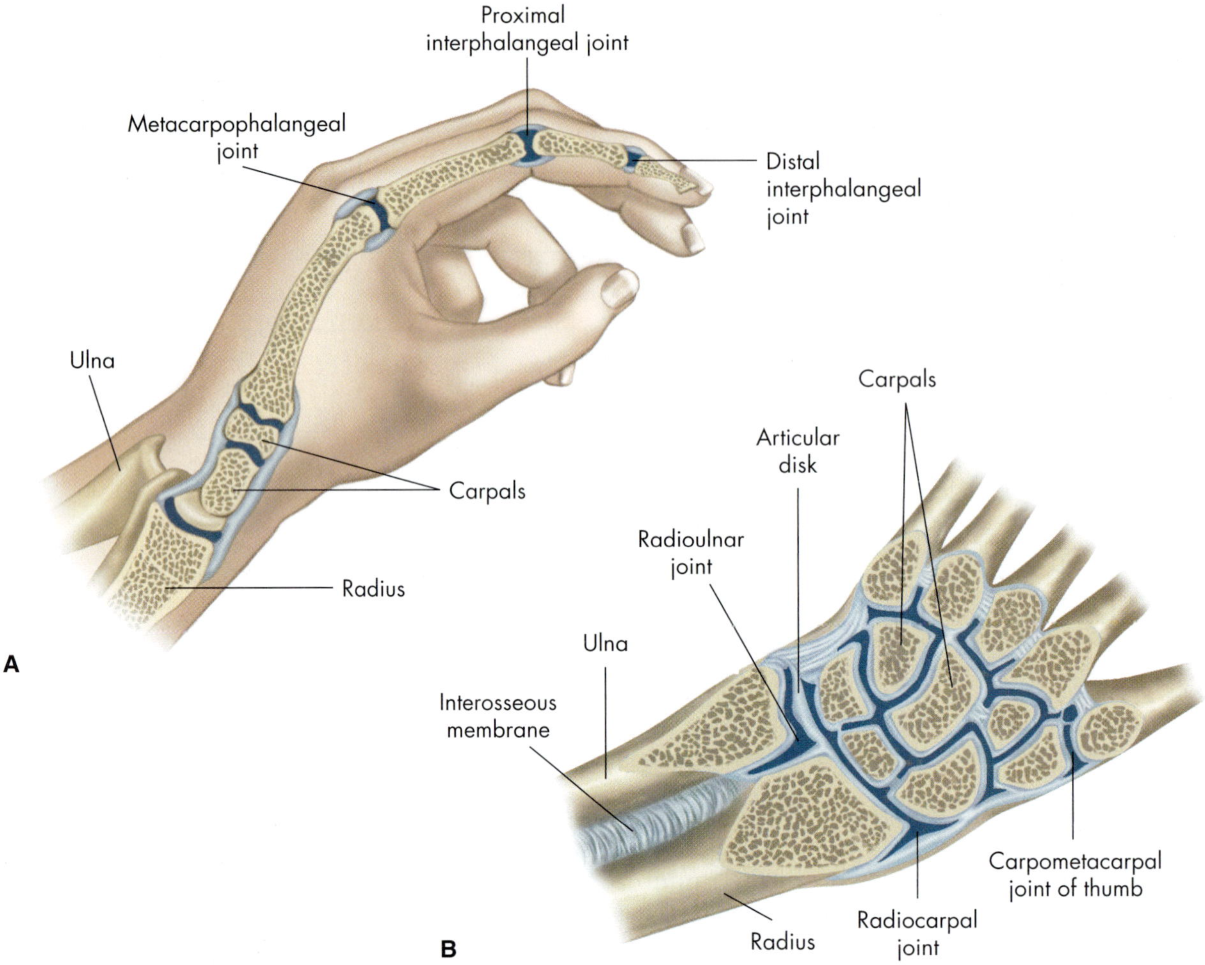

Proximal interphalangeal joint
Metacarpophalangeal joint
Distal interphalangeal joint
Ulna
Carpals
Radius
A
Carpals
Articular disk
Radioulnar joint
Ulna
Interosseous membrane
Carpometacarpal joint of thumb
Radiocarpal joint
Radius
B

FIGURE 10.2 Wrist and hand joint structures

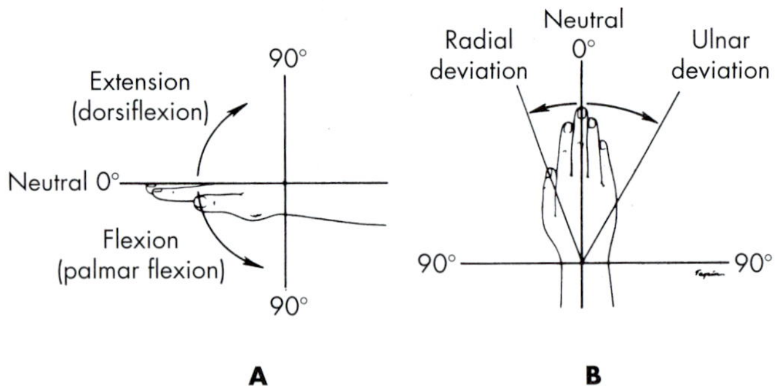

FIGURE 10.3 Range of motion of the wrist

little fingers occurs when they move medially toward the ulnar side of the hand. Movement medially of the index and middle fingers toward the ulnar side of the forearm is adduction. Ring and little-finger adduction occurs when these fingers move laterally toward the radial side of the hand. The thumb is abducted when it moves away from the palm, and it is adducted when it moves toward the palmar aspect of the second metacarpal. These movements, together with pronation and supination of the forearm, make possible the many fine, coordinated movements of the forearm, wrist, and hand.

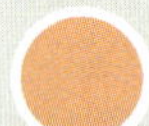

FLEXIBILITY & STRENGTH

Movements of the Wrist

Flexion (palmar flexion)
Movement of the palm of the hand and/or the phalanges toward the anterior or volar aspect of the forearm.

Extension (dorsiflexion)
Movement of the back of the hand and/or the phalanges toward the posterior or dorsal aspect of the forearm; sometimes referred to as *hyperextension.*

Abduction (radial deviation, radial flexion)
Movement of the thumb side of the hand toward the lateral aspect or radial side of the forearm; also movement of the fingers away from the middle finger.

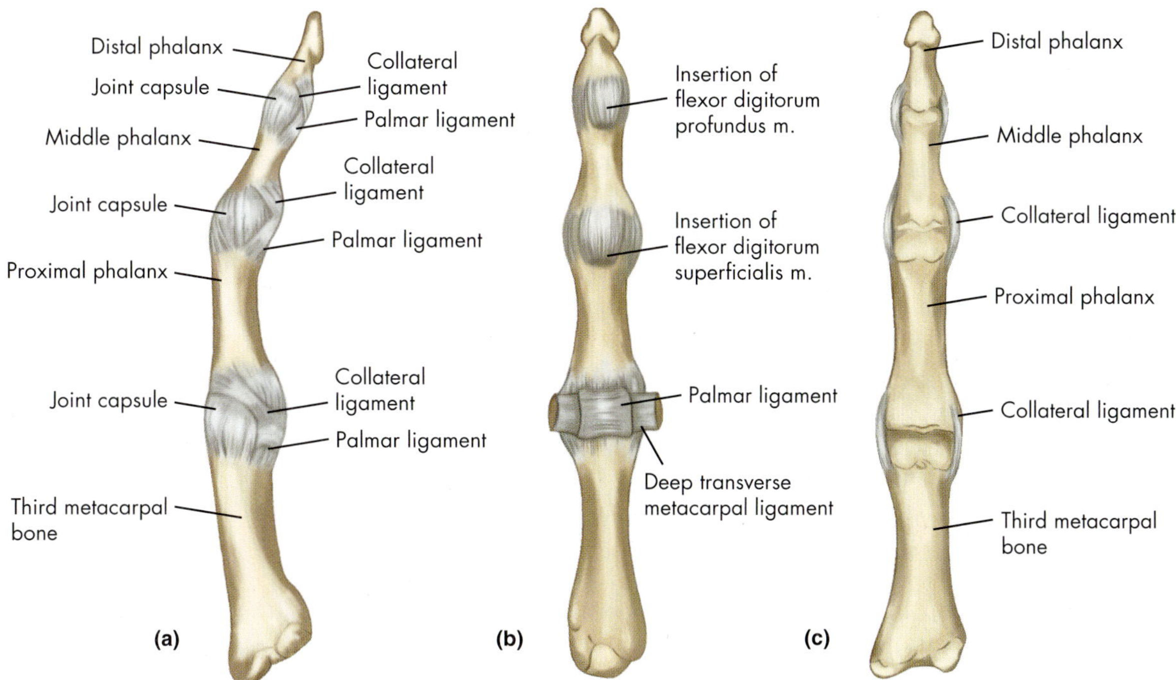

FIGURE 10.4 Finger joints and ligaments

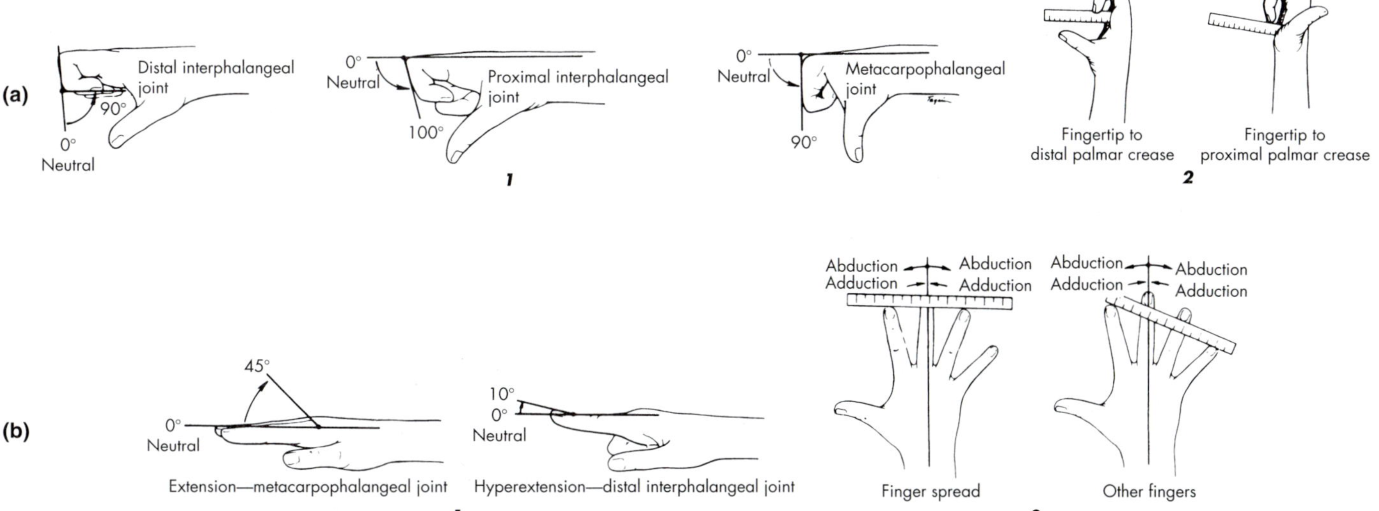

FIGURE 10.5 Range of motion of the fingers

Adduction (ulnar deviation, ulnar flexion)
Movement of the little-finger side of the hand toward the medial aspect or ulnar side of the forearm; also movement of the fingers back together toward the middle finger.

Opposition
Movement of the thumb across the palmar aspect to oppose any or all of the phalanges.

Reposition
Movement of the thumb as it returns to the anatomical position from opposition with the hand and/or fingers.

Muscles

The extrinsic muscles of the wrist and hand can be grouped according to function and location, as listed in table 10.1. There are six muscles that move the wrist but that do not cross the hand to move the fingers and thumb. The three wrist flexors in this group are the **flexor carpi radialis, flexor carpi ulnaris,** and **palmaris longus**—all of which have their origin on the medial epicondyle of the humerus (figure 10.8). The wrist extensors have their origin on the lateral epicondyle and include the **extensor carpi radialis longus,**

TABLE 10.1 The Extrinsic Muscles of the Wrist and Hand

Name of Muscle	Origins	Insertion	Actions	Innervations
Palmaris longus	Medial epicondyle of humerus	Palmaris aponeurosis of 2nd, 3rd, 4th, and 5th metacarpals	Assists in flexion of wrist, weak flexion of elbow joint	Median nerve (C6, C7)
Flexor carpi radialis	Medial epicondyle of humerus	Base of 2nd and 3rd metacarpals, palmar surface	Flexion of hand, abduction of hand at wrist, weak flexion of elbow	Median nerve (C6, C7)
Flexor carpi ulnaris	Medial epicondyle of humerus via common tendon, posterior aspect of proximal ulna	Base of 5th metacarpal, pisiform (hamate)	Flexion and adduction of wrist, weak flexion of elbow	Ulnar nerve (C8, T1)
Flexor digitorum superficialis	Medial epicondyle of humerus via common tendon *Ulna:* medial coronoid process of ulna *Radial:* oblique line of radius	Sides of shafts of middle phalanges of four fingers	Flexion of four fingers at PIP joint and MP joint, flexion of hand and wrist, weak flexion of elbow	Median nerve (C7, C8, T1)
Flexor digitorum profundus	Proximal three-fourths of anterior and medial ulna	Base of distal phalanges of four fingers	Flexion of four fingers at distal interphalangeal joints, PIP joints, and MP joints, flexion of wrist	Median nerve (C8, T1) to the 2nd and 3rd fingers Ulnar nerve (C8, T1) to the 4th and 5th fingers
Flexor pollicis longus	Middle anterior radius, anterior medial border of the ulna just distal to the coronoid process, interosseous membrane	Distal phalanx of thumb	Flexion of thumb carpometacarpal, metacarpophalangeal, and interphalangeal joints, assists flexion and abduction of wrist	Median nerve, palmar interosseous branch (C8, T1)
Extensor carpi ulnaris	Lateral epicondyle of humerus (common extensor tendon), middle two-fourths of posterior border of ulna	Base of 5th metacarpal	Extension of wrist, adduction of wrist, weak extension of forearm	Radial nerve (C6–C8)
Extensor carpi radialis brevis	Lateral epicondyle of humerus (common extensor tendon)	Base of 3rd metacarpal (dorsal)	Extension of wrist, abduction of wrist, weak flexion of elbow	Radial nerve (C6, C7)
Extensor carpi radialis longus	Lower third of lateral supracondylar ridge of humerus and lateral epicondyle of humerus	Base of 2nd metacarpal (dorsal)	Extension and abduction of wrist, weak flexion of elbow, weak pronation from supination	Radial nerve (C6, C7)
Extensor digitorum	Lateral epicondyle of humerus	Base of middle phalanges of four fingers, extensor expansion of four fingers, dorsal surface	Extension of MP joints of four fingers (phalanges of fingers), extension of wrist, extension of elbow	Radial nerve (C6–C8)

TABLE 10.1 (Continued)

Name of Muscle	Origins	Insertion	Actions	Innervations
Extensor indicis	Middle to distal third of posterior ulna, interosseous membrane	Head of 2nd metacarpal and joins the extensor expansion at proximal phalanx	Extension of index finger at metacarpophalangeal joint, weak wrist extension, weak supination for forearm from pronation	Radial nerve (C6–C8)
Extensor digiti minimi	Lateral epicondyle of humerus	Joins extensor expansion on proximal phalanx of 5th phalange (dorsal)	Extension of little finger at metacarpophalangeal joint, weak wrist extension, weak elbow extension	Radial nerve (C6–C8)
Extensor pollicis longus ("anatomical snuffbox")	Posterior middle to lower ulna and interosseous membrane	Base of distal phalanx of thumb (dorsal)	Extension of thumb at IP, MP, and CMP joints, extension of wrist, abduction of wrist, weak supination for the forearm	Radial nerve (C6–C8)
Extensor pollicis brevis	Posterior surface of lower middle radius	Base of proximal phalanx of thumb (dorsal)	Extension of thumb at CMP and MP joints, weak wrist extension, wrist abduction	Radial nerve (C6, C7)
Abductor pollicis longus	Posterior aspect of radius and midshaft of ulna	Base of 1st metacarpal (dorsal)	Abduction and extension of thumb at CMP, abduction of wrist, weak supination of forearm, weak flexion of wrist	Radial nerve (C6, C7)

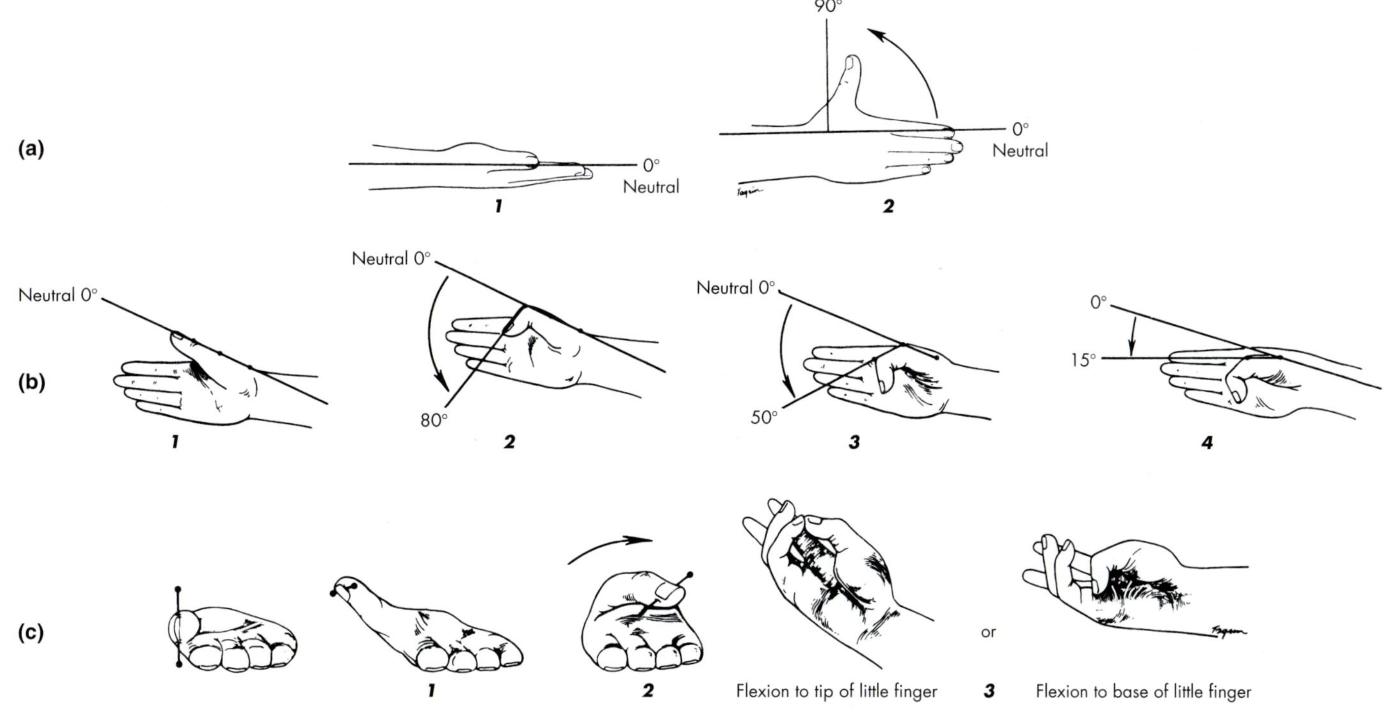

FIGURE 10.6 Range of motion of the thumb

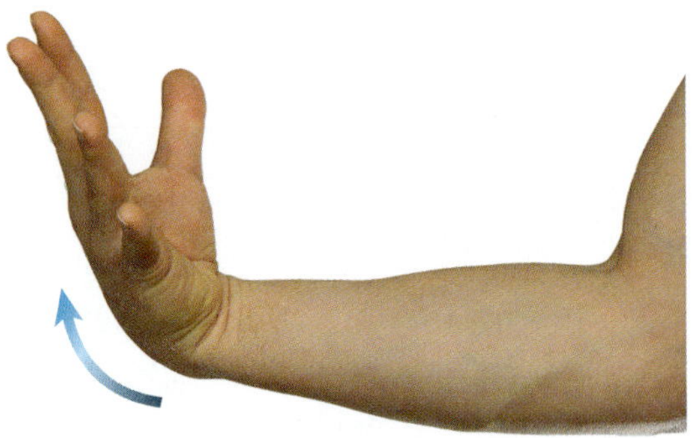

Wrist flexion

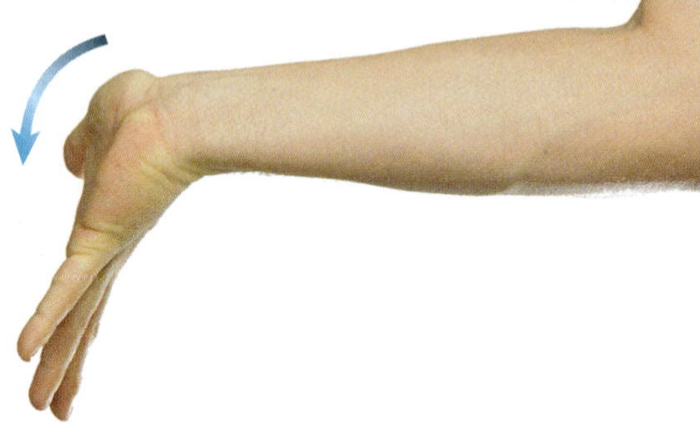

Wrist extension

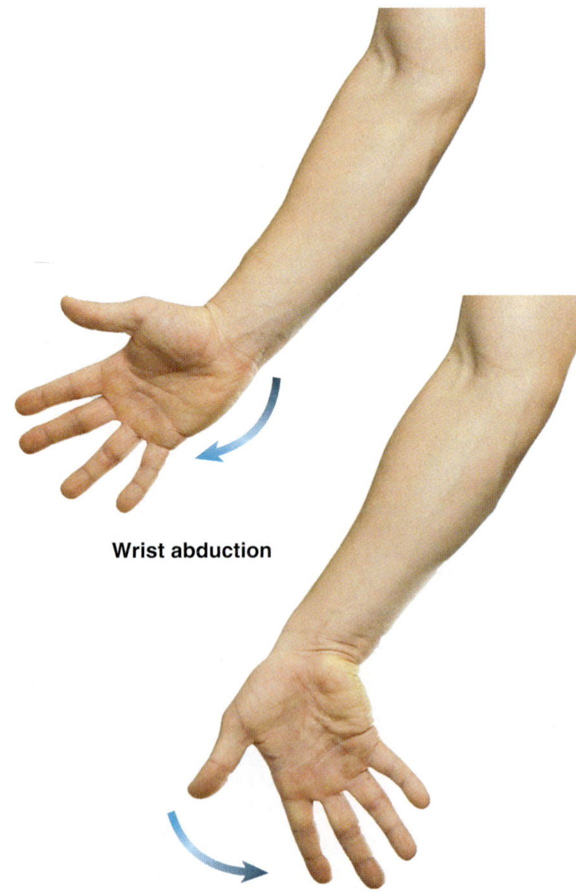

Wrist abduction

Wrist adduction

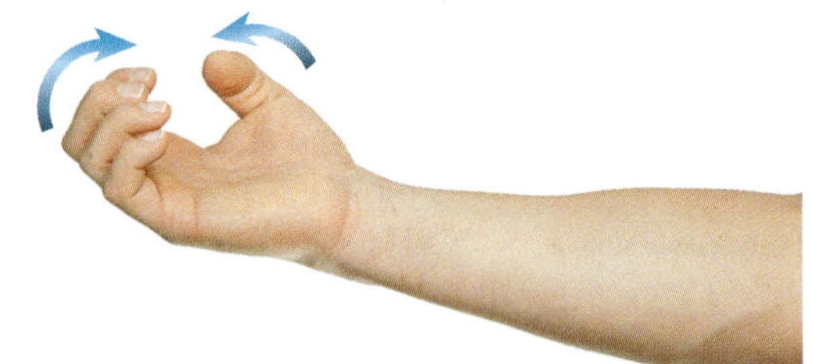

Flexion of fingers and thumb

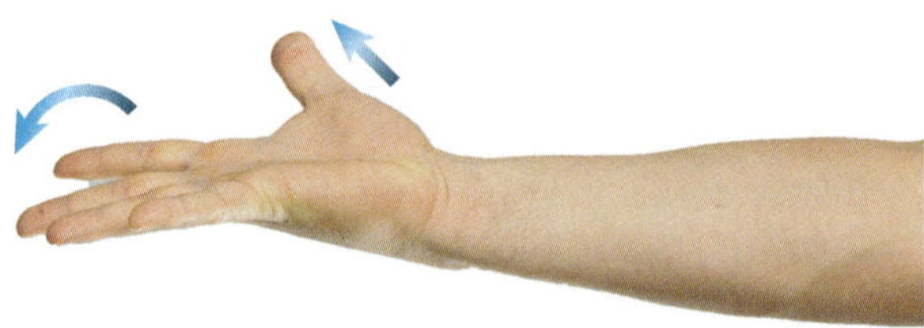

Extension of fingers and thumb

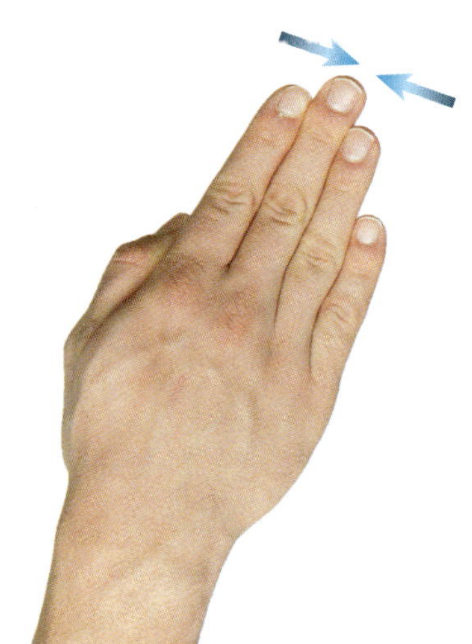

Adduction of metacarpophalangeal

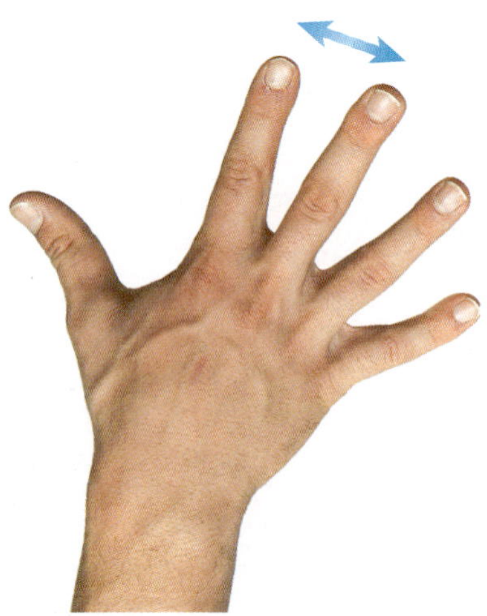

Abduction of metacarpophalangeal

FIGURE 10.7 Wrist and hand movements

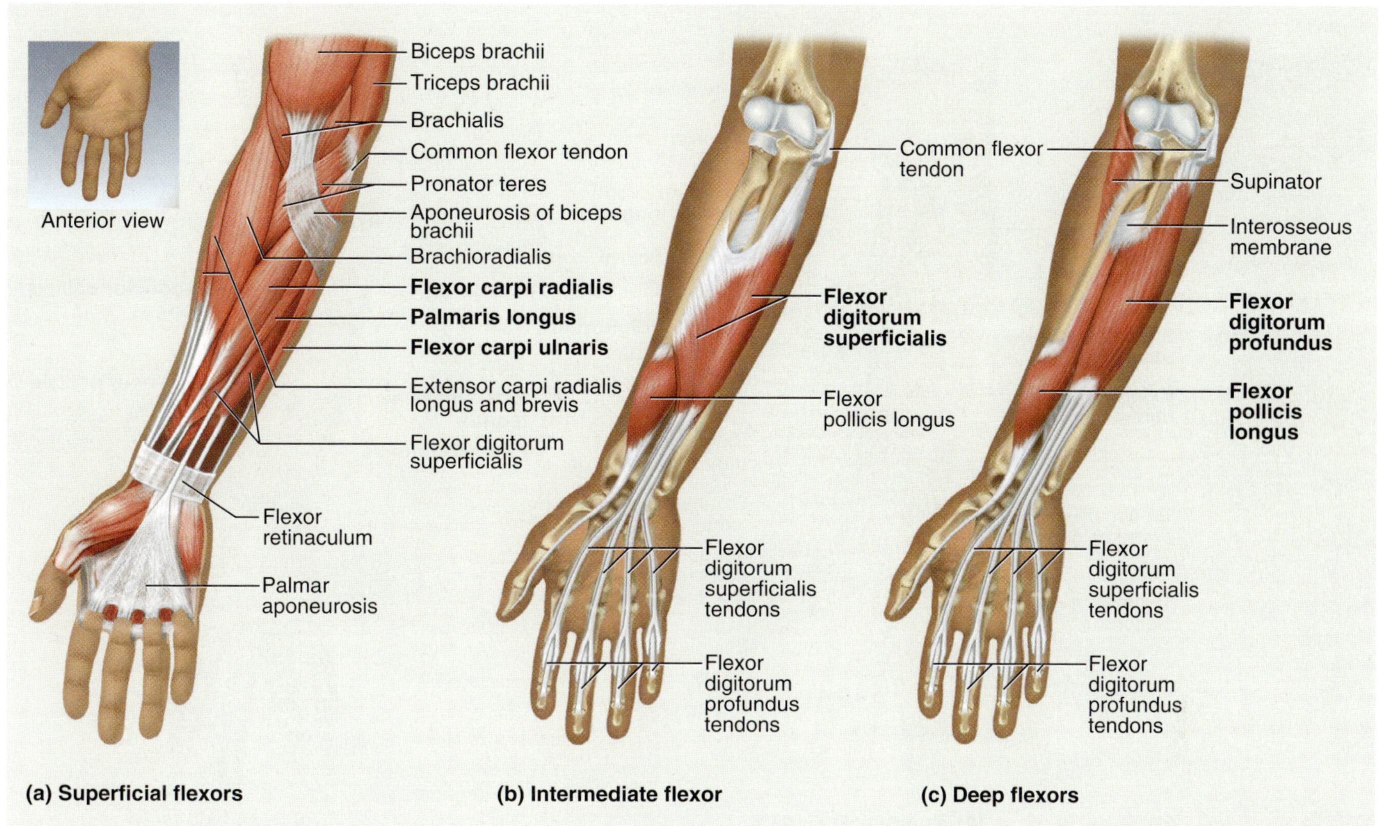

FIGURE 10.8 Flexor muscles of the wrist and hand, anterior view

extensor carpi radialis brevis, and **extensor carpi ulnaris** (figure 10.9).

There are another nine muscles that function primarily to move the phalanges. They also are involved in wrist joint actions because they originate on the forearm and cross the wrist. These muscles generally are weaker in their actions on the wrist. The **flexor digitorum superficialis** and the **flexor digitorum profundus** are finger flexors; however, they also assist in wrist flexion along with the **flexor pollicis longus,** which is a thumb flexor. The **extensor digitorum,** the **extensor indicis,** and the **extensor digiti minimi** are finger extensors, but they also assist in wrist extension, along with the **extensor pollicis longus** and the **extensor pollicis brevis,** which extends the thumb. The **abductor pollicis longus** abducts the thumb and assists in wrist abduction.

All the wrist flexors generally have their origins on the anteromedial aspect of the proximal forearm and medial epicondyle of the humerus, whereas their insertions are on the anterior aspect of the wrist and hand. All the flexor tendons, except for the flexor carpi ulnaris and palmaris longus, pass through the carpal tunnel, along with the median nerve. Conditions leading to swelling and inflammation in this area can result in increased pressure in the carpal tunnel. This can interfere with the normal function of the median nerve, leading to reduced motor and sensory function of its distribution (figure 10.10), which is known as *carpal tunnel syndrome.* This condition is commonly caused by activities that require the repetitive use of the hand and wrist and is frequently found in those who play musical instruments, perform manual labor, and perform clerical work such as typing. Modifications in work habits, including ergonomics and hand and wrist positions during activities, are useful preventive measures. Additionally, flexibility exercises for the wrist, finger flexors, and neck may be helpful. See Chapter 13 for more information on the importance of flexibility for the neck and brachial plexus.

The wrist extensors generally have their origins on the posterolateral aspect of the proximal forearm and the lateral humeral epicondyle, whereas their insertions are located on the posterior aspect of the wrist and hand. The flexor and extensor tendons at the distal forearm immediately proximal to the wrist are held in place on the palmar and dorsal aspects by transverse bands of tissue. These bands, respectively known as the *flexor* and *extensor retinaculum* (antebrachial fascia), prevent these

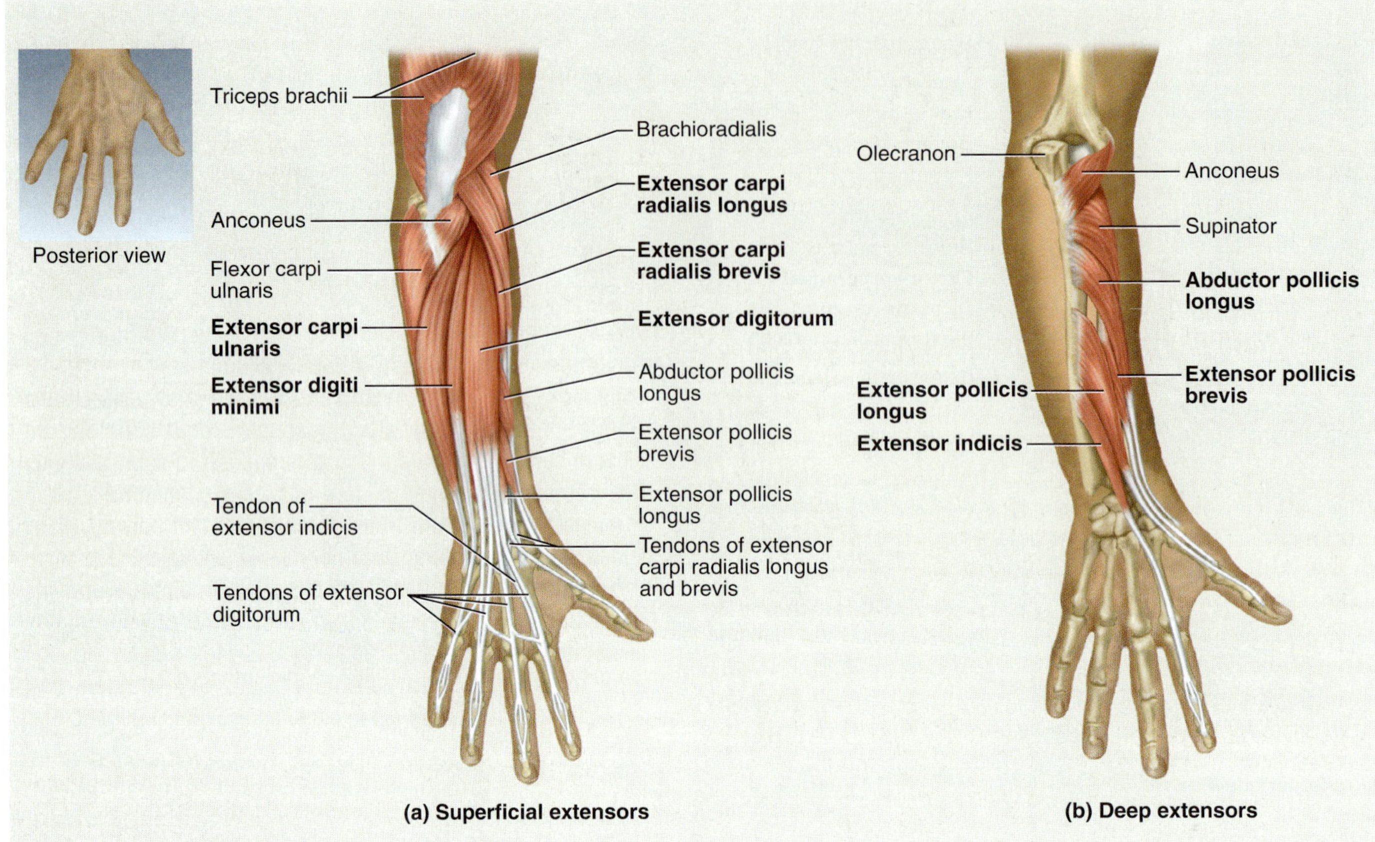

FIGURE 10.9 Extensor muscles of the wrist and hand, posterior view

tendons from bowstringing during flexion and extension.

The wrist abductors are the flexor carpi radialis, extensor carpi radialis longus, extensor carpi radialis brevis, abductor pollicis longus, extensor pollicis longus, and extensor pollicis brevis. These muscles generally cross the wrist joint anterolaterally and posterolaterally to insert on the radial side of the hand. The flexor carpi ulnaris and extensor carpi ulnaris adduct the wrist and cross the wrist joint anteromedially and posteromedially to insert on the ulnar side of the hand. All of these muscles should be considered in treatment for epicondyle conditions, since some of their origins are on the lateral and medial aspect of the forearm, as well as on the epicondyles.

The intrinsic muscles of the hand, listed in table 10.2, have their origins and insertions on the bones of the hand. Organizing the intrinsic muscles into three groups according to location is helpful in understanding and learning these muscles. On the radial side, there are four muscles of the thumb—the opponens pollicis, the abductor pollicis brevis, the flexor pollicis brevis, and the adductor pollicis. On the ulnar side, there are three muscles of the little finger—the opponens digiti minimi, the abductor digiti minimi, and the flexor digiti minimi brevis. In the remainder of the hand, there are 11 muscles, which can be further grouped as the 4 lumbricals, the 3 palmar interossei, and the 4 dorsal interossei.

Wrist and Hand Muscles—Location

MUSCLE SPECIFIC

Anteromedial *is at the elbow and forearm and anterior at the hand. (See figure 10.8.)*

Primarily wrist flexion
- Flexor carpi radialis
- Flexor carpi ulnaris
- Palmaris longus

Primarily phalangeal flexion, assists in wrist flexion
- Flexor digitorum superficialis
- Flexor digitorum profundus
- Flexor pollicis longus

Posterolateral *is at the elbow and forearm and posterior at the hand. (See figure 10.9.)*

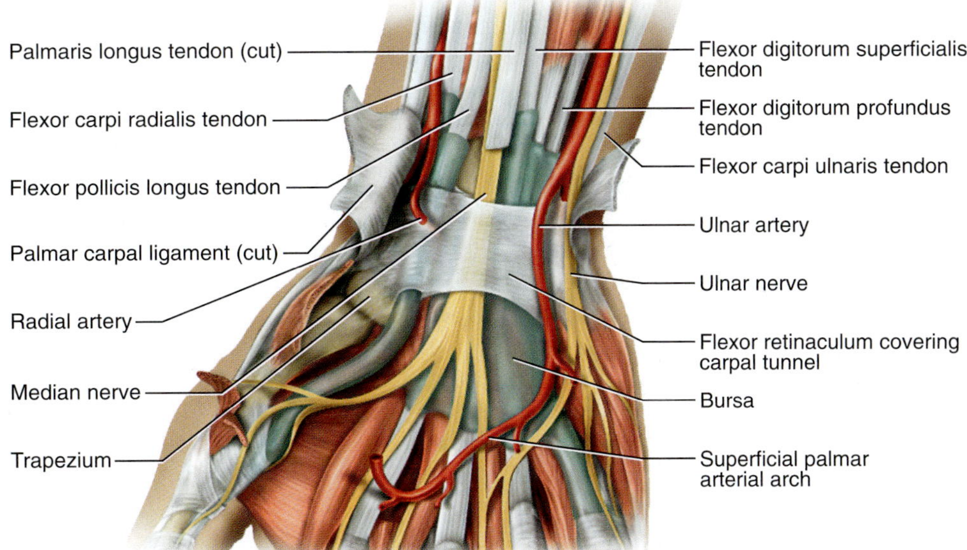

(a) Anterior view

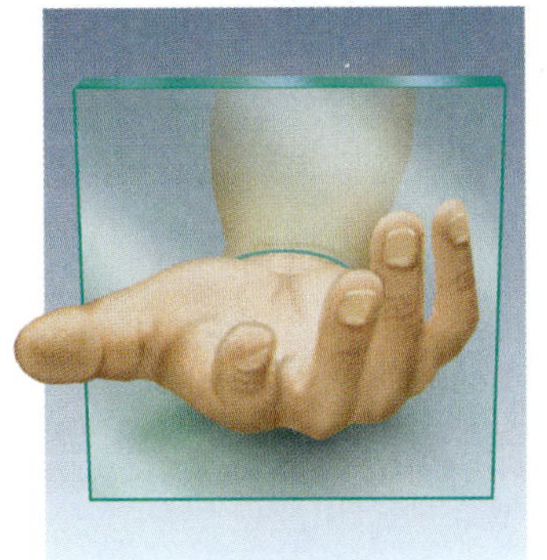

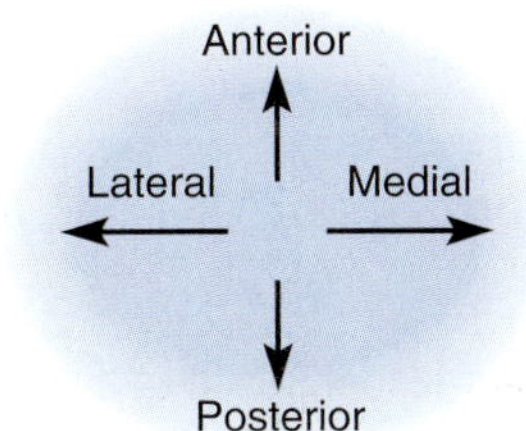

Flexor retinaculum
Median nerve
Flexor carpi radialis tendon
Abductor pollicis longus tendon
Extensor pollicis brevis tendon
Flexor pollicis longus tendon
Ulnar bursa
Trapezium
Trapezoid
Capitate
Palmaris longus tendon
Ulnar nerve
Flexor digitorum superficialis tendons
Pisiform
Carpal tunnel
Flexor digitorum profundus tendons
Triquetrum
Hamate
Extensor digitorum tendons

(b) Cross section

FIGURE 10.10 Carpal tunnel

Primarily wrist extension

- Extensor carpi radialis longus
- Extensor carpi radialis brevis
- Extensor carpi ulnaris

Primarily phalangeal extension, assists in wrist extension

- Extensor digitorum
- Extensor indicis
- Extensor digiti minimi
- Extensor pollicis longus
- Extensor pollicis brevis
- Abductor pollicis longus

Nerves

The muscles of the wrist and hand are all innervated from the radial, median, and **ulnar nerves** of the brachial plexus, as illustrated in figure 10.11. Also see figures 8.9 and 8.10 on pages 160 and 162. The radial nerve, originating from C6, C7, and C8, provides innervation for the extensor carpi radialis brevis and extensor carpi radialis longus. It then branches to become the posterior interosseous nerve, which supplies the extensor carpi ulnaris, extensor digitorum, extensor digiti minimi, abductor pollicis longus, extensor pollicis longus, extensor pollicis brevis, and extensor indicis. The median nerve, arising from C6, C7, C8, and T1, innervates the flexor carpi radialis, palmaris longus, and flexor digitorum superficialis. It then branches to become the anterior interosseous nerve, which innervates the flexor digitorum profundus for the index and long finger as well as for the flexor pollicis longus. Regarding the intrinsic muscles of the hand, the median nerve innervates the abductor pollicis brevis, flexor pollicis brevis (superficial head), opponens pollicis, and the 1st and 2nd lumbricals. The ulnar nerve, branching from C8 and T1, supplies the flexor digitorum profundus for the 4th and 5th fingers and the flexor carpi ulnaris. Additionally, it innervates the remaining intrinsic muscles of the hand (the deep head of the flexor pollicis brevis, adductor pollicis, palmar interossei, dorsal interossei, 3rd and 4th lumbricals, opponens digiti minimi, abductor digiti minimi, and flexor digiti minimi brevis). Sensation to the ulnar side of the hand, the ulnar half of the ring finger, and the entire little finger is provided by the ulnar nerve (figure 10.11).

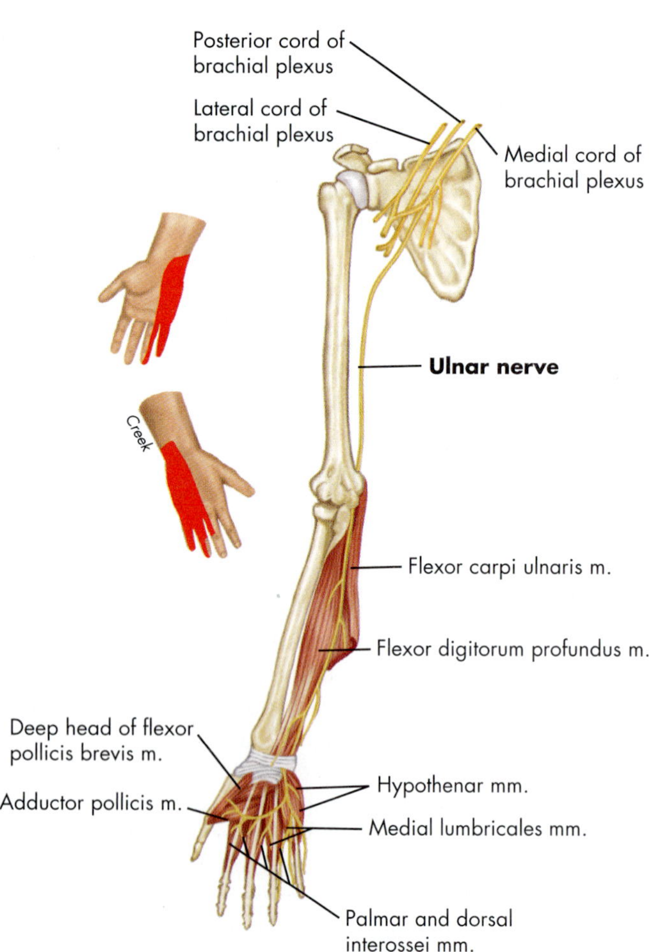

FIGURE 10.11 Ulnar nerve

CLINICAL NOTES **Entrapped Nerves**

Since the median, radial, and ulnar nerves are so important to the hand and wrist muscles, it is prudent to mention that the nerves can get entrapped by soft tissue on their route to the hand and wrist. The radial nerve can be entrapped by the triceps and supinator, for example, and the median nerve can be entrapped by the pectoralis minor or pronator teres or both. This reduction of nerve supply to the muscles of the hand and wrist could be interpreted as a problem of the hand and wrist. A good treatment protocol includes checking the upper kinetic chain before treating the hand and wrist muscles. Releasing the neck, shoulder, and arm muscles before the forearm makes an efficient treatment.

Individual Muscles of the Wrist and Hand—Flexors

PALMARIS LONGUS MUSCLE

Palpation

Palpate the palmaris longus on the anteromedial and central aspect of the anterior forearm just proximal to the wrist, particularly with slight wrist flexion and opposition of the thumb to the 5th finger.

CLINICAL NOTES **Tendon Repair**

The palmaris longus often is used for tendon repair in surgery, probably because it is superficial, it does not go through the carpal tunnel, and it is not crucial to wrist flexion. The palmaris longus is absent in either one or both forearms in some people. It seems to be an extra bonus for those who have this muscle. See Chapter 11 for information of Dupuytren's contracture.

Muscle Specifics

Unlike the flexor carpi radialis and flexor carpi ulnaris, which are not only wrist flexors but also abductors and adductors, respectively, the palmaris longus is involved only in weak wrist flexion from the anatomical position because of its central location on the anterior forearm and wrist. It can, however, assist in abducting the wrist from an extremely adducted position back to neutral and can assist in adducting the wrist from an extremely abducted position back to

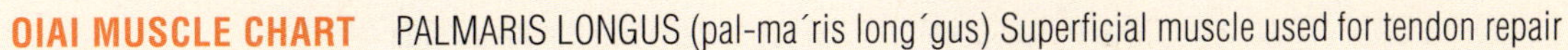

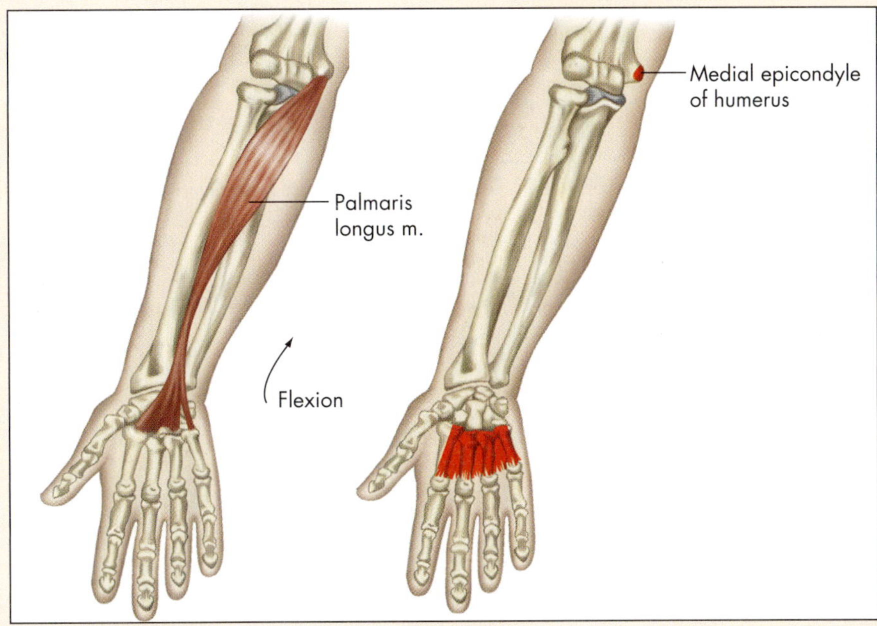

Name of Muscle	Origins	Insertion	Actions	Innervations
Palmaris longus	Medial epicondyle of humerus	Palmaris aponeurosis of 2nd, 3rd, 4th, and 5th metacarpals	Assists in flexion of wrist, weak flexion of elbow joint	Median nerve (C6, C7)

neutral. It may also assist slightly in forearm pronation because of its slightly lateral insertion in relation to its origin on the medial epicondyle.

Clinical Flexibility

Maximal elbow and wrist extension stretches the palmaris longus. Try placing one hand under the elbow and extending the involved elbow and wrist completely, palm up. Take the wrist into extreme hyperextension while allowing the fingers to remain in relaxed flexion. Hold 2 seconds, and completely flex the elbow to perform another set. This also helps stretch the brachialis. *Contraindications:* This exercise is safe with controlled movements.

Strengthening

This exercise is excellent for all the flexor muscles affecting the wrist and forearm. It is helpful for carpal tunnel and elbow epicondylitis, and, because of its simplicity, it is easy to teach. Please refer to this exercise as noted for other muscles in this chapter. On a wrist roller (a 13-inch PVC pipe with a hole drilled in the middle and a 5-foot rope attached), attach a small weight (1 to 3 pounds to start). Extend the arms directly out in front of you. Begin rolling the pipe *clockwise* to wrap the rope around the pipe and bring the weight slowly up. Be sure to use full wrist flexion and extension. When the weight reaches the pipe, drop the arms and rest, and then bring them back into the extended position. Now roll the pipe *counterclockwise* to slowly lower the weight. This downward movement forces the flexors to eccentrically contract, while the upward movement is a concentric contraction. Repeat 10 times with 2 to 3 sets. *Contraindications:* This exercise is safe with controlled movements. If it is painful to use the wrists, start with no weight first and add more weight slowly.

OIAI MUSCLE CHART FLEXOR CARPI RADIALIS (fleks´or kar´pi ra´di-a´lis) Wrist flexor on the radial side

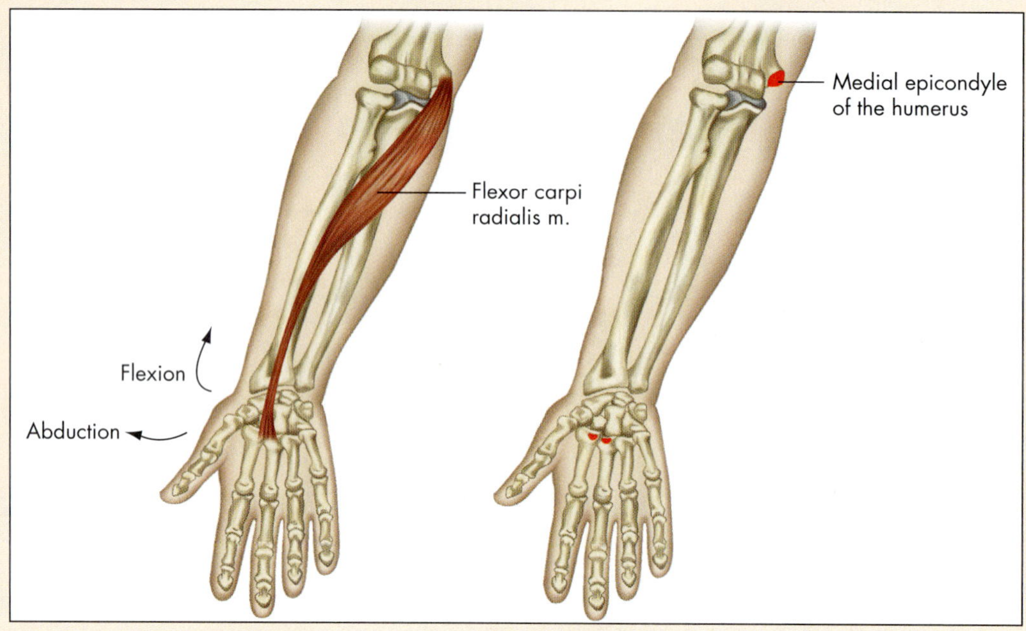

Name of Muscle	Origins	Insertion	Actions	Innervations
Flexor carpi radialis	Medial epicondyle of humerus	Base of 2nd and 3rd metacarpals, palmar surface	Flexion of hand, abduction of hand at wrist, weak flexion of elbow	Median nerve (C6, C7)

FLEXOR CARPI RADIALIS MUSCLE

Palpation

Palpate the flexor carpi radialis on the anterior surface of the wrist, slightly lateral, in line with the 2nd and 3rd metacarpals with resisted flexion and abduction.

CLINICAL NOTES **Overused Muscle**

The wrist should not be hyperflexed, hyperextended, or held in either position for long periods of time. Repetitive actions of hyperflexion or hyperextension can lead to symptoms of carpal tunnel syndrome. The flexor carpi radialis travels through the carpal tunnel and should be addressed as a co-contributor to the syndrome in a hypertonic state. Regardless of the presence of carpal tunnel syndrome, there could be tenderness at the medial epicondyle area as well as at its attachments at the 2nd and 3rd metacarpals. See Chapter 11 for more details on soft-tissue conditions and technique solutions.

Muscle Specifics

The flexor carpi radialis and flexor carpi ulnaris are the most powerful of the wrist flexors. The palmaris longus is much weaker by design and often absent, as discussed above. Both are brought into play during any activity that requires wrist curling or wrist stabilization against resistance, particularly if the forearm is supinated.

Clinical Flexibility

To stretch the flexor carpi radialis, the elbow must be fully extended with the forearm supinated. The stretch for palmaris longus can be performed for this muscle.

Strengthening

The wrist roller exercise for palmaris longus can be performed for this muscle.

OIAI MUSCLE CHART FLEXOR CARPI ULNARIS (fleks´or kar´pi ul-na´ris) Wrist flexor on the ulnar side

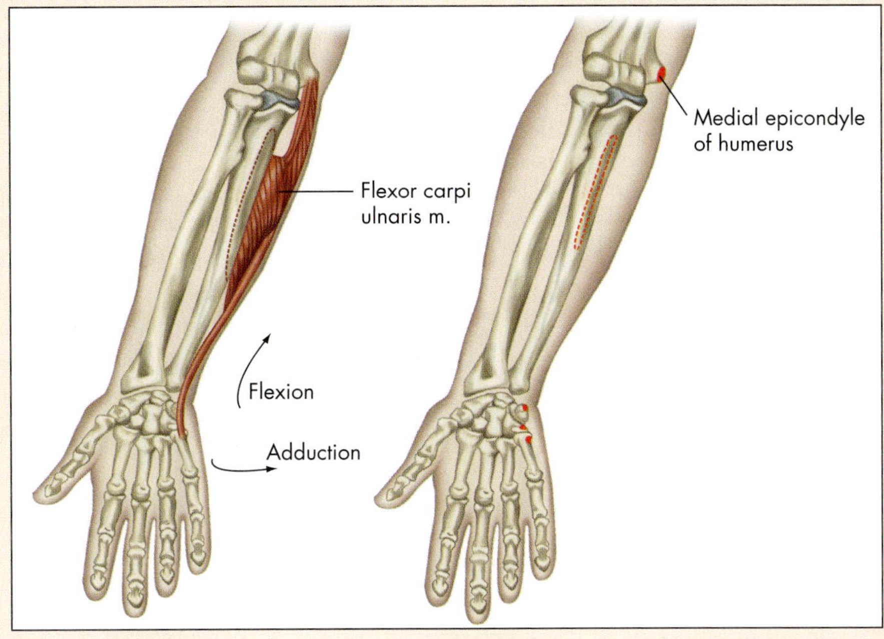

Name of Muscle	Origins	Insertion	Actions	Innervations
Flexor carpi ulnaris	Medial epicondyle of humerus via common tendon, posterior aspect of proximal ulna	Base of 5th metacarpal, pisiform (hamate)	Flexion and adduction of wrist, weak flexion of elbow	Ulnar nerve (C8, T1)

FLEXOR CARPI ULNARIS MUSCLE

Palpation

Palpate the flexor carpi ulnaris on the anteromedial surface of the forearm, a few inches below the medial epicondyle of the humerus to just proximal to the wrist, with resisted flexion and adduction.

CLINICAL NOTES **Strain at Attachments**

It is crucial for manual therapists to keep their wrists in alignment with their forearms when they perform massage techniques. Leaning into radial flexion can strain the flexor carpi ulnaris and its synergist, extensor carpi ulnaris. Other overuse movements might include using a trowel on cement, painting with a brush, or scrubbing a floor pushing into radial flexion. Tenderness can appear at the attachments of the flexor carpi ulnaris or at the extensor insertions at the wrist. Injuries range from tenderness to variable levels of strains. All of this should be considered for treatment of epicondyle issues. Ice, rest, stretching, strengthening, and other clinical solutions may be necessary to help relieve symptoms.

Muscle Specifics

The flexor carpi ulnaris is important in wrist flexion or curling activities. In addition, it is one of only two muscles involved in wrist adduction or ulnar flexion. As stated above, this muscle can be strained at the wrist by repetitive wrist actions. Include the flexor carpi ulnaris for a complete treatment of flexors of the hand and wrist.

Clinical Flexibility

To stretch the flexor carpi ulnaris, the elbow must be fully extended with the forearm supinated. See the stretch for palmaris longus. *Contraindications:* This stretch is safe with controlled movements.

Strengthening

The flexor carpi ulnaris may be strengthened with any type of wrist-curling activity against resistance, such as the activities described for the palmaris longus muscle. *Contraindications:* Strengthening is safe with controlled movements.

FLEXOR DIGITORUM SUPERFICIALIS MUSCLE

Palpation

Palpate the flexor digitorum superficialis in the depressed area between the palmaris longus and flexor carpi ulnaris tendons, particularly when making a fist. Extend the distal interphalangeal with slightly resisted wrist flexion, and palpate the flexor digitorum superficialis on the anterior midforearm.

CLINICAL NOTES **Sleep Postures**

Poor sleep positions persistently contribute to soft-tissue and inflammatory nerve conditions. In extreme flexion, the wrist can compress the median nerve. Many people sleep with their hands in flexed positions as a habit. This is probably not a good idea if, on waking, the hands experience numbness, tingling, or pins-and-needles sensations. Propping a pillow under the hand and forearm can help prevent abduction of the scapulae and help prevent wrist hyperflexion during sleep.

OIAI MUSCLE CHART FLEXOR DIGITORUM SUPERFICIALIS (fleks´or dij-i-to´rum su´per-fish-e-al´is) Superficial flexor of the fingers

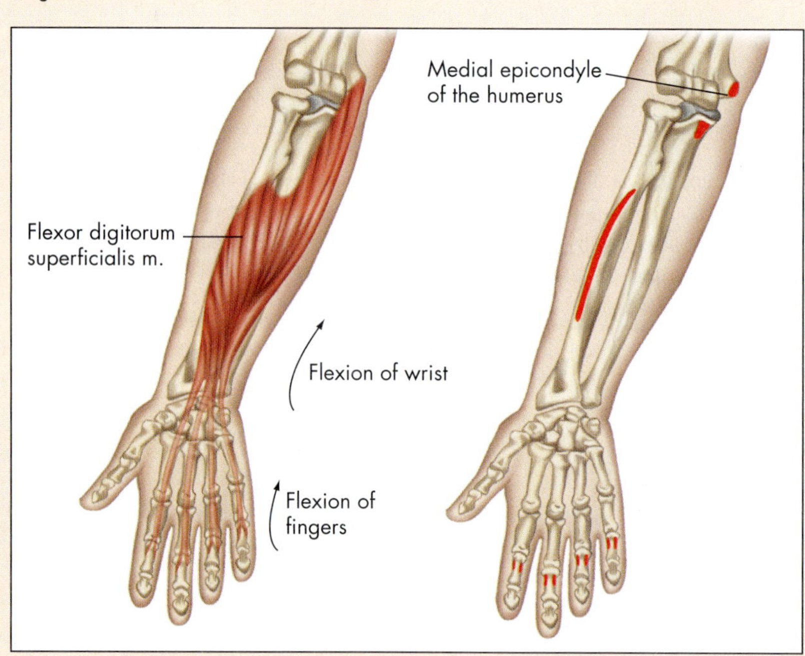

Name of Muscle	Origins	Insertion	Actions	Innervations
Flexor digitorum superficialis	Medial epicondyle of humerus via common tendon *Ulna*: medial coronoid process of ulna *Radial:* oblique line of radius	Sides of shafts of middle phalanges of four fingers	Flexion of four fingers at PIP joint and MP joint, flexion of hand and wrist, weak flexion of elbow	Median nerve (C7, C8, T1)

Muscle Specifics

The flexor digitorum superficialis muscle divides into four tendons on the palmar aspect of the wrist and hand to insert on each of the four fingers. The flexor digitorum superficialis and the flexor digitorum profundus are the only muscles involved in flexion of all four fingers. Both of these muscles are vital in any type of gripping activity.

Clinical Flexibility

The flexor digitorum superficialis is stretched by passively extending the elbow, wrist, metacarpophalangeal, and proximal interphalangeal joints while maintaining the forearm in full supination. The stretch for the palmaris can be applied here. *Contraindications:* Stretching is safe with controlled movements.

Strengthening

Since the flexor digitorum helps produce digit flexion, it is important to strengthen the gripping motion of the four fingers; this can be done by squeezing a small therapy ball. Hold the ball between the 1st finger and the thumb with the elbow extended. Squeeze the ball as able and slowly release. Do this for all four fingers, especially the 4th finger. Using resistance on the 4th finger will challenge the flexor digitorum at the epicondyle, and if inflammation is present (golfer's elbow), the client usually feels discomfort as the thumb and pinky finger squeeze the ball. This is a good exercise to include in any prescribed exercise program for carpal tunnel and epicondylitis. It helps to use a ball that has spring to it for eccentric contraction; putties and other soft tools do not work as well. *Contraindications:* This exercise is safe with controlled movements.

FLEXOR DIGITORUM PROFUNDUS MUSCLE

Palpation

The flexor digitorum profundus is difficult to distinguish deep to the flexor digitorum superficialis, but it can be palpated on the anterior midforearm while flexing the distal interphalangeal joints and keeping the proximal

OIAI MUSCLE CHART FLEXOR DIGITORUM PROFUNDUS (fleks´or dij-i-to´rum pro-fun´dus) Deep flexor of the fingers

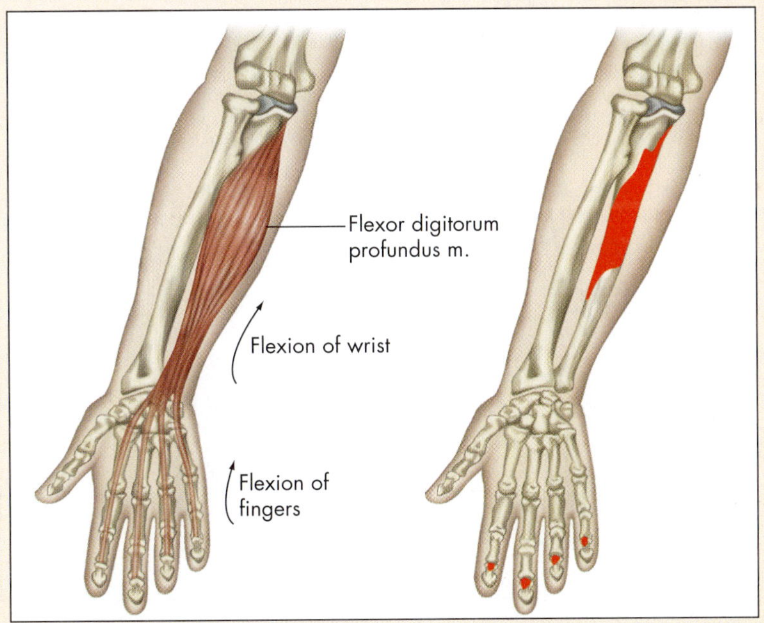

Name of Muscle	Origins	Insertion	Actions	Innervations
Flexor digitorum profundus	Proximal three-fourths of anterior and medial ulna	Base of distal phalanges of four fingers	Flexion of four fingers at distal interphalangeal joints, PIP joints, and MP joints, flexion of wrist	Median nerve (C8, T1) to 2nd and 3rd fingers Ulnar nerve (C8, T1) to 4th and 5th fingers

interphalangeal joints in extension and felt over the palmar surface of the 2nd, 3rd, 4th, and 5th metacarpophalangeal joints during finger flexion against resistance.

CLINICAL NOTES **Distal Phalanx Flexor and Gross Closure**

The insertion of the flexor digitorum profundus enables the hand to have a secure grip and gross closure. Picking up a pencil or holding on to a rope in a tug-of-war requires that the distal phalanx flex. Constant gripping causes overuse and soreness in the anterior forearm area and often a weakness of grip. The flexor digitorum profundus could be involved with medial epicondylitis and should be strengthened at the fingers.

Muscle Specifics

Both the flexor digitorum profundus muscle and the flexor digitorum superficialis muscle assist in wrist flexion because of their palmar relationship to the wrist. The flexor digitorum profundus is used in any type of gripping, squeezing, or hand-clenching activity, such as gripping a racket or climbing a rope.

Clinical Flexibility

The flexor digitorum profundus is stretched similarly to the flexor digitorum superficialis, except that the distal interphalangeal joints must be passively extended in addition to the elbow, wrist, metacarpophalangeal, and proximal interphalangeal joints while maintaining the forearm in full supination. The palmaris stretch is effective for this muscle.

Strengthening

The flexor digitorum profundus muscle is strengthened using the exercises described for the flexor digitorum superficialis muscle.

OIAI MUSCLE CHART FLEXOR POLLICIS LONGUS (fleks´or pol´i-sis long´gus) Long flexor of the thumb

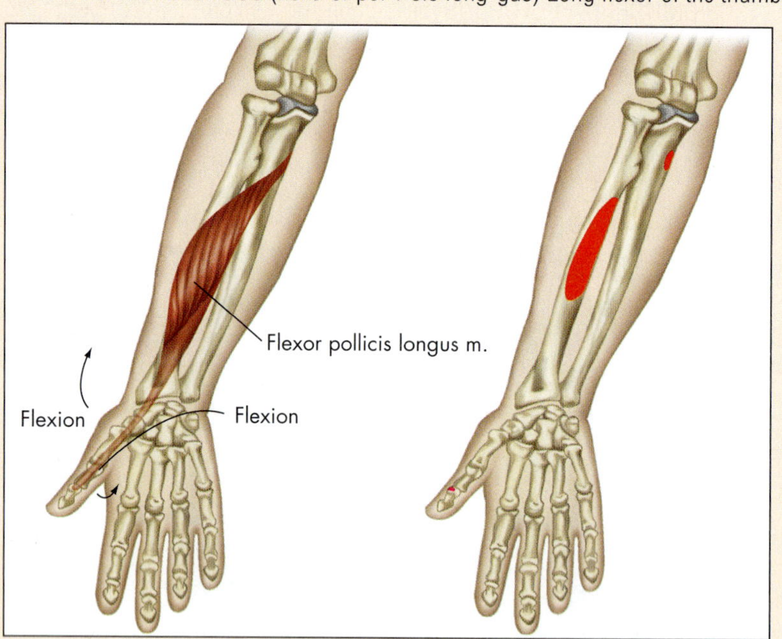

Name of Muscle	Origins	Insertion	Actions	Innervations
Flexor pollicis longus	Middle anterior radius, anterior medial border of the ulna just distal to the coronoid process, interosseous membrane	Distal phalanx of thumb	Flexion of thumb carpometacarpal, metacarpophalangeal, and interphalangeal joints, assists flexion and abduction of wrist	Median nerve, palmar interosseous branch (C8, T1)

FLEXOR POLLICIS LONGUS MUSCLE

Palpation

Palpate the flexor pollicis longus on the anterior surface of the thumb on the proximal phalanx, and just lateral to the palmaris longus and medial to the flexor carpi radialis on the anterior distal forearm, especially during active flexion of the thumb interphalangeal joint.

CLINICAL NOTES — **Weeder's Thumb**

Spring and summer bring out the gardeners, and where there is a garden, there are weeds. Grasping a weed and pulling is an activity that could affect the flexor pollicis longus. A repetitive action condition, aptly called *weeder's thumb*, could result. There are other intrinsic muscles involved in the hand, but the condition usually causes tenderness within the forearm muscles as well as at the radial side of the hand and wrist.

Muscle Specifics

The primary function of the flexor pollicis longus muscle is flexion of the thumb, which is vital in gripping and grasping activities of the hand. Because of its palmar relationship to the wrist, it provides some assistance in wrist flexion. Although the muscle attaches to the middle anterior surface of the radius and the anterior medial border of the ulna just distal to the coronoid process, occasionally a small "slip," or head, is present attaching on the medial epicondyle of the humerus.

Clinical Flexibility

The flexor pollicis longus is stretched by actively extending the entire thumb while simultaneously maintaining maximal wrist extension. To achieve this, extend the elbow and wrist palms up. Grasp the thumb with the other hand and actively move it into hyperextension. Apply a gentle 2-second stretch at the end movement. *Contraindications:* This stretch is safe with controlled movements. Tenderness might exist if de Quervain's tenosynovitis is present.

Strengthening

The flexor pollicis longus may be strengthened by using the ball again. Place the ball in the palm, toward and just below the pinky finger. Flex the thumb into the ball, pressing it down. Slowly release and repeat. *Contraindications:* Strengthening is safe with controlled movements. Tenderness might exist if de Quervain's tenosynovitis is present.

Individual Muscles of the Wrist and Hand—Extensors

EXTENSOR CARPI ULNARIS MUSCLE

Palpation

Palpate the extensor carpi ulnaris just lateral to the ulnar styloid process and crossing the posteromedial wrist, particularly with wrist extension and adduction.

CLINICAL NOTES — **Sideways Accomplice**

The expression "It takes two to tango" is useful in describing the extensor carpi ulnaris. Although there are many muscles involved in wrist extension, the two ulnar deviators, flexor carpi ulnaris and extensor carpi ulnaris, could both be strained in the wrist's sideways repetitive action. (See "Flexor Carpi Ulnaris," above.) Coming from the lateral epicondyle, the extensor carpi ulnaris is also likely to be involved in tendon conditions of that area. Look for tenderness at the lateral epicondyle and at its base on the 5th metacarpal of the little finger. See Chapter 11 for more information about lateral epicondylitis.

Muscle Specifics

The extensor carpi ulnaris, the extensor carpi radialis brevis, and the extensor carpi radialis longus are the most powerful of the wrist extensors. Any activity requiring wrist extension or stabilization of the wrist against resistance, particularly if the forearm is pronated, depends greatly on the strength of these muscles. They often are brought into play with the backhand in racquet sports and thus need to be included in treatment for lateral epicondyle soft-tissue conditions.

Clinical Flexibility

Stretching the extensor carpi ulnaris requires that the elbow be extended with the forearm pronated while the wrist is passively flexed and slightly abducted. A good stretch for this muscle is one used in the martial art aikido. Extend the elbow, palm down. Actively radial flex the open hand; with the other hand, grip it from underneath. Apply a gentle, rotary-type stretch for 2 seconds, and repeat. *Contraindications:* This stretch is safe with controlled movements. Tenderness at the wrist might exist if inflammation is present.

Strengthening

The extensor carpi ulnaris may be developed by performing the roller exercise used for the flexors.

OIAI MUSCLE CHART EXTENSOR CARPI ULNARIS (eks-ten´sor kar´pi ul-na´ris) Wrist extensor on the ulnar side

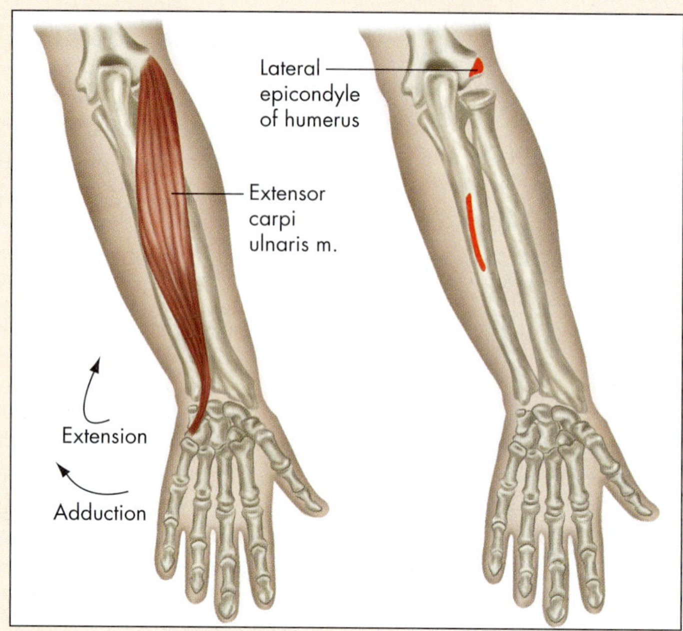

Name of Muscle	Origins	Insertion	Actions	Innervations
Extensor carpi ulnaris	Lateral epicondyle of humerus (common extensor tendon), middle two-fourths of the posterior border of ulna	Base of 5th metacarpal	Extension of wrist, adduction of wrist, weak extension of forearm	Radial nerve (C6–C8)

This time, roll the weight *counterclockwise* to challenge this muscle. Remember to keep the arms extended in front, and rest between sets. *Contraindications:* Strengthening is safe with controlled movement.

EXTENSOR CARPI RADIALIS BREVIS MUSCLE

Palpation

Palpate the extensor carpi radialis brevis on the dorsal side of the forearm; it is difficult to distinguish between the extensor carpi radialis longus and the extensor digitorum. Just proximal to the dorsal aspect of the wrist and approximately 1 centimeter medial to the radial styloid process, the tendon may be felt during extension and traced to the base of the 3rd metacarpal, particularly when making a fist. It is located proximally and posteriorly, just medial to the bulk of the brachioradialis.

CLINICAL NOTES **Common Extensor Tendon Partner**

Extensor carpi radialis brevis is often part of the repetitive misuse at the lateral epicondyle. As part of the common extensor tendon, it contributes to tendonitis, tendonosis, strains, and other soft-tissue problems. Powerful wrist extension comes with its drawbacks for long-term use. Stretching and strengthening this muscle specifically can help offset the misuse of this muscle and its counterparts—the extensor radialis longus and extensor digitorum.

Muscle Specifics

The extensor carpi radialis brevis is important in any sports activity that requires powerful wrist extension, such as golf or tennis.

Clinical Flexibility

Stretching the extensor carpi radialis brevis and longus requires that the elbow be extended with the fore-

OIAI MUSCLE CHART EXTENSOR CARPI RADIALIS BREVIS (eks-ten´sor kar´pi ra´di-a´lis bre´vis) Short wrist extensor on radial side

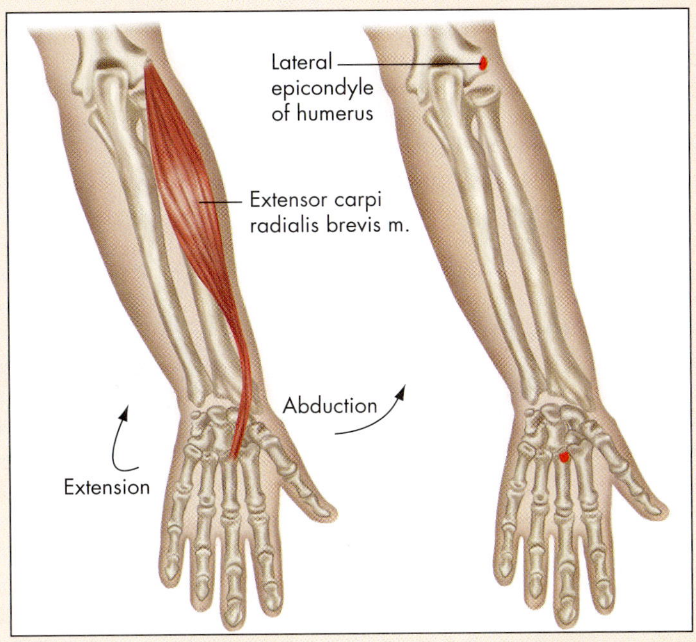

Name of Muscle	Origins	Insertion	Actions	Innervations
Extensor carpi radialis brevis	Lateral epicondyle of humerus (common extensor tendon)	Base of 3rd metacarpal (dorsal)	Extension of wrist, abduction of wrist, weak flexion of elbow	Radial nerve (C6–C7)

arm pronated while the wrist is passively flexed and slightly adducted. Place one hand under the elbow, and fully extend the involved elbow. Ulnar flex the hand at the end movement for a gentle 2-second stretch. This also stretches the brachialis. *Contraindications:* This stretch is safe with controlled movement.

Strengthening

Wrist extension exercises, such as those described for the extensor carpi ulnaris, are appropriate for muscle development. The extensor carpi radialis brevis can also be strengthened using a dumbbell sleeve. Stand with the arm holding the sleeve at the side, and use the other hand to secure it at the wrist against the hip. Radially flex the sleeve, and slowly lower it to the start position. This is a good exercise for epicondylitis dysfunctions. Take care not to flex or extend the wrist as you perform this exercise. *Contraindications:* This exercise is safe with controlled movements.

EXTENSOR CARPI RADIALIS LONGUS MUSCLE

Palpation

Palpate the extensor carpi radialis longus just proximal to the dorsal aspect of the wrist and approximately 1 centimeter medial to the radial styloid process; the tendon may be felt during extension and traced to the base of the 2nd metacarpal, particularly when the hand is closed into a fist. The extensor carpi radialis longus is located proximally and posteriorly, just medial to the bulk of the brachioradialis.

CLINICAL NOTES **Tennis Elbow**

Lateral epicondylitis is the technical term for tennis elbow syndrome. Because its origin is so close to the brachioradialis

OIAI MUSCLE CHART EXTENSOR CARPI RADIALIS LONGUS (eks-ten´sor kar´pi ra´di-a´lis long´gus) Long wrist extensor on radial side

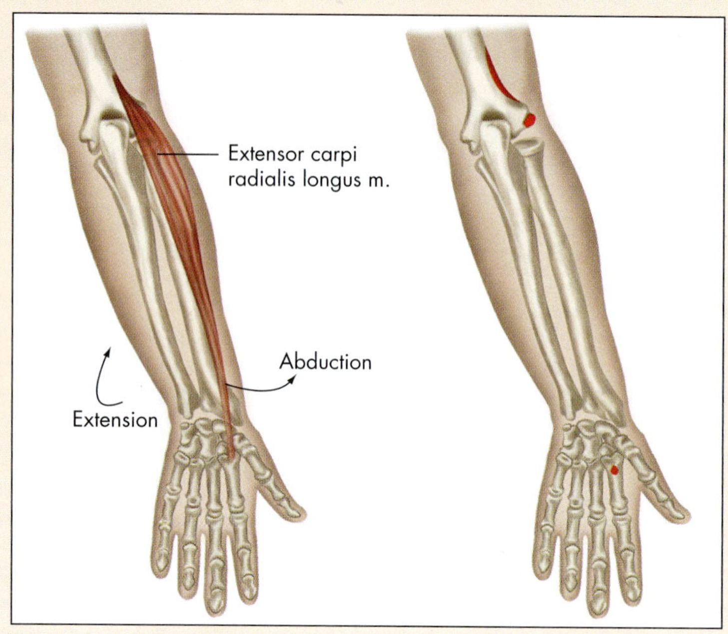

Name of Muscle	Origins	Insertion	Actions	Innervations
Extensor carpi radialis longus	Lower third of lateral supracondylar ridge of humerus and lateral epicondyle of humerus	Base of 2nd metacarpal (dorsal)	Extension and abduction of wrist, weak flexion of elbow, weak pronation from supination	Radial nerve (C6, C7)

and other lateral epicondyle tendons, the extensor carpi radialis longus is involved in this overuse problem. Tennis is no longer the sole cause of tennis elbow. Carpenters, musicians, massage therapists, and keyboard operators share common complaints in the upper forearm muscles. See Chapter 11 for additional details.

Muscle Specifics

The extensor carpi radialis longus, like the extensor carpi radialis brevis, is also important in any sports activity that requires powerful wrist extension. In addition, both muscles are involved in abduction of the wrist. The extensor carpi radialis longus also helps in functioning weak pronation to the neutral from a fully supinated position.

Clinical Flexibility

The extensor carpi radialis longus is stretched in the same manner as the extensor carpi radialis brevis.

Strengthening

The extensor carpi radialis longus may be developed with the wrist extension exercises described for the extensor carpi ulnaris muscle.

EXTENSOR DIGITORUM MUSCLE

Palpation

With all four fingers extended, palpate extensor digitorum on the posterior surface of the distal forearm immediately medial to the extensor pollicis longus tendon and lateral to the extensor carpi ulnaris and extensor digiti minimi; extensor digitorum then divides into four separate tendons that are over the dorsal aspect of the hand and metacarpophalangeal joints.

OIAI MUSCLE CHART EXTENSOR DIGITORUM (eks-ten´sor dij-i-to´rum) Finger extensor

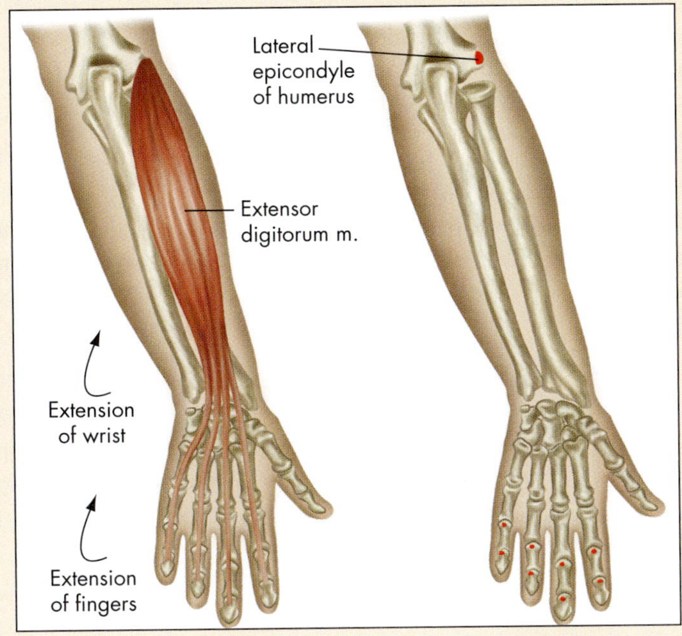

Name of Muscle	Origins	Insertion	Actions	Innervations
Extensor digitorum	Lateral epicondyle of humerus	Base of middle phalanges of four fingers, extensor expansion of four fingers, dorsal surface	Extension of MP joints of four fingers (phalanges of fingers), extension of wrist, weak extension of elbow	Radial nerve (C6–C8)

CLINICAL NOTES **Overused Extenders**

Unlike the eight flexor tendons, the extensor digitorum is on its own to extend the four fingers. It is easy to rationalize why the extensor digitorum is involved in overuse activities. For example, massage students sometimes extend their fingers instead of relaxing the digits and shaping to the structure. The constant repetitive action takes a toll on the entire muscle and at the lateral epicondyle area. When this muscle is not functioning properly, it cannot contribute to a powerful grip. See Chapter 11 for techniques to unwind the forearm muscles.

Muscle Specifics

The extensor digitorum is the only muscle involved in extension of all four fingers. This muscle divides into four tendons on the dorsum of the wrist that insert on each of the fingers. It also assists with wrist extension movements.

Clinical Flexibility

To stretch the extensor digitorum, the fingers must be maximally flexed at the metacarpophalangeal, proximal interphalangeal, and distal interphalangeal joints while the wrist is fully flexed. Extend the elbow, palm down. Actively flex the fingers and hand while keeping the elbow extended. Use the other hand to stretch for 2 seconds. Try making a fist with the thumb inside, and then perform the same movement. This targets the carpal bone area and will isolate the extensor tendons as they emerge from the wrist. *Contraindications:* These stretches are safe with controlled movements. If carpal tunnel is present, there may be sensitivity at the wrist. Adjust the stretch for comfort.

Strengthening

While the wrist roller may be used to strengthen this muscle, the fingers should also be addressed. Wrap a rubber band around all the fingers and the thumb. With the arm extended, "open" the hand and thumb by maximally extending. Return to the closed position, and repeat. This is an easy exercise to do in the car, and it will help strengthen extension in the hand and wrist. It is also a good exercise for epicondylitis issues. *Contraindications:* This exercise is safe with controlled movements. Tenderness might exist if de Quervain's tenosynovitis is present.

EXTENSOR INDICIS MUSCLE

Palpation

With the forearm pronated, palpate the extensor indicis on the posterior aspect of the distal forearm and dorsal surface of the hand just medial to the extensor digitorum tendon of the index finger, with extension of the index fingers and flexion of the 3rd, 4th, and 5th fingers.

CLINICAL NOTES **Contributor to Overuse Keyboard Practices**

The index finger is strengthened through support from the extensor digitorum in pointing and reaching or in typing on a keyboard. The extensor indicis will contribute to overuse keyboarding practices. The index finger also has control of the left mouse clicker and can become an overuse syndrome in those who use the feature frequently. The forearm muscles, especially the extensors, may develop soreness in the lateral epicondyle areas. Ice, ergonomic practices, massage techniques, and stretching will all help dysfunctions of this muscle.

OIAI MUSCLE CHART EXTENSOR INDICIS (eks-ten´sor in´di-sis) Index finger extensor

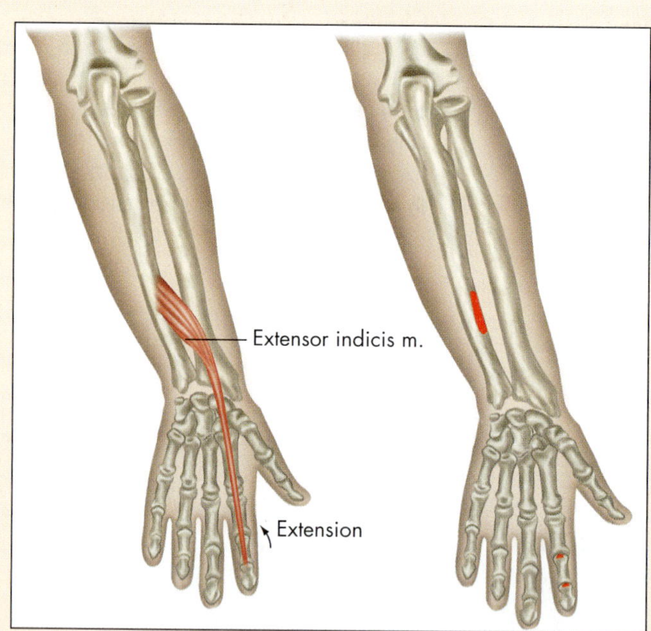

Name of Muscle	Origins	Insertion	Actions	Innervations
Extensor indicis	Middle to distal third of posterior ulna, interosseous membrane	Head of 2nd metacarpal and joins the extensor expansion at proximal phalanx	Extension of index finger at the metacarpophalangeal joint, weak wrist extension, weak supination for forearm from pronation	Radial nerve (C6–C8)

Muscle Specifics

The extensor indicis muscle is the pointing muscle. That is, it is responsible for extending the index finger, particularly when the other fingers are flexed. It also provides weak assistance to wrist extension and may be developed through exercises similar to those described for the extensor digitorum.

Clinical Flexibility

The extensor indicis is stretched by passively taking the index finger into maximal flexion at its metacarpophalangeal, proximal interphalangeal, and distal interphalangeal joints while fully flexing the wrist. The exercise for the extensor digitorum can be applied to this muscle, yet it also can be stretched separately. Flex the elbow, palm toward the navel, and actively flex the wrist. Use the other hand to place pressure at the dorsal side of the 1st finger, gently stretching as the hand and finger are in flexion. *Contraindications:* Stretching is safe with controlled movements.

Strengthening

This muscle can be strengthened by isolating the 1st finger. Wrap a rubber band around the thumb and 1st finger. Slowly extend the 1st finger while securing the band with the thumb. Return to the closed position, and repeat. The other fingers can be flexed and relaxed during this movement. *Contraindications:* Strengthening is safe with controlled movements.

EXTENSOR DIGITI MINIMI MUSCLE

Palpation

Locate extensor digiti minimi as it passes over the dorsal aspect of the distal radioulnar joint, particularly with relaxed flexion of the other fingers and alternating 5th-finger extension and relaxation. Palpate the extensor digiti minimi on the dorsal surface of the forearm immediately medial to the extensor digitorum and lateral to the extensor carpi ulnaris.

OIAI MUSCLE CHART EXTENSOR DIGITI MINIMI (eks-ten´sor dij´i-ti min´im-i) Little-finger extensor

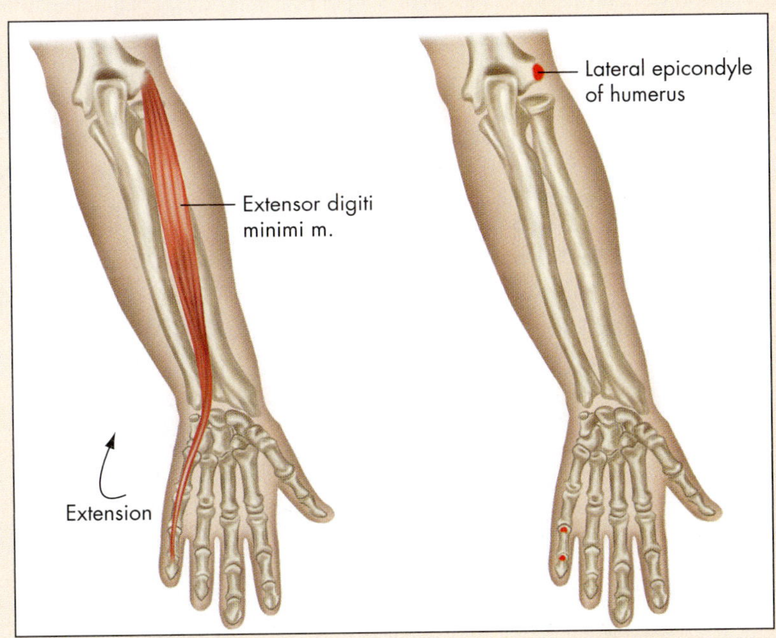

Name of Muscle	Origins	Insertion	Actions	Innervations
Extensor digiti minimi	Lateral epicondyle of humerus	Joins extensor expansion on proximal phalanx of 5th phalange (dorsal)	Extension of little finger at the metacarpophalangeal joint, weak wrist extension, weak elbow extension	Radial nerve (C6–C8)

CLINICAL NOTES **Excessive Stretch**

For computer programmers and pianists, stretching the little finger to its maximum length can be a repetitive action that results in hand pain and discomfort. A combination of little-finger extension and abduction contributes to this overuse condition, which plagues manual therapists. The extensor digitorum lends its support to extend the little finger, making its efforts and abilities larger than they should be for such a little digit. Because this muscle begins at the lateral epicondyle, it should be included in treatment of any overuse conditions.

Muscle Specifics

The primary function of the extensor digiti minimi muscle is to assist the extensor digitorum in extending the little finger. Because of its dorsal relationship to the wrist, it also provides weak assistance in wrist extension.

Clinical Flexibility

The extensor digiti minimi is stretched by passively taking the little finger into maximal flexion at its metacarpophalangeal, proximal interphalangeal, and distal interphalangeal joints while fully flexing the wrist. The stretch for extensor digitorum applies here.

Strengthening

The extensor digiti minimi is strengthened with the exercises described for the extensor digitorum. The 4th finger also can be isolated with a rubber band.

EXTENSOR POLLICIS LONGUS MUSCLE

Palpation

Palpate the extensor pollicis longus on the dorsal aspect of the hand to its insertion on the base of the distal phalanx. Also palpate the muscle on the posterior surface of the lower forearm between the radius and the ulna, just proximal to the extensor indicis and

OIAI MUSCLE CHART EXTENSOR POLLICIS LONGUS (eks-ten´sor pol´i-sis long´gus) Long thumb extensor

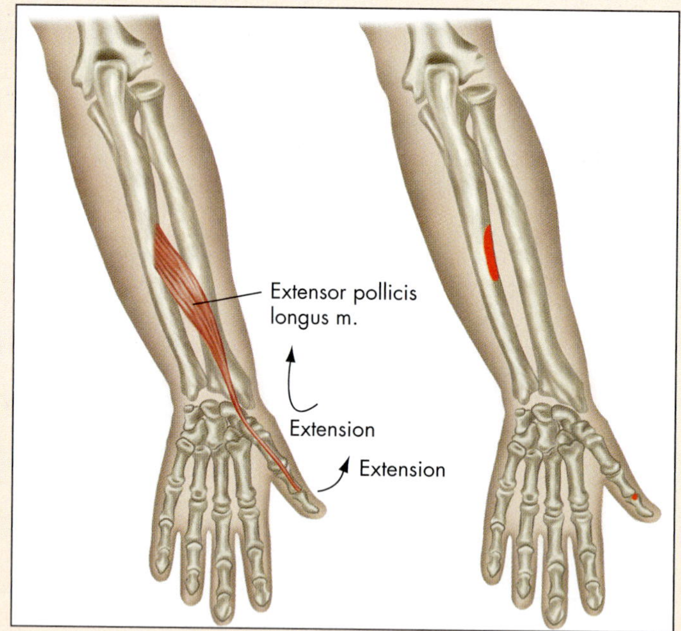

Name of Muscle	Origins	Insertion	Actions	Innervations
Extensor pollicis longus ("anatomical snuffbox")	Posterior middle to lower ulna and interosseous membrane	Base of distal phalanx of thumb (dorsal)	Extension of thumb at IP, MP, and CMP joints, extension of wrist, abduction of wrist, weak supination for forearm	Radial nerve (C6–C8)

medial to the extensor pollicis brevis and abductor pollicis longus, with the forearm pronated and fingers in relaxed flexion while actively extending the thumb.

CLINICAL NOTES — **Overused Thumbs**

It is hard to imagine life without thumbs. Thumbs perform many activities, such as pressing the spacebar on the keyboard automatically. Massage therapists use the thumb on a regular basis to apply constant pressure. Overuse in extension develops tightness in the tendon itself as well as at the attachments in the forearm. Many individuals have a hyperextendable thumb. Passed down genetically, the thumb bends to almost a right angle to itself. Massage therapists must take care not to overstretch their thumbs. Hyperextendable thumbs should be strengthened using resistance for both flexors and extensors.

Muscle Specifics

The primary function of the extensor pollicis longus muscle is thumb extension, although it does provide weak assistance in wrist extension. It supports weak supination of the forearm from a pronated position.

The tendons of the extensor pollicis longus and extensor pollicis brevis, along with the tendon of the abductor pollicis brevis, form the anatomical snuffbox, which is the small depression that develops between these two tendons when they contract. The name "anatomical snuffbox" originates from tobacco users placing their snuff in this depression. Deep in the snuffbox, the scaphoid bone can be palpated and is often a site of point tenderness when it is fractured.

Clinical Flexibility

The extensor pollicis longus is stretched by passively taking the entire thumb into maximal flexion at its carpometacarpal, metacarpophalangeal, and interphalangeal joints while fully flexing and adducting the wrist. Extend the elbow and hold the arm in front of you. With the other hand, position the fingers over the involved thumb, and move the thumb into flexion. Press gently and stretch for 2 seconds. *Contraindications:* Stretching is safe with controlled movements. Tenderness might exist if de Quervain's tenosynovitis is present.

Strengthening

The extensor pollicis longus may be strengthened by extending the flexed thumb against manual resistance. Wrap a rubber band around the thumb, and secure the other end with the 4th finger. With the palm down, extend the thumb, and repeat. *Contraindications:* Strengthening is safe with controlled movements. Tenderness might exist if de Quervain's tenosynovitis is present.

EXTENSOR POLLICIS BREVIS MUSCLE

Palpation

Palpate the extensor pollicis brevis just lateral to the extensor pollicis longus tendon on the dorsal side of the hand to its insertion on the proximal phalanx, with extension of the thumb carpometacarpal and metacarpophalangeal and flexion of the interphalangeal joints.

CLINICAL NOTES — **Extensor Assistant**

The extensor pollicis brevis contributes to the misuse of the thumb by its assistance to the extensor pollicis longus. Massage therapists hold the thumb in extension when applying ischemic pressure. Practicing good body mechanics helps prevent injury by properly using body weight and leaning into the soft tissue. Holding the thumb in extension and pressing into the tissues can irritate the joint and soft tissues.

Muscle Specifics

The extensor pollicis brevis assists the extensor pollicis longus in extending the thumb. Because of its dorsal relationship to the wrist, it also provides weak assistance in wrist extension.

Clinical Flexibility

The extensor pollicis brevis is stretched by passively taking the first carpometacarpal joint and the metacarpophalangeal joint of the thumb into maximal flexion while fully flexing and adducting the wrist. The stretch described for extensor pollicis applies here. *Contraindications:* These stretches are safe with controlled movements. Tenderness might exist if de Quervain's tenosynovitis is present.

Strengthening

The extensor pollicis brevis may be strengthened through the exercises described for the extensor pollicis longus muscle. *Contraindications:* Strengthening is safe with controlled movements. Tenderness might exist if de Quervain's tenosynovitis is present.

OIAI MUSCLE CHART EXTENSOR POLLICIS BREVIS (eks-ten´sor pol´i-sis bre´vis) Short thumb extensor

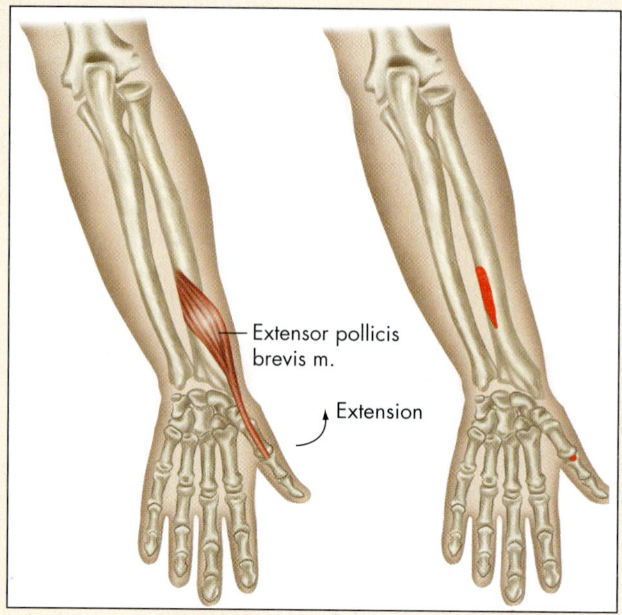

Name of Muscle	Origins	Insertion	Actions	Innervations
Extensor pollicis brevis	Posterior surface of lower middle radius	Base of proximal phalanx of the thumb (dorsal)	Extension of thumb at CMP and MP joints, weak wrist extension, wrist abduction	Radial nerve (C6, 7)

ABDUCTOR POLLICIS LONGUS MUSCLE

Palpation

With the forearm in neutral pronation and supination, palpate abductor pollicis longus on the lateral aspect of the wrist joint, just proximal to the 1st metacarpal during active thumb and wrist abduction.

CLINICAL NOTES **Tenosynovitis**

The abductor pollicis longus has a tendon sheath that, when used repetitively, can be irritated and become inflamed. This often is diagnosed as *de Quervain's tenosynovitis.* To test for this problem, draw the thumb across the palm and flex the fingers over the thumb. In this position, ulnar flex the hand at the wrist. If pain, soreness, or restricted action is present, this may indicate a positive test, which is called *Finkelstein's test.*

Muscle Specifics

The primary function of the abductor pollicis longus muscle is abduction of the thumb, although it does provide some assistance in wrist abduction.

Clinical Flexibility

Stretching of the abductor pollicis longus is accomplished by fully flexing and adducting the entire thumb across the palm with the wrist fully adducted, as during Finkelstein's test. To achieve this, make a tight fist with the thumb tucked inside the fingers. Extend the elbow, and use the other hand to clasp the involved fist. Actively move the hand into ulnar flexion, and stretch at the end movement for 2 seconds. *Contraindications:* This stretch is safe with controlled movements. Tenderness might exist if de Quervain's tenosynovitis is present.

Strengthening

This muscle is best strengthened with the dumbbell sleeve used previously. Stand clasping it with

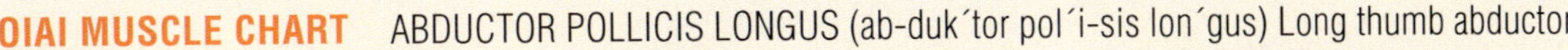

OIAI MUSCLE CHART ABDUCTOR POLLICIS LONGUS (ab-duk´tor pol´i-sis lon´gus) Long thumb abductor

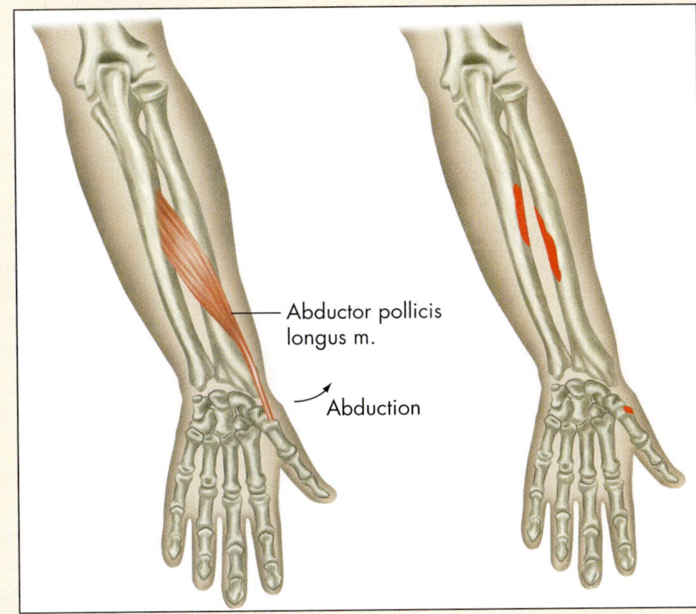

Name of Muscle	Origins	Insertion	Actions	Innervations
Abductor pollicis longus	Posterior aspect of radius and midshaft of ulna	Base of 1st metacarpal (dorsal)	Abduction and extension of thumb at CMP, abduction of the wrist, weak supination of forearm, weak flexion of wrist	Radial nerve (C6, 7)

the thumb forward. Secure the involved hand with the other hand to stabilize it. Lift the weight of the sleeve into radial flexion, and slowly return to the start position. This is an excellent movement to help treat de Quervain's tenosynovitis. *Contraindications:* Strengthening is safe with controlled movements. Tenderness might exist if de Quervain's tenosynovitis is present.

Intrinsic Muscles of the Hand

The intrinsic hand muscles may be grouped according to location as well as to the parts of the hand they control (figure 10.12). The abductor pollicis brevis, opponens pollicis, flexor pollicis brevis, and adductor pollicis make up the *thenar eminence*—the muscular pad on the palmar surface of the first metacarpal. The *hypothenar eminence* is the muscular pad that forms the ulnar border on the palmar surface of the hand; it is made up of the abductor digiti minimi, flexor digiti minimi brevis, and opponens digiti minimi. The intermediate muscles of the hand consist of three palmar interossei, four dorsal interossei, and four lumbrical muscles.

Four intrinsic muscles act on the carpometacarpal joint of the thumb. The opponens pollicis is the muscle that causes opposition in the thumb metacarpal. The abductor pollicis brevis abducts the thumb metacarpal and is assisted in this action by the flexor pollicis brevis, which also flexes the thumb metacarpal. The metacarpal of the thumb is adducted by the adductor pollicis. Both the flexor pollicis brevis and the adductor pollicis flex the proximal phalanx of the thumb.

The three palmar interossei are adductors of the 2nd, 4th, and 5th phalanges. The four dorsal interossei

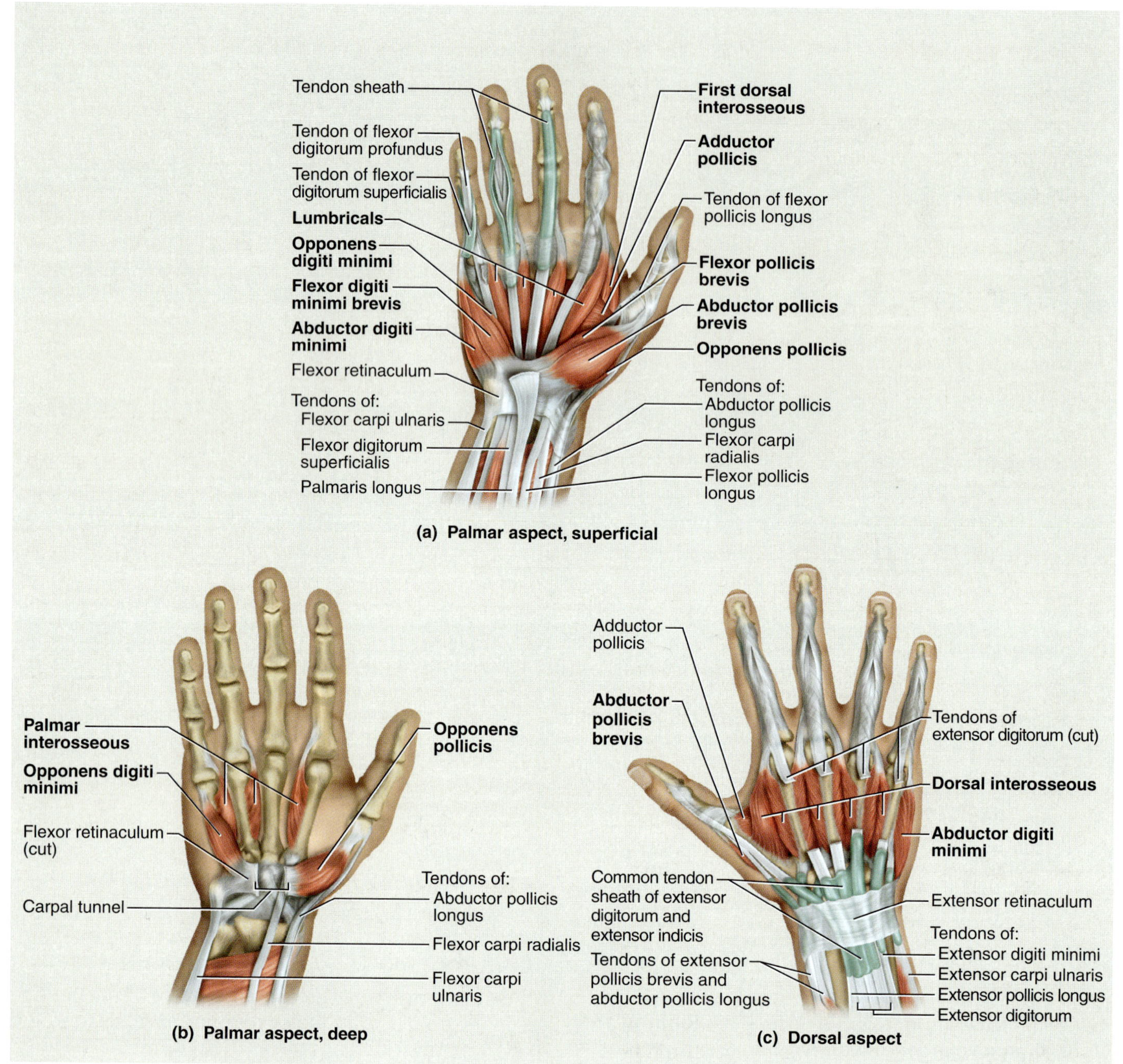

FIGURE 10.12 Intrinsic hand muscles

both flex and abduct the index, middle, and ring proximal phalanxes, in addition to assisting with extension of the middle and distal phalanxes of these fingers. The 3rd dorsal interossei also adducts the middle finger. The four lumbricals flex the index, middle, ring, and little proximal phalanxes, as well as extend the middle and distal phalanxes of these fingers.

Three muscles act on the little finger. The opponens digiti minimi causes opposition of the little finger metacarpal. The abductor digiti minimi abducts the little finger metacarpal, and the flexor digiti minimi brevis flexes this metacarpal.

Refer to table 10.2 for further details regarding the intrinsic muscles of the hand.

TABLE 10.2 Intrinsic Muscles of the Hand

	Muscle	Origin	Insertion	Action	Palpation	Innervation
Thenar muscles	Opponens pollicis	Anterior surface of transverse carpal ligament, trapezium	Lateral border of 1st metacarpal	CMC opposition of thumb	Palmar aspect of 1st metacarpal with opposition of fingertips to thumb	Median nerve (C6, C7)
	Abductor pollicis brevis	Anterior surface of transverse carpal ligament, trapezium, scaphoid	Base of 1st proximal phalanx	CMC abduction of thumb	Radial aspect of palmar surface of 1st metacarpal with 1st CMC abduction	Median nerve (C6, C7)
	Flexor pollicis brevis	*Superficial head:* trapezium and transverse carpal ligament *Deep head:* ulnar aspect of 1st metacarpal	Base of proximal phalanx of 1st metacarpal	CMC flexion and abduction; MCP flexion of thumb	Medial aspect of thenar eminence just proximal to 1st MCP joint with 1st MCP flexion against resistance	*Superficial head:* median nerve (C6, C7) *Deep head:* ulnar nerve (C8, T1)
Intermediate muscles	Adductor pollicis	*Transverse head:* anterior shaft of 3rd metacarpal *Oblique head:* base of 2nd and 3rd metacarpals, capitate, trapezoid	Ulnar aspect of base of proximal phalanx of 1st metarcapal	CMC adduction; MCP flexion of thumb	Palmar surface between 1st and 2nd metacarpal with 1st CMC adduction	Ulnar nerve (C8, T1)
	Palmar interossei	Shaft of 2nd, 4th, and 5th metacarpals and extensor expansions	Bases of 2nd, 4th, and 5th proximal phalanxes and extensor expansions	MCP adduction of 2nd, 4th, and 5th phalanges	Cannot be palpated	Ulnar nerve (C8, T1)
	Dorsal interossei	Two heads on shafts on adjacent metacarpals	Bases of 2nd, 3rd, and 4th proximal phalanxes and extensor expansions	MCP flexion and abduction; PIP/DIP extension of 2nd, 3rd, and 4th phalanges; MCP adduction of 3rd phalange	Dorsal surface between 1st and 2nd metacarpals, between shafts of 2nd through 5th metacarpals with active abduction/adduction of 2nd, 3rd, and 4th MCP joints	Ulnar nerve, palmar branch (C8, T1)
	Lumbricals	Flexor digitorum profundus tendon in center of palm	Extensor expansions on radial side of 2nd, 3rd, 4th, and 5th proximal phalanxes	MCP flexion and PIP/DIP extension of 2nd, 3rd, 4th, and 5th phalanges	Cannot be palpated	*1st and 2nd:* median nerve (C6, C7) *3rd and 4th:* ulnar nerve (C8, T1)

(Continued)

TABLE 10.2 (Continued)

	Muscle	Origin	Insertion	Action	Palpation	Innervation
Hypothenar muscles	Opponens digiti minimi	Hook of hamate and adjacent transverse carpal ligament	Medial border of 5th metacarpal	MCP opposition of 5th phalange	On radial aspect of hypothenar eminence with opposition of 5th phalange to thumb	Ulnar nerve (C8, T1)
	Abductor digiti minimi	Pisiform and flexor carpi ulnaris tendon	Ulnar aspect of base of 5th proximal phalanx	MCP abduction of 5th phalange	Ulnar aspect of hypothenar eminence with 5th MCP abduction	Ulnar nerve (C8, T1)
	Flexor digiti minimi brevis	Hook of hamate and adjacent transverse carpal ligament	Ulnar aspect of base of 5th proximal phalanx	MCP flexion of 5th phalange	Palmar surface of 5th metacarpal, lateral to opponens digiti minimi with 5th MCP flexion against resistance	Ulnar nerve (C8, T1)

CHAPTER summary

Introduction

- ✔ The distal end of the upper extremity enables multifaceted movements. Overusing the muscles of the forearm, hand, and wrist with repetitive actions may lead to soft-tissue dysfunction.

Bones

- ✔ There are 29 bones that make up the complexity of the hand and wrist, including 8 carpals, 5 metacarpals, 14 phalanges, and the radius and ulna. Bony landmarks provide muscular attachment to make movement possible.

Joints

- ✔ The wrist is classified as a condyloid joint. The carpal joints are gliding joints, and the metacarpophalangeal joints are classified as condyloid, like those in the wrist. The phalanges have ginglymus, or hinge, joints. The thumb has a saddle joint at its metacarpal base to provide opposition.

Movements of the Wrist and Hand

- ✔ The wrist provides movement in two planes that includes flexion, extension, abduction (radial flexion), and adduction (ulnar flexion). The metacarpophalangeal joints, or knuckles, also provide flexion, extension, abduction, and adduction. The phalanges only flex and extend. The specialized thumb provides flexion, extension, abduction, and adduction. The ability to touch the thumb to other fingers is called opposition.

Muscles

- ✔ Anteriorly, the palmaris longus is the most superficial muscle and is supported by flexor carpi radialis and flexor carpi ulnaris on both sides. The flexor digitorum superficialis and flexor digitorum profundus cause flexion of the fingers. Flexor pollicis longus flexes the thumb. Most flexors originate on or near the medial epicondyle of the humerus.
- ✔ Posteriorly, the extensors stem from the lateral epicondyle area of the humerus. The extensor carpi radialis longus and extensor radialis brevis run side by side to the hand. The extensor carpi ulnaris occupies the ulnar side to the base of the metacarpal of the little finger. Extensor digitorum governs extension of the fingers. Extensor indicis helps point the index finger. Extensor digiti minimi holds up the little finger by itself. Extensor pollicis longus and extensor pollicis brevis extend the thumb. Abductor pollicis longus inserts on the base of the 1st metacarpal and abducts the thumb.
- ✔ There are many intrinsic muscles of the hand that add to movement of the thumb and fingers.

Nerves

- ✔ The nerves for the hand and wrist muscles stem primarily from the brachial plexus. They include the radial, ulnar, and median nerves.

Individual Muscles of the Wrist and Hand—Flexors

- ✔ *Palmaris longus* is a superficial muscle that does not go through the carpal tunnel. It comes from the medial epicondyle and inserts into the palm of the hand. It is sometimes used for tendon repair and may even be absent on some people.
- ✔ *Flexor carpi radialis* spans from the medial epicondyle and inserts on the radial side of the wrist at the base of the 2nd and 3rd metacarpals. It is a strong flexor of the wrist and radially flexes the wrist.
- ✔ *Flexor carpi ulnaris* comes from the medial epicondyle and runs down the ulnar side of the forearm to the base of the 5th metacarpal. Its functions are flexion and ulnar flexion of the wrist. This tendon does not go through the carpal tunnel.
- ✔ *Flexor digitorum superficialis* is an anterior forearm muscle that has multiple attachments to the radius, the ulna, and the medial epicondyle of the humerus. It inserts distally to the sides of four fingers and flexes the fingers and wrist. All four tendons go through the carpal tunnel.
- ✔ *Flexor digitorum profundus* is a deep muscle that supports the superficialis as a foundation, but it has attachment only to the ulna and not to the humerus. It inserts on the base of the distal phalanxes of the four fingers and gives only the ability to flex the distal phalanxes. All four tendons go through the carpal tunnel.
- ✔ *Flexor pollicis longus* is a thumb flexor and assists in flexion of the wrist. This tendon also goes through the carpal tunnel.

Individual Muscles of the Wrist and Hand—Extensors

- ✔ *Extensor carpi ulnaris* comes from the lateral epicondyle and runs down the ulnar side of the forearm to the base of the 5th metacarpal on the dorsal side of the hand. Its functions are extension and ulnar flexion of the wrist.
- ✔ *Extensor carpi radialis brevis* spans from the lateral epicondyle and inserts at the base of the 3rd metacarpal on the dorsal side of the hand. It extends the wrist and assists in radial flexion of the wrist.
- ✔ *Extensor carpi radialis longus* is a posterior forearm muscle that spans from the lateral epicondyle to the dorsal side of the hand at the base of the 2nd metacarpal. It is a strong extensor of the wrist and radially flexes the wrist.
- ✔ *Extensor digitorum* is a large muscle of the posterior forearm that runs from the lateral epicondyle to the dorsal base of the distal phalanxes of the four fingers. It extends the fingers and wrist.
- ✔ *Extensor indicis* does not come from the lateral epicondyle. It is a smaller muscle that originates from the ulna and inserts at the index finger on the dorsal side. It helps to extend the index finger.
- ✔ *Extensor digiti minimi* begins at the lateral epicondyle and runs down the posterior forearm to the dorsal side of the little finger. It supports extension of the little finger.
- ✔ *Extensor pollicis longus* is a posterior forearm thumb muscle. It begins on the ulna and inserts at the base of the distal phalanx of the thumb. It is a fairly strong muscle that extends the thumb and wrist and assists in abduction of the wrist.
- ✔ *Extensor pollicis brevis* comes from the posterior radius to insert on the dorsal base of the proximal phalanx of the thumb. It assists the extensor pollicis longus to extend the thumb.
- ✔ *Abductor pollicis longus* crosses the posterior forearm from the ulna and radius to the base of the dorsal 1st metacarpal of the thumb. It abducts the thumb and wrist and assists in extension of the thumb.

Intrinsic Muscles of the Hand

- ✔ The intrinsic hand muscles may be grouped according to location as well as to the parts of the hand they control.

CHAPTER *review*

Worksheet Exercises

As an aid to learning, for in-class or out-of-class assignments, or for testing, tear-out worksheets are found at the end of the text, on pages 531–534.

True or False

Write true *or* false *after each statement.*

1. The pronator teres can entrap the radial nerve.
2. There are 10 carpal bones in the hand.
3. The radial nerve goes through the carpal tunnel.
4. The wrist is a condyloid joint that performs flexion, extension, abduction, and adduction.
5. The palmaris longus is a superficial muscle and performs weak flexion of the wrist.
6. The capitate can sometimes depress the carpal tunnel.
7. The flexor digitorum profundus controls flexion at the distal end of the four phalanxes.

8. The tendons of extensor pollicis longus and brevis and the abductor pollicis longus form a depression in the hand called the anatomical snuffbox.
9. The thumb extensors assist in wrist adduction.
10. The extensor digiti minimi assists in extension of the wrist as well as of the little finger.
11. Flexor carpi ulnaris does not go through the carpal tunnel.
12. Flexors and extensors of the wrist work together to cause wrist abduction and adduction.

Short Answers

Write your answers on the lines provided.

1. Discuss why the thumb is the most important part of the hand.

2. What muscles work together to complete ulnar flexion of the wrist?

3. Name a common origin of many flexors of the hand and wrist.

4. What extensor muscles work together to complete radial flexion of the wrist?

5. Name the common origin of many extensors of the hand and wrist.

6. What muscle of the forearm could be used for tendon repair?

7. Name three nerves that primarily innervate the muscles that have action on the hand and wrist.

8. Name the nerve that goes through the carpal tunnel.

9. What special function does the saddle joint allow the thumb to perform?

10. How many bones are in the hand and wrist, including the ulna and radius? Name them, and give the number of each in the cases of multiple similar bones.

11. Name the two muscles that are the *strongest* flexors of the wrist.

Multiple Choice

Circle the correct answers.

1. The distal interphalangeal joints are which classification of joint?
   a condyloid
   b. ginglymus
   c. saddle
   d. pivot

2. The metacarpophalangeal joints are which classification of joint?
   a. ginglymus
   b. saddle
   c. condyloid
   d. ball and socket
3. The carpometacarpal joint of the thumb is a ________ joint.
   a. ginglymus
   b. condyloid
   c. pivot
   d. saddle
4. The nerves that innervate the flexors and extensors of the hand and wrist include:
   a. radial, median, and ulnar nerves
   b. radial and ulnar
   c. sciatic
   d. ulnar only
5. The muscles that flex the finger include:
   a. flexor carpi radialis, flexor digitorum superficialis, and flexor carpi ulnaris
   b. flexor digitorum superficialis and flexor digitorum profundus
   c. flexor carpi radialis and flexor carpi ulnaris
   d. extensor digitorum and flexor digitorum superficialis
6. The muscle that attaches to the dorsal base of the distal phalanx of the thumb is called:
   a. extensor pollicis brevis
   b. abductor pollicis longus
   c. flexor hallucis longus
   d. extensor pollicis longus
7. The base of the 2nd and 3rd metacarpal on the palmar side is the insertion for:
   a. extensor carpi radialis
   b. palmaris longus
   c. flexor carpi radialis
   d. flexor carpi ulnaris
8. Abductor pollicis longus can perform:
   a. abduction of the thumb
   b. abduction and extension of the thumb
   c. abduction of the thumb and weak flexion of the elbow
   d. abduction of the thumb and weak extension of the elbow joint
9. Primary wrist extensors include:
   a. extensor carpi radialis longus, brevis, and ulnaris
   b. extensor carpi radialis brevis and longus and flexor carpi radialis
   c. flexor digitorum superficialis and extensor pollicis longus
   d. extensor carpi radialis longus only
10. Superficial to deep flexors of the forearm include:
    a. flexor digitorum profundus, flexor digitorum superficialis, flexor carpi radialis and ulnaris, and palmaris longus
    b. flexor digitorum superficialis and palmaris longus
    c. palmaris longus, flexor carpi ulnaris and radialis, flexor digitorum superficialis, and flexor digitorum profundus
    d. flexor carpi ulnaris, flexor digitorum profundus, palmaris longus, flexor carpi radialis, and flexor digitorum superficialis

EXPLORE & *practice*

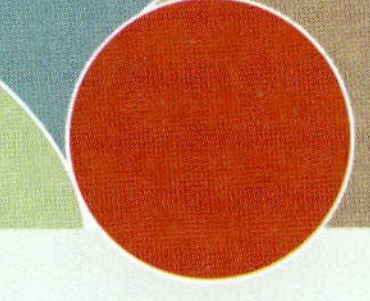

1. Locate the following parts of the humerus, radius, ulna, carpals, and metacarpals on a human skeleton and on a partner.

   a. Skeleton:
   1. Medial epicondyle
   2. Lateral epicondyle
   3. Lateral supracondylar ridge
   4. Trochlea
   5. Capitulum
   6. Coronoid process
   7. Tuberosity of the radius
   8. Styloid process—radius
   9. Styloid process—ulna
   10. 1st and 3rd metacarpals
   11. Carpal bones
   12. 1st phalanx of the 3rd metacarpal

b. Partner:

1. Medial epicondyle
2. Lateral epicondyle
3. Lateral supracondylar ridge
4. Pisiform, hook of hamate, capitate
5. Scaphoid (navicular), trapezium
6. Metacarpal bones

2. How and where can the following muscles be palpated on a partner?
   a. Flexor pollicis longus
   b. Flexor carpi radialis
   c. Flexor carpi ulnaris
   d. Extensor digitorum longus
   e. Extensor pollicis longus
   f. Extensor carpi ulnaris

3. Demonstrate the following actions, and list the muscles primarily responsible for these movements at the wrist joint.
   a. Flexion
   b. Extension
   c. Abduction
   d. Adduction

4. Locate on a partner all the origins and insertions of each muscle listed in this chapter.

5. How should boys and girls be taught to do push-ups? Justify your answer.
   a. Hands flat on the floor
   b. Fingertips

6. With a laboratory partner, determine how and why maintaining full flexion of all the fingers is impossible when passively moving the wrist into maximal flexion. Is it also difficult to maintain maximal extension of all the finger joints while passively taking the wrist into full extension?

7. *Muscle analysis chart:* Fill in the chart below by listing the muscles primarily involved in each movement.

Wrist and hand	
Flexion	Extension
Adduction	Abduction
Fingers—metacarpophalangeal joints	
Flexion	Extension
Abduction	Adduction
Fingers—proximal interphalangeal joints	
Flexion	Extension
Fingers—distal interphalangeal joints	
Flexion	Extension
Thumb	
Flexion	Extension
Abduction	Adduction

8. Describe the importance of the intrinsic muscles in the hand in turning a doorknob.

9. Determine the kind of flexibility exercises that would be indicated for a patient with carpal tunnel syndrome, and explain in detail how they should be performed.

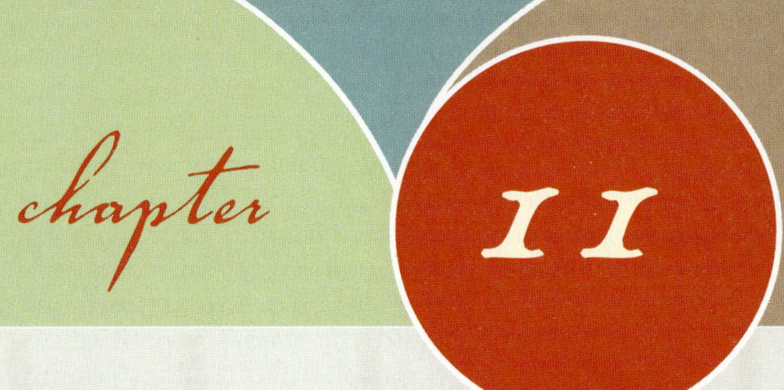

Unwinding the Soft Tissues of the Forearm: Dimensional Massage Techniques for the Muscles of the Hand and Wrist

LEARNING OUTCOMES

After completing this chapter, you should be able to:

- **11-1** Define key terms.
- **11-2** Describe the difference between entrapment and compression.
- **11-3** Discuss how posture and sleep positions can contribute to soft-tissue conditions.
- **11-4** List several potential causes of carpal tunnel syndrome.
- **11-5** Determine safe treatment protocols and refer clients to other health professionals when necessary.
- **11-6** Review general pathologies and conditions of the muscles of the hand and wrist.
- **11-7** Develop a treatment protocol for conditions of the lateral and medial epicondyle areas.
- **11-8** Demonstrate safe body mechanics.
- **11-9** Practice specific techniques on the hand and wrist muscles.
- **11-10** Incorporate dimensional massage therapy techniques in a regular routine or use them when needed.

KEY TERMS

Adhesion
Arthritis
Collagen
Degenerative disk disease
Dupuytren's contracture
Ganglion
Osteoarthritis
Sprains
Spurs
Strains
Subluxation
Tendon sheath

Introduction

The distal end of the upper extremity enables people to perform a number of detailed actions, including gripping, pushing, grasping, and letting go of objects. Yet the muscles that control these abilities are not just in the hands. The forearm and arm provide the bony attachments for the muscles that span the territory to the hand and wrist. The entire kinetic chain of the upper extremity provides the body with the mechanism to utilize the hand and wrist to their maximum capacities.

There are many complicated issues associated with the wrist, which performs only four actions:

flexion, extension, abduction, and adduction. There is no rotary action at the wrist; the wrist simply goes along for the supination and pronation "ride," because the radioulnar joint performs these actions. Flexor muscles originating from the medial epicondyle area of the humerus offer powerful support to flexion. The extensors oppose flexion with an appropriate number of muscles and matched strength that perform extension. The extensor muscles begin on the contralateral side of the forearm on or near the lateral epicondyle region of the humerus. Although the flexor and extensor anatomy seems perfectly reasonable for appropriate actions, there is a problem with the design in the actual structures that make up the hand and forearm.

As discussed in Chapter 10, the anatomy of the forearm and the hand and wrist is a combination of many muscles and tendons in a compact package. The carpal tunnel provides a limited area for 10 flexor tendons, blood vessels, and the median nerve and its branches to traverse through without developing inflammation or friction. Unfortunately, because of the tunnel's structure, this creates a recipe for potential injury and overuse syndromes. Extreme positions and the wrist's repetitive actions add torque on muscles and tendons coming from proximal positions and attachments, and this often results in tenderness at those origins. The hand commonly performs sideways actions (ulnar flexion or radial flexion). Applying pressure with the palm while the hand is in ulnar or radial flexion can develop tendonitis or soreness at the tendinous points of insertion in the hand. Structure, positions of the hand, and repetitive actions are all at fault for overuse syndromes and soft-tissue dysfunctions. Additionally, physical trauma to the region often results in injury and possible hand and wrist structural problems.

Injuries and Overuse Syndromes

FRACTURES AND TRAUMATIC INJURIES TO THE HAND AND WRIST

A variety of soft-tissue problems and bony injuries can occur in the hand and wrist. Carpenters, manual laborers, and fishermen often sustain hand injuries from myriad sources. Chefs and cooks perform job-related repetitive hand actions that can potentially lacerate tendons or cause other hand and wrist injuries. Athletic injuries, car accidents, or falls on an icy sidewalk also can result in traumatic injuries to the hand and wrist. In short, throughout life, the hand and wrist rarely escape injuries and accidents unscathed.

Like any joint in the body, the hand and wrist joints are susceptible to dislocation and fracture from trauma. Usually, a person's natural reaction to a slip and fall is to use his hand to break the fall. Landing on the hand with the entire weight of the body, however, is often harmful. The force of the fall can fracture the radius and ulna at the wrist; dislocate and fracture fingers, metacarpals, and/or carpals; tear or avulse ligaments; and cause sprains and strains. **Sprains** are injuries with various levels of severity that often tear ligaments and soft tissue and bruise nerves. All signs and symptoms of inflammation are present, and x-rays often are required to rule out fractures. **Strains** are injuries to the soft tissue, such as a stretch or tear of a tendon or muscle; like sprains, they also have various levels of severity. For broken bones and dislocations, medical attention is needed to appropriately set and realign fingers. Improperly treated bone injuries can lead to arthritic buildup around joints that can limit motion sooner than the natural aging process would, although these arthritic conditions may be inevitable even with proper treatment.

Laceration of tendons in the hand are problematic and require surgical tendon repair. Tendons that are cut in the hand recede like a rubber band that has lost its elasticity. If the tendon is a flexor, the surgeon may have to thread the tendon back through the carpal tunnel and reattach it to its insertion. Injuries of this nature require physical therapy and massage therapy in the rehabilitation phase for the best results in maintaining or restoring maximum range of motion and grip.

Tendonitis, Tendonosis, and Tenosynovitis

Repetitive injuries frequently result in humeral epicondyle conditions, including tendonitis, tendonosis, and tenosynovitis. *Tendonitis* is defined as an inflammation of a tendon. There are different types of tendonitis that require diagnoses. The worst cases of tendonitis usually involve the tendon pulling the periosteum away from the bone. This could be a partial tear, but it will still require a clinical evaluation and diagnosis. Sometimes tendons develop a lesion in the body of the tendon from constant-use, injury, or certain-use patterns. (See the *adhesion* definition below.) What separates tendonitis from tendonosis is that with tendonitis inflammation is present at the injury site.

The immediate physical responses at an injury site, such as a tear in a tendon, are inflammation and repair. The connective tissue binds the wound in an attempt to rapidly begin the repair process, but this does not begin to return the area to its preinjured state or original structure. The result is not always optimal and may leave a painful scar or **adhesion.** Ice is a first-aid measure and is applicable for tears. Deep transverse friction has long been a technique to help with adhesive tissue, but what if the condition is not tendonitis but, rather, tendonosis?

Tendonosis is defined as a breakdown in **collagen** fibers in the tissue. Collagen is made up of mostly protein and is composed of the white fibers of connective tissue. Tendonosis may be more common than otherwise expected, as tendonitis has been used as a catchall term of diagnosis for some time. In tendonosis, there is a lack of vascularity in the tendon structure as well as a "fray" in the fibers. This condition causes the tendon structure to lack integrity and strength, and it produces chronic pain and soreness. Unwinding the forearm in a logical sequential pattern and using circular friction on the offending site is an appropriate treatment option for massage therapy. See the techniques and treatment protocols of the forearm, hand, and wrist, discussed later in the chapter, for additional information.

Tenosynovitis is an inflammation of a tendon sheath. Flexor and extensor tendons have "common" tendons that originate on the medial and lateral epicondyles, respectively. **Tendon sheaths,** plastic wrap–like connective tissue, surround these individual groups and can become inflamed from the repetitive action and continual torque received in this region. As previously stated, the flexor group in the carpal tunnel also has a tendon sheath, as does the flexor pollicis longus in the thumb.

These three conditions are difficult to distinguish from each other and certainly require diagnosis. Generally, tenosynovitis occurs only where tendon sheaths are located. Orthopedic tests can help determine the diagnosis. Clinical solutions include ice, bracing, and corticosteroids. Practitioners should use extreme caution with acute conditions. Follow careful treatment protocols for these painful injuries, and refer clients to medical practitioners when necessary.

Other Soft-Tissue Issues

A lump on the dorsal side of the wrist often is a **ganglion.** A wrist ganglion is a cyst that usually protrudes on the dorsal side of the wrist. It sometimes comes from the tendon sheath or from a joint capsule. Ganglions are annoying, slightly painful growths that occasionally impair range of motion. Physicians tend to drain the fluid contained in a ganglion. Ganglions should not be massaged directly; however, the area around the growth can be worked, as long as inflammation is not present.

Dupuytren's contracture is a debilitating hand condition that can inhibit normal hand and finger functions. Named after French surgeon Guillaume Dupuytren (1777–1835), this condition involves the palmar aponeurosis or fascia and nodules that develop in the fibrous tissue and cause a permanent flexion of mostly the 4th or 5th fingers in one or both hands. The muscle that inserts into the palm is the palmaris longus. Although this condition is thought to be hereditary, it is common in clam diggers and lobster fishermen, whose hands are submerged in cold water in flexed positions performing repetitive actions, and in carpenters, who use tools that press into the palm. Caught at the onset, this condition might be helped with paraffin baths and massage to the palm, the palmaris longus, and other wrist flexors. Stretching is a necessary maintenance tool for this condition. Should the problem proceed to permanent flexion, surgical intervention is a known alternative.

Nerve Complaints

CARPAL TUNNEL REVISITED

Chapters 9 and 10 defined *carpal tunnel syndrome* as an inflammatory condition of the median nerve in the carpal tunnel that distributes pain and discomfort to distal fingers. There are many causes of this condition. Anything that diminishes the area in the carpal tunnel can be a causative factor. Small tumors and/or a ganglion can reduce the room in the carpal tunnel. Fluid retention during pregnancy can decrease available space. The shape of the tunnel is an important factor, and it cannot have any depressions that deprive its "occupants" of available room. A depressed capitate bone can reduce space in the carpal tunnel. Tenosynovitis of the flexor digitorum superficialis and flexor digitorum profundus can increase swelling and add friction in this confined area, which could in turn press against the median nerve.

Outside the tunnel itself, the median nerve is at risk of entrapment by the pronator teres and/or pectoralis minor soft tissues. Bony compression of the brachial plexus can reduce innervation, eventually irritate the median nerve, and produce distal symptoms. Many factors, in addition to repetitive actions and extreme wrist positions, can contribute to carpal tunnel syndrome and/or distal sensations. Diagnosis may include a nerve conduction test to determine the exact cause of the distal sensations, whether it is indeed carpal tunnel syndrome or is a median nerve entrapment at a different site. Conservative measures include releasing soft-tissue entrapment, wearing wrist braces, and correcting any sleep postures. Surgery of the flexor retinaculum might be a necessary solution, but it should be considered a last resort.

ENTRAPMENT VERSUS COMPRESSION

Not all nerve complaints in the hand and wrist involve the carpal tunnel and/or the median nerve. Entrapment of the radial nerve in the triceps can translate to decreased innervation, inadequate ability to apply pressure between the thumb and the index finger, and painful sensations. Ulnar nerve entrapment in the arm and flexor carpi ulnaris can cause weakness and discomfort in the 4th and 5th fingers. The ulnar nerve also can be compressed by the cubital tunnel, as previously discussed. Nerve transposition is a surgical solution for ulnar nerve compression. In an ulnar nerve transposition, the surgeon reroutes the ulnar nerve. Dropping of objects and weakness of grip are typical symptoms of this compression problem. Passive movement of the involved joints of the upper extremity will help to confirm or negate pain, numbness, or tingling. Undiagnosed positive pain results with passive movement should be a reason to refer the client to the appropriate health professional. Massage therapy is beneficial when the soft tissue is involved.

SLEEP POSITIONS AND POSTURE

Sleep positions and posture play a part in distal nerve sensation problems. Sleeping with the upper extremity above the head helps the pectoralis minor entrap the brachial plexus and possibly impede blood supply to the hand and wrist. The individual will awaken with a numb extremity and will have to use the other hand to pull the affected body part back to an anatomical position. (See Chapters 4 and 5 on the shoulder girdle.) Sleeping in a fetal position with rounded, collapsed shoulders can contribute to entrapment of the brachial plexus. Some people sleep with the wrists in extreme flexion, and this can cause numbness and tingling to the whole hand and wrist. Remedies for these troublesome habits may range from using multiple pillows to help prevent bad sleep postures to wearing a brace to prevent bending the wrist joint.

Posture can contribute to nerve complaints. Abducted scapulae (rounded shoulders) and the repetitive action of leading with a pronated forearm engage the pronator teres to possibly entrap the median nerve.

The position of the body while asleep or awake can have a long-term effect on the musculoskeletal structure. The body grows accustomed to sleeping positions; it "learns" and remembers repeated poor postural habits. Therapists should routinely examine their clients' postures. Is one shoulder higher? Does the dominant arm round forward and sit in front of the body in a pronated area on the thigh? The answers to these questions will provide clues to the client's shortened muscles, compensating antagonists, and learned posture. It is beneficial for the therapist to use a visual cue chart or diagram of the body for jotting down observations and then to share the information with the client and develop a meaningful goal of treatment based on the total information.

Arthritis, Osteoarthritis, Degenerative Disk Disease, and Cervical Subluxations

Compression of nerves at the cervical level may involve arthritis, osteoarthritis, degenerative disk disease, and/or cervical subluxations. **Arthritis** is an inflammation of a joint and is common in the aging process. More common in the cervical and lumbar spine is osteoarthritis. **Osteoarthritis** is a degenerative joint disease that in the spine can add to the bony growth size of individual vertebrae and fray the edges in a jagged manner. **Spurs,** or bony growths on the side of the vertebrae, can grow together, sometimes virtually linking the vertebrae in what is called "kissing spurs." The additional bony growth inhibits neck movement and innervation. Nerves that are inhibited by bony growths may result in muscle atrophy and twitching in the upper extremity. Osteoarthritis has no cure and often resides in bones and joints that have experienced previous injuries.

Degenerative disk disease is often present in individuals who have osteoarthritis; it also may be included in the definition of osteoarthritis. Degenerative disk disease is the literal depletion of the disk space between the vertebrae. The disk itself degenerates and reduces in size. The disk is needed to separate the vertebrae and allow space for nerves to travel safely out of the area.

Anyone who has visited a chiropractor or a manipulative osteopath may understand the definition of a **subluxation.** With the exception of the C1 and C2 relationship, most of the vertebrae are classified as gliding joints. A subluxation is a joint that is slightly ajar. It is not dislocated, but it has articular surfaces that are somewhat out of alignment. The chiropractor will "adjust" the vertebrae to realign the bones in an optimum placement. Massage therapy and chiropractic and/or manipulative adjustors complement each other. Massage therapy can relax the soft tissue, thereby assisting in the success of adjustments and maintenance, and may decrease the number of further subluxations.

Pain, numbness, and tingling with passive movement may help distinguish a problem in the cervical region. If the massage therapist suspects cervical involvement and/or nerve compression, it is appropriate to refer the client to a medical practitioner.

This book is not meant to be a complete pathology text. Students are urged to take required pathology courses to become knowledgeable about a variety of pathologic conditions and problems of the whole body. Contraindications for each condition should be reviewed. After confirming local and general contraindications, the therapist can proceed with caution, care, and appropriate applications to injured areas as well as to compensating regions. Often, the rest of the body needs massage as it tries to deal with its injured parts.

Unwinding the Forearm Muscles

In Swedish massage, therapists are taught to start with effleurage at the wrist and apply the technique to the entire upper extremity. Many therapists perform stripping immediately following effleurage to the forearm tendons and muscles. Therapeutically, however, this is not necessarily an appropriate sequence for the forearm muscles. Only techniques that allow the tissue to respond without undue discomfort should be applied. Using the stripping technique too soon in a sequence may feel like trying to push cement through a tube. If the muscles are tight and overworked, it will be difficult to push through the knots. Instead, the therapist needs to unwind the tissue methodically and apply the appropriate technique for the right purpose. It is important for the therapist to reflect on what the technique actually does and how it works.

Chapter 9 stated that it would be prudent to start on the shoulder girdle muscles to set the stage and treat the muscles that are holding on to the upper extremity. Relaxing the shoulder girdle muscles that have had a compensating tension establishes a positive response pattern. Because the client is seeking pain relief, it is important not to start on the most painful site first.

POSSIBLE SEQUENCE FOR THE LATERAL AND MEDIAL EPICONDYLE AREAS

A client presents with diagnosed tendonosis or tendonitis in the lateral epicondyle area, which is uncomfortable and tender at the origin sites of the common extensor tendons. Depending on the repetitive action and how long the tissues have been overworked, there may be a number of involved muscles in this overuse condition. The therapist should take a dimensional approach and apply techniques to the involved muscles, compensating soft tissue, and muscles associated with similar joint activity. The probable muscles in this example could include:

- Brachioradialis, extensor carpi radialis longus and brevis, extensor digitorum, possibly extensor carpi ulnaris and extensor digiti minimi, triceps and anconeus, supinator, biceps, and brachialis.
- Among the medial epicondyle muscles, the pronator teres, flexor carpi ulnaris and radialis, flexor digitorum superficialis, and flexor digitorum profundus, even though it does not attach to the medial epicondyle. Do not overlook the biceps and brachialis in the arm.

Therapists must remember that overuse and repetitive soft-tissue problems are created over time; however, massage therapy does not "fix" people. Instead, it allows the body to process the benefits of the techniques applied and help itself toward healing. It usually takes more than one session to unwind a problematic forearm—it may even take months. Therapists must be patient and stay positive. Additionally, massage therapy is just one facet of the teamwork involved in the healing process. The client may well need other professionals to assist in rehabilitation with stretching and strengthening. She will have to take responsibility for her journey to wellness by repeating the recommended exercises and stretches and performing any repetitive actions more safely with better body mechanics or in a more ergonomic setting.

The following techniques can be used as a complete sequence or be incorporated into other treatment sequences. As stated earlier, these techniques support the therapist's purpose to reduce hypertonicities, lengthen fibers, separate tissues, reduce soreness and pain levels, increase flexibility, and increase movement to restricted action.

Dimensional Massage Therapy for the Hand and Wrist Muscles

When practicing dimensional massage techniques, remember that the parts of the upper extremity are connected. To properly treat the whole, it is necessary to manipulate the shoulder, elbow, wrist, and hand soft tissues. If there is referring distal soft-tissue discomfort, investigate the infraspinatus, subscapularis, scalenes, and pectoralis major and minor. See Chapters 13 and 14 for more about the scalenes and possible entrapment syndrome.

TREATMENT PROTOCOL FOR THE MUSCLES OF THE FOREARM, HAND, AND WRIST

How do you approach these problems in a sequence?

- Always use treatment protocols to determine the sequence of a therapeutic session.
- Palpate tissues.
- Follow a dimensional approach, and critically think about the involved joints and kinetic chain.
- Determine pressure intelligently.
- Start on the shoulder girdle muscles to unwind compensating tissues.
- Move to the arm muscles and attachments to rule out any muscles that are assisting repetitive actions or entrapment issues.
- Unwind the soft tissue in the elbow joint area.
- Start superficially to deep on the forearm muscles. Use elliptical movement and techniques to unwind the brachioradialis. Use dry techniques first on the forearm.
- Visit all the muscles possibly involved in the problem.
- Visit all the attachments of the involved muscles.
- Use ice when appropriate.
- Work on the uninjured or less injured extremity first.
- Passively shorten the muscles whenever possible with techniques to decrease tension.
- Administer stripping and compressive effleurage at appropriate times when the tissue is ready for increased circulation.
- Be careful of the thumb muscles on the dorsal side of the forearm when you are "stripping" tendons. See Chapter 10 for the direction of fibers of the thumb muscles.
- Use active engagement techniques toward the end of the sequence. They are performed by asking the client to move the hand in flexion or extension while you are administering a particular technique. Active engagement techniques increase the neuromuscular mechanisms in the tissues and reinforce movement patterns.
- Do not ignore the flexor muscles just because the condition is an extension or lateral epicondyle issue. Remember, muscles work in groups and in paired opposition.
- Do not overwork sore areas. It is better to allow the extremity to process the treatment naturally and in its own time rather than to overwork it.
- See the techniques in the section below for additional suggestions.

Additionally, make sure you release the muscles of the posterior neck and shoulder girdle. Review and utilize the techniques from the previous chapter, as they overlap liberally in this routine. Use ice, when necessary, before administering massage and deep-tissue techniques, and use plenty of warm-up techniques before deep-tissue work. Intersperse elliptical movements to facilitate loosening of tissue. Use the techniques intelligently. Sink into the tissues, and they will respond by melting.

SUPINE BODY POSITION: FOREARM, HAND, AND WRIST

Compression of the Forearm Muscles

Use the palm of one hand to effectively compress the muscles of the client's forearm. Apply the technique to the extensors as well as to the flexors. Make sure your hands are relaxed; use your body weight as you compress. Use a pumping motion beginning closer to the elbow joint area, and work distally. (See figure 11.1.)

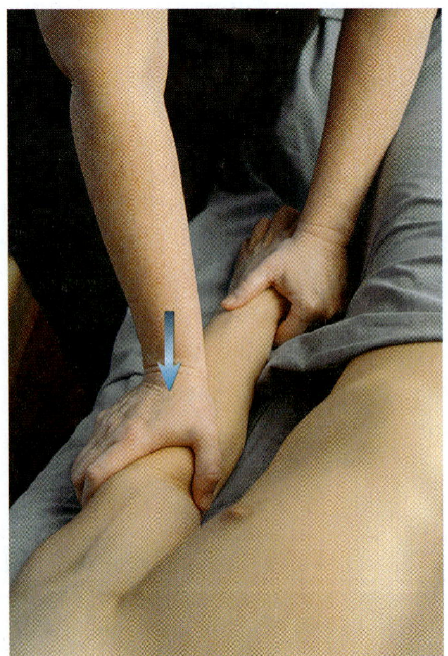

FIGURE 11.1 Compression of the forearm muscles

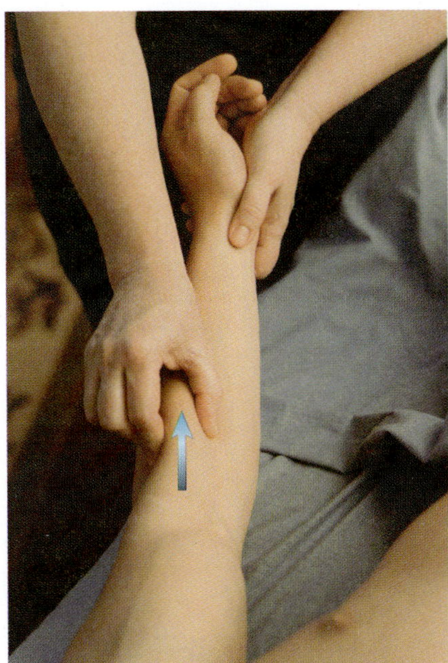

FIGURE 11.2 Jostling the brachioradialis

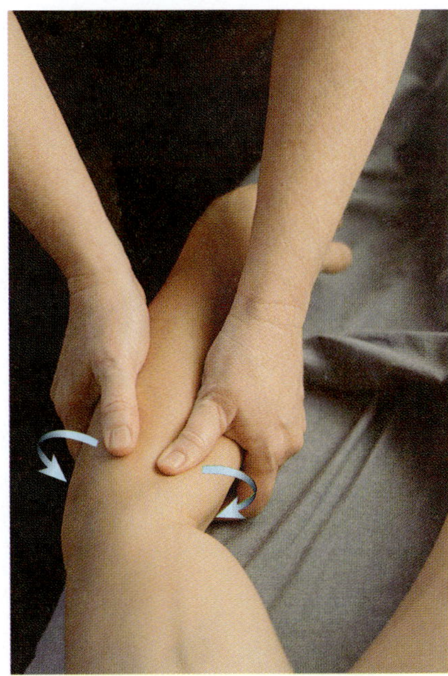

FIGURE 11.3 Elliptically moving the forearm muscles

Jostle of the Brachioradialis

Make sure the elbow joint is slightly flexed. Pick up the bulk of the muscle close to the elbow joint, apply a bit of a stretch, and jostle the brachioradialis toward the wrist. Repeat several times. (See figure 11.2.)

Elliptically Move the Forearm Muscles

Pick up the client's forearm (palm down) and grasp the muscles on both sides with your thumbs top-side-up and your fingers on the other side of the forearm. Elliptically move the forearm muscles. Notice how the radius shows movement. Move your hands in a variety of positions from proximal to distal. Repeat on the flexor side. (See figure 11.3.) This technique can be used liberally throughout the routine. *Note:* Lubrication will make it too difficult to grasp and hold the soft tissue.

Myofascial Stretch of the Brachioradialis

At a right angle to the client's forearm, pick up the belly of the muscle and draw the tissue over your thumbs. Start close to the elbow joint, and work toward the wrist. Repeat. (See figure 11.4.)

Parallel Thumbs on the Brachioradialis

At a right angle to the client's forearm, pick up the tissue with a thumb-over-thumb technique, moving from the elbow to the wrist. (See figure 11.5.)

Skin Rolling

How loose the fascia is will determine how comfortable this technique will feel. Grasp a small amount of fascia between the thumbs and forefingers. Roll it along in a strip. Obtain feedback from the client regarding comfort levels. Repeat in a different section of tissue. On the forearm, it is best to pick up the tissue at a right angle to the tendons and go across the tendons with the skin rolling. This is an optional warm-up technique.

Locate and Palpate the Forearm Tendons

Locate the belly of the muscles and tendons to determine necessary technique requirements. Assess

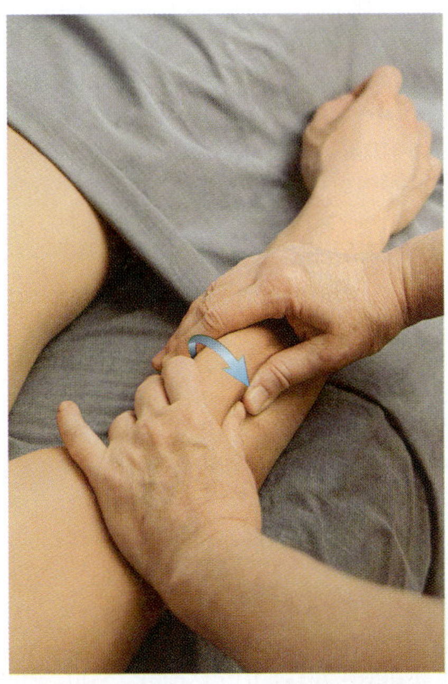

FIGURE 11.4 Myofascial stretch of the brachioradialis

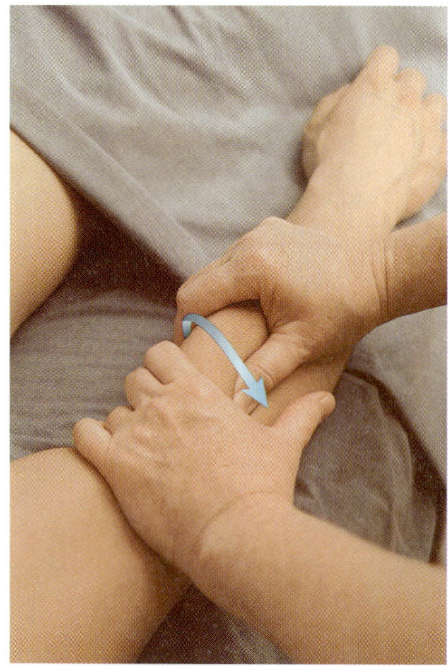

FIGURE 11.5 Parallel thumbs on the brachioradialis

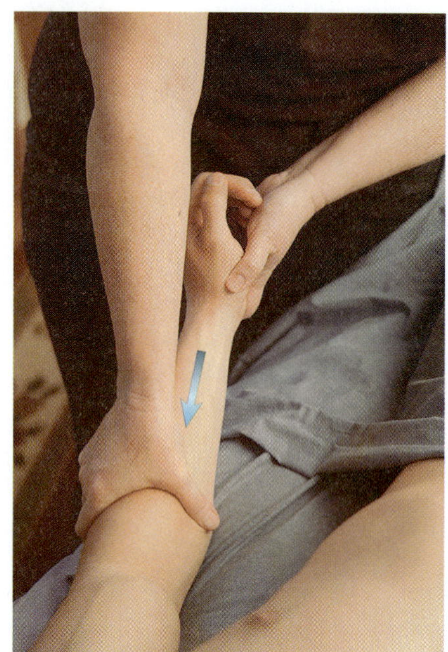

FIGURE 11.6 Compressive effleurage

hypertonicities, tenderness, and pain tolerance level at attachment sites.

Compressive Effleurage

Perform long strokes on the forearm. Hold the ulnar side of the client's hand. With your other hand, straddle the brachioradialis muscle in neutral. Mold your hand to the structure. Using your body weight and momentum, stroke from the distal end toward the elbow with a soft, compressive hand instead of hard hand pressure. Repeat several times. Switch hands to hold the client's hand on the radial side of the wrist. Straddle the forearm, and stroke the flexors and extensors distal to proximal. Repeat several times. Do not underestimate the benefits of compressive effleurage. (See figure 11.6.)

Alternating Petrissage of the Forearm Muscles

Slightly flex the client's elbow joint to help passively shorten the muscles. Petrissage the forearm muscles at a right angle to the tendons. Lift and separate the fibers. Relax your hands, and keep them in alignment with your forearms. Grasp the tissue with only enough grip to hold the tissue. Relax your hands between strokes. (See figure 11.7.)

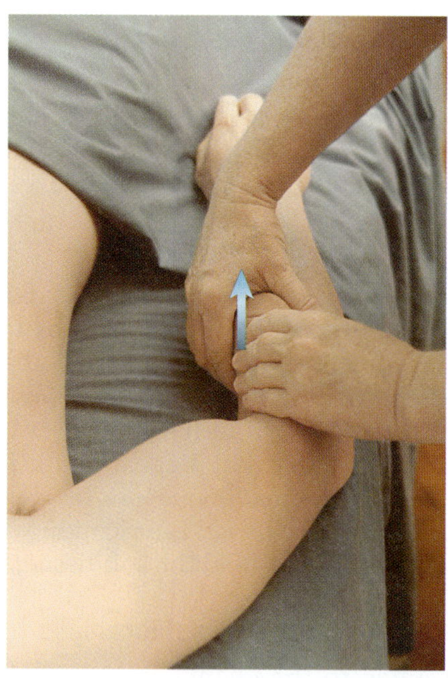

FIGURE 11.7 Alternating petrissage of the forearm muscles

Broadening of the Forearm Muscles

Broaden the brachioradialis, extensors, and flexors. For broadening the brachioradialis, place the client's forearm in a neutral position. Place your hands proximal to the elbow joint, and begin lifting and spreading the brachioradialis with your thumbs and the thenar side of your palms. Move distally toward the wrist. Repeat. Reposition the forearm, and apply the same technique to the extensors and then to the flexors. (See figure 11.8.)

Myofascial Humeral Twist

Stand at the side of the table at the client's side. With your inferior hand, grasp the client's wrist and

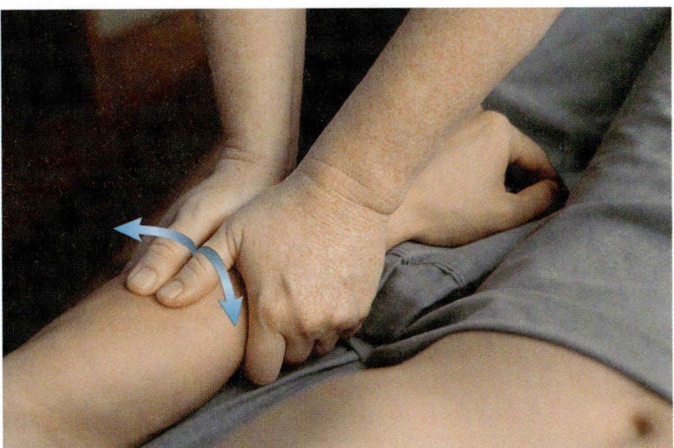

FIGURE 11.8 Broadening of the forearm muscles

flex the elbow joint. Passively move the arm into lateral rotation with the forearm flexed at a right angle. The arm should remain on the table next to the client. While moving the forearm toward the body, grasp the tissue above the medial epicondyle area with your superior hand and myofascially drag the tissue in a wringing fashion from medial to lateral. Repeat several times. This will help unwind the tissues going into the medial epicondyle region and can be used in the elbow and radioulnar techniques. (See figure 11.9.)

Petrissage Elbow Joint Muscles with Distraction Movement

With the client's elbow slightly flexed, lightly grasp the distal end of the triceps with one hand, and grasp the brachioradialis and forearm muscles with the other hand. Petrissage the triceps and the forearm muscles as you slightly flex and extend the elbow repeatedly. This stretches the soft tissues at the elbow joint as you massage the muscles. (See figure 11.10.)

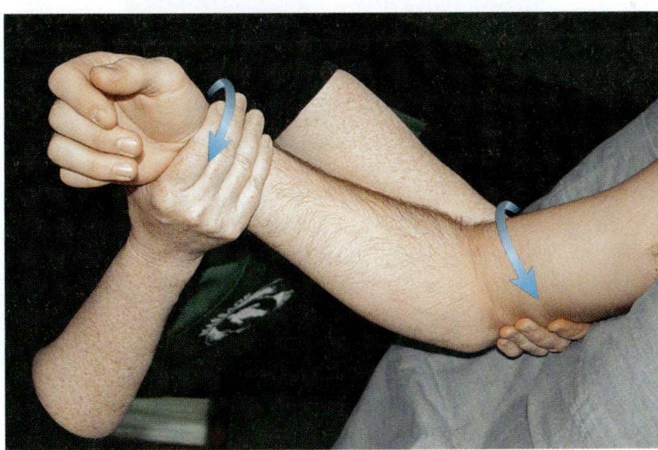

FIGURE 11.9 Myofascial humeral twist

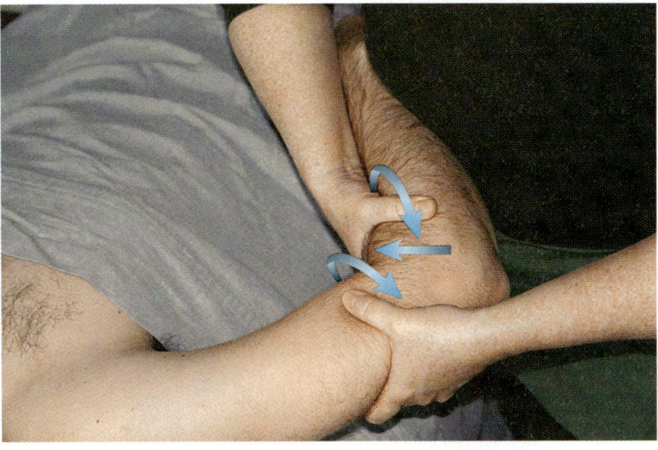

FIGURE 11.10 Petrissage elbow joint with distraction movement

Friction and Vibration of Tendons

Use circular friction and vibration on tendinous attachments and to the muscles and tendons. Intersperse the techniques liberally throughout your routine.

Elliptically Move the Carpals and Metacarpals

Grasp the client's wrist with your thumbs on the dorsal side of the hand and fingers on the palm side; elliptically move the muscles of the hand as you move the wrist in an alternating sideways fashion (ulnar flexion and radial flexion). Locate the carpals individually to slightly separate them with elliptical motion. Move to the carpometacarpal joints, and repeat the elliptical motion there. (See figure 11.11.)

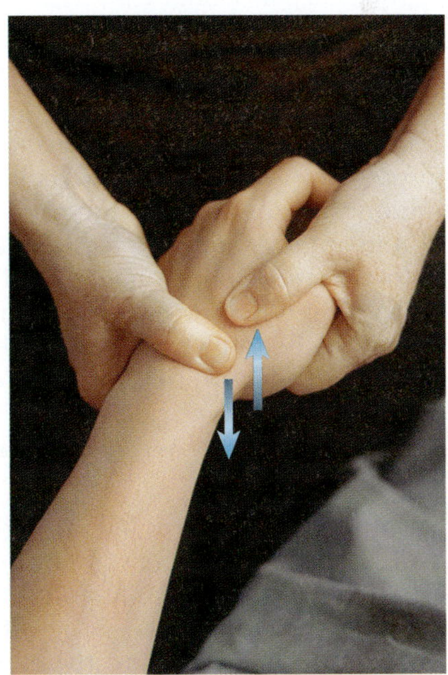

FIGURE 11.11 Elliptically moving the carpals and metacarpals

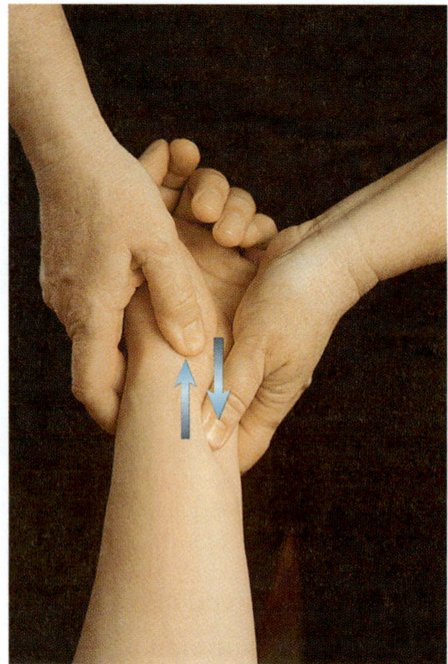

FIGURE 11.12 Short cross stroke to the antebrachial fascia

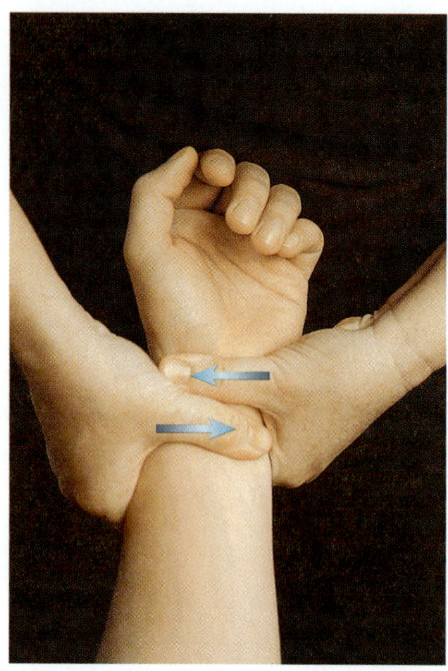

FIGURE 11.13 Thumb stripping to the antebrachial fascia

Note: Perform regular hand massage. Work deep into the palm, and pin and stretch the palmar aponeurosis at the metacarpophalangeal joint.

Locate Insertions of Flexor and Extensor Carpi Tendons in the Hand

As part of your hand massage, locate the attachments of the flexor carpi tendons in the palm and on the dorsal side of the hand. Apply circular friction to the attachments. On the dorsal side of the hand, stroke between the metacarpals from distal to proximal.

Short Strokes to the Antebrachial Fascia and Flexor Retinaculum

The antebrachial fascia is virtually invisible and improbable to palpate. Locate the antebrachial fascial area surrounding tendons on the anterior and posterior wrist, and apply a short cross stroke at a right angle to the tissues. (See figure 11.12.) Strip the tissue in opposing directions with your thumbs. (See figure 11.13.) Apply the same strokes to the flexor retinaculum. (See figure 11.14.) *Caution:* It is contraindicated to work over the flexor retinaculum in clients suffering from acute carpal tunnel syndrome.

Strip the Forearm Tendons

Passively shorten the client's wrist joint by placing the hand in slight flexion or extension, depending on which tendons and muscles you are stripping. Start at the wrist, and strip toward the elbow joint. Figure 11.15 shows the flexor digitorum superficialis in supported slight flexion. Make sure you strip in the direction of the tendons. Repeat with other tendons. Be careful of the thumb muscles and tendons on the extensor side. They should be stripped individually.

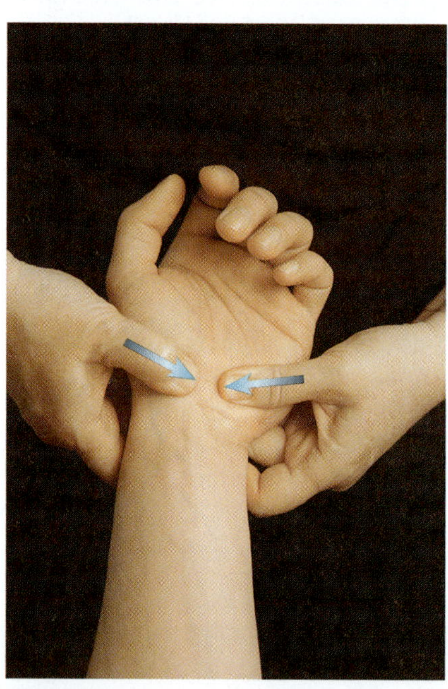

FIGURE 11.14 Thumb stripping to the flexor retinaculum

Flex, Extend, and Strip the Flexor Carpi Radialis and Flexor Carpi Ulnaris

Passively shorten the client's wrist, and as you are stripping the tendon, stretch the wrist at the same time. Perform short strokes, and repeat several times,

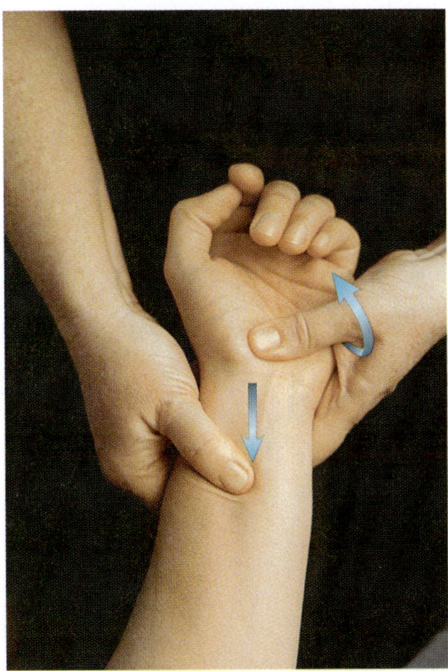

FIGURE 11.15 Stripping the flexor digitorum

moving the wrist as you stroke. (See figure 11.16.) The same process can be applied to the extensors of the wrist and to thumb muscles and tendons with accompanying passive stretching.

Treatment for Attachments at the Lateral and Medial Epicondyles

Locate the lateral and medial epicondyles for the tendinous attachments. With your superior hand (thumb), apply deep transverse friction or circular friction as needed to the attachments; move the forearm from supine to prone while using your inferior hand at the wrist. This is a dual-hand distraction technique with passive movement. (See figures 11.17 and 11.18.)

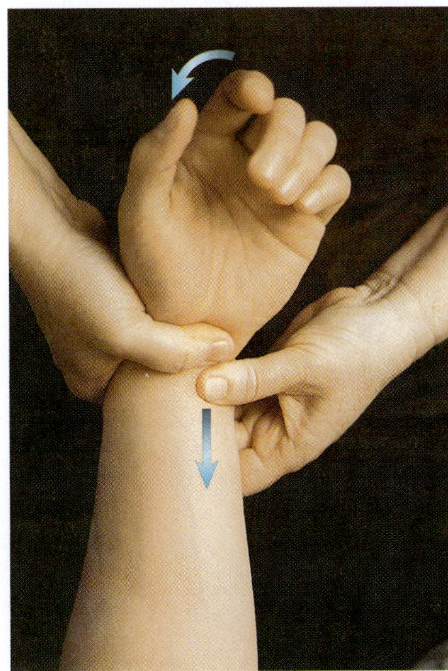

FIGURE 11.16 Flexing, extending, and stripping the wrist flexors

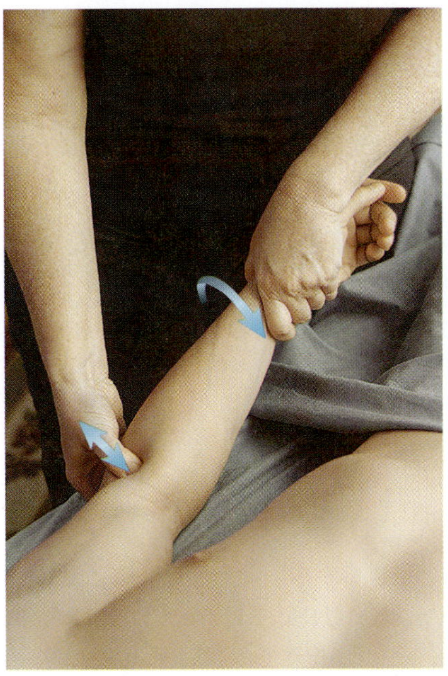

FIGURE 11.17 Lateral attachments

Broadening the Extensors with Active Engagement

Prop the client's wrist and hand with a rolled towel. Broaden the extensors proximal to distal as the client shortens the fibers by actively extending the hand from flexion. Stop when the hand is fully extended, and

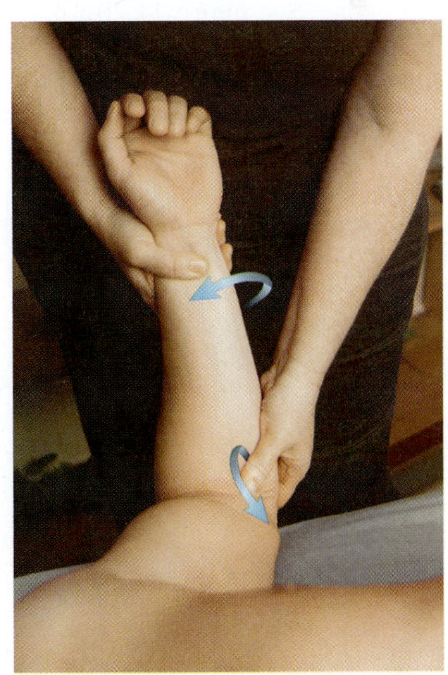

FIGURE 11.18 Medial attachments

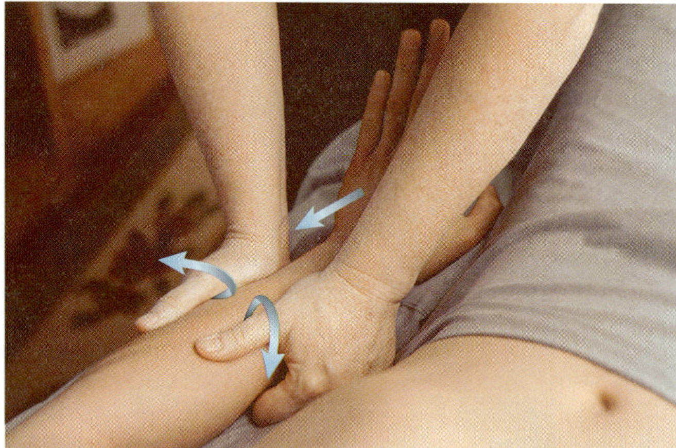

FIGURE 11.19 Broadening with active engagement of the extensor muscles

repeat the process. (See figure 11.19.) For the flexors, reverse the hand movement to extension to flexion as you broaden the flexors proximal to distal.

Lengthen the Extensors with a Loose Fist and/or Thumbs

Extensors and flexors can be lengthened with a loose fist or with the thumbs. Start distal at the wrist, and move proximal as the client stretches the tendons. For extensors, position the hand in extension and move toward flexion. Stop when the hand is in full flexion, and start over again. Repeat until you reach the elbow area. Watch the thumb muscles on the extensor side. Reverse the process for the flexors. Start with the hand in full flexion, and strip distal to the medial epicondyle region, repeating the hand movement as necessary. (See figure 11.20 for lengthening extensors with a loose fist and figure 11.21 for lengthening extensors with thumbs.) Stripping and active lengthening can easily be applied to the extensor pollicis muscles.

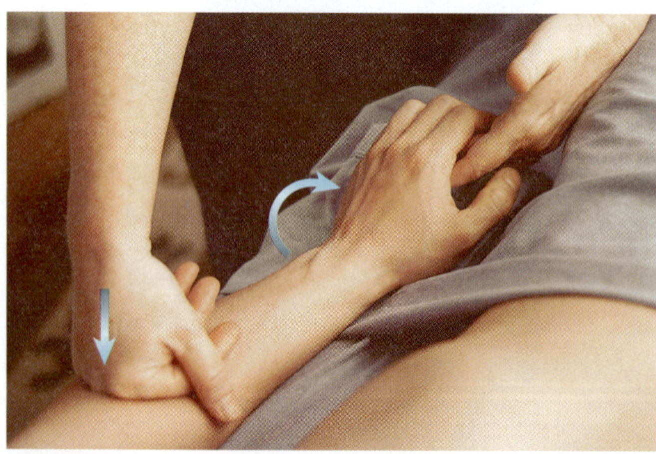

FIGURE 11.20 Lengthening the extensors with a loose fist

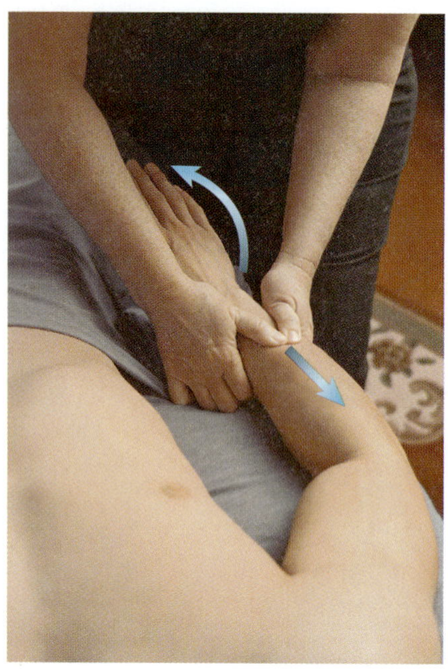

FIGURE 11.21 Lengthening the extensors with thumbs

Tapotement—Light Hacking

Stimulate nerves with light hacking to the forearm muscles. Use only your fingers and not the ulnar side of your hand. Keep the strikes close together, and use your wrist for the action. Hacking can be accomplished by using one hand if the other hand "refuses" to work. It is applied in the direction of the fibers. (See figure 11.22.)

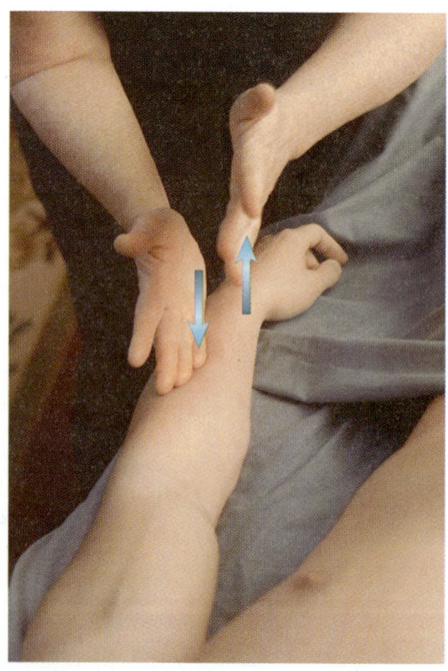

FIGURE 11.22 Light hacking to the forearm muscles

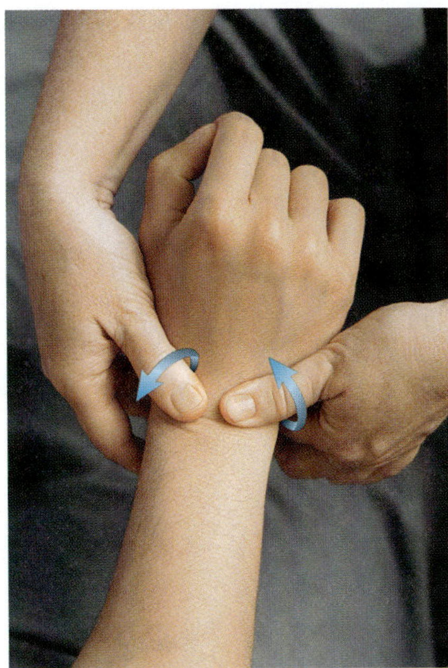

FIGURE 11.23 Flipping the hand

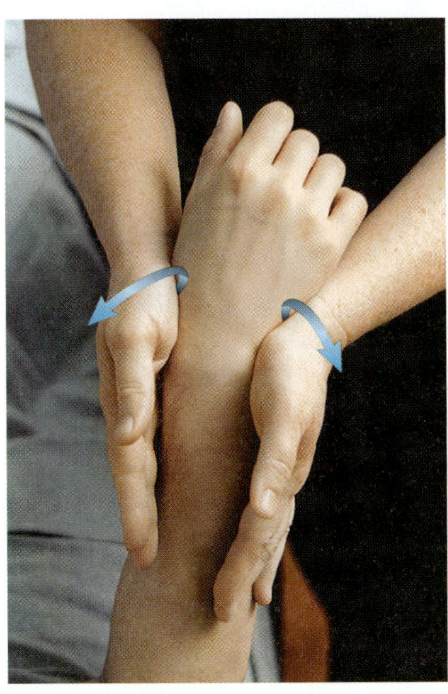

FIGURE 11.24 Ulnar and radial flexion shake

Sample Range of Motion of Hand and Wrist

Flipping the Hand Place your thumbs on the dorsal side of the client's wrist at the joint. Put your index fingers on the palm side of the hand. Gently extend and flex the hand at the wrist using thumbs and fingers alternately. (See figure 11.23.)

Shake the Wrist Place the medial portion of your palms on either side of the client's wrist, with your fingers facing toward the forearm. Alternately shake the wrist laterally and back. (See figure 11.24.)

CHAPTER *summary*

Introduction

- ✔ The hand and wrist are at the end of the upper-extremity kinetic chain.
- ✔ The hand, wrist, and forearm are a compact package with muscles, tendons, bones, and nerves in close quarters.
- ✔ Structure, positions of the hand, and repetitive actions are at fault for overuse syndromes and soft-tissue dysfunctions.
- ✔ Physical trauma also causes problems for the hand and wrist.

Injuries and Overuse Syndromes

- ✔ Fractures, dislocations, sprains, and strains are common to the hand and wrist.
- ✔ Lacerations in the hand and to tendons may require surgical tendon repair.

Tendonitis, Tendonosis, and Tenosynovitis

- ✔ Tendonitis, tendonosis, and tenosynovitis are conditions caused by repetitive injuries.
- ✔ Tendonitis is defined as inflammation of a tendon, which may develop a painful adhesion.
- ✔ Tendonosis is described as a breakdown of collagen fibers, causing chronic pain and soreness.
- ✔ Tenosynovitis is an inflammation of the tendon sheath surrounding tendons in specific areas.

Other Soft-Tissue Issues

- ✔ A ganglion is a cyst usually located on the dorsal side of the wrist.
- ✔ Dupuytren's contracture can permanently cause flexion of the 4th and 5th fingers.

Nerve Complaints

✔ Carpal tunnel syndrome has many causes.
✔ The radial nerve, ulnar nerve, and median nerve can be entrapped by soft tissue or compressed by bony structures and cause distal nerve sensations.
✔ Sleep positions and posture can cause numbness and tingling in the hand and wrist and contribute to overall nerve innervation problems.

Arthritis, Osteoarthritis, Degenerative Disk Disease, and Cervical Subluxations

✔ Arthritis, osteoarthritis, degenerative disk disease, and cervical subluxations can contribute to nerve complaints.

Unwinding the Forearm Muscles

✔ Shoulder girdle muscles contribute to compensatory soft-tissue discomforts.
✔ Work on the uninvolved upper extremity first.
✔ Follow a dimensional approach, and critically think about the involved joints and kinetic chain.
✔ Always use treatment protocols to determine the sequence of a therapeutic session.

Dimensional Massage Therapy for the Hand and Wrist Muscles

✔ The massage therapist's purpose is to reduce hypertonicities, lengthen fibers, separate tissues, reduce soreness and pain levels, increase flexibility, and increase restricted movements.
✔ Approach techniques methodically, unwinding soft tissue superficially to deep.

CHAPTER *review*

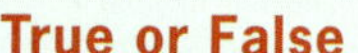

True or False

Write true *or* false *after each statement.*

1. All repetitive action problems at the lateral epicondyle result in tendonitis.
2. A subluxation is an actual dislocation of a vertebra.
3. Stripping is a technique that therapists can use right after effleurage to the whole extremity.
4. Carpal tunnel syndrome symptoms can be caused by soft-tissue entrapment outside the carpal tunnel.
5. Osteoarthritis has no cure.
6. The flexors digitorum superficialis and digitorum profundus share a tendon sheath.
7. Most extensors of the hand and wrist originate on or near the lateral epicondyle.
8. The hamate carpal can depress the carpal tunnel.
9. Collagen fibers are made up of mostly protein and make up the white fibers of connective tissue.
10. Elliptical movement is a good technique to start with on the forearm, as it is deep but at the same time does not hurt the client.

Short Answers

Write your answers on the lines provided.

1. Provide definitions for *tendonitis* and *tendonosis*.

___

___

___

2. What muscles might be involved in conditions of the lateral epicondyle area?

___

___

___

3. What muscles might be involved in conditions of the medial epicondyle area?

___

___

___

4. Why is it important to keep the hands in alignment with the forearms when completing techniques in massage?

___

___

___

5. Why are the hand and wrist prone to injury? What physical attributes contribute to injury in this area?

___

___

___

6. Where are tendon sheaths located?

____

____

____

7. Describe what happens in Dupuytren's contracture.

____

____

____

8. What is the difference between a sprain and a strain?

____

____

____

9. What is an adhesion?

____

____

____

10. Why is it important to work on the shoulder girdle muscles first?

____

____

____

11. What questions would a therapist ask of an individual who is complaining of numbness and tingling in the hand and/or wrist?

____

____

____

12. Why would a therapist work on the arm muscles and elbow joint before working on the forearm muscles?

____

____

____

Multiple Choice

Circle the correct answers.

1. A spur is:
   a. something you put on your boot if you are a cowboy
   b. an osteoarthritic bony growth on the side of the vertebra
   c. a thorn
   d. part of a nerve
2. Degenerative disk disease:
   a. can be responsible for distal nerve complaints
   b. is not something to ever worry about
   c. goes away very easily
   d. can be easily fixed
3. Possible causes of carpal tunnel syndrome include:
   a. fluid retention in pregnancy, repetitive actions, and compression of the ulnar nerve
   b. extreme wrist positions, sleep postures, and normal activity
   c. fluid retention in pregnancy, extreme wrist positions, sleep postures, and repetitive actions
   d. none of the above
4. Inflammation of a tendon sheath is described as:
   a. tenosynovitis
   b. carpal tunnel syndrome
   c. tendonosis
   d. tendonitis
5. If a client constantly pronates the forearm, what nerve especially could be entrapped by the repetitive action?
   a. ulnar nerve
   b. median nerve
   c. radial nerve
   d. none of the above
6. Some of the muscles involved in lateral epicondyle problems include:
   a. flexor carpi ulnaris, extensor carpi ulnaris, and flexor pollicis longus
   b. extensor carpi radialis longus and brevis, triceps, and extensor digitorum
   c. pronator teres
   d. none of the above
7. Treatment protocol for working on extensors of the forearm should include:
   a. only working on the forearm muscles
   b. working on the uninjured arm first
   c. working on the lower extremity first
   d. stripping forearm muscles and tendons first

8. Working directly on the flexor retinaculum when a client has carpal tunnel syndrome:
   a. is an accepted procedure
   b. is contraindicated
   c. should be done in a passively shortened manner
   d. should lengthen fibers
9. The muscles that work together to accomplish ulnar flexion are:
   a flexor carpi ulnaris and extensor carpi ulnaris
   b. flexor pollicis longus and abductor pollicis longus
   c. flexor carpi radialis and flexor carpi ulnaris
   d. none of the above
10. If a client presents with an undiagnosed condition and has numbness and tingling with passive flexion of the upper extremity, you would:
   a. massage the client and make repeated appointments
   b. massage the other extremity only
   c. discuss treatment possibilities and make an appropriate referral
   d. do nothing

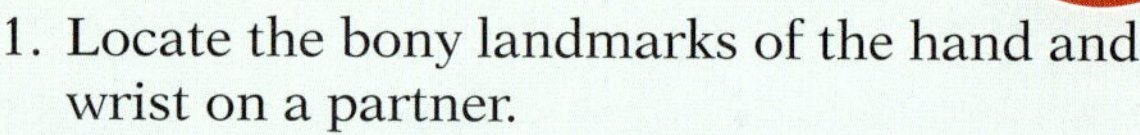

EXPLORE & practice

1. Locate the bony landmarks of the hand and wrist on a partner.
2. Locate the origins and insertions of the hand and wrist joint muscles on a partner.
3. Demonstrate how to passively shorten the flexors and extensors of the hand and wrist.
4. Demonstrate passive range of motion of the hand and wrist with a partner.
5. Demonstrate active range of motion of the hand and wrist with a partner.
6. Demonstrate passive range of motion of the thumb with a partner.
7. Demonstrate active range of motion of the thumb with a partner.
8. Locate the carpal tunnel on an individual. Locate all the muscles that go through the carpal tunnel.
9. In a client's medical history, you find that his current signs and symptoms are consistent with those he experienced when he fell from a horse 3 years ago. The client indicates that his hand goes to sleep as he holds a phone. What questions would you ask, and what simple tests might you perform? If the client had numbness with passive flexion of the upper extremity, would you refer him to a medical practitioner?
10. Demonstrate some principles of safe body mechanics while performing massage techniques.
11. Demonstrate warm-up techniques without lubrication.
12. Practice deep-tissue techniques individually and in a sequence on a partner.

chapter 12

Concepts of Muscular Analysis and Clinical Flexibility of the Upper Extremities

LEARNING OUTCOMES

After completing this chapter, you should be able to:

12-1 Analyze sports skills in terms of phases and the various joint movements occurring in those phases.

12-2 Compare various conditioning principles and apply them to strengthening major muscle groups.

12-3 Demonstrate specific clinical flexibility and strengthening exercises for the upper extremity.

12-4 Explain the concept of an open versus closed kinetic chain.

12-5 Recognize the actions of individual muscles that produce certain joint movements.

12-6 Describe specific exercises that increase the strength of individual muscle groups.

12-7 Discuss the concepts of analyzing and prescribing exercises to strengthen major muscle groups.

KEY TERMS

Breathing
Closed kinetic chain
Follow-through phase
Kinetic chain
Movement phase
Open kinetic chain
Overload principle
Periodization
Preparatory phase
Recovery phase
SAID (specific adaptations to imposed demands)
Specificity
Stance phase

Introduction

The upper extremity is capable of a wide range of dynamic movements. Natural, pain-free movement is critical for sports activities and daily living. Flexibility and strength in the upper extremity are essential for improved appearance and posture, as well as for more efficient skill performance. Unfortunately, the upper extremity is often one of the body's weaker areas because of the number of muscles involved. In addition, atrophy and muscle tightness in the neck and shoulder create imbalance that the lower extremity adapts to. Daily activities become painful because movement is deficient. Specific stretching and resistance exercises for conditions in this area can help keep natural movement optimal and assist in abating injury. If the therapist or trainer is qualified, she can teach individuals simple, yet specific, exercises that isolate groups of muscles and that ultimately can help those individuals maintain a better quality of life. Some of these simple, introductory exercises are included in this chapter.

The early analysis of human movement makes the study of structural kinesiology more meaningful, as students come to better understand the importance of individual muscles as they act on joints. Chapter 13 contains analyses of exercises for the entire body, with emphasis on the trunk and lower extremity. Contrary to what most beginning students in structural kinesiology believe, muscular analysis of activities is not difficult once the basic concepts are understood.

Upper-Extremity Activities

Children seem to have an innate desire to climb, swing, and hang. Such movements use the muscles of the hands, wrists, elbows, and shoulder joints. But the opportunity to continue to perform these types of activities is limited in our modern culture. Unless physical education teachers in elementary schools, for both boys and girls, emphasize development of this area of the body, it will continue to be muscularly the weakest area; moreover, continued maintenance of this area in adults should be reinforced in the health care field. Often, individuals reach a point in their lives when suddenly it hurts to do the things they love doing; this is a reduction in their quality of life. Weakness in the upper extremity can impair skill development and performance in many common, enjoyable recreational activities, such as golf, tennis, softball, and racquetball. However, people may continue to enjoy these and other activities if they learn how to increase the strength of this part of the body; therefore, adequate skill development built on an appropriate base of muscular strength and endurance is essential for enjoyment and prevention of injury.

American culture often is persuaded to learn typical strengthening exercises in a fitness club, with cosmetic focus on the larger, streamlined muscles, such as the pectoralis and biceps. Exercises for these muscles might include the bench press, overhead press, and biceps curl. While these exercises are beneficial, they concentrate primarily on the larger muscles of the anterior upper extremity. This can lead to overdevelopment with respect to the posterior, antigravity muscles. As a result, individuals may become strong and tight anteriorly and weak and flexible posteriorly. It also leads to posture dysfunctions, with the anterior chest collapsed and the posterior upper back rounded. For many weekend athletes, it is this overdevelopment in the large muscles and atrophy in the smaller intrinsic muscles that causes so many injuries. Thus, clinicians must be able to analyze specific strengthening and stretching exercises and subsequently determine the muscles involved so that overall muscular balance is addressed through appropriate exercise routines. In addition, individuals must always be educated on what they can do on their own to improve their quality of life.

Concepts for Analysis

In analyzing activities, it is important to understand that muscles are usually grouped according to their *concentric* (shortening contraction of muscle fibers) function and that they work in paired opposition to an antagonistic group. One example of an aggregate muscle group performing a given joint action is seen when all the elbow flexors work together to curl a dumbbell. In this example, the elbow flexors (biceps brachii, brachialis, and brachioradialis) are concentrically contracting as an agonist group to achieve flexion. As they flex the elbow, each muscle contributes significantly to the task, depending on the position of the hand. The muscles are working in opposition to their antagonists, the triceps brachii and anconeus. The triceps brachii and anconeus both work together as an aggregate muscle group to cause elbow extension, but in this example they are cooperating to allow the flexors to perform their task, elbow flexion. An often-confusing aspect of muscle contraction is that muscle groups can function to control the exact opposite actions by contracting *eccentrically* (lengthening of muscle fibers). During the return phase of a dumbbell curl (eccentric contraction of the biceps brachii from flexion), the triceps begins the movement and then acts as a stabilizer as the elbow moves into extension. Yet elbow extension is controlled by the flexors. Contrary to what some students believe, this eccentric movement (elbow extension) is not driven by the triceps.

Exercise professionals should be able to view an activity and not only determine which muscles are performing the movement but also know which type of contraction is occurring and what exercises are appropriate for developing the muscles. Chapter 2 provides a review of how muscles contract to work in groups that function in joint movement.

Analysis of Movement

Analyzing human movement is an important component to helping individuals improve dysfunction. In addition to sports activities, normal daily movements also can be analyzed. In analyzing various exercises and sports skills, it is essential to break down all the movements into phases. The number of phases, usually three to five, varies depending on the skill. Practically all sports skills have at least a preparatory phase, a movement phase, and a follow-through phase. Many also begin with a stance phase and end with a recovery phase. The names of the phases vary from skill to skill to fit in with the terminology used in various sports; they also may vary depending on which body part is involved. In some cases, these major phases may be divided further, as with baseball, where the preparatory phase for the pitching arm is divided into early cocking and late cocking.

The **stance phase** allows the athlete to assume a comfortable and appropriately balanced body position from which to initiate the sport skill. The emphasis is on setting the various joint angles in the correct positions with respect to one another and to the sport surface. Generally, with respect to the subsequent phases, the stance phase is a relatively static phase with fairly short ranges of motion involved. Due to the minimal amount of movement in this phase, the majority of the joint position maintenance throughout the body will be accomplished through isometric contractions.

The **preparatory phase,** often referred to as the *cocking* or *wind-up phase,* is used to lengthen the appropriate muscles so that they will be in position to generate more force and momentum as they concentrically contract in the next phase. It is the most critical phase in leading toward the desired result of the activity, and it becomes more dynamic as the need for explosiveness increases. Generally, to lengthen the muscles needed in the next phase, concentric contractions occur in their antagonist muscles in this phase.

The **movement phase,** sometimes known as the *acceleration, action, motion,* or *contact phase,* is the action part of the skill. It is the phase in which the summation of force is generated directly to the ball, sport object, or opponent, and it is usually characterized by near-maximal concentric activity in the involved muscles.

The **follow-through phase** begins immediately after the climax of the movement phase, in order to bring about negative acceleration of the involved limb or body segment. In this phase, often referred to as the *deceleration phase,* the velocity of the body segment progressively decreases, usually over a wide range of motion. The velocity decrease is usually attributed to high eccentric activity in the muscles that were antagonistic to the muscles used in the movement phase. Generally, the greater the acceleration in the movement phase, the greater the length and the importance of the follow-through phase. Occasionally, some athletes may begin the follow-through phase too soon, thereby cutting short the movement phase and having a less-than-desirable result in the activity.

The **recovery phase** is used after follow-through to regain balance and positioning so that the muscles can be ready for the next sport demand. To a degree, the muscles used eccentrically in the follow-through phase to decelerate the body or the body segment will be used concentrically in recovery to bring about the initial return to a functional position.

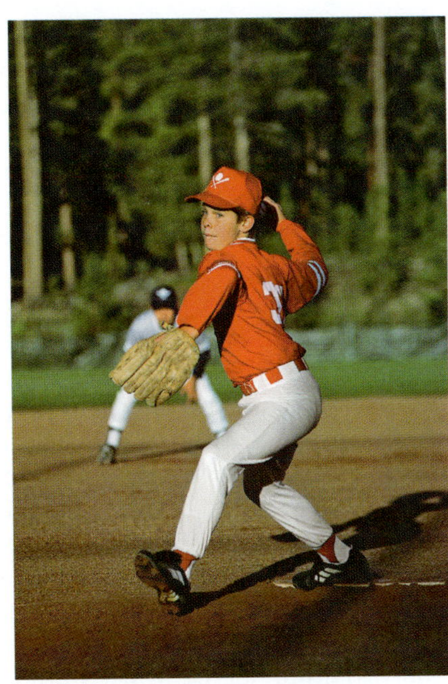

FIGURE 12.1 Pitcher throwing baseball

Skill analysis can be demonstrated with the example of a baseball pitch (figure 12.1). The stance phase begins when the player assumes a position with the ball in the glove before receiving the signal from the catcher. The pitcher begins the preparatory phase by extending the throwing arm posteriorly and rotating the trunk to the right in conjunction with left-hip flexion. The right shoulder girdle is fully retracted in combination with abduction and maximum external rotation of the glenohumeral joint to complete this phase. Immediately following, the movement phase begins with forward movement of the arm and continues until ball release. At ball release, the follow-through phase begins as the arm continues moving in the same direction established by the movement phase until the velocity decreases to the point that the arm can safely change movement direction. This deceleration of the body, and especially the arm, is accomplished by high amounts of eccentric activity. At this point, the recovery phase begins, enabling the player to reposition to field the batted ball. In this example, reference has been made briefly only to the throwing arm, but there are many similarities in other overhand sports skills, such as the tennis serve, javelin throw, and volleyball serve. In actual practice, the movements of each joint in the body should be analyzed in the various phases.

The Kinetic Chain Concept

As discussed earlier, the extremities consist of several bony segments linked by a series of joints. These bony segments and their linkage system of joints may be likened to a chain. Just as with a chain, any one link in the extremity may be moved individually without significantly affecting the other links if the chain is open or not attached at one end. However, if the chain is securely attached or closed, substantial movement of any one link cannot occur without substantial and subsequent movement of the other links. This is known as a **kinetic chain.**

In the body, an extremity may be seen as representing an **open kinetic chain** if the distal end of the extremity is not fixed to any surface. This arrangement allows any one joint in the extremity to move or function separately without necessitating movement of other joints in the extremity. Examples in the upper extremity of such single-joint exercises are a shoulder shrug, deltoid raise (shoulder abduction), or biceps curl. Lower-extremity examples include seated hip flexion, knee extension, and ankle dorsiflexion exercises. In all of these examples, the core of the body and the proximal segment are stabilized while the distal segment is free to move in space through a single plane. These types of exercises are known as *joint-isolation exercises* and are beneficial in isolating a particular joint to concentrate on specific muscle groups; however, they are not very functional in that most physical activity, particularly with the lower extremity, requires multiple-joint activity involving numerous muscle groups simultaneously. Furthermore, since the joint is stable proximally and loaded distally, shear forces are acting on the joint with potential negative consequences.

If the distal end of the extremity is fixed, as in a push-up, dip, squat, or dead lift, the extremity represents a **closed kinetic chain.** In this closed system, movement of one joint cannot occur without causing predictable movements of the other joints in the extremity. Closed-chain activities are very functional and involve the body moving in relation to the relatively fixed distal segment. The advantage of these multiple-joint exercises is that several joints are involved, and numerous muscle groups must participate in causing and controlling the multiple-plane movements, which strongly correlate to most physical activities. Additionally, the joint is more stable due to the joint compressive forces from weight bearing.

To state the differences another way, open-chain exercises involve the extremity being moved to or from the stabilized body, whereas closed-chain exercises involve the body being moved to or from the stabilized extremity. Table 12.1 provides a comparison of variables that differ with open- versus closed-chain exercises, and figure 12.2 provides examples of each.

TABLE 12.1 Differences between Open- and Closed-Chain Exercises

Variable	Open-chain exercise	Closed-chain exercise
Distal end of extremity	Free in space and not fixed	Fixed to something
Movement pattern	Characterized by rotary stress in the joint (often nonfunctional)	Characterized by linear stress in the joint (functional)
Joint movements	Occur in isolation	Multiple occur simultaneously
Muscle recruitment	Isolated (minimal muscular co-contraction)	Multiple (significant muscular co-contraction)
Joint axis	Stable during movement patterns	Primarily transverse
Movement plane	Usually single	Multiple (triplanar)
Proximal segment of joint	Stable	Mobile
Distal segment of joint	Mobile	Mobile, except for most distal aspect
Motion occurs	Distal to instantaneous axis of rotation	Proximal and distal to instantaneous axis of rotation
Functionality	Often nonfunctional, especially lower extremity	Functional
Joint forces	Shear	Compressive
Joint stability	Decreased due to shear and distractive forces	Increased due to compressive forces
Stabilization	Artificial	Not artificial, realistic and functional
Loading	Artificial	Physiological, provides for normal proprioceptive and kinesthetic feedback

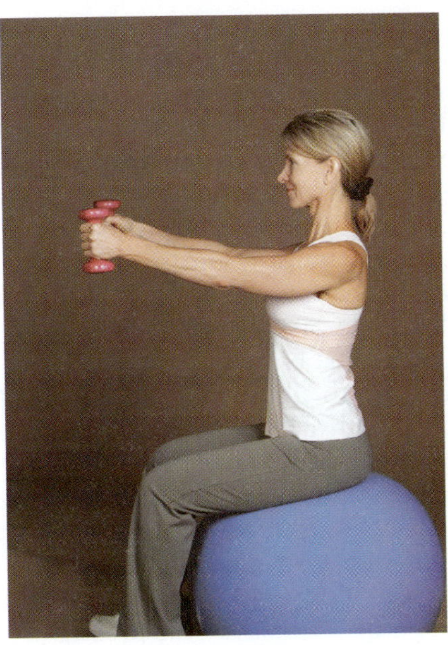

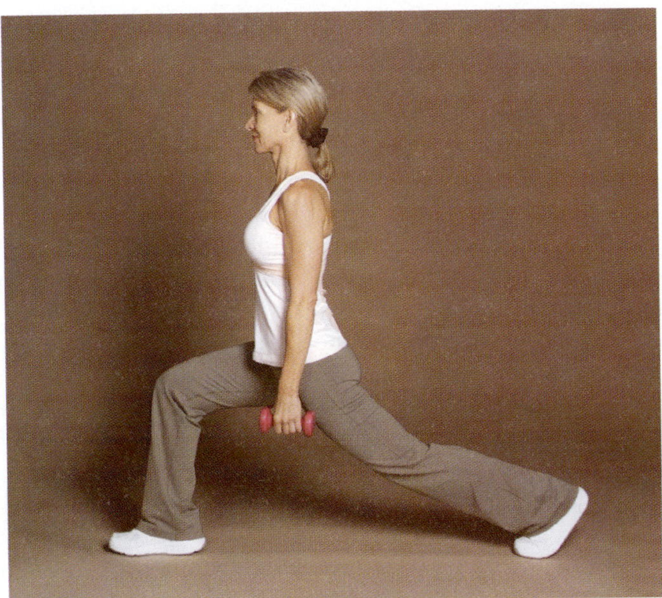

FIGURE 12.2 Open-and closed-chain exercises

Not every exercise or activity can be classified totally as either an open- or closed-chain exercise. For example, walking and running are both open and closed due to their swing and stance phases, respectively. Another case is bicycle riding, which is mixed in that the pelvis on the seat is the most stable segment but the feet are attached to movable pedals.

Consideration of the open versus closed kinetic chain is important in determining both the muscles and their types of contractions when analyzing sports activities. Realizing the relative differences in demands on the musculoskeletal system through detailed analyses of skilled movements is critical for determining the most appropriate conditioning exercises to improve performance. Generally, closed kinetic chain exercises are more functional and applicable to the demands of sports and physical activities. Most sports involve closed-chain activities in the lower extremities and open-chain activities in the upper extremities; however, there are many exceptions, and closed-chain conditioning exercises may be beneficial for extremities primarily involved in open-chain sporting activities. Open-chain exercises are useful in concentrating on the development of a specific muscle group at a single joint.

Conditioning Considerations

OVERLOAD PRINCIPLE

A basic physiologic principle of exercise is the **overload principle.** It states that, within appropriate parameters, a muscle or muscle group increases in strength in direct proportion to the overload placed on it. While it is beyond the scope of this text to fully explain specific applications of the overload principle for each component of physical fitness, some general concepts are mentioned. To improve the strength and functioning of major muscles, this principle should be applied to every large muscle group in the body, progressively throughout each year, at all age levels. In actual practice, the amount of overload applied varies significantly depending on several factors. For example, an untrained person beginning a strength-training program will usually make significant gains in the amount of weight she is able to lift in the first few weeks of the exercise program. Most of this increased ability is due to a refinement of neuromuscular function, rather than an actual increase in muscle-tissue strength. Similarly, a well-trained person will see relatively minor improvements in the amount of weight that can be lifted over a much longer period of time. Therefore, the amount and rate of progressive overload are extremely variable and must be adjusted to match the specific needs of the individual's exercise objectives.

Overload may be modified by changing any one or a combination of three exercise variables—frequency, intensity, and duration. *Frequency* is usually the number of times per week. *Intensity* is usually a certain percentage of the absolute maximum, and *duration* is usually the number of minutes per exercise bout. Ways to modify these variables and apply the overload principle include increasing the speed of doing the exercise, the number of repetitions, the weight, and the length of exercise bouts. All of these factors are important in determining the total exercise volume.

Overload is not always progressively increased. In certain periods of conditioning, the overload should actually be prescriptively reduced to improve the total results of the entire program. This intentional variance in a training program at regular intervals is known as **periodization,** and it is done to bring about optimal gains in physical performance. One reason for periodization is so that the athlete will be at her peak level during the most competitive part of the season. To achieve this, a number of variables may be manipulated, including the number of sets per exercise, number of repetitions per set, types of exercises, number of exercises per training session, rest periods between sets and exercises, resistance used for a set, type of muscle contraction, and number of training sessions per day and per week.

SAID PRINCIPLE

The **specific adaptations to imposed demands (SAID)** principle should be considered in all aspects of physiologic conditioning and training. This principle, which states that the body will gradually, over time, adapt very specifically to the various stresses and overloads to which it is subjected, is applicable in every form of muscle training, as well as to the other systems of the body. For example, if an individual were to undergo several weeks of strength-training exercises for a particular joint through a limited range of motion, the specific muscles involved in performing the strengthening exercises would improve primarily in the ability to move against increased resistance through the specific range of motion used. There would be, in most cases, minimal strength gains beyond the range of motion used in the training. Additionally, other components of physical fitness—such as flexibility, cardiorespiratory endurance, and muscular endurance—would be enhanced minimally, if at all. In other words, to achieve specific benefits, exercise programs must be specifically designed for the adaptation desired.

It should be recognized that adaptation may be positive or negative, depending on whether the correct techniques are used and stressed in the design and administration of the conditioning program. Inappropriate or excessive demands placed on the body in too short a time span can result in injury. If the demands are too minimal or administered too infrequently over too long a time period, less-than-desired improvement will occur. Conditioning programs and the exercises included in them should be analyzed to determine whether they are using the specific muscles for which they were intended in the correct manner.

SPECIFICITY

Specificity is a concentrated approach in a specific area of focus. The components of physical fitness—such as muscular strength, muscular endurance, and flexibility—are not general body characteristics. They are specific to each body area and muscle group; therefore, an individual's specific needs must be addressed when the therapist is designing an exercise program. This includes muscular flexibility and strength. Quite often, it will be necessary to analyze an individual's exercise and skill technique, as well as potential exercises, to design an appropriate program. The goals of the exercise program should be determined on the basis of specific areas of the body, preferred time to physically peak, and physical fitness needs, such as strength, muscular endurance, flexibility, cardiorespiratory endurance, and body composition. After establishing goals, a regimen incorporating the overload variables of frequency, intensity, and duration may be prescribed to include the entire body or specific areas in a manner that addresses the improvement of the preferred physical fitness components. Regular observation and follow-up exercise analysis is necessary to ensure proper adherence to correct technique.

MUSCULAR DEVELOPMENT

For years it was thought that a person developed adequate muscular strength, endurance, and flexibility through participation in sports activities. While there is a well-adapted philosophy in athletics that one needs to develop muscular strength, endurance, and flexibility in order to participate safely and effectively in sports activities, there is a deficit of knowledge among the general public regarding maintenance for daily movements. Simple activities such as getting out of a chair, lifting a child, or doing household chores all require the same muscle groups as those used in sports; however, because some individuals are not athletic, maintaining proper strength and flexibility rarely comes to mind. Unlike a training program for a serious athlete, conditioning for daily living is simple and does not require membership in a fitness club.

Adequate muscular strength, endurance, and flexibility of the entire body should be developed through the correct use of the appropriate exercise principles. The individuals responsible for this development need to prescribe specific exercises that will meet these objectives.

In schools, this development should start at an early age and continue throughout the formative years. Sit-ups, the standing long jump, the mile run, and other tests all indicate fitness deficiencies among children in the United States. Adequate muscular strength and endurance are important in the adult years for daily living, as well as for job-related requirements and recreational activities. Ergonomic backpacks should be mandatory, as heavy and overloaded packs cause postural changes in young children. Many back problems and other physical ailments can be avoided completely through proper maintenance of the musculoskeletal system.

THE IMPORTANCE OF BREATHING

Many people do not know how to breathe properly when they perform simple resistance exercises. Breathing is often shallow and/or limited, and some people even hold air in the lungs. It is not uncommon to see recent stroke patients holding their breath during exercise. Indeed, many people in the Western world in particular often have breathing deficits, even during regular breathing at rest. Proper **breathing,** however, has many benefits, and it is important for exercise and health. The "art" of proper breathing has a long history; the ancients believed that breathing powered the energy that is the "life force," and in many cultures this philosophy is paramount to living a healthy life. Yoga enthusiasts understand the great importance of breathing techniques; every yoga posture has a specific breathing pattern. In martial arts, proper breathing is vital for delivering effective techniques and for preventing injury.

Every clinician should reinforce the importance of proper breathing during exercise. Stroke patients, especially, must be monitored during treatment, as holding the breath is extremely dangerous during stroke recovery. During exertion, all air should be exhaled. Inhalation occurs during the rest or preparatory phase. While there are many breathing techniques, air should be expelled by contracting the stomach muscles, in effect sucking the navel in. The individual should visualize the air moving from the navel in toward the spine and then up and out through the open mouth. Ideally, inhalation should pass through the nasal passages, and the air should be visualized as moving in and up through the diaphragm.

A common bad habit for many athletes or weight lifters is bearing down by holding the breath when attempting to lift something heavy. This bearing down, known as the *Valsalva maneuver,* is accomplished by trying to exhale against a closed epiglottis (the flap of cartilage behind the tongue that shuts the air passage when swallowing) and is thought by many to enhance one's lifting ability. The maneuver is mentioned here to caution against its use due to the dramatic increase in blood pressure followed by the equally dramatic drop in blood pressure it causes. Using the Valsalva maneuver can cause lightheadedness and fainting and can lead to complications in people with heart disease. Instead of using the Valsalva maneuver, one should use rhythmic and consistent breathing.

Analysis of Clinical Flexibility and Therapeutic Exercise of the Upper Extremity

As discussed in Chapter 4, Clinical Flexibility and Therapeutic Exercise movements can be used in a clinical setting for increasing the range of motion in specific muscles. Presented over the next several pages are some of these movements. Following the stretches, strengthening is shown for the muscle group that was stretched (antagonists) so that students can understand functional anatomy better. Please see the tables after each resistance exercise to better understand agonist, joint, and muscle action. The client should exhale deeply on the work phase and inhale on the relaxation phase for all of these movements. Generally, 10 repetitions and 2 to 3 sets are performed for these exercises. Please review the components of *Active Isolated Stretching* in Chapter 4 before proceeding.

FLEXIBILITY ANALYSIS: HORIZONTAL FLEXION (ADDUCTION)

Stretching the Rhomboid Major, Rhomboid Minor, and External Rotators

This exercise lengthens the antigravity muscles of the upper shoulder, muscles that often hold tension. These muscles have an enormous responsibility in that they must keep the scapula retracted (shoulders back) against gravity. This stretch helps provide oxygen to this area, as it lengthens muscle fibers gently. Although the movement can be done sitting or standing, sitting on a balance ball is recommended because it helps encourage core posture muscles to contract. Beginning with arms at the sides (figure 12.3), lift one arm, elbow extended, across the midline (horizontal adduction) to the opposite shoulder contracting the agonist muscles listed below. Using the other hand, apply a gentle 2-second stretch just above the elbow. Return to the starting position each time, and perform 8 to 10 repetitions (figure 12.4). Be sure that the elbow remains extended. The shoulder should remain relaxed with no contraction of the upper trapezius (shoulder shrug), and the torso should not rotate as the arm is brought into horizontal adduction. *Contraindications:* Arthroplasty clients should avoid this movement. (*Muscles contracted:* pectoralis major, anterior deltoid, and coracobrachialis.)

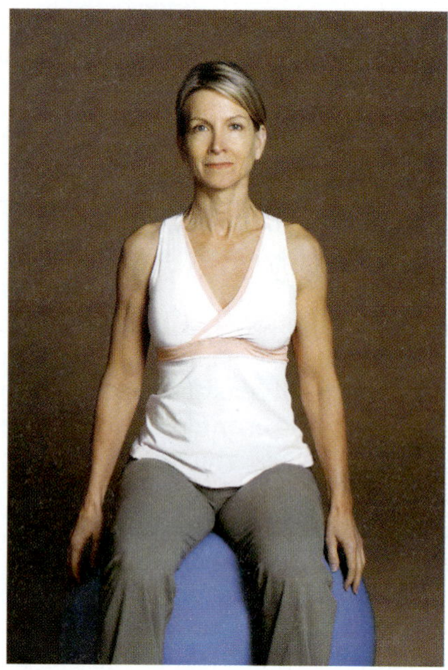

FIGURE 12.3 Horizontal adduction start

STRENGTHENING ANALYSIS: SCAPULAR ADDUCTION

Strengthening the Rhomboid Major, Rhomboid Minor, Trapezius, and Middle and Posterior Deltoid

This is an important exercise to help strengthen the antigravity muscles of the scapular region, as it isolates the rhomboid major and makes it work against gravity. Like many of the smaller muscles in the body, the rhomboid major is often overlooked in strength routines because it is not isolated enough for strengthening. Performing this exercise will help kyphotic postures and chronic cervical stiffness and pain and will improve overall movement of scapular adduction. It should be included in any weight-training program, especially if the pectoralis major is worked in multiple sets. Anyone involved in bodywork that entails pushing and pulling would do well to perform this exercise a few times each week. This exercise is best performed on a therapy table or bench, but a balance ball also can be used. In a prone position, drop the head to relax the upper trapezius, and maintain the elbow at a 95- to 100-degree angle (figure 12.5). The wrists should be flexed while clasping the dumbbells. Beginning in the lower position, start the movement at the scapulae, squeezing them together while bringing the elbows toward the ceiling (figure 12.6). Gently hold for 2 to 3 seconds, and then slowly lower the dumbbells back to the start position. The elbows and wrists should remain in their rounded position throughout the exercise, and the head should stay

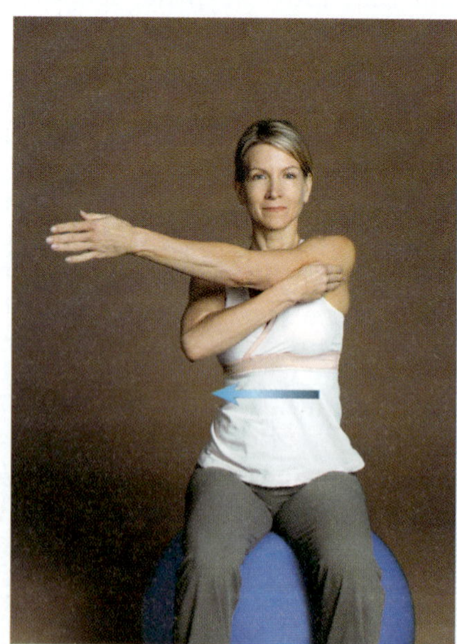

FIGURE 12.4 Horizontal adduction finish

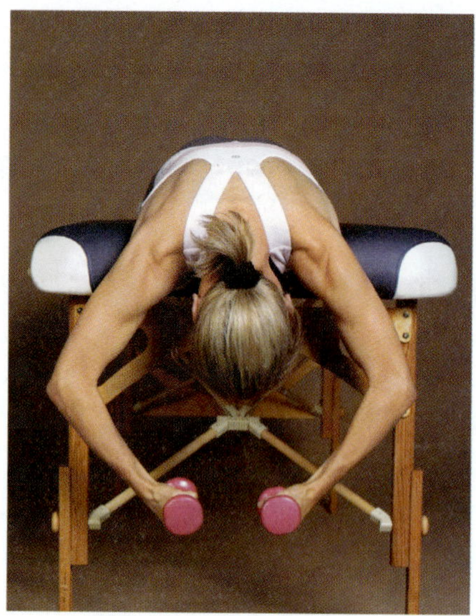

FIGURE 12.5 Scapular adduction start

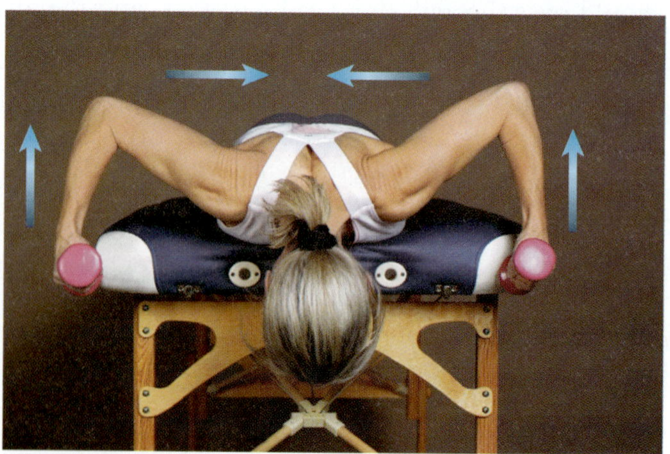

FIGURE 12.6 Scapular adduction finish

TABLE 12.2 Scapular (Shoulder Girdle) Adduction—Agonist, Joint, and Muscle Action

	Lifting Phase		Lowering Phase	
Joint	**Action**	**Agonists**	**Action**	**Agonists**
Wrist and hand*	Remain in flexion (isometric)	Wrist and hand flexors, flexor carpi radialis, flexor carpi ulnaris, palmaris longus, flexor digitorum profundus, flexor digitorum superficialis, flexor pollicis longus	Remain in flexion (isometric)	Flexor carpi radialis, flexor carpi ulnaris, palmaris longus, flexor digitorum profundus, flexor digitorum superficialis, flexor pollicis longus
Elbow*	Remains in flexion (isometric)	Biceps brachii, brachialis, brachioradialis	Remains in flexion (isometric)	Biceps brachii, brachialis, brachioradialis
Shoulder	Horizontal abduction, extension (humeral)	Rhomboid major, posterior deltoid, latissimus, teres major	Abduction, slight flexion	Pectoralis major, pectoralis minor, anterior deltoid
Shoulder girdle	Adduction	Rhomboid major, trapezius	Abduction	Serratus anterior, pectoralis minor

* The wrist, hand, and elbow muscles remain in an isometric contraction throughout the movement.

down to prevent the upper trapezius from engaging. (See table 12.2.) Perform 3 sets of 10 repetitions. *Contraindications:* This exercise is safe with controlled movements.

FLEXIBILITY ANALYSIS: HYPEREXTENSION

Stretching the Biceps Brachii, Anterior Deltoid, Anterior Serratus, and Lower Pectoralis Major

This movement stretches the anterior capsule of the shoulder, especially the biceps brachii. It is a necessary stretch to help adhesive capsulitis and bicipital tendonitis. The proximal portion of the long head of the biceps is frequently weak and undertrained, and this area lacks proper blood flow; poor habits such as sleeping on an inflamed shoulder only exacerbate the condition. Specific, active stretching of this area with a full range of shoulder joint movement is a powerful way to help improve shoulder function. Begin with the arms at the side, and contract the posterior shoulder muscles to reach into hyperextension (figure 12.7). Lean forward and stretch gently for 2 seconds at the end movement (figure 12.8). By returning to the start position for each repetition, full range of motion in the shoulder joint provides blood and oxygen into the anterior capsule. *Contraindications:* Use caution for anterior-capsule conditions. (*Muscles contracted:* triceps brachii and posterior deltoid.)

STRENGTHENING ANALYSIS: THUMBS-UP FLEXION

Strengthening the Anterior Deltoid and the Clavicular Head of the Pectoralis Major

This exercise helps strengthen the anterior capsule of the shoulder. It should be performed with any upper-extremity routine, as it targets the underworked and

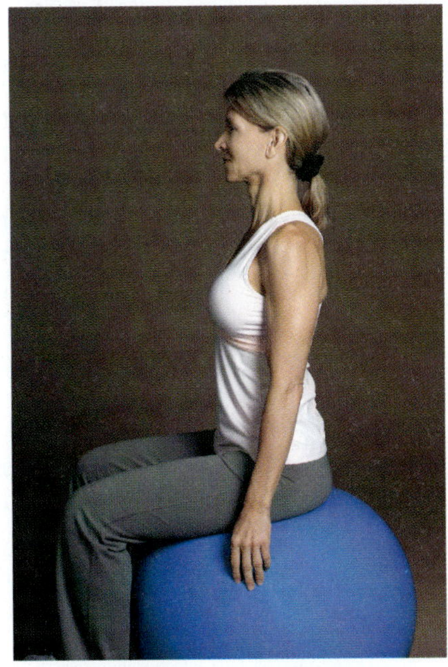

FIGURE 12.7 Shoulder hyperextension start

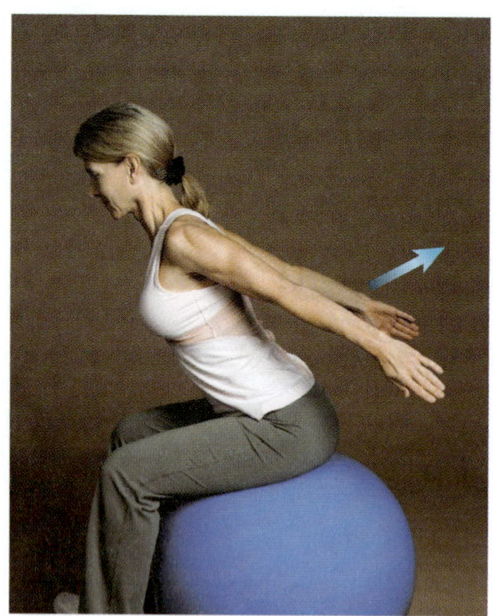

FIGURE 12.8 Shoulder hyperextension finish

often-weak smaller muscles. It also can help keep the long head of the biceps stabilized in the bicipital groove. Begin with the arms at the sides holding dumbbells (figure 12.9). Lift the arms, thumbs up, into flexion to shoulder level; pause and slowly return to the start position (figure 12.10). As in any resistance exercises, the returning movement is most important, as it challenges the muscles eccentrically.

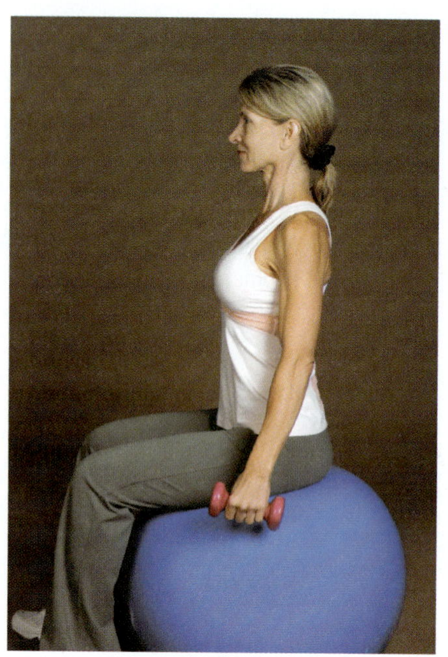

FIGURE 12.9 Arms at side

This return phase should always be slow and controlled; counting slowly while lowering the weight will help decelerate the movement. (See table 12.3.) *Contraindications:* This exercise is safe with controlled movement.

TABLE 12.3 Thumbs-Up Flexion—Agonist, Joint, and Muscle Action

	Lifting Phase		Lowering Phase	
Joint	**Action**	**Agonists**	**Action**	**Agonists**
Wrist and hand*	*Hand:* flexion (isometric contraction of fingers) *Wrist:* neutral	Wrist and hand flexors, flexor carpi radialis, flexor carpi ulnaris, palmaris longus, flexor digitorum profundus, flexor digitorum superficialis, flexor pollicis longus	*Hand:* flexion (isometric contraction of fingers) *Wrist:* neutral	Flexor carpi radialis, flexor carpi ulnaris, palmaris longus, flexor digitorum profundus, flexor digitorum superficialis, flexor pollicis longus
Elbow*	Extension (isometric)	Triceps brachii	Extension (isometric)	Triceps brachii
Shoulder	Flexion (concentric)	Anterior deltoid, clavicular head of pectoralis major	Extension (concentric; eccentric anterior shoulder muscles)	Triceps brachii, posterior deltoid, teres major, latissimus dorsi
Shoulder girdle	Protraction, upward rotation	Serratus anterior, pectoralis minor	Adduction, downward rotation	Rhomboids, upper and middle trapezius

* The wrist, hand, and elbow muscles remain in a neutral position throughout the movement.

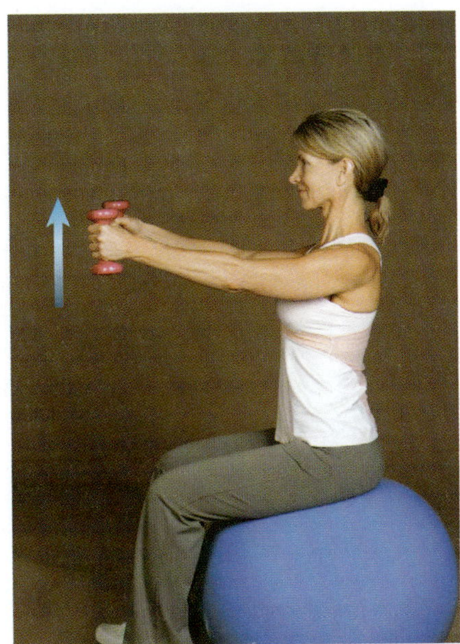

FIGURE 12.10 Arms lifted—flexion of shoulder

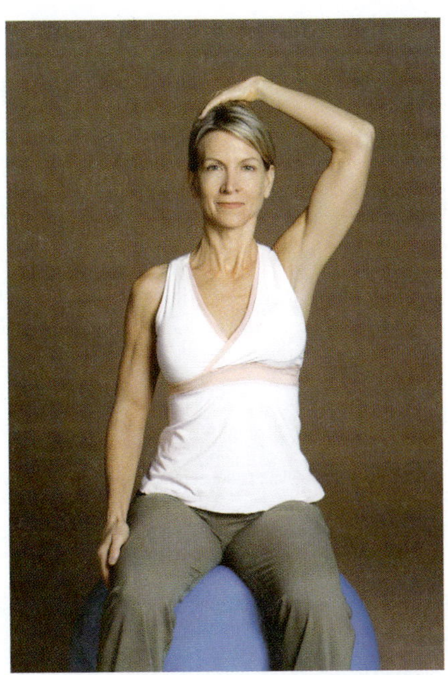

FIGURE 12.11 Lateral cervical flexion start

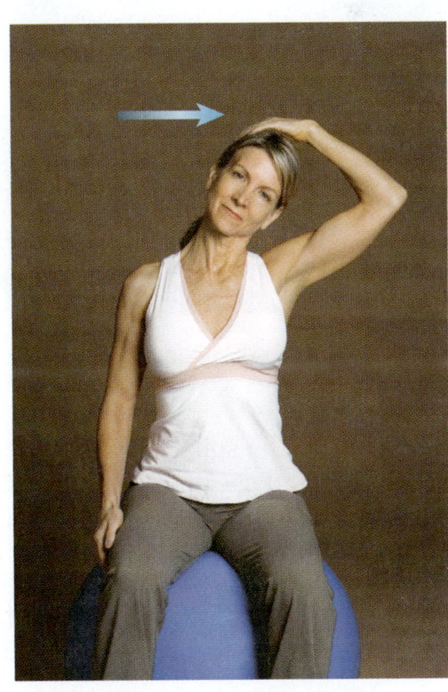

FIGURE 12.12 Lateral cervical flexion finish

FLEXIBILITY ANALYSIS: LATERAL CERVICAL FLEXION

Stretching the Upper Trapezius, Levator Scapulae, Semispinalis Capitis, Longissimus Capitis, Erector Spinae, and Middle and Posterior Scalenes

Stretching the neck specifically has many advantages, especially for those with chronic cervical conditions. Loss of natural range of motion in the neck is common with injuries. Arthritis and poor postures cause muscle tightness because of pain and lack of movement. When pain is present, cervical movement can become unbearable. Something as simple as backing out of the driveway becomes a compensatory movement; the torso must rotate because the cervical rotation is absent or impossible. Yet flexibility in the shoulder and cervical area can be improved regardless of age or disk condition. Begin in a neutral position with the chin in toward the spine, eyes straight ahead, and abdominals contracted. Raise one hand above the head to assist in the stretch movement (figure 12.11). Contract the opposite-side cervical muscles to bring the ear to the opposite shoulder (figure 12.12). Using the hand, apply a gentle stretch for 2 seconds. Bring the head back to the start position, and repeat. *Contraindications:* Cervical conditions such as herniation and arthritis should not prevent one from performing this movement, but the range of motion should be adjusted for comfort. It is important that an individual with chronic conditions be supervised carefully when performing this stretch.

STRENGTHENING ANALYSIS: LATERAL CERVICAL FLEXION

Strengthening the Anterior, Middle, and Posterior Scalenes, Sternocleidomastoid, Erector Spinae, and Paraspinal Muscles

Another common failure in the structure of the neck is its gradual weakness against gravity. Dysfunction can develop if the muscles that support the head against daily forces cannot work the way they were designed to. The antigravity muscles of the upper back and the

TABLE 12.4 Lateral Cervical Flexion—Agonist, Joint, and Muscle Action

	Lifting Phase		Lowering Phase	
	Action	Agonists	Action	Agonists
Head movement	Lateral flexion	Anterior, middle, and posterior scalenes, sternocleidomastoid, erector spinae, and paraspinals (concentric)	Lateral flexion* (opposite side)	Anterior, middle, and posterior scalenes, sternocleidomastoid, erector spinae, and paraspinals (concentric)

*In the return phase, the lateral flexors are contracting *eccentrically* while the agonists contract *concentrically*.

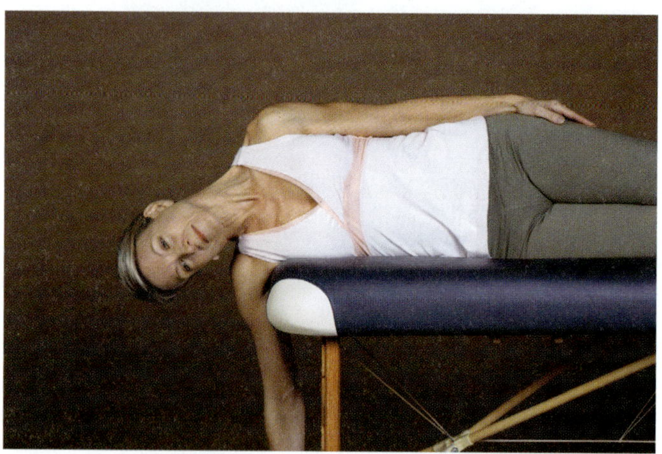

FIGURE 12.13 Lateral cervical flexion start

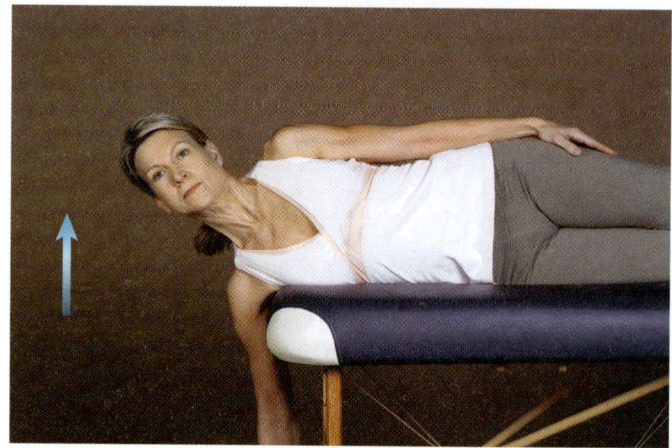

FIGURE 12.14 Lateral cervical flexion finish

paraspinal muscles of the spine must be strengthened to help support head and neck movement. This exercise is an excellent way to strengthen the cervical muscles using only the weight of the head and gravity. Begin by lying on the side, either on a table or bed, with the arm and head off the edge (figure 12.13). Secure the arm by grasping the bed or table; this helps stabilize the spine. Focus vision on an object directly in front at eye level. Begin the movement by contracting the opposite cervical muscle and flexing the head up to the opposite side (figure 12.14). The returning movement is slow and controlled. (See table 12.4.) *Contraindications:* Individuals who have cervical conditions can perform this movement without hanging the head off the edge.

CHAPTER *summary*

Introduction

- ✔ The upper extremity is capable of a wide range of dynamic movements. Natural, pain-free movement is critical for sports activities as well as activities of daily living. Flexibility and strength in the upper extremity are essential for improved appearance and posture, as well as for more efficient skill performance.

Upper-Extremity Activities

- ✔ Children seem to have an innate desire to climb, swing, and hang. Such movements use the muscles of the hands, wrists, elbows, and shoulder joints. Unless educators emphasize development of the upper extremity, for both boys and girls, it will continue to be muscularly the weakest area of our bodies. Also, continued maintenance of this area in adults must be reinforced in the health care field. Individuals often reach a point in their lives when suddenly it hurts to do the things they love doing. This is a reduction of quality of life.

Concepts for Analysis

- ✔ In analyzing activities, it is important to understand that muscles are usually grouped according to their concentric function and work in paired opposition to an antagonistic group.
- ✔ An example of an aggregate muscle group performing a given joint action is seen when all the elbow flexors work together.

Analysis of Movement

- ✔ In analyzing various exercises and sports skills, it is essential to break down all the movements into phases.
- ✔ The number of phases, usually three to five, varies depending on the skill.
- ✔ Practically all sports skills have at least a preparatory phase, a movement phase, and a follow-through phase.
- ✔ Many also begin with a stance phase and end with a recovery phase.
- ✔ The names of the phases vary from skill to skill to fit in with the terminology used in various sports, and they may also vary depending on the body part involved.
- ✔ In some cases, these major phases may be divided further, as with baseball, where the preparatory phase for the pitching arm is divided into early cocking and late cocking.

The Kinetic Chain Concept

- ✔ The extremities consist of several bony segments linked by a series of joints.
- ✔ The bony segments and their linkage system of joints may be likened to a chain.
- ✔ Just as with a chain, any one link in the extremity may be moved individually without significantly affecting the other links if the chain is open or not attached at one end.
- ✔ If the chain is securely attached or closed, substantial movement of any one link cannot occur without substantial and subsequent movement of the other links.

Conditioning Considerations: Overload Principle

- ✔ A basic physiologic principle of exercise is the overload principle.
- ✔ The overload principle states that, within appropriate parameters, a muscle or muscle group increases in strength in direct proportion to the overload placed on it.
- ✔ To improve the strength and functioning of major muscles, this principle should be applied to every large muscle group in the body, progressively throughout each year, at all age levels.
- ✔ The amount of overload applied varies significantly depending on several factors.

Conditioning Considerations: SAID Principle

- ✔ The specific adaptations to imposed demands (SAID) principle should be considered in all aspects of physiologic conditioning and training.
- ✔ It states that the body will gradually, over time, adapt very specifically to the various stresses and overloads to which it is subjected; it is applicable in every form of muscle training, as well as to the other systems of the body.

Conditioning Considerations: Specificity

- ✔ Specificity of exercise strongly relates to the SAID principle.
- ✔ The components of physical fitness—such as muscular strength, muscular endurance, and flexibility—are not general body characteristics.
- ✔ They are specific to each body area and muscle group.
- ✔ The specific needs of the individual must be addressed when designing an exercise program.

Conditioning Considerations: The Importance of Breathing

- ✔ Every clinician should reinforce the importance of proper breathing during exercise.
- ✔ Stroke patients, in particular, must be monitored during treatment, as holding the breath is extremely dangerous during recovery following a stroke.
- ✔ During exertion, all air should be exhaled from the lungs.
- ✔ Inhalation occurs during the rest or preparatory phase.

Analysis of Clinical Flexibility and Therapeutic Exercise of the Upper Extremity

- ✔ Clinical Flexibility and Therapeutic Exercise consists of exercises that can be used in a clinical setting for increasing the range of motion and strengthening the muscles of the upper extremity.

True or False

Write true *or* false *after each statement.*

1. Strengthening of the rhomboids and upper trapezius will not help neck dysfunction.
2. Eccentric contractions are extremely important in resistance training because they challenge the muscle fibers.
3. Ballistic stretching is a bouncing movement that is safe for herniated-disk patients.
4. A good example of a closed-chain exercise is one in which the distal end is fixed, such as a lunge.
5. Working the belly of the biceps femoris will help keep the long head of the biceps in the bicipital groove.
6. In the horizontal flexion Active Isolated Stretch, the antagonists are the rhomboids and trapezius.
7. When performing a seated weight curl, a person can improve the results by holding his breath during the exercise.
8. Active Isolated Stretching is beneficial for stroke patients because it supports muscle reeducation.
9. Posture in the upper extremity is not affected by limited flexibility and muscle weakness.
10. Specificity of exercise strongly relates to the SAID principle.
11. Active Isolated Stretching uses only antagonist muscles.

Short Answers

Write your answers on the lines provided.

1. In what plane do most golf swings take place?

____

____

____

2. A patient presents with bicipital tendonitis. What strength exercise would help?

____

____

____

3. Name three muscles that are stretched in horizontal flexion.

____

____

____

4. What muscles produce cervical lateral flexion?

____

____

____

5. What breathing recommendations should a therapist give to a stroke patient?

____

____

____

6. What muscles produce horizontal flexion?

____

____

____

7. Explain why the cervical and posterior upper-extremity muscles often develop issues.

____

____

____

8. How should a therapist strengthen the lateral neck flexors?

____

____

____

9. Briefly explain the concept of the kinetic chain.

____

____

____

Multiple Choice

Circle the correct answers.

1. What is the proper form of breathing during exercise?
   a. inhale on the work phase
   b. hold the breath throughout
   c. blow out repeatedly in succession
   d. exhale on the work phase
2. Which of the following is an agonist during the horizontal flexion stretch?
   a. rhomboids
   b. triceps
   c. pectoralis major
   d. serratus anterior
3. Dropping the head during scapular adduction exercises allows for:
   a. contraction of the upper trapezius
   b. specific isolation of the rhomboids
   c. a safer technique
   d. relaxation of the rhomboids
4. Strengthening the rhomboids can help improve which of the following?
   a. thoracic posture
   b. bursitis
   c. bicipital tendonitis
   d. epicondylitis
5. Anterior shoulder raises (shoulder flexion) with resistance help stabilize what area?
   a. shoulder girdle
   b. antigravity muscles
   c. long head of the biceps
   d. brachialis
6. Specificity pertains to what component of prescribed exercise?
   a. individual exercises for specific conditions
   b. general exercises
   c. arm curls on the affected side
   d. correct exercise posture
7. The SAID principle is important in exercise prescription because:
   a. programs should be specific and challenging for optimal results
   b. it is required by all licensed therapists
   c. it prevents muscle atrophy
   d. it prevents muscle tears
8. An example of closed-chain exercise is:
   a. a knee extension machine
   b. biceps curl
   c. dips
   d. shoulder shrugs
9. The overload principle states that:
   a. muscles get stronger only if trained twice each week
   b. muscles increase in strength in direct proportion to the overload placed on them
   c. after age 50, muscles cannot be overloaded as much
   d. muscles increase in strength in an amount equal to how fast repetitions are performed
10. Analyzing human movement has what great benefit in kinesiology?
    a. It has no benefit unless it is done in a clinic.
    b. It helps improve endurance.
    c. Forces against gravity can be calculated.
    d. It allows for greater understanding of dysfunctions for proper exercise prescription.

EXPLORE & practice

1. Analyze other conditioning exercises that might help strengthen the rhomboids and upper trapezius. List how you would perform the exercises.
2. Observe and analyze a rowing exercise at a gym. What muscles are the agonists and antagonists?
3. Describe an open-chain resistance exercise for the biceps brachii.
4. Describe a closed-chain resistance exercise for the latissimus dorsi.
5. What is the importance of understanding the myotatic reflex arc in stretching?

6. Compare the different types of stretching on a partner, and make a journal record of your findings. Which type do you feel would be the safest for someone with a herniated cervical disk?

7. Stand slightly farther than arm's length from a wall with your hands facing forward at shoulder-level height. Push your hand straight in front of your shoulder until the elbow is extended fully by performing each of the following movements before proceeding to the next:
   - Glenohumeral flexion to 90 degrees
   - Full elbow extension
   - Wrist extension to 70 degrees

   Analyze the movements and the muscles responsible for each movement at the shoulder girdle, glenohumeral joint, elbow, and wrist. Include the type of contraction for each muscle for each movement.

8. Now face a wall and stand about 6 inches from it. Place both hands on the wall at shoulder level, and put your nose and chest against the wall. Keeping your palms in place on the wall, slowly push your body from the wall as in a push-up until your chest is as far away from the wall as possible without removing your palms from the wall surface. Analyze the movements and the muscles responsible for each movement at the shoulder girdle, glenohumeral joint, elbow, and wrist. Include the type of contraction for each muscle for each movement.

9. Go to a public place and observe people passing by. Looking at their upper-body postures, design a series of exercises that will help correct the postures.

10. How would you strengthen the pectoralis major so that an imbalance with other muscle groups does not occur?

part 3

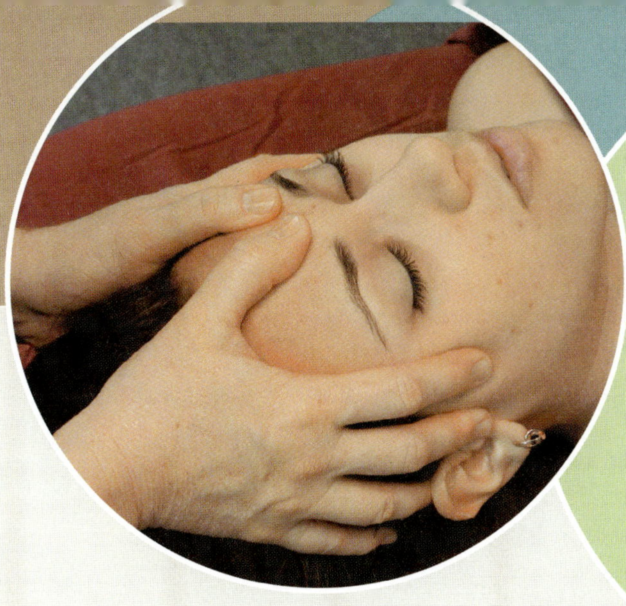

TRUNK

chapter 13

The Trunk and Spinal Column

LEARNING OUTCOMES

After completing this chapter, you should be able to:

13-1 Define key terms.

13-2 Identify the different types of vertebrae in the spinal column.

13-3 Label on a skeletal chart the types of vertebrae and their important features.

13-4 Draw and label on a skeletal chart the muscles of the trunk and spinal column outlined in this chapter.

13-5 Demonstrate all the active and passive movements of the head, neck, and trunk with a partner.

13-6 Palpate on a partner the muscles of the trunk and spinal column emphasized in this chapter.

13-7 Explore the origins and insertions of the muscles emphasized in this chapter.

13-8 Organize and list the muscles that produce the primary movements of the head, neck, and trunk.

13-9 Practice flexibility and strengthening exercises for each muscle group.

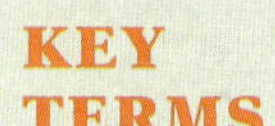

- Atlantoaxial joint
- Atlanto occipital joint
- Atlas
- Axis
- Cervical vertebrae
- Erector spinae
- External oblique
- Internal oblique
- Interspinales
- Intertransversarii
- Intervertebral disks
- Kyphosis
- Linea alba
- Lordosis
- Lumbar vertebrae
- Manubrium
- Quadratus lumborum
- Rectus abdominis
- Scoliosis
- Splenius capitis
- Splenius cervicis
- Sternocleidomastoid (SCM)
- Suboccipitals
- Tendinous inscriptions
- Thoracic vertebrae
- Transversus abdominis
- Xiphoid process

Introduction

The trunk houses the spinal column, supports the head and neck, provides a home for the internal organs, and acts as attachments for the upper and lower extremities. The trunk is the body's core that enables—or at least should enable—balanced movement in physical activity. If the body's weight is not evenly distributed during activity, the trunk muscles that attach to the spine can be jeopardized and the upper and lower extremities can be exposed to injury. Lifting injuries are prevalent in work-related activities. The human body is not designed for the trunk muscles to perform dynamic lifts while the lower extremities provide static stability. Instead, the trunk muscles provide static stability to the area while the larger lower-extremity muscles perform the majority of the work in lifting. Healthy movement occurs when the upper and lower extremities are in perfect balance. Poor body mechanics, faulty ergonomics, or lifting too much weight often results in strains, herniated disks, vertebral subluxations, and/or multiple hypertonicities.

The anterior portion of the trunk is, put simply, the front of the back, but the body is not flat; it has depth and dimension forming more of an oval shape. The abdominal muscles must be in harmony with the back muscles to support and oppose the extensor muscles. Ideally, the abdominal muscles should be strong and well toned. It is not necessary for everyone to have "six-pack" abs; however, weak abdominals allow adipose tissue to protrude, which in turn adds more weight for the back muscles to support. This extra anterior force pulls directly on fibers of lumbar fascia and the back muscles. Healthy abdominal muscles support a balanced lumbar curve and a positive anterior-posterior pelvic position. The sides of the abdomen are also the sides of the back. Abdominal muscles wrap around the crest and support the foundation of the lumbar muscles.

Like a patchwork quilt, the abdominal muscles cover the internal organs from the ribs to the pubis, inguinal ligament, and crest. These muscles are different from others in that some sections are linked by fasciae and tendinous bands, instead of attaching bone to bone. They provide compression on the organs to keep them contained in the abdominal cavity and assist women during childbirth. The abdominal muscles actively function in respiration, and the transversus abdominis has fibers that directly attach to the diaphragm. The rectus abdominis has superior fibers that attach to the inferior fibers of the pectoralis major. The external oblique interdigitates with the serratus anterior and latissimus dorsi. These attachments support the chest and back muscles and provide a connection for stretching.

All the posterior spinal column muscles bilaterally from the sacrum to the back of the head are designed to counteract trunk flexion. Extension is a constant action to prevent the body from falling into flexion. Whether standing or sitting, if the extensor muscles are not working, the head will fall forward and the trunk will collapse to the ground. The cervical spine supports the head, which weighs 10 to 12 pounds. Head posture affects the contraction or strain on the extensors and flexors. The posterior cervical muscles control the cervical curve, oppose flexion, and support lateral flexion and rotation in combination with the anterior cervical muscles.

This chapter reviews the bones and joints of the spinal column and thorax. It covers the primary agonists and nerves of the trunk and some of the primary muscles of the head and neck. The reader is urged to review the trapezius and levator scapulae in Chapter 4, as they are part of the head and neck functional area. Intrinsic muscles of the head, neck, and spinal column are covered, but not in the same depth as the primary muscles. Some of these muscles are highlighted, however, because they are important to the development of or treatment for specific conditions, such as the suboccipitals for headaches and the scalenes for potential entrapment of the brachial plexus.

Bones

VERTEBRAL COLUMN

The intricate and complex bony structure of the vertebral column consists of 24 articulating vertebrae not including the 9 that are fused together to make up the sacrum and coccyx (figure 13.1). The column is further divided into the 7 **cervical** (neck) **vertebrae,** 12 **thoracic** (chest) **vertebrae,** and 5 **lumbar** (lower-back) **vertebrae.** The sacrum (posterior pelvic girdle) consists of five fused vertebrae, and the coccyx (tailbone) consists of four fused vertebrae. The first two cervical vertebrae are unique because their shapes allow for extensive rotary head movements from side to side, as well as forward and backward. The spine has three normal curves within its movable vertebrae. The thoracic spine curve is concave anteriorly and convex posteriorly, whereas the cervical and lumbar curves are concave posteriorly and convex anteriorly. The normal curves of the spine enable it to absorb blows and shocks from the body's regular movement patterns.

The bones in each region of the spine have slightly different sizes and shapes to allow for various functions (figure 13.2). The vertebrae increase in size from the cervical region to the lumbar region, primarily because they have to support more weight in the lower back than in the neck. The first two cervical vertebrae are known as the **atlas** and **axis,** respectively. The vertebrae C2 through L5 have similar architecture: Each has a bony block anteriorly, known as the *body;* a vertebral foramen centrally for the spinal cord to pass through; a transverse process projecting out laterally to each side; and a spinous process projecting posteriorly that is easily palpable.

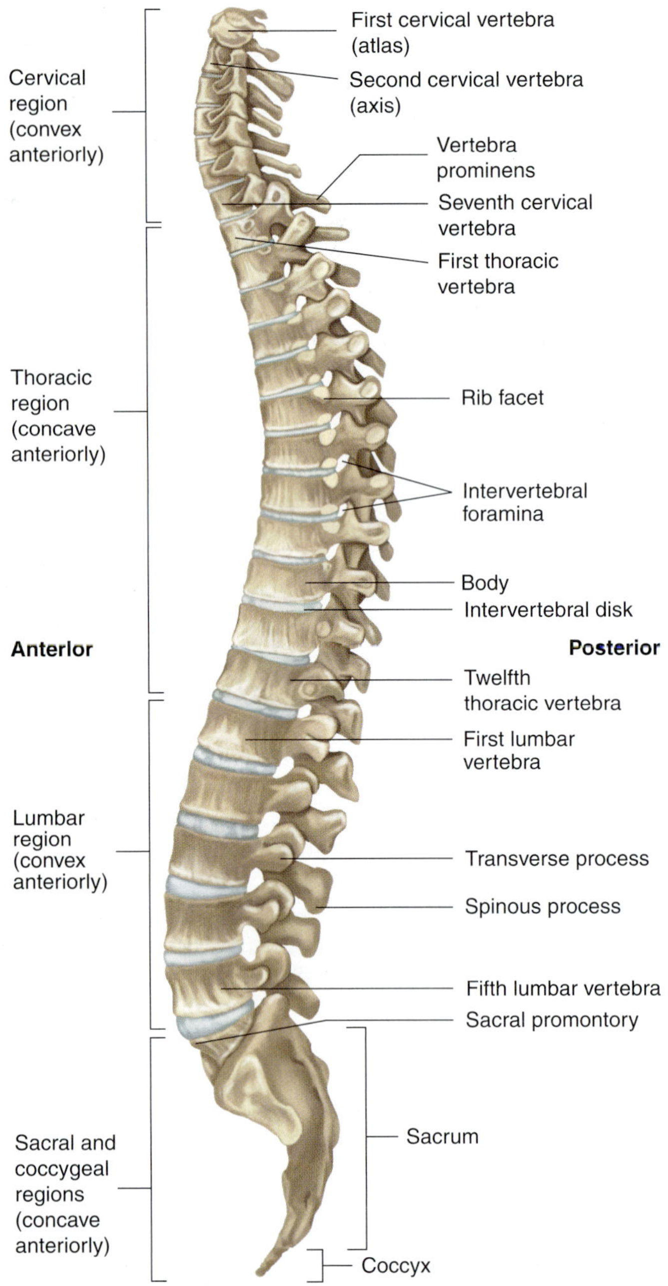

FIGURE 13.1 Bones of the vertebral column

CLINICAL NOTES

Curvatures of the Spine

Undesirable deviations from the normal curvatures occur for a number of reasons. Increased posterior concavity of the lumbar and cervical curves is known as **lordosis,** while increased anterior concavity of the normal thoracic curve is known as **kyphosis.** The lumbar spine may have a reduction of its normal lordotic curve, resulting in a flat-back appearance, referred to as *lumbar kyphosis.* **Scoliosis** refers to lateral curvatures, or sideward deviations of the spine. Most common are the S curve and the C curve. Curvatures of the spine can be genetic (structural or fixed), but they also can be caused by contracted muscles that pull on the spine unilaterally (functional). Postural distortions, especially kyphosis, are enhanced by rounded shoulders and a head-forward posture. Pregnancy weight, especially with the predominance of the baby in the last trimester, plays havoc with lordosis in the lower back. The body tends to adapt to permanent genetic curves, but soft-tissue problems and pain often develop from short- or long-term postural conditions. Scoliosis can be helped by proper specific stretching of the contracted side, as well as strengthening of the weaker side. Massage is also helpful in relieving pain associated with scoliosis.

THORAX

The skeletal foundation of the thorax is formed by 12 pairs of ribs (figure 13.3). Seven pairs are true ribs, attaching directly to the sternum. Five pairs are considered false ribs. Of these, three pairs attach indirectly to the sternum and two pairs are floating ribs with free ends. The **manubrium,** the body of the sternum, and the **xiphoid process** are the other bones of the thorax. All the ribs are attached posteriorly to the thoracic vertebrae.

Key bony landmarks for locating the muscles of the neck include the mastoid process, transverse and spinous processes of the cervical spine, spinous processes of the upper four thoracic vertebrae, manubrium of the sternum, and medial clavicle. The spinous and transverse processes of the thoracic spine and the posterior ribs are key areas of attachment for the posterior muscles of the spine. The anterior trunk muscles have attachments on the borders of the lower eight ribs, the costal cartilages of the ribs, the iliac crest, and the pubic crest. The transverse processes of the upper four lumbar vertebrae also serve as points of insertion for the quadratus lumborum, along with the lower border of the 12th rib.

Joints

The first joint in the axial skeleton is the **atlanto-occipital joint.** It is formed by the occipital condyles of the skull sitting on the articular fossa of the 1st vertebra and allows flexion and extension of the head on the neck. The atlas (C1), in turn, sits on the axis (C2) to form the **atlantoaxial joint** (figure 13.4). Except for the atlantoaxial joint, there is not a great deal of movement possible between any two vertebrae. However, the cumulative effect

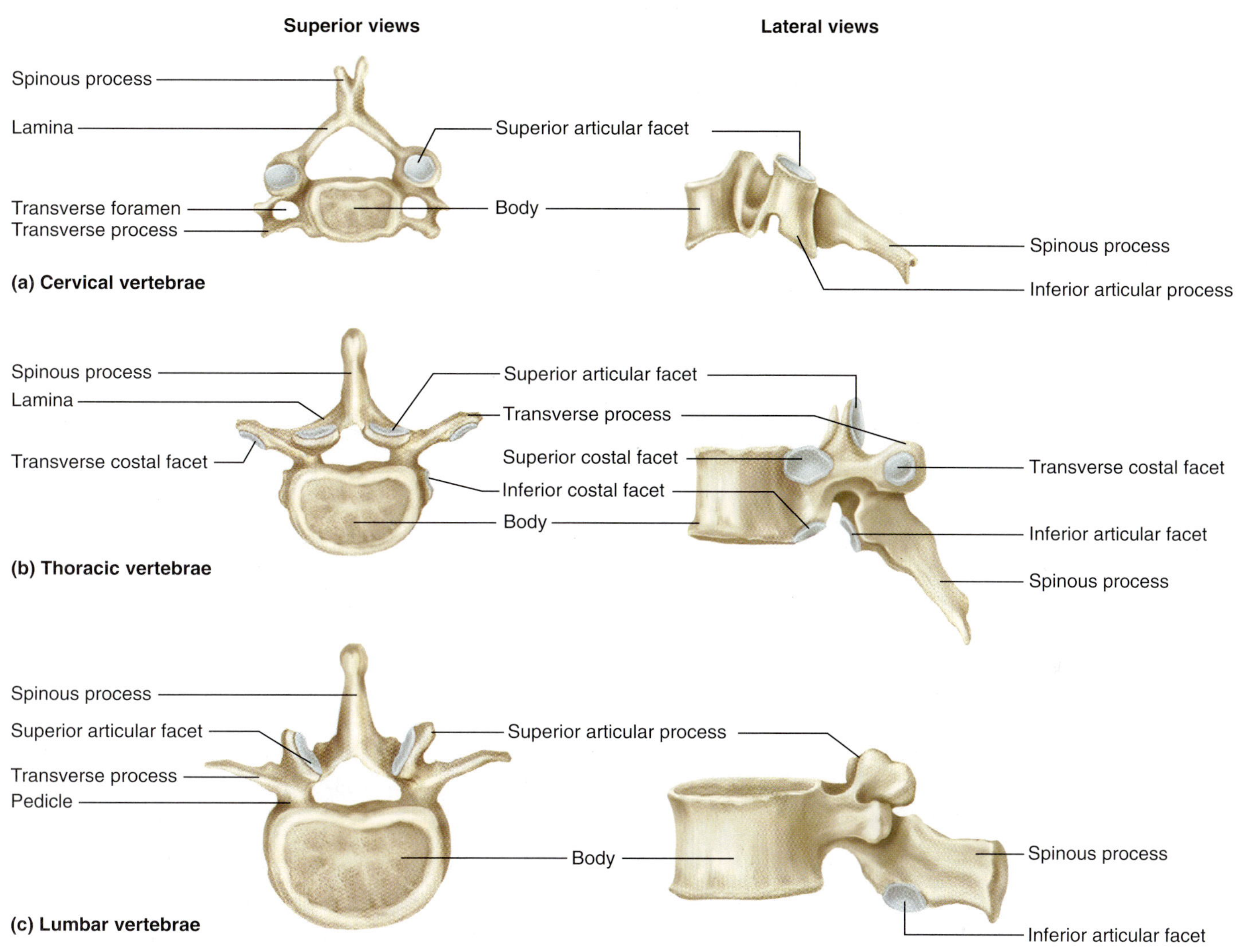

FIGURE 13.2 Bone shapes of the spine

of combining the movement from several adjacent vertebrae allows substantial movements within a given area. Most of the rotation within the cervical region occurs in the atlantoaxial joint, which is classified as a trochoid, or pivot-type, joint. The remaining vertebral articulations are classified as arthrodial, or gliding-type, joints, because of their limited gliding movements.

Gliding movement occurs between the superior and inferior articular processes that form the facet joints of the vertebrae, as depicted in figure 13.5. Located in between and adhering to the articular cartilage of the vertebral bodies are the **intervertebral disks** (figure 13.6). These disks are composed of an outer rim of dense fibrocartilage known as the *annulus fibrosus* and a central gelatinous, pulpy substance known as the *nucleus pulposus*. This arrangement of compressed elastic material allows compression in all directions, along with torsion. With age, injury, or improper use of the spine, the intervertebral disks become less resilient, resulting in a weakened annulus fibrosus. Substantial weakening combined with compression can result in the nucleus protruding through the annulus, which is known as a *herniated nucleus pulposus*. Commonly referred to as a herniated or "slipped" disk, this protrusion can put pressure on the spinal nerve root, causing a variety of symptoms, including radiating pain, tingling, numbness, and weakness in the dermatomes and myotomes of the extremity supplied by the spinal nerve (figure 13.7).

A substantial number of low-back problems are caused by improper use of the back over time. Improper mechanics often result in acute strains and muscle spasm of the lumbar extensors and chronic mechanical changes leading to disk herniation. Many problems occur from using the relatively small back muscles to lift objects from a lumbar spine–flexed

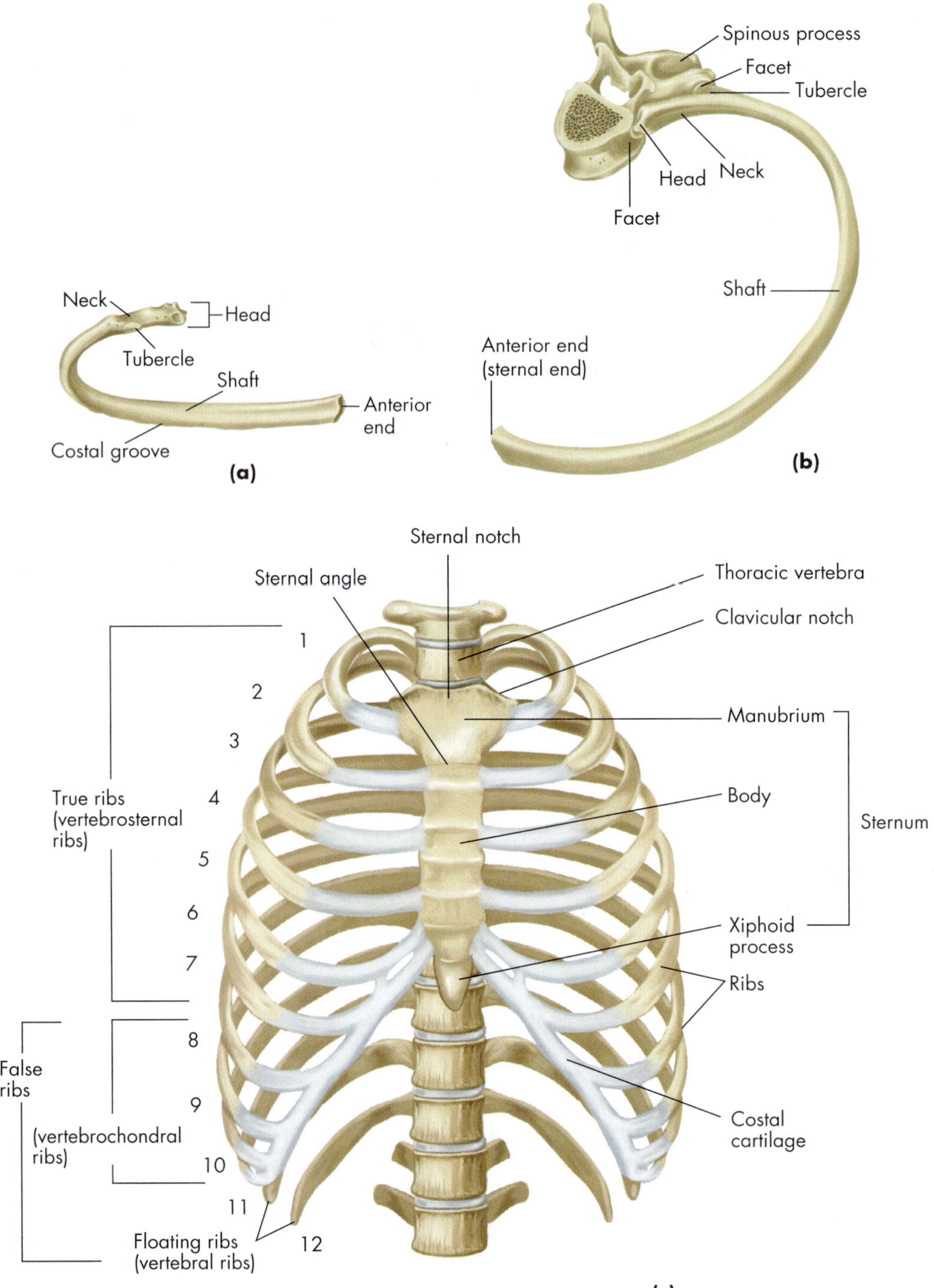

FIGURE 13.3 Thorax: **(a)** Posterior view of typical rib; **(b)** articulations of a rib with a thoracic vertebra (superior view); and **(c)** the thoracic cage, including the thoracic vertebra, the sternum, the ribs, and the costal cartilages that attach the ribs to the sternum.

position instead of keeping the lumbar spine in a neutral position while squatting and using the larger, more powerful muscles of the lower extremity. Additionally, a shortened psoas can chronically place the back in lumbar flexion, which over time leads to a gradual loss of lumbar lordosis. This "flat-back syndrome" results in increased pressure on the lumbar disk and intermittent or chronic low-back pain.

The majority of spinal column movement occurs in the cervical and lumbar regions. There is, of course, some thoracic movement, but it is slight in comparison with that of the neck and low back. In discussing

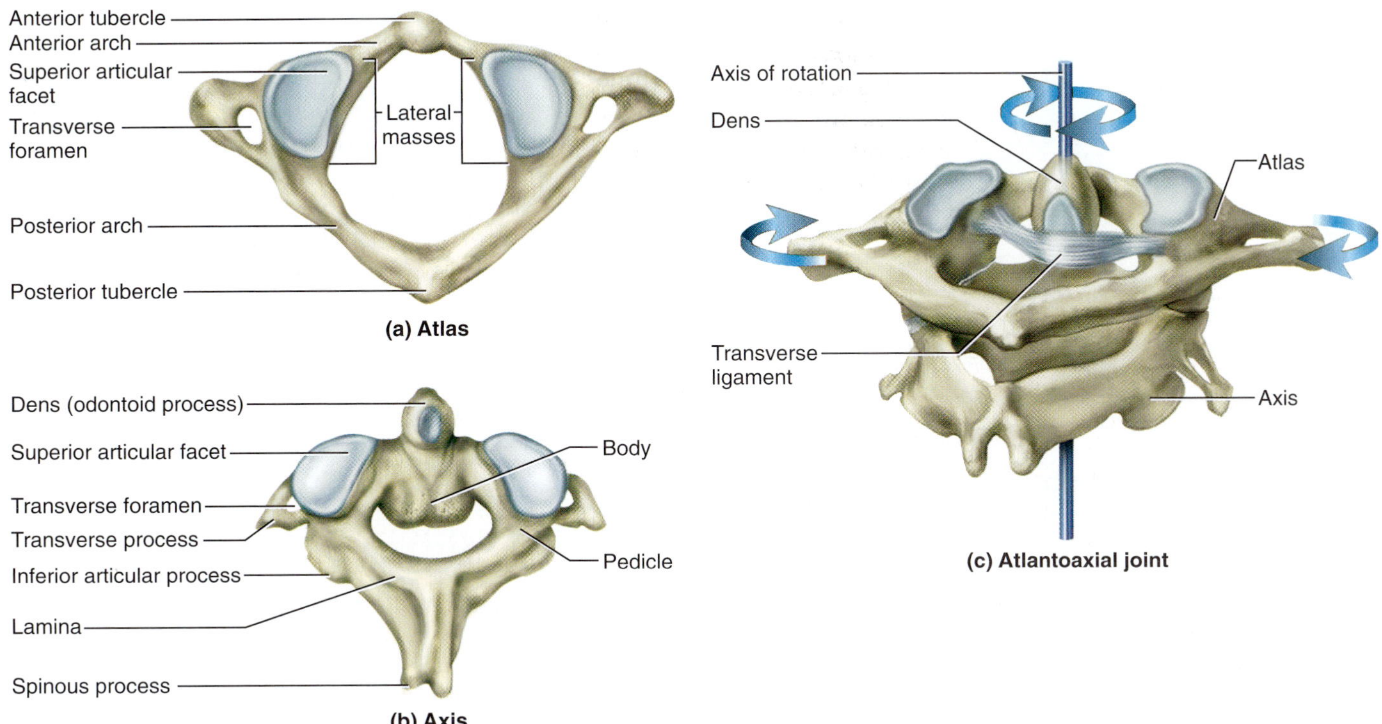

FIGURE 13.4 Atlas and axis, cervical vertebrae C1 and C2

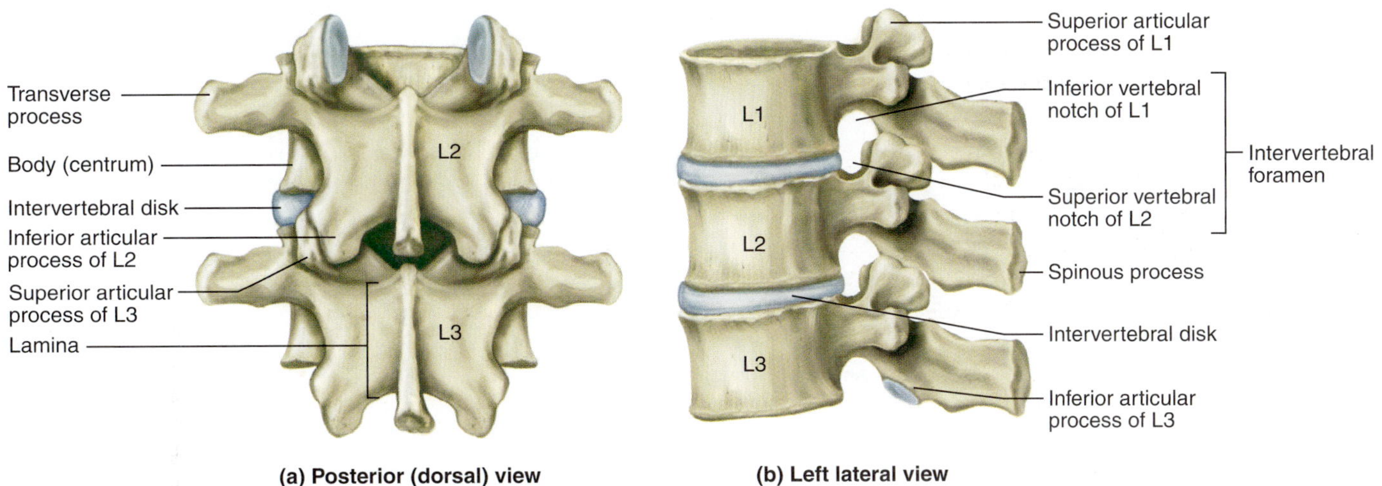

FIGURE 13.5 Articulated vertebrae

movements of the head, it must be remembered that these movements occur between the cranium and the 1st cervical vertebra, as well as within the cervical vertebrae. With the understanding that these motions usually occur together, this text, for simplification purposes, refers to all movements of the head and neck as cervical movements. Similarly, in discussing trunk movements, lumbar motion terminology is used to describe the combined motion that occurs in both the thoracic and lumbar regions. A closer investigation of specific motion between any two vertebrae is beyond the scope of this text.

The cervical region (figure 13.8) can flex 45 degrees and extend 45 degrees. The cervical area laterally flexes 45 degrees and can rotate approximately 60 degrees. The lumbar spine, accounting for most of the trunk movement (figure 13.9), flexes approximately 80 degrees and extends 20 to 30 degrees. Lumbar lateral flexion to each side is usually within 35 degrees, and approximately 45 degrees of rotation occurs to the left and right.

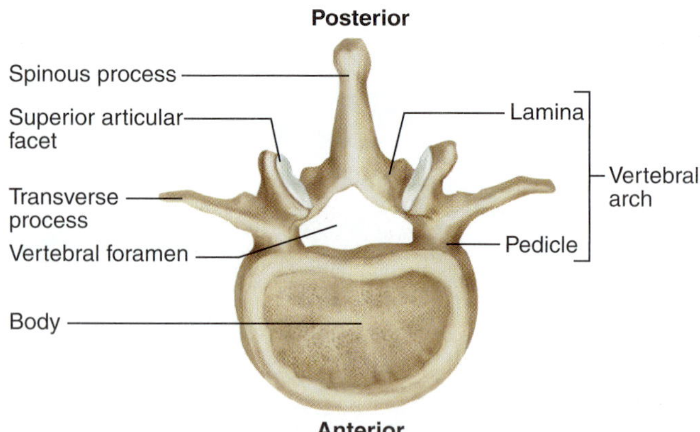

(a) 2nd lumbar vertebra (L2)

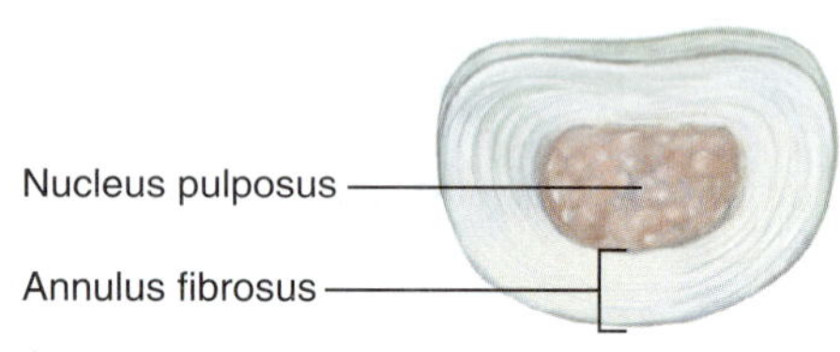

(b) Intervertebral disk

FIGURE 13.6 Structure of the vertebrae and intervertebral disk, superior view

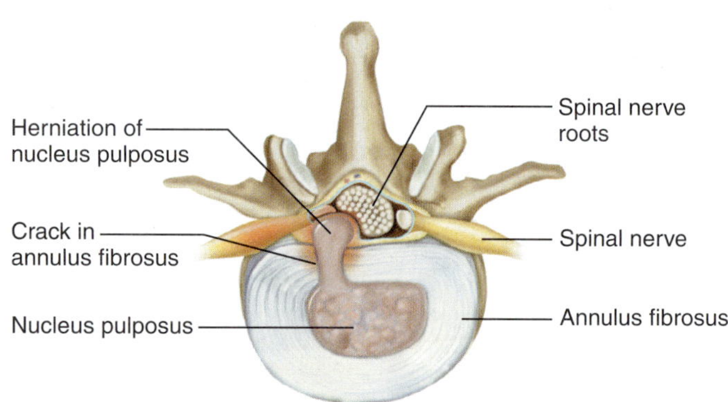

FIGURE 13.7 Herniated disk

Movements of the Trunk and Head

Spinal movements are often preceded by the name given to the region of movement. See figure 13.10 for these movements. For example, flexion of the trunk at the lumbar spine is known as *lumbar flexion,* and extension of the neck is often referred to as *cervical extension.* Additionally, the pelvic girdle rotates as a unit due to movement that occurs in the hip joints and the lumbar spine. This is discussed in Chapter 15.

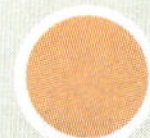

FLEXIBILITY & STRENGTH

Movements of the Trunk and Head

Spinal flexion
Anterior movement of the spine in the sagittal plane. In the cervical region, the head moves toward the chest; in the lumbar region, the thorax moves toward the pelvis.

Spinal extension
Return from flexion; posterior movement of the spine in the sagittal plane. In the cervical spine, the head moves away from the chest; in the lumbar spine, the thorax moves away from the pelvis. Sometimes referred to as *hyperextension.*

Lateral flexion (left or right)
The head moves laterally toward the shoulder, and the thorax moves laterally toward the pelvis—both in the frontal plane. Sometimes referred to as *side bending.*

Spinal rotation (left or right)
Rotary movement of the spine in the transverse plane. The chin rotates from neutral toward the shoulder, and the thorax rotates toward one iliac crest.

Reduction
Return movement from lateral flexion to neutral in the frontal plane.

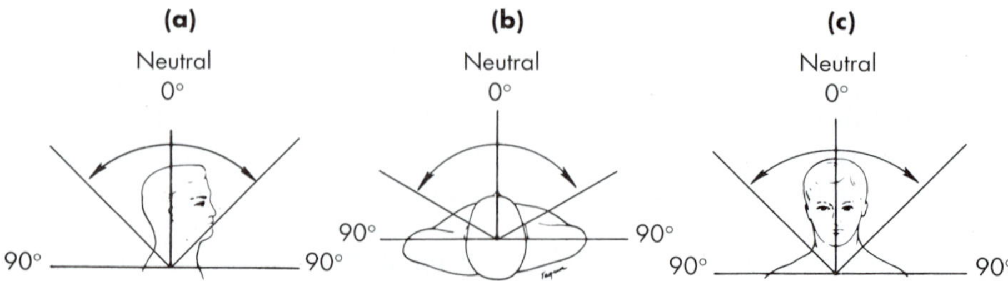

FIGURE 13.8 Active ROM of the cervical spine

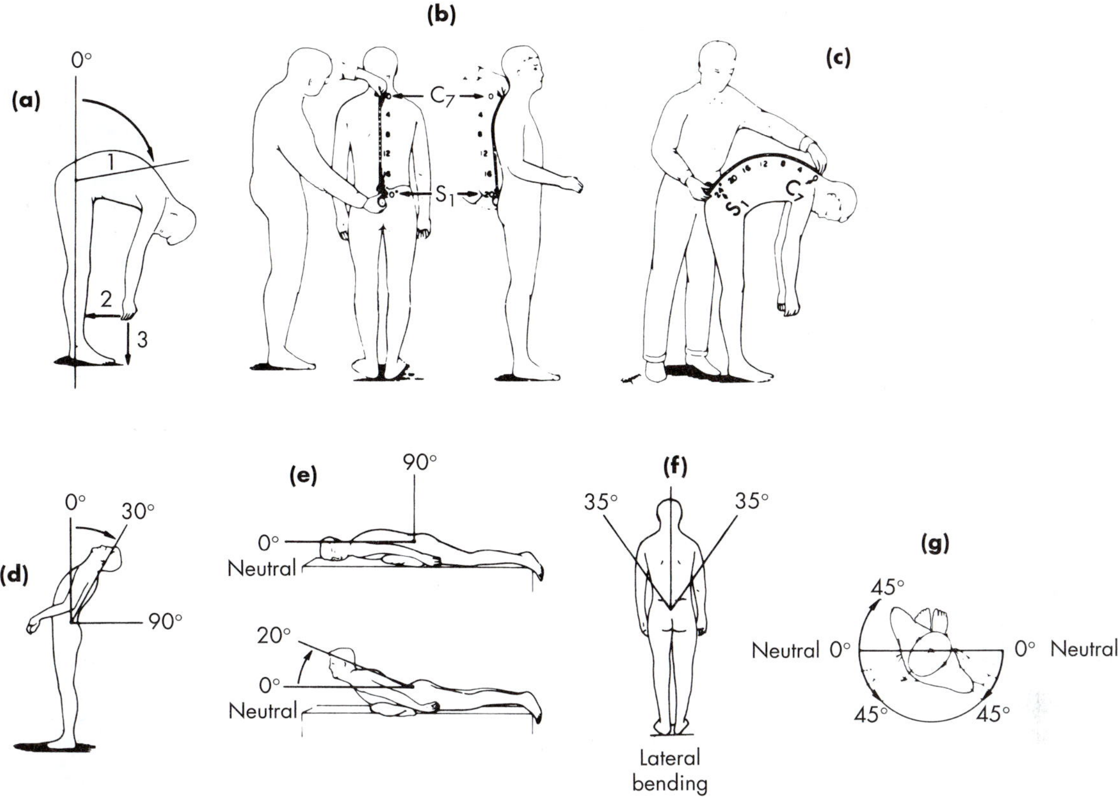

FIGURE 13.9 Active ROM of the thoracic and lumbar spine

Trunk and Spinal Column Muscles

The largest muscle group in this area is the **erector spinae** (sacrospinalis), listed in table 13.1, which extends on each side of the spinal column from the sacrum to the occiput. It is divided into three muscles: the spinalis, the longissimus, and the iliocostalis. From the medial to the lateral side, it has attachments in the lumbar, thoracic, and cervical regions. Thus, the erector spinae group is actually made up of nine muscles. Additionally, the **sternocleidomastoid (SCM), splenius cervicis,** and **splenius capitis** muscles are large muscles involved in cervical and head movements. Large abdominal muscles involved in lumbar movements include the **rectus abdominis, external oblique,** and **internal oblique.** Deep in the posterior lumbar region, the **quadratus lumborum** is also involved in lumbar movements and spinal stabilization.

Numerous small muscles are located in the spinal column region. Many of them originate on one vertebra and insert on the next vertebra. They are important in the functioning of the spine, but this discussion focuses on the larger muscles primarily involved in trunk and spinal column movements. Table 13.3 page 276 emphasizes some of these smaller functional spinal muscles.

Muscles of the trunk and spinal column are grouped according to both location and function for better comprehension. Some muscles have multiple segments. As a result, one segment of a particular muscle may be located and perform movement in one region, while another segment of the same muscle may be located in another region to perform movements in that region. Many of the trunk and spinal column muscles function by moving the spine, as well as in aiding respiration. All the thorax muscles are primarily involved in respiration. The abdominal wall muscles are different from the other muscles that have been studied. They do not attach from bone to bone but, rather, mesh with an aponeurosis (fascia) around the rectus abdominis area. They are the external oblique abdominal, internal oblique abdominal, and **transversus abdominis.**

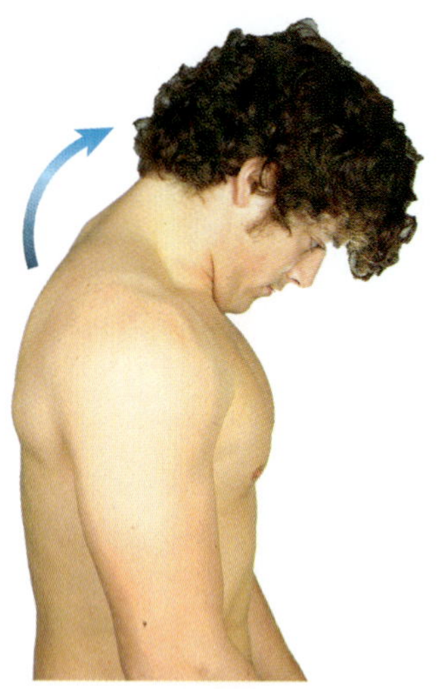
(a) Cervical flexion

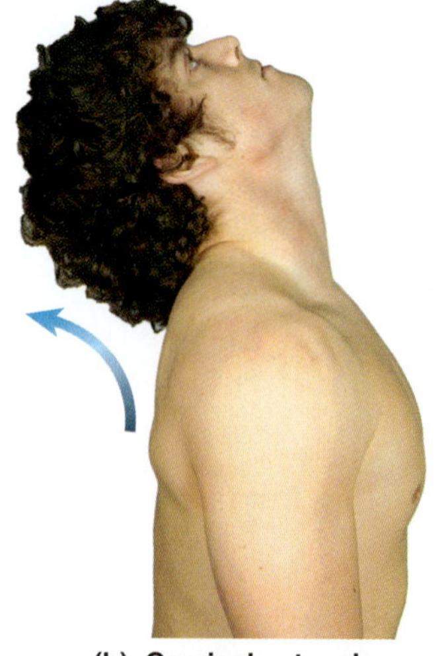
(b) Cervical extension (hyperextension)

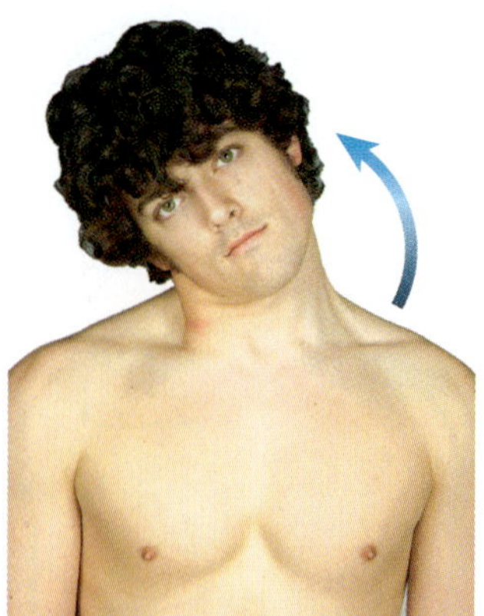
(c) Cervical lateral flexion to the right

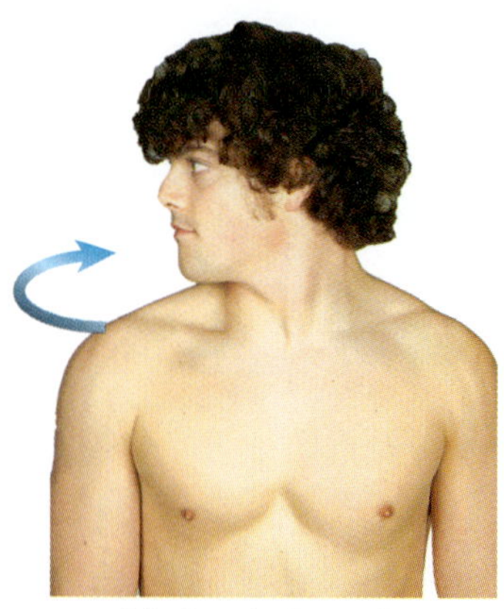
(d) Cervical rotation to the right

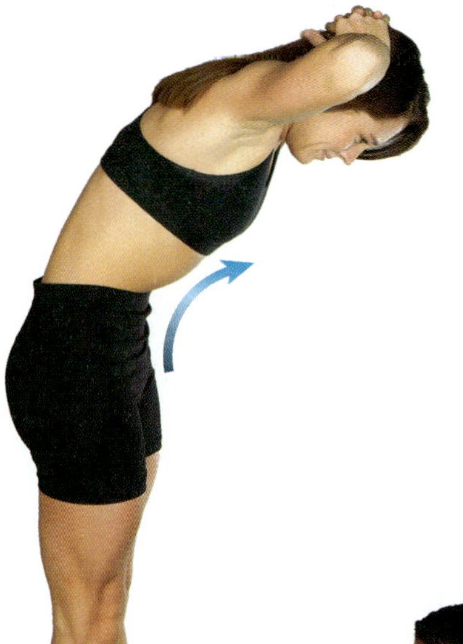
(e) Lumbar flexion

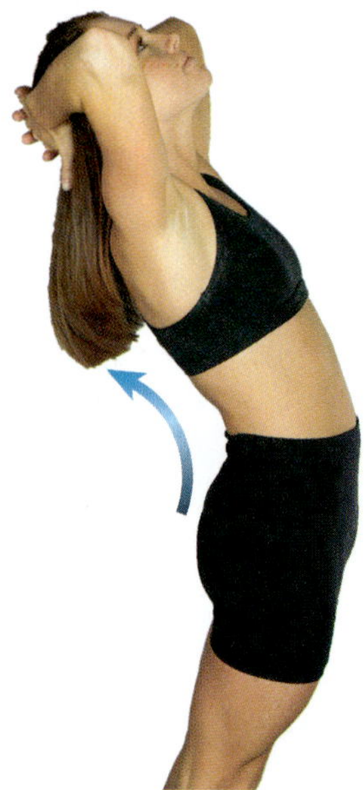
(f) Lumbar extension (hyperextension)

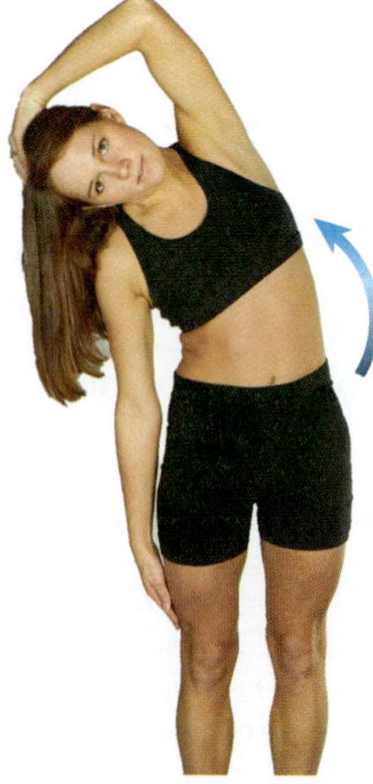
(g) Lumbar lateral flexion to the right

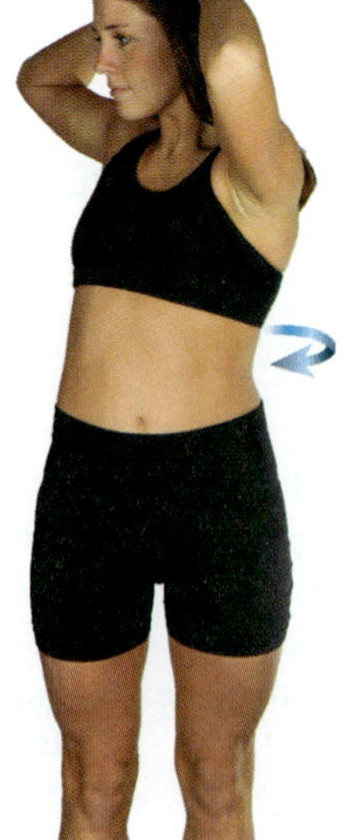
(h) Lumbar rotation to the right

FIGURE 13.10 Movements of the spine

TABLE 13.1 Muscles of the Trunk and Spinal Column

Name of Muscle	Origins	Insertion	Actions	Innervations
Muscles That Move the Head				
Sternocleidomastoid	Manubrium of sternum, anterior superior surface of medial clavicle	Mastoid process	*Both sides:* cervical flexion *Right side:* rotation to left and lateral flexion to right *Left side:* rotation to right and lateral flexion to left, bilateral extension of head at atlantooccipital joint	Accessory nerve (CN XI, C2–C3)
Splenius capitis	Below ligamentum nuchae, lower cervical, spinous process of C7, spinous processes of T1, T2, T3, T4	Mastoid bone and occipital bone	Face rotation to one side and chin up, rotation of head and neck and extension of head and neck bilaterally, lateral flexion same side	Posterior lateral branches of C4–C8
Splenius cervicis	Spinous processes of T3–T6	Transverse processes of C1, C2, C3	Face rotation to one side and chin up, rotation of head and neck and extension of neck bilaterally, lateral flexion same side	Posterior lateral branches of C4–C8
Muscles of the Vertebral Column				
Erector spinae: Iliocostalis	Medial iliac crest, thoracolumbar aponeurosis from sacrum, posterior ribs 3–12	Posterior ribs, 1–12, cervical transverse processes 4–7	Extension of spine bilaterally *Unilateral:* lateral flexion of spine, ipsilateral rotation of spine and head, anterior pelvic rotation to contralateral side	Posterior branches of spinal nerves
Longissimus dorsi	Medial iliac crest, thoracolumbar aponeurosis from sacrum, lumbar 1–5 and thoracic transverse processes, cervical 5–7 articular processes	Cervical and spinous processes 2–6 and thoracic transverse processes 1–12, lower nine ribs, mastoid process	Same	Same
Spinalis dorsi	Ligamentum nuchae; 7th cervical and thoracic spinous processes 11, 12; lumbar 1, 2 spinous processes	2nd cervical and thoracic spinous processes 5–12, occipital bone	Same	Same

(Continued)

TABLE 13.1 (Continued)

Name of Muscle	Origins	Insertion	Actions	Innervations
		Muscles of the Vertebral Column		
Quadratus lumborum	Posterior inner lip of iliac crest and transverse processes of the lower four lumbar vertebrae	Transverse processes of upper four lumbar vertebrae and lower border of 12th rib	Lateral flexion to ipsilateral side, "guy wires," stabilization of pelvis and lumbar spine, bilateral extension of lumbar spine, anterior pelvic rotation, lateral pelvic rotation to contralateral side	Branches of T12, L1
		Muscles of the Abdominal Wall		
Rectus abdominis	Crest of pubis	Cartilage of 5th, 6th, 7th ribs and xiphoid	Flexion of trunk, compression of abdominal contents, lateral flexion same side, posterior pelvic rotation	Intercostal nerves (T7–T12)
External oblique	Lower eight ribs, interdigitating with serratus anterior and latissimus dorsi	Abdominal aponeurosis and anterior iliac crest, inguinal ligament, crest of pubis	Compression of abdominal contents, bilateral flexion of spine, lateral flexion *Unilateral:* rotation of trunk to opposite side, pelvic rotation to opposite side	Intercostal nerves (T8–T12), iliohypogastric nerve (T12, L1), ilioinguinal nerve (L1)
Internal oblique	Inguinal ligament and anterior iliac crest, lumbar fascia	Costal cartilage of last three or four ribs, abdominal aponeurosis	Bilateral flexion of spine, compression of abdominal contents *Unilateral:* lateral flexion, rotation of trunk to same side, posterior pelvic rotation, opposite-side pelvic rotation	Intercostal nerves (T8-12), iliohypogastric nerve (T12, L1), ilioinguinal nerve (L1)
Transversus abdominis	Inguinal ligament, iliac crest, thoracolumbar aponeurosis, lower margin of rib cage (lower six ribs), lumbar fascia	Abdominal aponeurosis and linea alba, crest of pubis, iliopectineal line	Interdigitates with fibers of diaphragm and compression of abdominal contents, increases intra-abdominal pressure, helps in forced expiration	Intercostal nerves (T7–T12), iliohypogastric nerve (T12, L1), ilioinguinal nerve (L1)

Muscles That Move the Head—Location

MUSCLE SPECIFIC

Anterior
- Rectus capitis anterior
- Longus capitis

Posterior
- Suboccipitals:
  - Obliquus capitis superior
  - Obliquus capitis inferior
  - Rectus capitis posterior—major and minor
- Longissimus capitis
- Trapezius, superior fibers
- Splenius capitis
- Semispinalis capitis

Lateral
- Rectus capitis lateralis
- Sternocleidomastoid

Muscles of the Vertebral Column—Location

MUSCLE SPECIFIC

Superficial
- Erector spinae (sacrospinalis)
- Spinalis—capitis, cervicis, thoracis
- Longissimus—capitis, cervicis, thoracis
- Iliocostalis—cervicis, thoracis, lumborum
- Splenius cervicis

Deep
- Longus colli—superior oblique, inferior oblique, vertical
- Interspinales—entire spinal column
- Intertransversarii—entire spinal column
- Multifidi—entire spinal column
- Psoas minor
- Rotatores—entire spinal column
- Semispinalis—cervicis, thoracis

Muscles of the thorax
- Diaphragm
- Intercostalis—external, internal
- Levator costarum
- Subcostalis
- Scalenes—anterior, middle, posterior
- Serratus posterior—superior, inferior
- Transversus thoracis

Muscles of the abdominal wall
- Rectus abdominis
- External oblique
- Internal oblique
- Transversus abdominis
- Quadratus lumborum

Nerves

There are 31 pairs of spinal nerves emerging from the spinal column. Cranial nerve XI and the spinal nerves of C2 and C3 innervate the sternocleidomastoid. The posterior lateral branches of C4 through C8 innervate the splenius muscles. The entire erector spinae group is supplied by the posterior branches of the spinal nerves, whereas the intercostal nerves of T7 through T12 innervate the rectus abdominis. Both the internal and external oblique abdominal muscles receive innervation from the intercostal nerves (T8 through T12), the iliohypogastric nerve (T12, L1), and the ilioinguinal nerve (L1). The same innervation is provided to the transversus abdominis, except that innervation begins with the T7 intercostal nerve. Branches from T12 and L1 supply the quadratus lumborum.

Muscles That Move the Head

All the muscles featured in this section originate on the cervical vertebrae and insert on the occipital bone of the skull, as implied by their "capitis" name (figures 13.11 and 13.12). Table 13.2 lists the muscles that move the head. Three muscles make up the anterior vertebral muscles—the longus capitis, the rectus capitis anterior, and the rectus capitis lateralis. All are flexors of the head and upper cervical spine. The rectus capitis lateralis laterally flexes the head, in addition to assisting the rectus capitis anterior in stabilizing the atlantooccipital joint.

The rectus capitis posterior major and minor and the obliquus capitis superior and inferior are known as **suboccipitals** and are located posteriorly deep to the semispinalis capitis. All are extensors of the head, except the obliquus capitis inferior, which rotates the atlas. The obliquus capitis superior assists the rectus capitis lateralis in lateral flexion of the head. In addition to providing extension, the rectus capitis posterior major is responsible for head rotation to the ipsilateral side. It is assisted by the semispinalis capitis, which rotates the head to the contralateral side. The splenius capitis and the sternocleidomastoid are much larger and more powerful in moving the head and cervical spine, and they are covered in detail on the following pages. The suboccipitals are discussed further in Chapter 14. The remaining muscles that act on the cervical spine are addressed with the muscles of the vertebral column.

TABLE 13.2 Muscles That Move the Head

Muscle	Origins	Insertion	Actions	Innervations
Rectus capitis anterior	Anterior surface of lateral mass of atlas	Basilar part of occipital bone anterior to foramen magnum	Flexion of head and stabilization of atlantooccipital joint	C1–C3
Rectus capitis lateralis	Superior surface of transverse processes of atlas	Jugular process of occipital bone	Lateral flexion of head and stabilization of atlantooccipital joint	C1–C3
Rectus capitis posterior (major)	Spinous process of axis	Lateral portion of inferior nuchal line of occipital bone	Extension and rotation of head to ipsilateral side	Posterior rami of C1
Rectus capitis posterior (minor)	Spinous process of atlas	Medial portion of inferior nuchal line of occipital bone	Extension of head	Posterior rami of C1
Longus capitis	Transverse processes of C3–C6	Basilar part of occipital bone	Flexes head and cervical spine	C1–C3
Obliquus capitis superior	Transverse process of atlas	Occipital bone between inferior and superior nuchal line	Extension and lateral flexion of head	Posterior rami of C1
Obliquus capitis inferior	Spinous process of axis	Transverse process of atlas	Rotation of atlas	Posterior rami of C1
Semispinalis capitis	Transverse processes of C4–T7	Occipital bone, between superior and inferior nuchal lines	Extension and contralateral rotation of head	Posterior primary divisions on spinal nerves

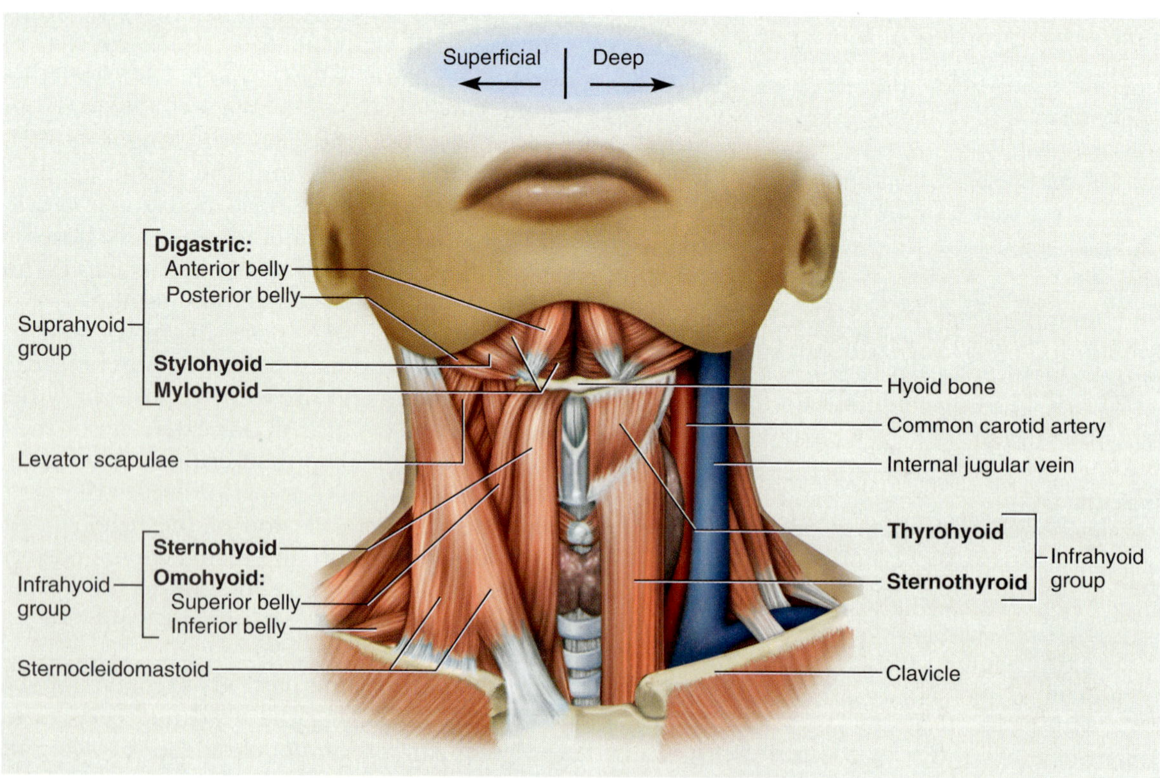

FIGURE 13.11 Anterior muscles of the neck

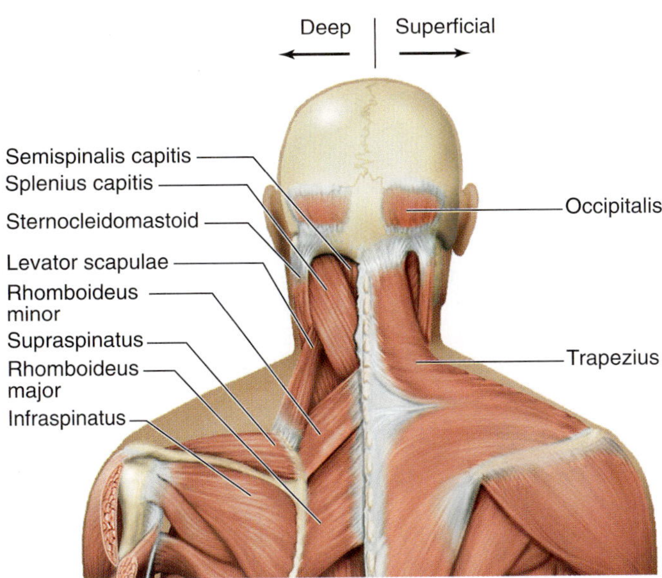

FIGURE 13.12 Deep muscles of the posterior neck and upper-back regions

Individual Muscles of the Trunk and Spinal Column—Muscles That Move the Head and Neck

STERNOCLEIDOMASTOID MUSCLE

Palpation

Palpate the sternocleidomastoid (SCM) on the anterolateral side of the neck, diagonally between the origin and insertion, particularly with rotation to the contralateral side.

> **CLINICAL NOTES** **Neck Problems**
>
> Prolonged positions of a flexed head can contract and shorten the sternocleidomastoid. Bilaterally, the muscle opposes posterior cervical muscles, including the trapezius, suboccipitals, erector spinae, splenius capitis, semispinalis, and others. Although gravity does not place extreme force on this muscle because it helps move the head in the transverse plane, the sternocleidomastoid is shaped and attached for lateral flexion of the head and neck; no other muscle in the body performs actions as unique as does the SCM. In addition to performing flexion, it laterally flexes and rotates to the opposite side. Sleeping postures and awkward head positions can lead to a stiff neck in the morning. The sternocleidomastoid is very important to respect and treat accordingly for a variety of soft-tissue complaints from whiplash to postural issues. It should be stretched and strengthened in every way that it moves the head.

Muscle Specifics

The sternocleidomastoid is primarily responsible for head and neck flexion and rotation. Each side of this muscle may be easily visualized and palpated when rotating the head to its opposite side. Remember that the accessory nerve can be entrapped by contracted fibers of sternocleidomastoid. Congenital absence of the sternocleidomastoid muscle on one side is present in some people.

Clinical Flexibility

Since the SCM performs many actions, it should be stretched by each action individually.

To stretch it as a lateral flexor, begin with the eyes focused ahead in the neutral position and slightly retract the chin. Contract the opposite-side flexors, and move the ear to the opposite shoulder. Raise the other hand above the head to help stretch gently for 2 seconds. To stretch it as a rotator, begin in the same position. This time begin moving the eyes first, and contract the SCM to rotate the head to the opposite shoulder. Use both hands to help with the stretch. Position one hand at the back of the head and the other hand at the mandible. Stretch gently for 2 seconds. *Contraindications:* Use caution on clients with cervical disk herniations.

Strengthening

To strengthen the SCM, apply the rules for isolating a muscle's actions. Lie on the side on a bed or table, allowing the head to hang off the side. If the neck is painful, keep the head on the table and do not allow it to hang without support. Hang the bottom arm off the table, and secure it on the table leg. Start by looking down; then contract the SCM to rotate the head to the opposite shoulder. Repeat. To strengthen the SCM as a lateral flexor, start in the same position, but this time with the ear to the bottom shoulder. Contract the opposite lateral flexors, and lift the ear to the shoulder. Take care not to contract the trapezius. Repeat. *Contraindications:* Use caution on clients with cervical disk herniations; proceed with gentle improvement of ROM first.

SPLENIUS CAPITIS MUSCLE

SPLENIUS CERVICIS MUSCLE

Palpation

Palpate the splenius capitis deep to the trapezius inferiorly and the sternocleidomastoid superiorly; with the client seated. It also can be palpated in the posterior triangle of the neck between the upper trapezius and the sternocleidomastoid with resisted rotation to the ipsilateral side.

Palpate the splenius cervicis in the lower posterior cervical spine just medial to the inferior levator scapulae with resisted ipsilateral rotation.

OIAI MUSCLE CHART STERNOCLEIDOMASTOID (ster´no-kli-do-mas-toyd) Named for its attachments

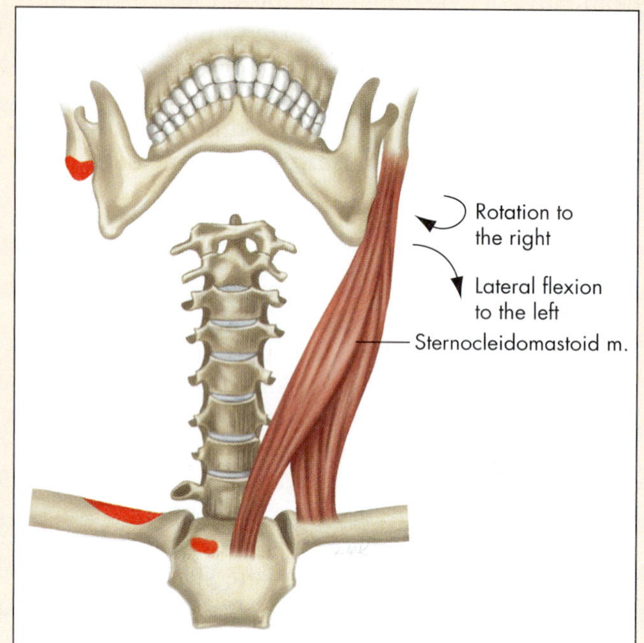

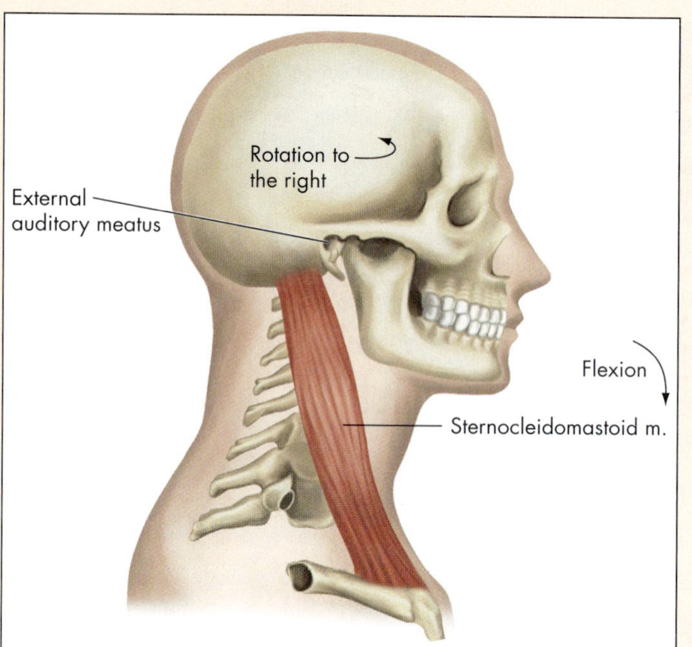

Name of Muscle	Origins	Insertion	Actions	Innervations
Sternocleidomastoid	Manubrium of sternum, anterior superior surface of medial clavicle	Mastoid process	*Both sides:* cervical flexion *Right side:* rotation to left and lateral flexion to right *Left side:* rotation to right and lateral flexion to left, bilateral extension of head at atlantooccipital joint	Accessory nerve (CN XI, C2–C3)

CLINICAL NOTES

Chronic Tension

Chronic tension in the back of the neck can contribute to headaches, and splenius capitis assists posterior cervical muscles in the act of chronic tension. The posterior cervical muscles work all the time to combat ongoing flexion. Supporting the weight of the head against gravity is a chore. If the head is in partial flexion, the posterior neck muscles have to work harder, thus putting more stress on these muscles. Releasing the posterior cervical muscles from mastoid process to mastoid process helps relieve chronic tension from the neck area. See Chapter 14 for more on this topic.

CLINICAL NOTES

Stabilization of the Upper Cervicals

The splenius cervicis attaches to the most movable vertebrae, which gives it some distinction and allows for possible subluxation and hypertonicity. Bilaterally, the splenius cervicis has attachments to the C1 through C3 transverse processes. Along with the levator scapulae, which attaches to the C1 through C4 transverse processes, and the scalenes, which also attach to vertebrae, the splenius cervicis provides an intricate stabilization of the spine. Should the neck be in a rotated position and sustain whiplash, damage to the fibers in a variety of neck muscles could occur in an extreme lateral flexion. Hypertonic fibers on either side of the upper cervicals pull on the spine and cause the dreaded stiff neck.

OIAI MUSCLE CHART SPLENIUS CAPITIS (sple´ni-us kap´i-tis) Bandage to the head

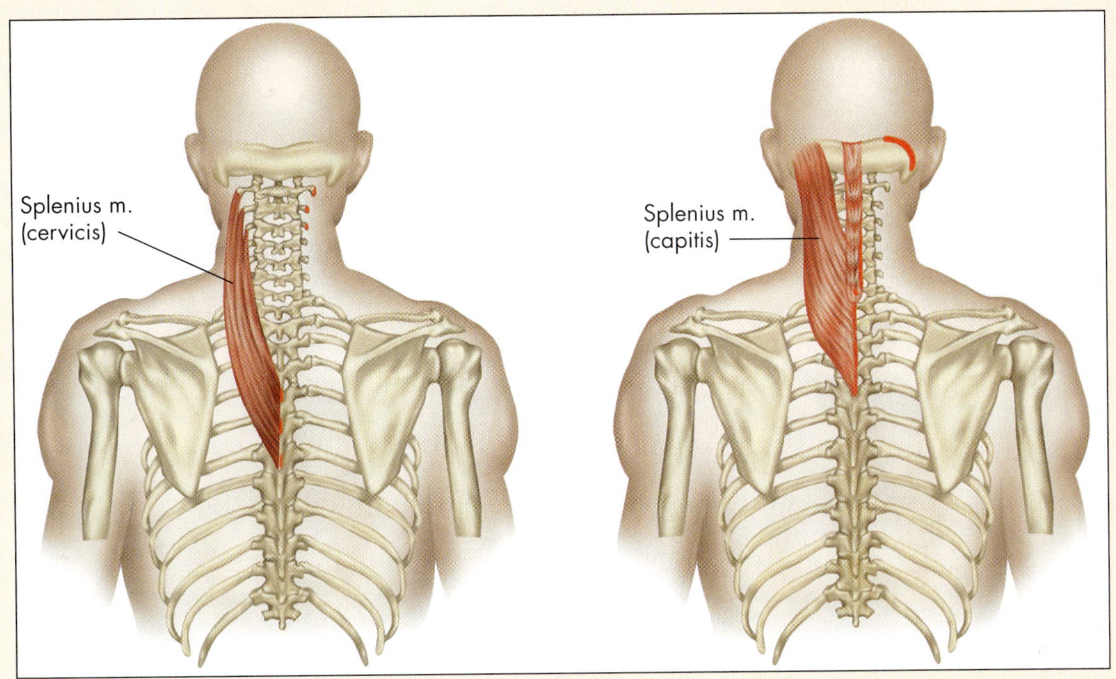

Name of Muscle	Origins	Insertion	Actions	Innervations
Splenius capitis	Below ligamentum nuchae, lower cervical, spinous process of C7, spinous processes of T1, T2, T3, T4	Mastoid bone and occipital bone	Face rotation to one side and chin up, rotation of head and neck and extension of head and neck bilaterally, lateral flexion same side	Posterior lateral branches of C4–C8

Muscle Specifics

Any movement of the head and neck into extension, particularly extension and rotation, brings the splenius capitis and cervicis muscles strongly into play, together with the erector spinae and the upper trapezius muscles. Tone in both the splenius muscles tends to hold the head and neck in proper posture position.

Clinical Flexibility

Splenius capitis and cervicis may be stretched with maximal flexion of the head and cervical spine. See the stretch for the sternocleidomastoid.

Strengthening

The strength exercises for the sternocleidomastoid apply here.

Muscles of the Vertebral Column

In the cervical area, the longus colli muscles are located anteriorly and flex the cervical and upper thoracic vertebrae. Posteriorly, the erector spinae group, the transversospinal group, the interspinal-intertransverse group, and the splenius all run vertically parallel to the spinal column (figures 13.13 and 13.14). Table 13.3 lists the muscles of the vertebral column. This location enables them to extend the spine as well as assist in rotation and lateral flexion. The splenius and erector spinae group are addressed in detail later in this chapter. The transversospinal group consists of the semispinalis, multifidi, and rotatores muscles. These muscles all originate on the transverse processes of their respective vertebrae

OIAI MUSCLE CHART SPLENIUS CERVICIS (sple´ni-us ser´vi-sis) Bandage to the cervicals

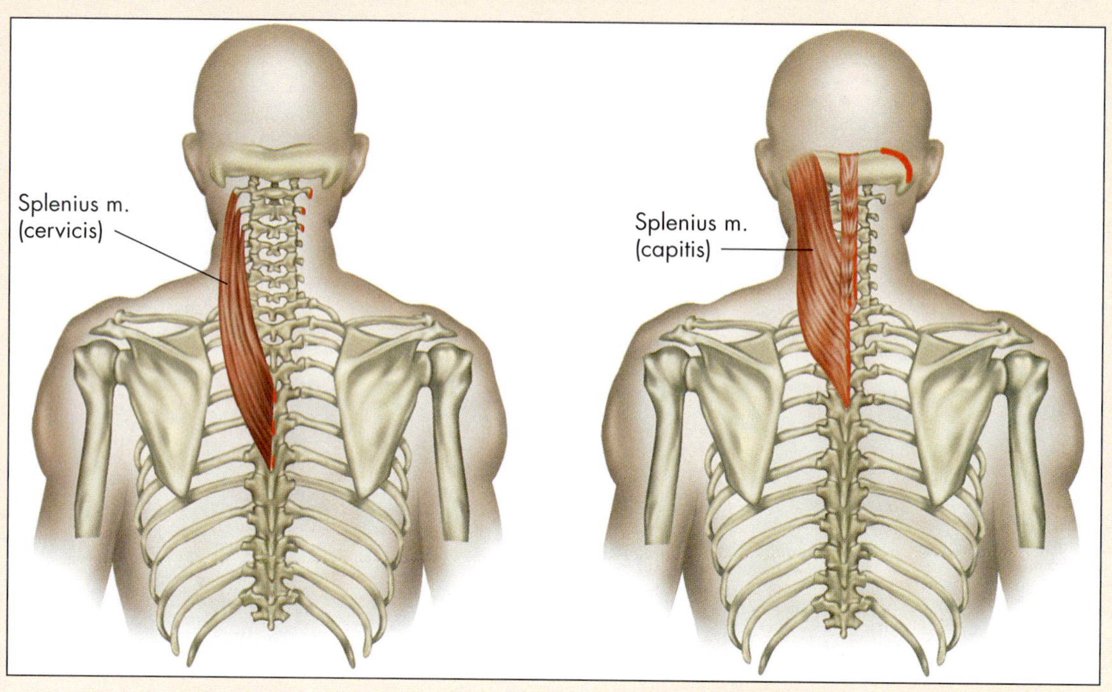

Name of Muscle	Origins	Insertion	Actions	Innervations
Splenius cervicis	Spinous processes of T3–T6	Transverse processes of C1, C2, C3	Face rotation to one side and chin up, rotation of head and neck and extension of neck bilaterally, lateral flexion same side	Posterior lateral branches of C4–C8

and generally run posteriorly to attach to the spinous processes on the vertebrae just above their vertebrae of origin. All are extensors of the spine and contract to rotate their respective vertebrae to the contralateral side. The interspinal-intertransverse group lies deep to the rotatores and consists of the interspinales and the intertransversarii muscles. As a group, they laterally flex and extend but do not rotate the vertebrae. The **interspinales** are extensors that connect from the spinous process of one vertebra to the spinous process of the adjacent vertebra. The **intertransversarii** muscles flex the vertebral column laterally by connecting to the transverse processes of adjacent vertebrae.

Individual Muscles of the Trunk and Spinal Column—Muscles That Move the Vertebral Column

ERECTOR SPINAE MUSCLES (SACROSPINALIS)

Palpation

The erector spinae muscles are deep and difficult to distinguish from other muscles in the cervical and thoracic regions; with the client prone, palpate the longissimus dorsi group immediately lateral to the spinous processes in the lumbar region with active extension.

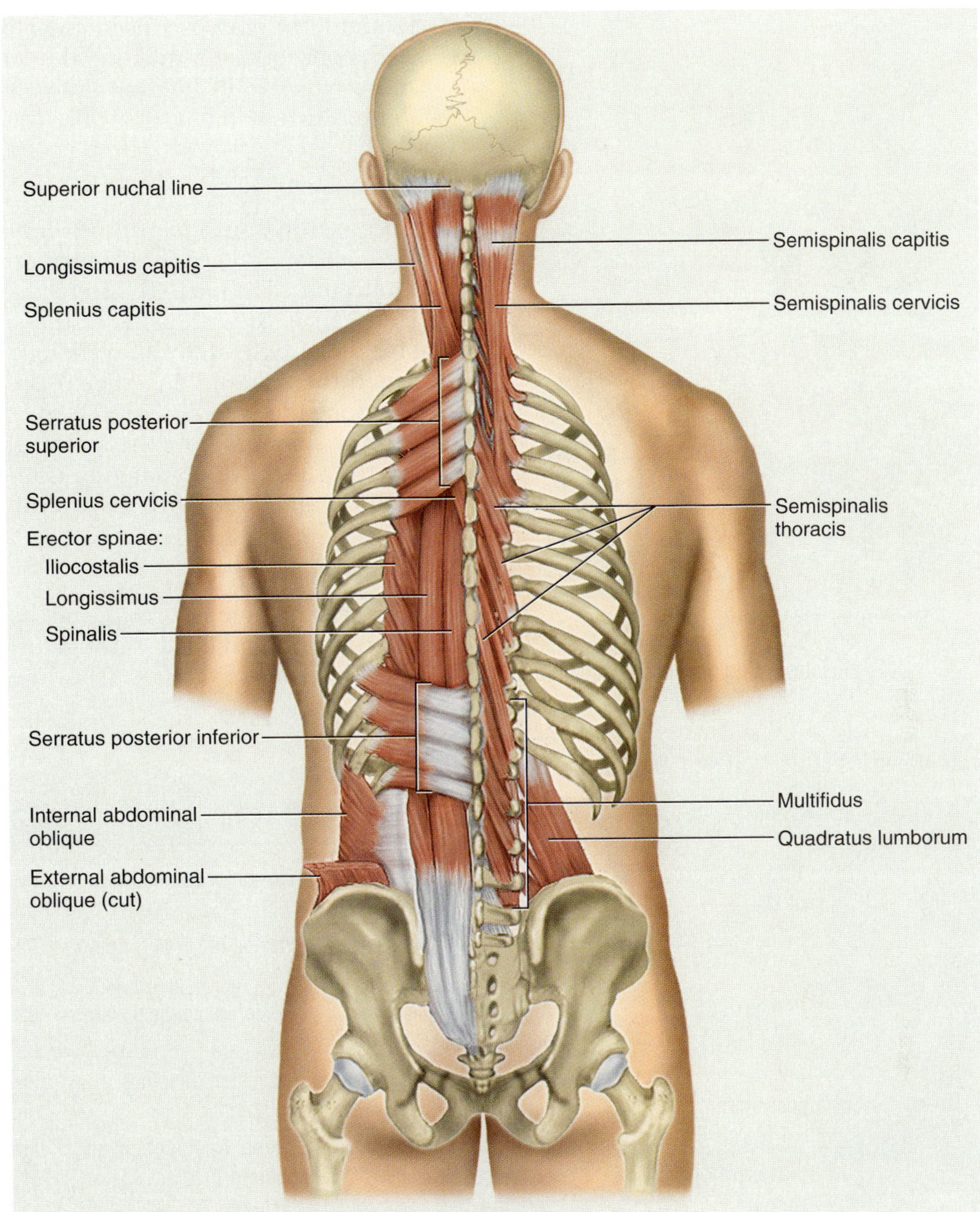

FIGURE 13.13 Muscles acting on the vertebral column

CLINICAL NOTES

Long-Range Communication System

The nine muscles on both sides of the spine create a useful "communication" system. Should the lumbar section of the erector spinae become strained, it does not take long to experience tension throughout the muscle mass right up to the neck. Unwinding the erector spinae requires having knowledge of the different sections and their attachments, understanding the actions of the different segments, and knowing which muscles are working in tandem or in opposition to the actions. Remember that if the spine is being laterally flexed or rotated, the opposite side is being lengthened.

Muscle Specifics

The erector spinae muscles function best when the pelvis is posteriorly rotated. This lowers the origin of the erector spinae and makes the muscles more effective in keeping the spine straight. As the spine is held

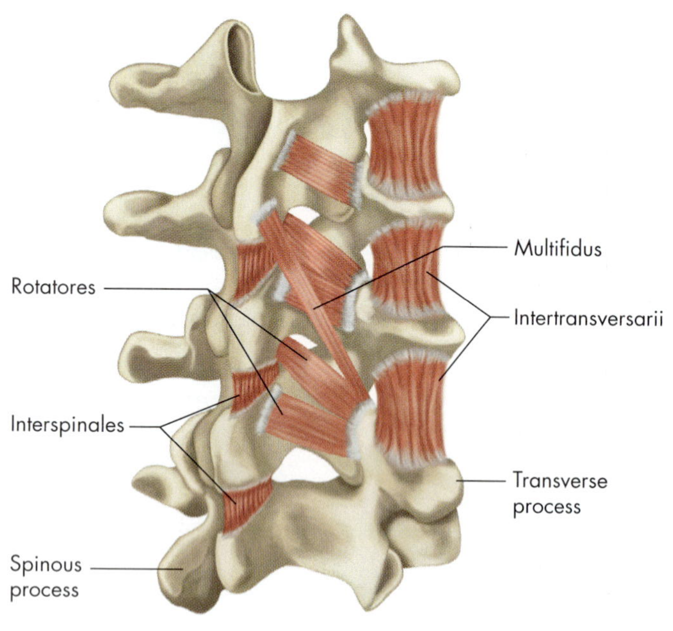

FIGURE 13.14 Deep muscles acting on the vertebral column

straight, the ribs are raised, thus fixing the chest high and consequently making the abdominal muscles more effective in holding the pelvis up in front and flattening the abdominal wall.

Clinical Flexibility

Because this muscle group is long and acts on both the lumbar and cervical spines, it must be separated to stretch each part. To stretch it as a lateral flexor, stand straight with arms at the sides. Contract one side and reach laterally, as though you were trying to touch the side of your knee. Feel for the stretch on the opposite side. To stretch the cervical portion of erector spinae, apply the stretches described earlier for the sternocleidomastoid. *Contraindications:* Use caution on clients with disk herniations.

Strengthening

The erector spinae group and its various divisions may be strengthened through numerous forms of back extension exercises. They are usually done in a

TABLE 13.3 Muscles of the Vertebral Column

Muscle	Origins	Insertion	Actions	Innervations
Longus colli (superior oblique)	Transverse processes of C3–C5	Anterior arch of atlas	Flexion of cervical spine	C2–C7
Longus colli (inferior oblique)	Bodies of T1–T3	Transverse processes of C5–C6	Flexion of cervical spine	C2–C7
Longus colli (vertical)	Bodies of C5–C7 and T1–T3	Anterior surface of bodies of C2–C4	Flexion of cervical spine	C2–C7
Interspinalis	Spinous process of each vertebra	Spinous process of next vertebra	Extension of spinal column	Posterior primary ramus of spinal nerves
Intertransversarii	Tubercles of transverse processes of each vertebra	Tubercles of transverse processes of next vertebra	Lateral flexion of spinal column	Anterior primary ramus of spinal nerves
Multifidus	Sacrum, iliac spine, transverse processes of lumbar, thoracic, and lower four cervical vertebrae	Spinous processes of 2nd, 3rd, or 4th vertebra above origin	Extension and contralateral rotation of spinal column	Posterior primary ramus of spinal nerves
Rotatores	Transverse process of each vertebra	Base of spinous process of next vertebra above	Extension and contralateral rotation of spinal column	Posterior primary ramus of spinal nerves
Semispinalis cervicis	Transverse processes of T1–T5 or T6	Spinous processes from C2–C5	Extension and contralateral rotation of vertebral column	All divisions, posterior primary ramus of spinal nerves
Semispinalis thoracis	Transverse processes of T6–T10	Spinous processes of C6–C7 and T1–T4	Extension and contralateral rotation of vertebral column	Posterior primary ramus of spinal nerves

OIAI MUSCLE CHART ERECTOR SPINAE (e-rek´tor spi´ne) Extensors of the spine

ILIOCOSTALIS (il´i-o-kos-ta´lis) Lateral layer

LONGISSIMUS (lon-jis´i-mus) Middle layer

SPINALIS (spi-na´lis) Medial layer

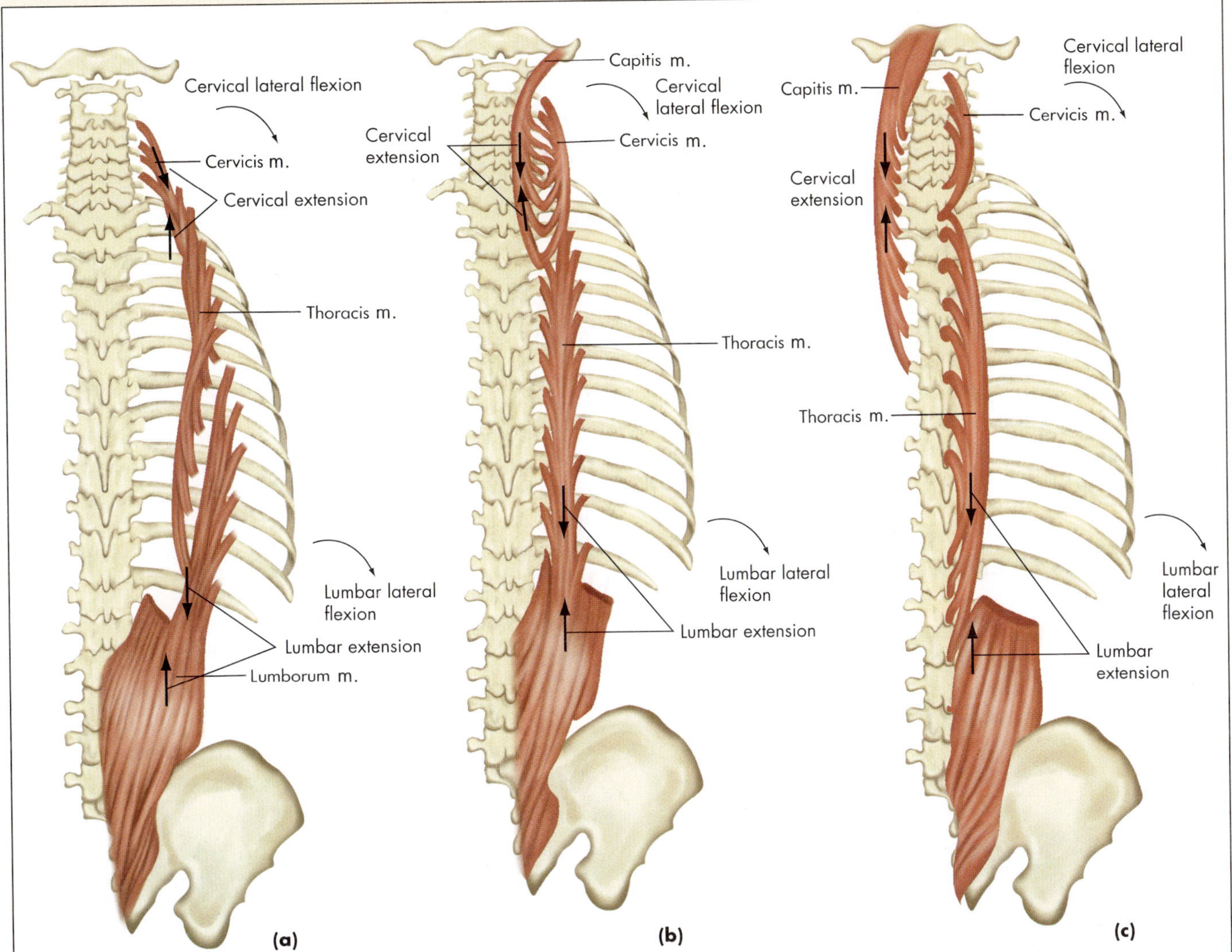

Name of Muscle	Origins	Insertion	Actions	Innervations
Iliocostalis	Medial iliac crest, thoracolumbar aponeurosis from sacrum, posterior ribs 3–12	Posterior ribs 1–12, cervical transverse processes 4–7	Extension of spine bilaterally *Unilateral:* lateral flexion of spine, ipsilateral rotation of spine and head, anterior pelvic rotation, lateral pelvic rotation to contralateral side	Posterior branches of spinal nerves

(Continued)

Longissimus dorsi	Medial iliac crest, thoracolumbar aponeurosis from sacrum, lumbar 1–5 and thoracic transverse processes 1–5, cervical 5–7 articular processes	Cervical and spinous processes 2–6 and thoracic transverse processes 1–12, lower nine ribs, mastoid process	Same	Same
Spinalis dorsi	Ligamentum nuchae; 7th cervical and thoracic spinous processes 11, 12; lumbar 1, 2 spinous processes	2nd cervical and thoracic spinous processes 5–12, occipital bone	Same	Same

prone or face-down position with the spine already in some state of flexion. Use these muscles to move part of or the entire spine toward extension against gravity. Hold a weight in the hands behind the head to increase resistance. *Contraindications:* Use caution on clients with disk herniations; avoid using added weight until the injury has healed.

QUADRATUS LUMBORUM MUSCLE

Palpation

With the client prone, palpate the quadratus lumborum just superior to the iliac crest and lateral to the lumbar erector spinae with isometric lateral flexion.

CLINICAL NOTES **Guy Wires**

The quadratus lumborum has the extremely important job of stabilizing the lower back. The layers of fibers allow this muscle to offset the action of the other side of the muscle. Unfortunately, if a person lifts a child, for example, using only one side of his body and does not use his lower extremities, the other side of his quadratus lumborum is then at risk. This muscle is often in a state of spasm in most people because of its constant overuse in daily movements and its constant action in gravity. Straining the deep fibers is a very painful problem. Contracted fibers pull on the spinal vertebrae and can cause a lateral lumbar curve and possible subluxations. Posture is often distorted when this muscle is in spasm, creating a bent-forward position because extension is so painful. Strong abdominals and psoas major muscles help support the quadratus lumborum. Safe lifting practices can help prevent injury. See the discussion on psoas major in Chapter 15.

Muscle Specifics

The quadratus lumborum is important in lumbar lateral flexion and in elevation of the pelvis on the same side in the standing position—an action often called *hip hiking.* Studies on cadavers have shown that this muscle has a varied presentation, depending on the space between the 12th rib and the iliac crest. What remains the same is that there are usually three different fiber directions:

- *Iliocostal fibers* run from the 12th rib to the crest and iliolumbar ligament in a vertical direction.
- *Lumbocostal fibers* run from the 12th rib to the transverse processes of the lumbar vertebrae.
- *Iliolumbar fibers* run from the transverse processes L1 through L4 to the crest of the ilium and iliolumbar ligament.

These fiber directions help provide a visual of how the quadratus lumborum acts as tension wires for stabilization of the lumbar spine.

Clinical Flexibility

Left lumbar lateral flexion while in lumbar flexion stretches the right quadratus lumborum, and vice versa. Spinal rotation with lumbar flexion will help isolate each side. The lateral stretch for the erector spinae applies here.

Strengthening

Trunk rotation and lateral flexion movements against resistance are good exercises for development of the quadratus lumborum muscle. Stand with a weight in one hand, with arms at the sides. Contract the involved side and reach laterally, lifting the weight with the lateral flexors. *Contraindications:* Tenderness may be felt on the involved side as muscle fibers shorten.

OIAI MUSCLE CHART QUADRATUS LUMBORUM (kwad-ra´tus lum-bo´rum) Guy wires for the lower back

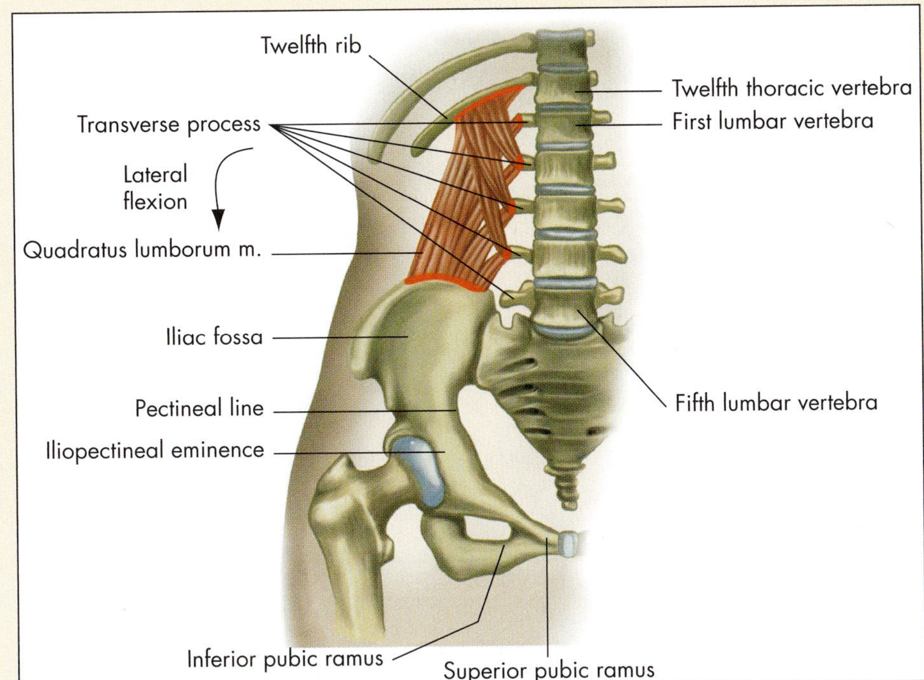

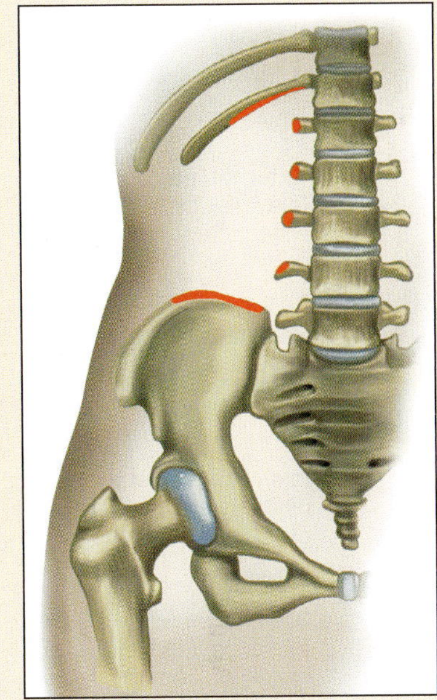

Name of Muscle	Origins	Insertion	Actions	Innervations
Quadratus lumborum	Posterior inner lip of iliac crest and transverse processes of lower four lumbar vertebrae	Transverse processes of upper four lumbar vertebrae and lower border of 12th rib	Lateral flexion to the ipsilateral side, "guy wires," stabilization of pelvis and lumbar spine, bilateral extension of lumbar spine, anterior pelvic rotation, lateral pelvic rotation to contralateral side	Branches of T12, L1

Muscles of the Thorax

The thoracic muscles are involved almost entirely in respiration (figure 13.15). During quiet rest, the diaphragm is responsible for breathing movements. As it contracts and flattens, the thoracic volume is increased and air is inspired to equalize the pressure. The other thoracic muscles take on a more significant role in inspiration when greater amounts of air are needed, such as during exercise. The scalene muscles elevate the first two ribs to increase the thoracic volume. (See more on the scalenes in Chapter 14.) Further expansion of the chest is accomplished by the external intercostals. Additional muscles of inspiration are the levator costarum and the serratus posterior. Forced expiration occurs with contraction of the internal intercostals, transversus thoracis, and subcostals. All of these muscles are detailed in table 13.4. (*Note:* The pectoralis minor and serratus anterior also serve as accessory respiratory muscles. Refer to Chapter 4 to review those muscles.)

Individual Muscles of the Abdominal Wall

Figures 13.16 and 13.17 show the abdominal wall muscles as a whole.

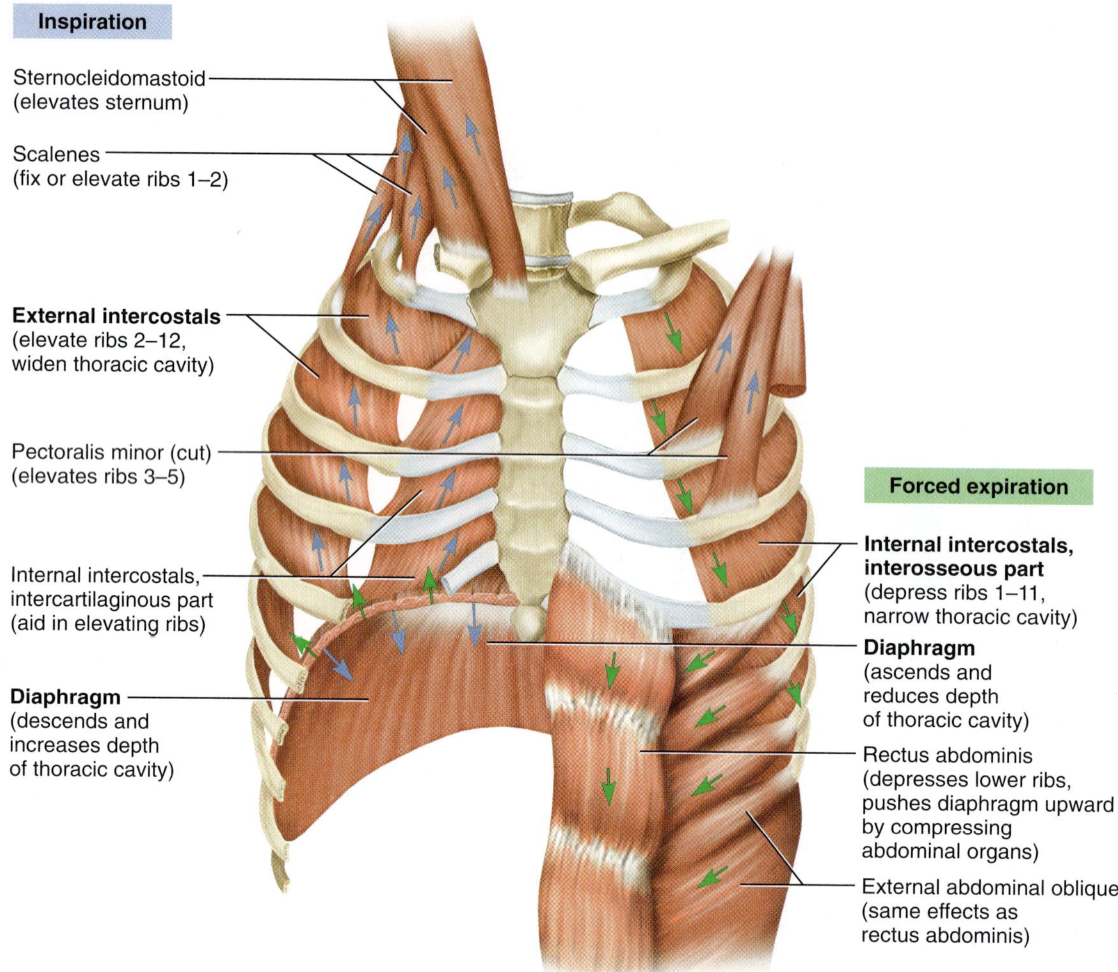

FIGURE 13.15 Muscles of respiration, anterior view

RECTUS ABDOMINIS MUSCLE

Palpation

Palpate the rectus abdominis on the anteromedial surface of the abdomen, between the rib cage and the pubic bone, with isometric trunk flexion.

CLINICAL NOTES **Front of the Back**

Sit forward and slump into a chair. This position makes it almost impossible to take a deep breath because it collapses the chest into the abdomen. Weak abdominals encourage the psoas major to assist in trunk flexion, an action that places strain on the psoas attachments on the lumbar spine. Although the rectus abdominis is the most superficial of the abdominal muscles, it has the most capability to tone due to its straight fibers and tendinous inscriptions. Keeping this muscle strong supports the lower back, assists posture, and promotes breathing from the abdomen.

Muscle Specifics

The rectus abdominis muscle controls the tilt of the pelvis and the consequent curvature of the lower spine. By rotating the pelvis posteriorly, the rectus abdominis flattens the lower back, making the erector spinae muscles more effective as an extensor of the spine and the hip flexors (the iliopsoas muscle, particularly) more effective in raising the legs.

In a relatively lean person with well-developed abdominals, three distinct sets of lines or depressions may be noted. Each represents an area of tendinous connective tissue connecting or supporting

TABLE 13.4 Muscles of the Thorax

Muscle	Origins	Insertion	Actions	Innervations
Diaphragm	Circumference of thoracic inlet from xiphoid process, costal cartilages 6–12, and lumbar vertebrae	Central tendon of diaphragm	Depresses and draws central tendon forward in inhalation, reduces pressure in thoracic cavity, and increases pressure in abdominal cavity	Phrenic nerve (C3–C5)
Internal intercostals	Longitudinal ridge on inner surface of ribs and costal cartilages	Superior border of next rib below	Elevates costal cartilages of ribs 1–4 during inhalation, depresses all ribs in exhalation	Intercostal branches of T1–T11
External intercostals	Inferior border of ribs	Superior border of next rib below	Elevates ribs	Intercostal branches of T1–T11
Levator costarum	Ends of transverse processes of C7, T2–T12	Outer surface of angle of next rib below origin	Elevates ribs, lateral flexion of thoracic spine	Intercostal nerves
Subcostales	Inner surface of each rib near its angle	Medially on the inner surface of 2nd or 3rd rib below	Draws the ventral part of the ribs downward, decreasing the volume of the thoracic cavity	Intercostal nerves
Scalenus anterior	Transverse processes of C3–C6	Inner border and upper surface of 1st rib	Elevates 1st rib, flexion, lateral flexion, and contralateral rotation of cervical spine	Ventral rami of C5–C6, sometimes C4
Scalenus medius	Transverse processes of C2–C7	Superior surface of 1st rib	Elevates 1st rib, flexion, lateral flexion, and contralateral rotation of cervical spine	Ventral rami of C3–C8
Scalenus posterior	Transverse processes of C5–C7	Outer surface of 2nd rib	Elevates 2nd rib, flexion, lateral flexion, and slight contralateral rotation of cervical spine	Ventral rami of C6–C8
Serratus posterior (superior)	Ligamentum nuchae, spinous processes of C7, T1, and T2 or T3	Superior borders lateral to angles of ribs 2–5	Elevates upper ribs	Branches from anterior primary rami of T1–T4
Serratus posterior (inferior)	Spinous processes of T10–T12 and L1–L3	Inferior borders lateral to angles of ribs 9–12	Counteracts inward pull of diaphragm by drawing last 4 ribs outward and downward	Branches from anterior primary rami of T9–T12
Transversus thoracis	Inner surface of sternum and xiphoid process, sternal ends of costal cartilages of ribs 3–6	Inner surfaces and inferior borders of costal cartilages 3–6	Depresses ribs	Intercostal branches of T3–T6

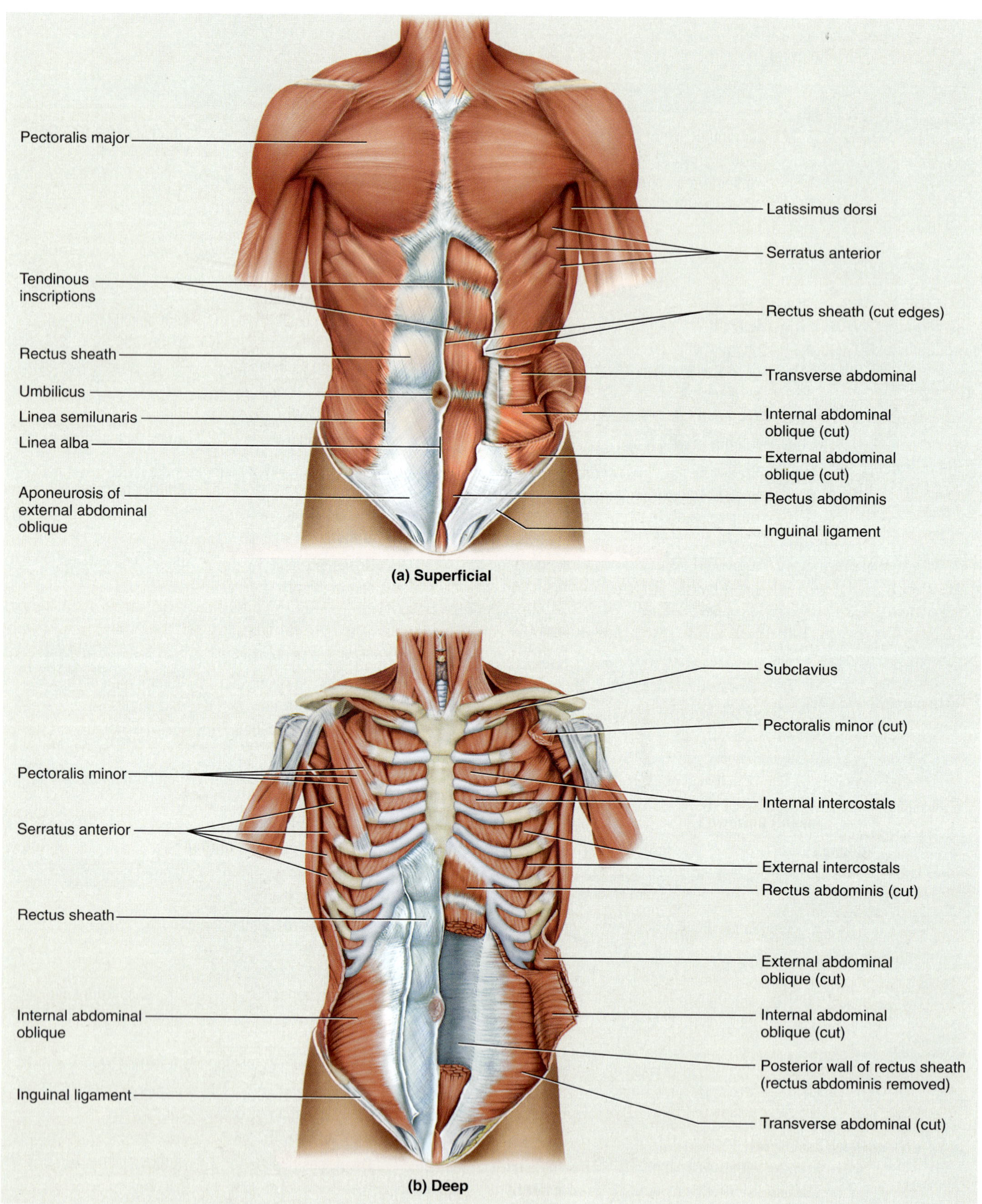

FIGURE 13.16 Muscles of the superficial and deep abdominal wall

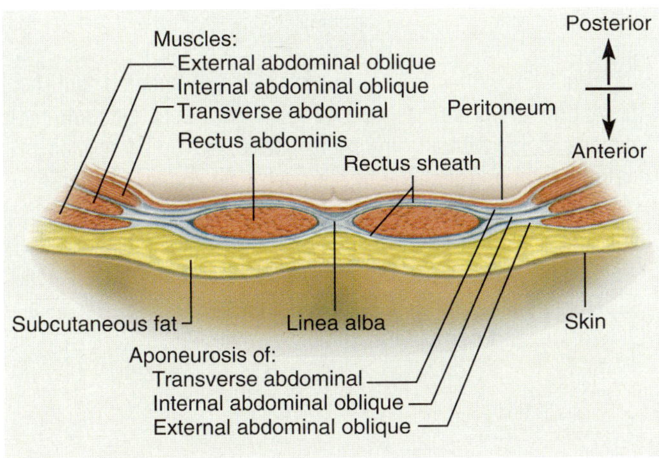

FIGURE 13.17 Cross section of the anterior abdominal wall

the abdominal arrangement of muscles in lieu of bony attachments. Running vertically from the xiphoid process through the umbilicus to the pubis is the **linea alba.** It divides each rectus abdominis and serves as its medial border. It is possible for the linea alba to divide the rectus abdominis into two sections, especially during pregnancy. Lateral to each rectus abdominis is the linea semilunaris, a crescent, or moon-shaped, line running vertically. This line represents the aponeurosis connecting the lateral border of the rectus abdominis and the medial border of the external and internal abdominal obliques. The **tendinous inscriptions** are horizontal indentations that transect the rectus abdominis at three or more locations, giving the muscle its segmented appearance. The tendinous inscriptions allow each section of the rectus abdominis to be strengthened.

OIAI MUSCLE CHART RECTUS ABDOMINIS (rek´tus ab-dom´i-nis) Flexor of the trunk—the six pack

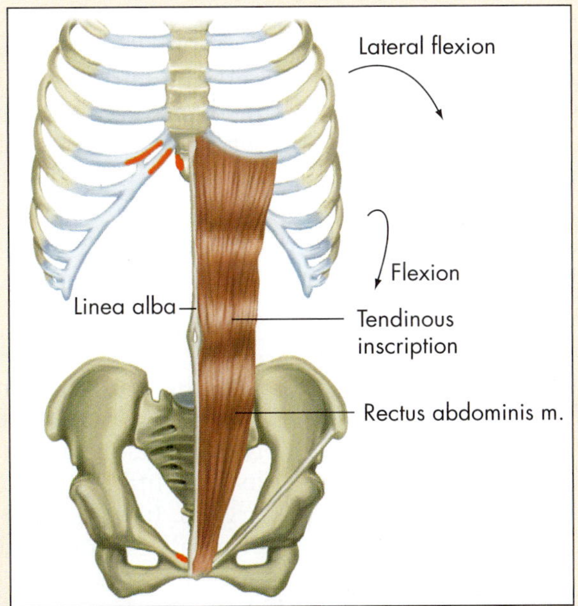

Name of Muscle	Origins	Insertion	Actions	Innervations
Rectus abdominis	Crest of pubis	Cartilage of 5th, 6th, 7th ribs and xiphoid	Flexion of trunk, compression of abdominal contents, lateral flexion same side, posterior pelvic rotation	Intercostal nerves (T7–T12)

Clinical Flexibility

The rectus abdominis is stretched by simultaneously hyperextending both the lumbar and thoracic spines. Stand and lift the arms overhead. Reach back into hyperextension, moving your arms back with your head. *Contraindications:* Use caution if disk issues are present. This exercise places pressure on the lower lumbar disks.

Strengthening

There are several exercises for the abdominal muscles, such as bent-knee sit-ups, crunches, and isometric contractions. To effectively challenge the muscles, these exercises should be done slowly—especially on the eccentric portion of the exercise. Bent-knee sit-ups with the arms folded across the chest are considered by many to be a safe and efficient exercise. Crunches are thought to be even more effective for isolating the work to the abdominals. Both of these exercises shorten the iliopsoas muscle and other hip flexors, thus reducing their ability to generate force. Twisting to the left and right brings the oblique muscles into more active contraction. In all of these exercises, it is important to use proper technique, which involves gradually moving to the up (flexed) position until the lumbar spine is actively flexed maximally and then slowly returning to the beginning position. The lower back should be flat against the floor. Jerking movements using momentum should be avoided. While crunches and other intense exercises are popular forms for defining the abdominals, simple pelvic tilts are also effective. This is accomplished by flattening the low back by tilting the pelvis posteriorly, with the knees bent. *Contraindications:* Movement beyond full lumbar flexion only exercises the hip flexors, which is not usually an objective. These exercises may be helpful in strengthening the abdominals; however, use careful analysis to determine which are indicated in the presence of various low-back injuries and problems.

EXTERNAL OBLIQUE MUSCLE

Palpation

With the client supine, palpate the external oblique lateral to the rectus abdominis between the iliac crest and the lower ribs, with active rotation to the contralateral side.

CLINICAL NOTES **Cross Crawl Muscle**

Touching the elbow to the opposite knee is often used for exercising the external oblique muscle, as any rotary movements engage its fibers. Like the rectus abdominis, this muscle is important for core strength for sports movements, such as the golf swing. The external oblique is not just an abdominal muscle; along with the internal oblique, it forms the side of the abdomen and the side of the back. The aponeurosis of the external oblique forms the inguinal ligament and interdigitates with the serratus anterior and latissimus dorsi, further connecting the abdomen to the side of the chest and to the back. Stretching and strengthening the obliques is important for stability of the entire trunk and spine.

Muscle Specifics

Working on each side of the abdomen, the external oblique abdominal muscles aid in rotating the trunk to the contralateral side when they work independently of each other. When they work together, they aid the rectus abdominis muscle in its described action.

Clinical Flexibility

Each side of the external oblique must be stretched individually. The right side is stretched by moving into extreme left lateral flexion combined with extension or by extreme lumbar rotation to the right combined with extension. Use the stretch described for the erector spinae here, but with a variation: Turn the torso so that one shoulder faces almost posteriorly, and reach back into lateral flexion and hyperextension. *Contraindications:* Use caution if disk issues are present.

Strengthening

The external oblique muscle is important to strengthen for core stability of the trunk and spine. Along with rectus abdominis, it is often weak in individuals, leaving little support for the low back and internal organs. It is strengthened using a medium-size exercise ball. Perform while seated on the edge of a table or bench or while seated on another large ball. Clasp the ball with both hands, and extend the arms out in front. Contracting the abdominals, begin moving slowly to the left or right. Rotate as far as possible; then rotate to the other side. The side obliques should "burn" slightly as they contract, and they should provide the rotary movement.

As an alternative, the left external oblique abdominal muscle contracts strongly during sit-ups when the trunk rotates to the right, as in touching the left elbow to the right knee. Rotating to the left brings the right external oblique into action. *Contraindications:* Use caution if disk issues are present.

OIAI MUSCLE CHART EXTERNAL OBLIQUE ABDOMINAL (ek-stur´nel o-bleek´ ab-dom´i-nel) Waist muscle

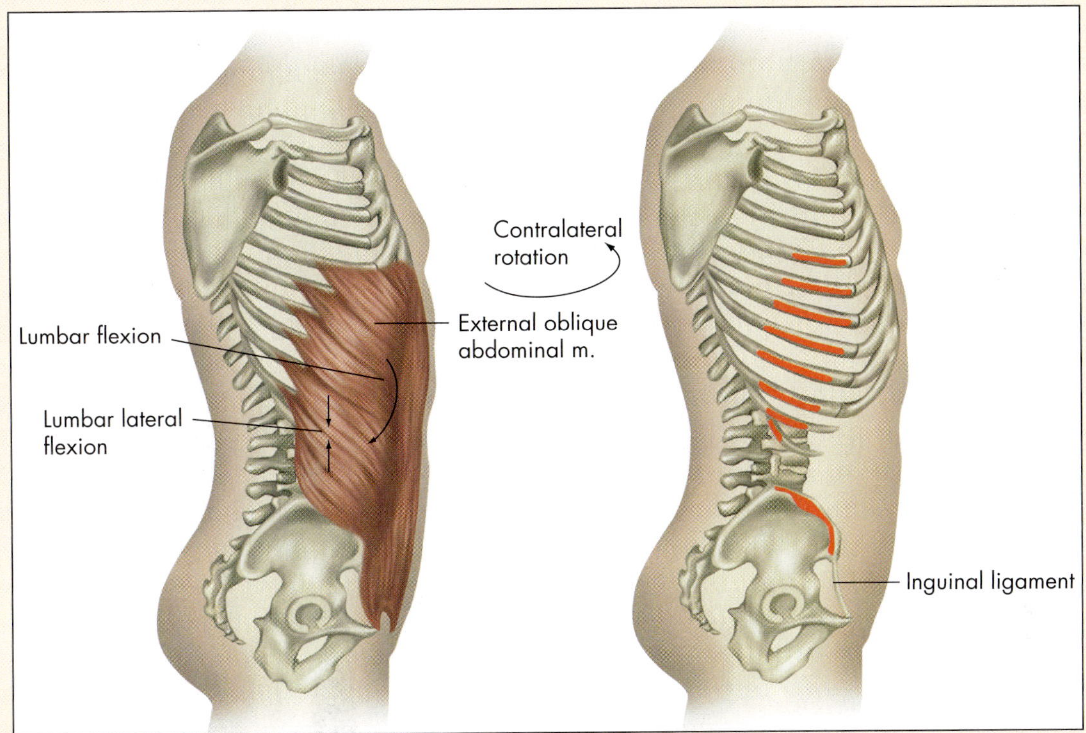

Name of Muscle	Origins	Insertion	Actions	Innervations
External oblique	Lower eight ribs, interdigitating with serratus anterior and latissimus dorsi	Abdominal aponeurosis and anterior iliac crest, inguinal ligament, crest of pubis	Compression of abdominal contents, bilateral flexion of spine, lateral flexion *Unilateral:* rotation of trunk to opposite side, pelvic rotation to opposite side	Intercostal nerves (T8–T12), iliohypogastric nerve (T12, L1), ilioinguinal nerve (L1)

INTERNAL OBLIQUE MUSCLE

Palpation

With the client supine, palpate the internal oblique on the anterolateral abdomen between the iliac crest and the lower ribs, with active rotation to the ipsilateral side.

CLINICAL NOTES **Opposites Attract**

The internal oblique gives strength to the layer of abdominal muscles by having fiber directions that are the opposite of those of the external oblique, much like an intricate patch. Together they create strong lateral flexors and trunk rotators. The internal oblique acts as an antagonist to the diaphragm, assisting in reducing the volume in the thoracic chest. Remember to work around the crest and sides of the abdomen to release hypertonic tissue.

Muscle Specifics

The internal oblique abdominal muscles run diagonally in the direction opposite that of the external obliques; when the muscles are working independently

OIAI MUSCLE CHART INTERNAL OBLIQUE ABDOMINAL (in-ter´nel o-bleek ab-dom´i-nel) Beneath the external oblique

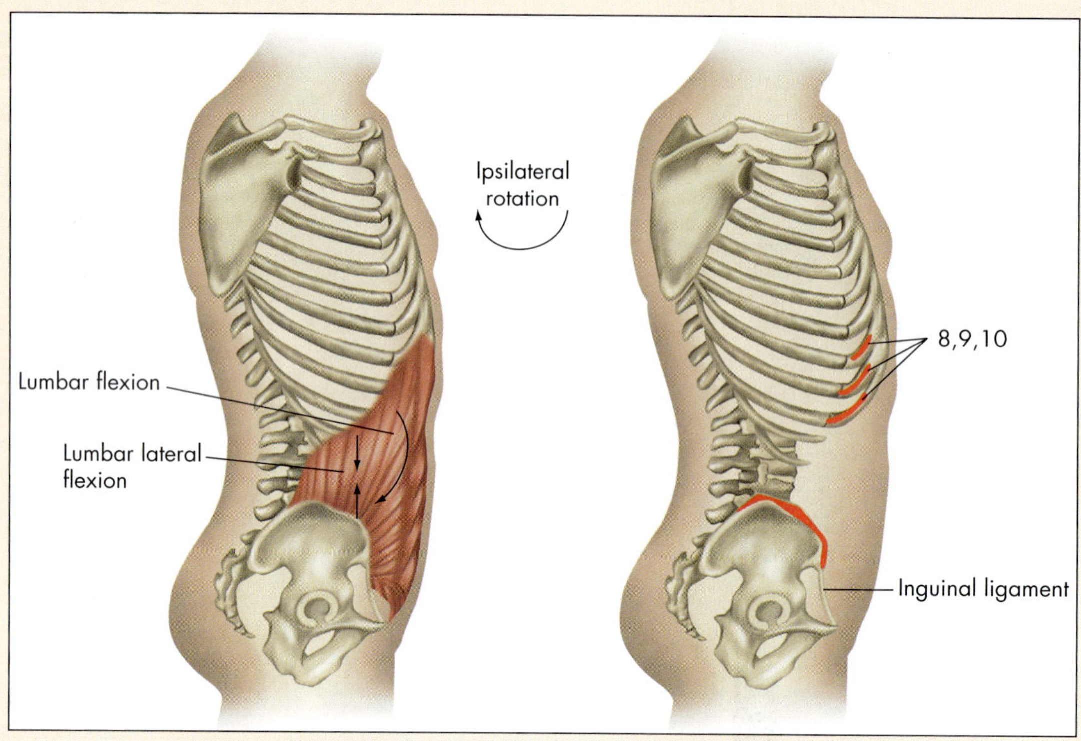

Name of Muscle	Origins	Insertion	Actions	Innervations
Internal oblique	Inguinal ligament and anterior iliac crest, lumbar fascia	Costal cartilage of last three or four ribs, abdominal aponeurosis	Bilateral flexion of spine, compression of abdominal contents *Unilateral:* lateral flexion, rotation of trunk to same side, posterior pelvic rotation, opposite-side pelvic rotation	Intercostal nerves (T8–T12), iliohypogastric nerve (T12, L1), ilioinguinal nerve (L1)

of each other, rotate the trunk to the ipsilateral side. The left internal oblique rotates to the left, and the right internal oblique rotates to the right.

Clinical Flexibility

As with the external oblique, each side of the internal oblique must be stretched individually. Stretch the right side in the manner used for the external oblique.

Strengthening

Strengthen the internal oblique muscle in the same way as strengthening the external oblique. In rotary movements, the internal oblique and the external oblique on opposite sides of each other always work together.

TRANSVERSUS ABDOMINIS MUSCLE

Palpation

With the client supine, palpate the transversus abdominis on the anterolateral abdomen between the iliac crest and the lower ribs during forceful exhalation. The transversus abdominis is very difficult to distinguish from the abdominal obliques.

OIAI MUSCLE CHART TRANSVERSUS ABDOMINIS (trans-vurs´us ab-dom´i-nis) Deepest abdominal muscle

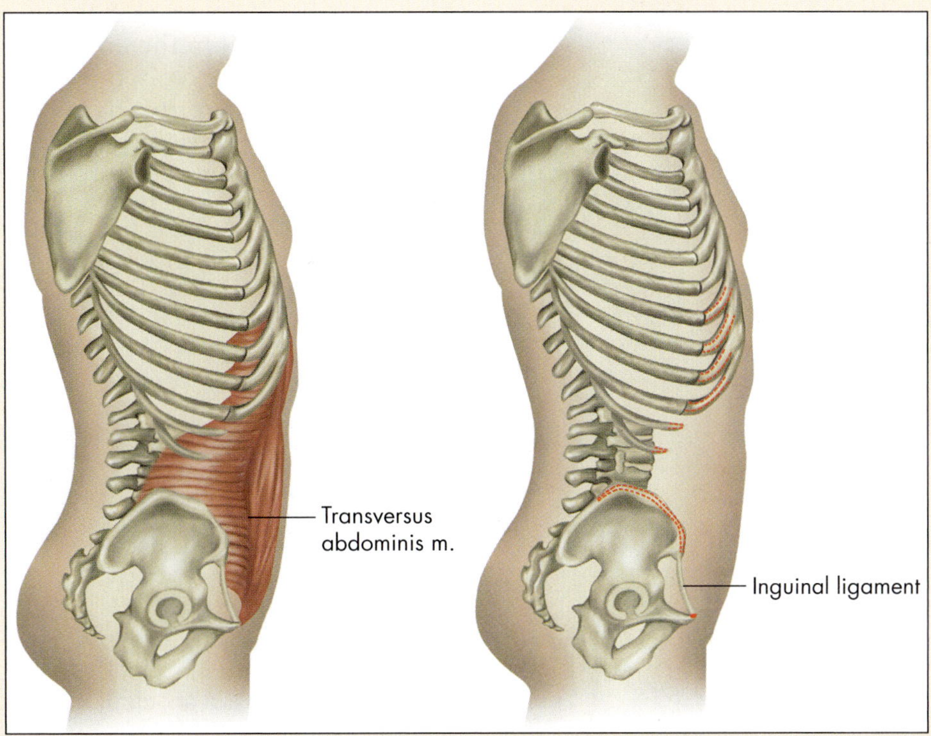

Name of Muscle	Origins	Insertions	Actions	Innervations
Transversus abdominis	Inguinal ligament, iliac crest, thoracolumbar aponeurosis, lower margin of rib cage (lower six ribs), lumbar fascia	Abdominal aponeurosis and linea alba, crest of pubis, iliopectineal line	Interdigitates with fibers of diaphragm and compression of abdominal contents, increases intra-abdominal pressure, helps in forced expiration	Intercostal nerves (T7–T12), iliohypogastric nerve (T12, L1), ilioinguinal nerve (L1)

CLINICAL NOTES

Pelvic Tilt

The transversus abdominis is one of the body's major core muscles, and part of the job of abdominal muscles is to compress the internal organs. This muscle forms a wall across the abdomen, keeping the internal organs secure. Should the abdominal muscles have poor tone, an abdominal hernia could develop, effectively allowing organs to penetrate the cavity. Additional adipose tissue helps gravity pull the abdominal contents forward. The importance of strong abdominal muscles cannot be overstated.

Muscle Specifics

The transversus abdominis is the chief muscle of forced expiration and is effective—together with the rectus abdominis, the external oblique abdominal, and the internal oblique abdominal muscles—in helping hold the abdomen flat. This abdominal flattening and forced expulsion of the abdominal contents is the only action of this muscle. It is also used to help push during childbirth. Pregnant women should begin strengthening all the abdominal muscles early to ease childbirth.

Clinical Flexibility

The transversus abdominis muscle is stretched by taking the torso into hyperextension. Stand and raise the arms overhead, and slowly move into hyperextension, feeling for a stretch in the abdominals. See the contraindications for stretching the rectus abdominis.

Strengthening

The transversus abdominis muscle is strengthened effectively by attempting to draw the abdominal contents back toward the spine. This may be done isometrically in the supine position or while standing. The pelvic tilt exercise assists building tone in all the abdominals. To perform the pelvic tilt, lay on a flat surface and flex the knees. Lift only the hips and pull in the abdomen, exhaling. Do not lift the lower back off the floor. Repeat as often as comfortable. *Contraindications:* Use caution if disk issues are present. This is a safe exercise for lower-back discomfort, but consult a physician if pain exists.

CHAPTER *summary*

Introduction

- ✔ The trunk contains the internal organs, houses the spinal column, and provides attachment for the upper and lower extremities.

Bones

- ✔ There are 24 articulating vertebrae in the spinal column, and 5 and 4 fused bones in the sacrum and coccyx, respectively. There are 7 cervical, 12 thoracic, and 5 lumbar vertebrae.
- ✔ Parts of the vertebra are the spinous process, transverse process, and body.
- ✔ The spine has three normal dynamic curves.
- ✔ Abnormal curves either are genetic or can develop for a variety of reasons. The curves include kyphosis, lordosis, and scoliosis.
- ✔ There are 12 pairs of ribs, 7 of which are true, attaching to the sternum; 5 pairs are false, and 2 of these pairs are floating ribs. The ribs attach to the vertebrae posteriorly.
- ✔ The manubrium of the sternum and the xiphoid process at the end of the sternum provide attachment sites. The clavicle is also an attachment site for the sternocleidomastoid.
- ✔ Abdominal muscles attach to pubic and iliac crest bones and to the inguinal ligament.
- ✔ The mastoid process and occiput provide attachment for lateral and posterior cervical muscles.

Joints

- ✔ The first joint is the atlantooccipital joint, allowing flexion and extension.
- ✔ The atlas and axis form a pivot joint (atlantoaxial joint), allowing rotation.
- ✔ The rest of the vertebrae are gliding joints.

Movements of the Trunk and Head

- ✔ The head moves forward with flexion, back with extension, and toward the shoulder in lateral flexion; the chin rotates toward the shoulder in rotation.
- ✔ The lumbar spine provides movement in flexion, extension, lateral flexion, reduction, and rotation.

Trunk and Spinal Column Muscles

- ✔ The sternocleidomastoid is located anteriorly and laterally.
- ✔ The splenius muscles connect the thoracic region to the head and upper cervical vertebrae.
- ✔ There are additional intrinsic muscles that move the head and neck, including the deep suboccipitals.
- ✔ Anteriorly, the rectus abdominis, external oblique, and internal oblique flex the trunk. The transversus abdominis assists in respiration and is the deepest abdominal muscle.
- ✔ The erector spinae muscles span the back from the sacrum to the occiput. This large group is divided into three groups of three muscles each, for nine muscles on each side of the spine.
- ✔ The quadratus lumborum is situated deep in the posterior lumbar region between the 12th rib and the iliac crest.

Nerves

- ✔ The accessory nerve and spinal nerves C2 and C3 innervate the sternocleidomastoid. Spinal nerves innervate the erector spinae and the quadratus lumborum. Intercostal nerves innervate abdominal muscles together with the iliohypogastric and ilioinguinal nerves.

Muscles That Move the Head

- ✔ There are many layers of muscles that surround the cervical spine, connect the head to the vertebrae and the vertebrae to the trunk, and provide movement on multiple levels. See table 13.2 on page 270 for additional muscles that move the head.

Individual Muscles of the Trunk and Spinal Column—Muscles That Move the Head and Neck

- ✔ *Sternocleidomastoid,* named for its attachments, begins at the sternum and clavicle and inserts at the mastoid process. It flexes the head forward, laterally flexes on the same side, and rotates the head to the opposite side.
- ✔ *Splenius capitis* and *cervicis* are bandage muscles that wrap around the neck. They connect the thoracic spine to the occiput and to the cervical vertebrae. They laterally flex and rotate the head and neck.

Muscles of the Vertebral Column

- ✔ Deep muscles of the vertebral column provide a network of muscles that connect the vertebra to vertebra and stability for the spine. See table 13.3 on page 276 for a listing of deep muscles of the vertebral column.

Individual Muscles of the Trunk and Spinal Column—Muscles That Move the Vertebral Column

- ✔ *Erector spinae* comprise nine muscles in three divisions; the group is a spinal extensor on either side of the vertebral column. This elaborate muscle group spans from the sacrum and attaches to ribs and vertebrae on its way to the mastoid process and the occiput. The three major divisions are the iliocostalis, longissimus, and spinalis. Although the erector spinae's primary action is extension of the whole spinal column, the divisions are involved in lateral flexion of the head and trunk and assist in other movements.
- ✔ *Quadratus lumborum* is a deep lower-back stabilizer. It spans from the 12th rib to the lumbar vertebrae and the iliac crest. It has multiple actions and is prone to soft-tissue injury when bearing the brunt of heavy lifting or incorrect body mechanics.

Muscles of the Thorax

- ✔ Muscles of the thorax assist in the process of respiration. See table 13.4 on page 281 for muscles of the thorax.

Individual Muscles of the Abdominal Wall

- ✔ *Rectus abdominis* spans from the ribs and xiphoid process to the pubis. It is a major trunk flexor.
- ✔ *External oblique* is located laterally to the rectus abdominis but connects to it through abdominal fascia. It interdigitates with the serratus anterior and with latissimus dorsi. It laterally flexes the trunk to the same side and will rotate to the opposite side.
- ✔ *Internal oblique* is located anteriorly and lateral to rectus abdominis. It is layered beneath the external oblique. It works with the external oblique to laterally flex to the same side and rotate the trunk.
- ✔ *Transversus abdominis* is the deepest abdominal muscle and is attached to lumbar fascia. It helps with forced expiration.

CHAPTER *review*

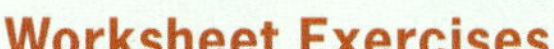

Worksheet Exercises

As an aid to learning, for in-class or out-of-class assignments, or for testing, tear-out worksheets are found at the end of the text, on pages 535–538.

True or False

Write true *or* false *after each statement.*

1. The sternocleidomastoid rotates the head to the same side.
2. The splenius capitis and cervicis attach to the thoracic vertebrae and connect the head and neck to the thoracic spine.
3. The sternocleidomastoid and splenius capitis and cervicis oppose each other in flexion and extension.
4. The most inferior division in the erector spinae muscles is the spinalis.
5. The suboccipitals are intrinsic muscles for the head and neck.
6. The rectus abdominis and the erector spinae both flex the trunk.
7. Tiny muscles located in between the spinous processes are called intertransversarii.
8. The vertebrae have a spinous process and a transverse process.
9. The atlas and axis do not rotate the head.
10. There are 25 pairs of spinal nerves.
11. The quadratus lumborum muscle is often related to lumbar dysfunctions.
12. Scoliosis can be caused by muscle imbalances.

Short Answers

Write your answers on the lines provided.

1. Which muscles assist in flexion of the trunk?

____

____

____

2. Which muscle is the primary flexor of the head and neck?

3. Which muscle of the abdomen has the primary function of respiration?

4. List the muscles of the abdomen superficial to deep.

5. Which muscle is made up of three groups of three muscles bilateral to the spine?

6. How does the quadratus lumborum act as a stabilizing guy wire?

7. What muscle might be contracted in a head-forward posture?

8. What does *rectus* mean?

9. What head flexor does the accessory nerve innervate?

10. What is the name of the line between the two sides of the rectus abdominis?

11. What is the name of the horizontal indentations in the rectus abdominis that give it the six-pack look?

12. How should the sternocleidomastoid be stretched and strengthened?

13. How would one stretch the quadratus lumborum?

Multiple Choice

Circle the correct answers.

1. The attachments for rectus abdominis are:
   a. xiphoid process; ribs 5, 6, 7; crest of pubis
   b. xiphoid process; ribs 8, 9, 10; crest of pubis
   c. sternum; ribs 5, 6, 7; iliac crest
   d. none of the above
2. The erector spinae muscles are divided into the following groups:
   a. longissimus, spinalis, quadratus lumborum
   b. spinalis, serratus posterior, longissimus
   c. iliocostalis, longissimus, spinalis
   d. none of the above
3. An increased posterior concavity of the lumbar spine is called what type of curve?
   a. kyphosis
   b. scoliosis
   c. lordosis
   d. bad back
4. The center of the intervertebral disk is called the:
   a. annulus fibrosus
   b. vertebral body

c. cavity for the spinal cord
d. nucleus pulposus

5. There are how many pairs of ribs?
   a. 12
   b. 10
   c. 8
   d. 9
6. There are how many articulating vertebrae?
   a. 12
   b. 36
   c. 24
   d. 48
7. The suboccipitals consist of:
   a. rectus capitis lateralis, obliquus capitis superior and inferior, semispinalis capitis
   b. rectus capitis posterior major and minor, obliquus capitis superior and inferior
   c. semispinalis, trapezius, splenius capitis, rectus capitis anterior
   d. none of the above
8. Muscles of the thorax that are located between ribs and assist in respiration are called the:
   a. scalenes
   b. intercostals
   c. sternocleidomastoid
   d. rectus abdominis
9. The muscles in the abdominal area connect to each other by:
   a. bone
   b. aponeurosis
   c. tendon
   d. adipose tissue
10. The ligament that attaches the iliac crest to the pubic bone and allows muscular attachment is called the:
    a. symphysis pubis
    b. iliotibial band
    c. inguinal ligament
    d. carpometacarpal ligament

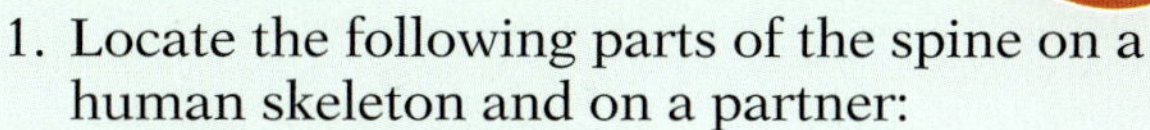

EXPLORE & *practice*

1. Locate the following parts of the spine on a human skeleton and on a partner:
   a. Cervical vertebrae
   b. Thoracic vertebrae
   c. Lumbar vertebrae
   d. Spinous processes
   e. Transverse processes
   f. Sacrum
   g. Manubrium
   h. Xiphoid process
   i. Sternum
   j. Rib cage (various ribs)
2. Palpate the following muscles on a partner:
   a. Rectus abdominis
   b. External oblique abdominal
   c. Internal oblique abdominal
   d. Erector spinae
   e. Sternocleidomastoid
3. Contrast crunches, bent-knee sit-ups, and straight-leg sit-ups. Which muscles are you feeling more in which exercise? Explain.
4. Have a partner stand and assume a position exhibiting good posture. What motions in each region of the spine does gravity attempt to produce? Which muscles are responsible for counteracting these motions against the pull of gravity?
5. Compare and contrast the spinal curves of a partner sitting erect with those of one sitting slouched in a chair. Which muscles are responsible for maintaining good sitting posture?
6. Which exercise is better for the development of the abdominal muscles—leg lifts or sit-ups? Analyze each one in regard to the activity of the abdominal muscles. Defend your answer.
7. Why is good abdominal muscular development so important? Why is this area so frequently neglected?
8. Why are weak abdominal muscles frequently blamed for lower-back pain?
9. Prepare an oral or a written report on abdominal or back injuries found in the literature.

10. *Muscle analysis chart:* Fill in the chart below by listing the muscles primarily involved in each movement.

Cervical spine	
Flexion	Extension
Lateral flexion right	Rotation right
Lateral flexion left	Rotation left
Lumbar spine	
Flexion	Extension
Lateral flexion right	Rotation right
Lateral flexion left	Rotation left

11. *Antagonistic muscle action chart:* Fill in the chart below by listing the muscle(s) or parts of muscles that are antagonistic in their actions to the muscles in the left column.

Agonist	Antagonist
Splenius capitis	
Splenius cervicis	
Sternocleidomastoid	
Erector spinae	
Rectus abdominis	
External oblique abdominal	
Internal oblique abdominal	
Quadratus lumborum	

chapter 14

The Balancing Act: Structural Perspectives of the Head and Neck and Dimensional Massage Techniques

Learning Outcomes

After completing this chapter, you should be able to:

14-1 Define key terms.

14-2 Explore on a partner the origins and insertions of the muscles of the head and neck specific to this chapter.

14-3 Organize and list the agonists and antagonists that produce and oppose the movements of the head and neck.

14-4 Review general pathologies and conditions of the muscles of the head and neck.

14-5 Discuss a treatment protocol for conditions of torticollis, stiff neck, whiplash, and tension headache.

14-6 Demonstrate safe body mechanics.

14-7 Practice specific techniques on the head and neck muscles.

14-8 Incorporate dimensional massage therapy techniques in a regular routine or use them when needed.

14-9 Determine safe treatment protocols and refer clients to other health professionals when necessary.

KEY TERMS

Headache
Occipital nerve entrapment
Occipitofrontalis
Stiff neck
Temporalis
Temporomandibular joint (TMJ) syndrome
Torticollis
Whiplash
Wry neck

Introduction

As people go about their daily activities, they often take for granted the ability to balance and move the head on the neck. The joints in the neck enable movement of the head, including rotation, flexion, and extension, and even lateral flexion to cradle a phone when the hands are occupied. However, a significant number of problems can interrupt one's ability to move the head freely. Injuries, disease, stiff necks, headaches, compensatory muscle tension due to postural positions of the shoulder girdle, and shoulder joint actions and entrapments contribute to head and neck soft-tissue dysfunction. Massage therapy can provide relief from much of the soft-tissue dysfunction causing reduced movement and discomfort in the head and neck region.

This chapter offers a close look at the structure and movement of the head and neck, specific information on the pertinent muscles in the region, and discussion about injuries, overuse syndromes, and nerve complaints. Treatment protocol and dimensional massage techniques are outlined and described for practice.

Note: Examination of the trunk and deep tissue of the lower back is included in Chapter 16, following discussion on the hip joint and pelvic girdle in Chapter 15.

Structural Perspectives of the Head and Neck

Picture a bowling ball balancing on a stick. This is similar to how the head, which weighs approximately 10 to 12 pounds, precariously perches on seven cervical vertebrae and disks and is supported only by a network of muscles, tendons, and ligaments. The cervical vertebrae connect to the thoracic and lumbar spines, and the trunk lends its bulk to supply a base for the neck. The muscles work constantly to support the head in its many positions. The posture of the shoulders, neck, and head influences the condition and tonicity of the muscles. When the shoulders are rounded forward from slumping in a chair, the head tries to compensate for the posture by assuming a forward position not unlike that of a turtle sticking its neck out of its shell. This does, however, present a problem. When located in front of the body, the head is perceived to weigh more than it does when balanced on top of the spine. Gravity assists the head-forward posture to cause more pressure on the cervical vertebrae and stress on the posterior cervical muscles. The results over time could be increased tension, headaches, muscular hypertonicity, trigger points, and postural acceptance of the head-forward posture.

Regardless of the head's actual position, all the muscles connected to the head and/or skeletal structure participate in its actions. The head can flex forward, side bend or laterally flex, rotate, extend, and hyperextend. Generally, muscles located anteriorly flex the head, and muscles located posteriorly extend the head. Muscles do not work alone; they work in collective groups. They are strategically placed to oppose each other perfectly to create balance, offset primary action, and support a strong structure.

Flexion is complicated by the weight of the head, gravity, and the position of the head as it flexes. For example, when a person flexes the head forward just a few degrees, such as when reading a book, and then extends the head back slowly, the posterior cervical muscles are hard at work. While the head is in flexion, the posterior cervical muscles are lengthened or stretched, acting as brakes to prevent the head from falling forward. Over time, while the head is in this slightly flexed forward position, the posterior cervical muscles play a continual tug-of-war with the head, building up tension in the muscles that work the hardest. In constant flexion, the flexors eventually get shortened in their contracted state. It takes more force or muscle power to extend the head and counteract the action of flexion and gravity in this sustained position. It is no wonder, then, that the posterior cervical muscles have so much tension constantly combating flexion.

The same principles hold true for lateral flexion. When the head laterally flexes, the opposite side prevents the head from staying in that lateral position. The muscles on the opposite side brake in their lengthened, or *eccentric,* state, already anticipating contraction, or *concentric* action, to return the head to extension or to laterally flex to the other side.

For these reasons, it is important to use massage techniques on all the head and neck muscles because they balance each other and are really part of the total joint action. Dimensional massage methods look at the actions of the client and then examine the opposing muscles: Which muscles are being stretched or lengthened (eccentric contraction) by the action? Which muscles are synergists (concentric contraction)? What are the primary actors or agonists, assistants or synergists, and opposing actors or antagonists, and which muscles are constantly stabilizing the joint? Remember, there may not be a lot of action. The position of the head when it is resting on a pillow or when the person is reading or working at a desk may stress the muscles that need to provide brakes, stability, or action for the head and neck. This particular aspect makes the joints and soft-tissue structures of the head and neck more complicated than others in the body.

The Muscles

The head's balancing act involves many muscles, some of which have been visited and studied in Chapter 4, on the shoulder girdle. These muscles are included here as a review so that students can visualize the movement and structure of the head and neck in a larger perspective. Please refer to the appropriate chapter to review additional information about specific muscles. Pay particular attention to each muscle's agonists, synergists, and antagonists in the review. Additional muscles involved in tension headaches, stiff necks, and postural problems are included to enable a closer examination of the structure and to provide the reader with more information.

TRAPEZIUS

The trapezius is complicated because it has three basic sections: the upper, middle, and lower divisions. The upper and lower sections oppose each other as agonist and antagonist—they perform opposite actions. The trapezius also provides a profound connection between the thoracic region and the head. As tension increases in the shoulders because of their repetitive action of holding up the skeleton, the likelihood of trigger points and referred pain patterns increases. The upper trapezius will work bilaterally to help extend the head and therefore oppose the action of flexion. The middle trapezius assists the rhomboids to resist protraction of the shoulders. The whole trapezius provides tremendous stability for the shoulder girdle because the upper extremities stress the structure with ball-and-socket joint movements. The trapezius can be involved in occipital nerve entrapment. It is a prominent superficial muscle that should be treated first in a protocol of the head and neck.

LEVATOR SCAPULAE

The levator scapulae elevates the scapula. If the levator scapulae is tight, it tends to pull on the scapula; however, its attachments at the cervical transverse processes are tendons hanging on with tenuous threads. Bilaterally it is fairly supportive of the structure; unilaterally it causes stiff neck and possible subluxations at the most movable vertebrae, C1 and C2. A repetitive action of elevating the scapula could result in a pull on the cervical vertebrae and affect the curve. The muscle's hypertonicity could contribute to many headaches. The levator scapulae should be included in the treatment of muscles for any stiff-neck syndrome.

RHOMBOIDS REVISITED

The rhomboids do a lot to prevent the scapulae from protracting off into space. Because people spend so much time these days in sedentary positions at the computer, in the office, or in front of the TV, many suffer from poor posture. Rounded shoulders collapse the chest, make it harder if not impossible to take a complete breath, and lengthen the rhomboids. Rounded shoulders lead to a head-forward posture, which places a lot of stress on the posterior cervical muscles. See Chapter 5 for techniques for the rhomboids and information about opposing contracted pectoralis minor and serratus anterior muscles.

SPLENIUS CAPITIS AND SPLENIUS CERVICIS

The splenius capitis and the splenius cervicis are two distinct muscles connecting the thoracic region to the cervical neck and head. They both work bilaterally and unilaterally. The splenius capitis attaches to the mastoid process underneath the sternocleidomastoid (SCM). It assists the sternocleidomastoid with laterally flexing the head to the same side, but, unlike the SCM, it will rotate the head to the same side. Bilaterally, it extends the head and therefore is in direct opposition to the forward flexion of the sternocleidomastoid. Although the splenius cervicis performs the same actions as the capitis does, its attachments cause a different torque on the spine as it contracts. All the components of both muscles affect posture and free movement of the head and neck. They have the unique ability to have one side rotate the head while the other side extends the head, elevating the chin. These muscles and others are heavily involved and frequently injured in whiplash injuries from automobile accidents, especially if the victim is looking out at the side-view mirror at the time of impact. Therapists must be sure to treat the attachments of these muscles at the spinous processes, as well as at the occiput for the splenius capitis, and treat the splenius cervicis with the levator scapulae.

LONGISSIMUS CAPITIS

The longissimus capitis is part of the erector spinae network. Although it bilaterally extends the head, it unilaterally flexes and rotates the head to the same side. Buried underneath the splenius capitis and sternocleidomastoid, it assists these muscles in their functions. This layering of muscles at the mastoid process and adjacent occipital bone provides a tender area to palpate on the lateral and posterior region of the head and neck. The splenius capitis should be released first.

SEMISPINALIS CAPITIS AND CERVICIS

These muscles are postural supports for the head. They provide a structural tetherline medially to prevent the head from forever being in flexion. The semispinalis capitis fills in the gaps attaching to the occiput between the splenius capitis and the trapezius, which it supports by cushioning the trapezius underneath. The semispinalis capitis can entrap the greater occipital nerve as it travels through the muscle to the trapezius and scalp. The semispinalis capitis and cervicis easily support the cervical spine by attaching to the skull and thoracic spine. If the head was a horse, these muscles would be considered the "reins."

ROTATORES AND MULTIFIDI

The rotatores and multifidi are deep paraspinal muscles. The rotatores connect each vertebra to each other from the transverse process to the superior spinous process. Bilaterally they help extend the spine, and unilaterally they help rotate the vertebrae to the opposite side. Sometimes tenderness can be felt by tapping on the spinous vertebra to which the muscle is attached. The rotatores begin on C2.

The multifidi are slightly longer muscles than the rotatores, and they skip a vertebra in their stretch from bone to bone. They also bilaterally extend the spine and support each other by their opposite attachments. Unilaterally, they contribute to lateral flexion and rotate the vertebrae to the opposite side. Both the rotatores and the multifidi make a good case for the massage therapist to spend time on the soft tissue connecting to the cervical vertebrae.

SUBOCCIPITALS

The suboccipitals provide posterior and medial support for the 1st and 2nd cervical vertebrae and the skull. Unfortunately, they are buried under the trapezius, semispinalis, splenius capitis, and part of the longissimus, so they are hard to palpate and must be treated through layers of these soft tissues. Because they are perched on the most movable of the cervical vertebrae, they are virtually in constant states of motion and repetitive action.

The rectus capitis posterior minor has the mammoth job of stabilization, as it extends the head bilaterally. It tries to oppose the action of flexion, but structurally it is too tiny for the job. It is a constant source of soreness and a probable source of postural tension headaches for many people. The rectus capitis posterior major rotates the head to the opposite side in addition to extending the head bilaterally. The obliquus capitis superior and inferior both rotate the head to the side of muscular activitiy and perform same-side lateral flexion. All of these muscles are very active with the rocking and tilting of the head. If the head is in a head-forward posture, the suboccipitals as a group are at risk and are highly strained. They are likely to be involved in any injury to the C1 and/or C2 regions, headaches, and postural dysfunction.

OCCIPITOFRONTALIS

The **occipitofrontalis** is a combination of the frontalis and occipitalis. The scalp from the front to the back of the head is a highway of connecting muscle fibers and possible referred pain discomfort. It is easy to visualize a "tight" scalp on a client who has a tension headache. Attached just above the eyebrows, the frontalis lifts the brow and wrinkles the forehead. Because the two muscles are so integrated, it is important to manipulate all the soft tissue of the scalp to release the tight fibers. Tight posterior cervical muscles pull on the back of the head and ultimately the occipitalis. It makes sense to treat the occipitofrontalis as a part of unwinding the neck muscles.

TEMPORALIS

The **temporalis** is an interesting muscle. It spans over the entire temporal fossa, which consists of the frontal, parietal, sphenoid, zygomatic, and temporal bones. It is shaped like a shell and covers the side of the head, extending superiorly above the ears. Because it inserts onto the mandible, it develops trigger points and pain patterns, especially in individuals who have **temporomandibular joint (TMJ) syndrome.** TMJ syndrome is a condition that causes pain in the jaw, headaches, and problems opening and closing the jaw. It is caused by trauma, teeth grinding, braces, dental procedures, the jaws being open too long, cervical traction, and other issues. If the capsule in the joint is injured or dislodged, the condition can be even more complicated. Individuals with TMJ may exhibit crepitus in the jaw and sideways movement of the jaw just by opening the mouth. The temporalis can harbor a horrific pain pattern for headache sufferers. It is also included in this chapter because of its proximity to the occipitofrontalis and its involvement with headaches.

STERNOCLEIDOMASTOID

The sternocleidomastoid is a powerful muscle located bilaterally on the anterior neck; it runs at an angle from the sternum and clavicle to the mastoid process. Bilaterally, it flexes the head forward. It laterally flexes to the same side and rotates to the opposite side. Because it attaches laterally at the mastoid process, it is capable of performing extension bilaterally at the atlantooccipital joint. It shares the same nerve as the trapezius and could possibly entrap the accessory nerve with constricted fibers. Students are often leery of treating the sternocleidomastoid because of its proximity to the carotid artery anteriorly. When the SCM is approached correctly, passively shortening the fibers and carefully working the muscle can make for a successful treatment of the soft tissue of the head, neck, and shoulders.

In addition to the individual muscles and structural perspectives, there are other problems that can contribute to head and neck issues. The following information offers a short list of conditions. Students are encouraged to enhance their education with a complete study in pathology.

Injuries and Overuse Syndromes

WHIPLASH

Whiplash is an injury resulting from a sudden impact that causes a violent hyperextension of the head and neck followed by hyperflexion and perhaps an additional hyperextension. Further injury from this condition can include fractures to the cervical vertebrae, subluxations, concussions, sprains, and strains to many neck muscles. Muscles involved can include the sternocleidomastoid, scalenes, longus colli, suboccipitals, splenius capitis and cervicis, levator scapulae, and many other posterior cervical muscles. Whiplash victims must have emergency care to rule out fractures, concussions, and damage to the spinal cord. Some accident victims do not immediately seek emergency care because they do not feel injured directly after the impact. Individuals who have not been diagnosed medically should be referred to a medical professional if they seek massage therapy before undergoing a physical examination by a doctor. Working with whiplash victims requires a team approach that includes diagnosis and clinical treatment, massage therapy, and likely physical therapy and chiropractic.

TORTICOLLIS

Another term for **torticollis** is **wry neck,** although the term *wry neck* often is mistaken as meaning a simple stiff neck. It refers to a spasmodic contraction of the neck muscles, mostly the trapezius and sternocleidomastoid, since they are supplied by the spinal accessory nerve. An individual who presents with this problem cannot move the head, which appears to be stuck in a rotated, somewhat laterally flexed position. This condition is not an ordinary stiff neck, nor is it caused by strained muscles, and it must be diagnosed. It can be caused by infection or central nervous system disorder, or it could be congenital. Massage may or may not be contraindicated, depending on severity and cause. It is best to work with a team of professionals from a holistic perspective to combat this disorder.

HEADACHES

A **headache** is defined as a diffuse pain in various areas of the head where the pain is not confined to the distribution of a nerve. It is, however, common for the neck muscles to be involved in causing headache pain. According to the International Headache Society, there are 13 different classifications of headaches and two basic categories. The primary category includes classifications of migraine, tension-type, and cluster headaches. The secondary category includes headaches associated with structural lesions, trauma, vascular disorders, nonvascular intracranial disorders, substances or withdrawal from them, metabolic disorder, facial and cranial pain, cranial neuralgias, and headaches not classifiable. Physicians use these classifications for diagnostic purposes. Massage therapists commonly see clients with headache complaints. This chapter focuses on the structural perspective of the head and neck and the result of the head-forward posture on the muscles. Tension headaches can be caused by shoulder tension as a result of repetitive action and/or posture. The techniques outlined in this chapter, especially the cranial holding techniques, can help relieve tension headaches. Research from the Touch Research Institute has shown that massage between headache episodes can reduce the number of headaches, decrease pain intensity, lower stress hormone levels, increase regular sleep patterns, and increase seratonin levels. Massage therapists should screen individuals with headaches carefully for contraindications and for referral. Headaches are symptoms of many diseases and conditions, as well as side effects of many medications.

Other Soft-Tissue Issues

STIFF NECK

Almost everyone has woken up from sleeping in a funny position with a "kink" in the neck. The term **stiff neck** is a catchall for limitations in neck movements. Causes include, but are not limited to, sleep positions, posture, repetitive actions, compensatory changes from other injuries, and postoperative and viral infections. Neck muscles on one side of the neck will be contracted and stuck. Massage therapy can provide tremendous relief for the everyday stiff neck.

Nerve Complaints

OCCIPITAL NERVE ENTRAPMENT

Occipital nerve entrapment occurs when the greater occipital nerve that innervates the scalp and in particular the occipitalis becomes entrapped by muscular tightness and/or spasm. To reach the scalp, the nerve usually traverses through the semispinalis capitis and subsequently through the trapezius. Individuals who have occipital nerve entrapment complain of numbness, pain, and tingling in the back of the head. This particular problem has been clinically treated with nerve blocks.

SCALENES

The scalenes are located on the anterior cervical spine and insert into the 1st and 2nd ribs. They are very involved in respiration, but the scalenes are also synergists to the sternocleidomastoid. Their biggest "claim to fame," however, is that the brachial plexus passes between the scalenus anterior and the scalenus medius. Entrapment of the brachial plexus can send a referred pain pattern spiraling down the upper extremity. For that reason, these muscles may be forgotten as important neck muscles to treat. The scalenes are stabilizers of the cervical spine and anterior neck. They are also often very involved in whiplash injuries.

Arthritis, Osteoarthritis, Degenerative Disk Disease, and Cervical Subluxations

Remember that compression of nerves at the cervical level may involve arthritis, osteoarthritis, degenerative disk disease, and/or cervical subluxations. Please read Chapter 11 for more information on these conditions. For further anatomy and pathology study, students may also want to review facet syndrome and neurologic disorders and be knowledgeable about neural pathways. As stated in Chapter 11, pain, numbness, and tingling with passive movement may help distinguish a problem in the cervical region. When the massage therapist suspects cervical involvement and/or nerve compression, it is appropriate to refer the client to a medical professional.

Unwinding the Muscles of the Head and Neck

Relieving the tension in the head, neck, and shoulders helps to balance the head on the neck, assists with appropriate postural alignment, supports chiropractic adjustments, increases range of motion, and reduces pain and/or soreness. How long it takes for this process to happen depends on each individual situation. The body needs natural time to heal and repair, and, unlike the extremities, the neck still has to hold up the head during this period. It may take several sessions to unwind a stiff neck. One session alone is unlikely to completely loosen a stiff neck, especially if any subluxations of the cervical vertebrae are present.

Headaches are a complete study unto themselves. There are so many causes of headaches that a complete and separate medical history should be used just for the headache history. Has the client kept a headache log previously to help understand and track the headaches? What other modalities and medical treatments has the client pursued? It is important for the therapist to distinguish between migraines and tension headaches. A client with a migraine may exhibit somatic symptoms of nausea, vomiting, and unilateral pain in the head. Once the client has progressed to these stages, it is unwise to increase circulation in the neck area. Most individuals who have a migraine do not want to be touched but, instead, seek dark, quiet areas. It is more beneficial to work on clients when they are not experiencing migraines and are not in the throes of severe pain. Therapists should not work on individuals who present with high blood pressure and a headache; they should refer such clients to a medical professional. Additionally, therapists should avoid working with a new client who is experiencing a headache. It would be torture for a client with a headache to complete medical history forms, think, and/or talk. Reschedule the client to a time when the appropriate health history information can be obtained and intelligent decisions about treatment goals can be made. Successfully working with clients with headaches requires a careful approach, complete information, good observation skills, critical thinking, excellent palpations, and appropriate techniques.

TREATMENT PROTOCOL

How do you unwind the neck muscles in a sequence?

- Take a careful medical history appropriate for the client, look for contraindications, and refer the client to appropriate professionals if necessary.
- Always use treatment protocols to determine the sequence of a therapeutic session; assess active and passive ranges of motion of the neck.
- Palpate tissues.
- Follow a dimensional approach, and critically think about the involved joints and muscles.
- Determine pressure intelligently; ask for feedback from the client.
- Work superficial to deep.
- Visit all the muscles possibly involved in the problem.
- Visit all the attachments of the involved muscles.
- Passively shorten muscles whenever possible with techniques to decrease tension.
- Do not overwork sore areas.
- Allow time for rest after the treatment.
- See the techniques below for additional suggestions.

Sequence for a Tension Headache

The environment of the treatment area is important when the therapist is seeing a client with a tension headache. There should be no heavy smells. Use unscented lubrication, and work in a room with clean air. Incense, sweet flowers, or scented oils or candles might make the headache sufferer nauseous. Make sure the room is fairly dark. Block out direct sunlight, and turn off fluorescent lights. Do not play music unless the client asks for it—you cannot guarantee that the client will like it, and the sound may reverberate with the throbbing of a headache. A cold washcloth over the eyes is a nice touch at the end of the treatment as the client rests with the cervical roll.

Dimensional Massage Therapy for the Muscles of the Head and Neck

The techniques presented below can be used as a complete sequence for a tension headache or be incorporated into other treatment sequences. Prepare well for working with someone with a headache. Wash your hands and forearms for several minutes. Take time for centering and grounding. Lay the person supine with a bolster under the knees and a cervical roll under the neck, if appropriate, when not working on the neck. Comfort and warmth are very important. Don't forget to breathe. Always ask the client where the discomfort or pain is located. Begin with soft, soothing strokes on the face.

SUPINE BODY POSITION

Check the shoulders for roundness, position, and unequal height. Reach under the back and pull the scapulae in a superior direction. Palpate for hypertonic muscles. Passively shorten area muscles whenever possible. Hold the client's head in your hands, and apply your fingers to below the occipital ridge. Push the chin up slightly with the palms of your hands. Palpate the whole ridge area. Follow the sequence below.

TECHNIQUES DURING A TENSION HEADACHE

Circular Friction on the Frontalis

A safe place to start is on the face. Apply soft, soothing strokes to activate the relaxation response. Try not to do anything startling or jerky; strokes must be sedative and rhythmic. Use circular friction on the frontalis over the frontal bone. Position the pads of your fingers on the frontalis just above the eyebrows. The pads of your right-hand fingers should go in a clockwise direction, while the pads of your left-hand fingers should travel in a counterclockwise direction. Work your way up toward the hairline with your strokes. (See figure 14.1.)

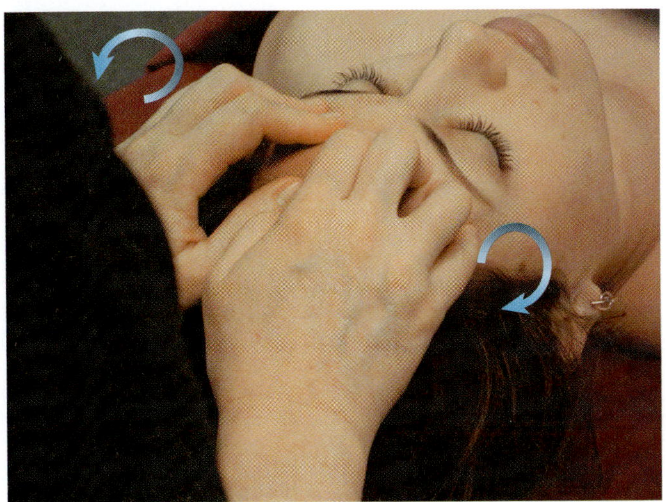

FIGURE 14.1 Circular friction on the frontalis

Circular Friction on the Temporalis

Lighten your pressure, and use a circular motion over the temple region with the pads of your fingers. Explore this region for tight fibers and tender areas. The temporalis is attached to the mandible and often is responsible for headaches. (See figure 14.2.)

Holding Techniques

Periodically during the treatment apply a gentle pull to the head superiorly. Place your fingers on the temporal region, straddling the client's ears on both sides of the head. Apply a good amount of pressure, and gently pull toward your body and hold. Ask the client

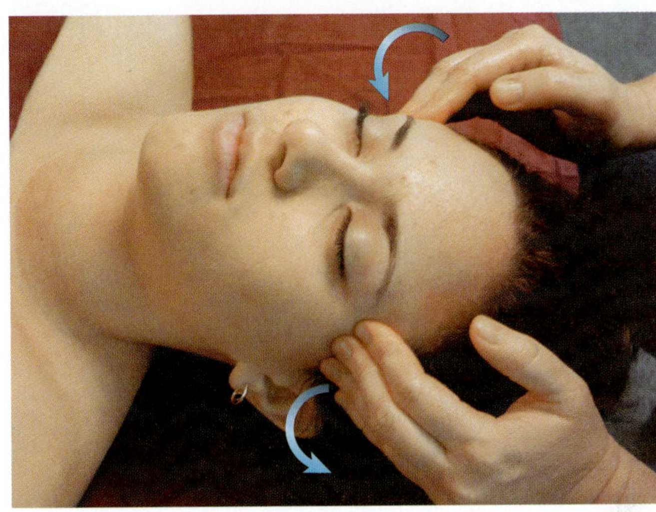

FIGURE 14.2 Circular friction on the temporalis

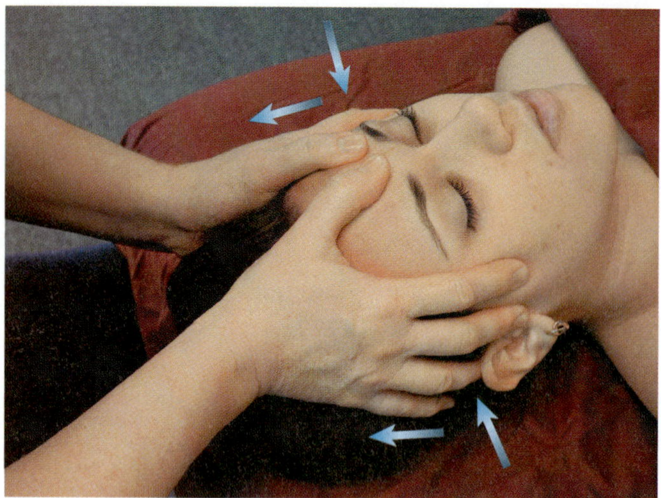

FIGURE 14.3 Gentle hold

if this relieves the pain in any way. Relax and reposition your hands during the treatment to relieve the stagnant position of your hands. (See figure 14.3.) Another way to help frontal pain is to place your thumb on one side of the temple just above and to the side of the eyebrow and place your middle-finger pad on the opposite side. From this position you can lift up and/or toward you superiorly. Your other hand should be cradling the occiput so that your palm is on one side of the head and the fingers are on the other. This is another holding technique. (See figure 14.4.) These techniques are a variation of an approach, not particular cranial techniques.

The amount of time you spend holding depends on the relief of pain the client feels. Speaking softly, check frequently with the client. Ask if your techniques change the pain or subdue it. Often the pain will travel and change locations. Continue to apply the techniques that relieve the client's pain.

Circular Friction on the Occipitofrontalis and Scalp Muscles

Use circular friction on the scalp muscles. Work all over the scalp muscles, front to back. Often the occipitofrontalis will be extremely tight. Start on the frontalis just over the eyebrows with circular friction, and work your way back over the whole area, including the temporalis. Make sure you are engaging the scalp muscles and not just "rubbing" hair. Strip and lengthen the fibers of the temporalis in its shell-like shape by drawing your fingers toward you from the ears. Start closest to the eyes, and work your way around the ears in a posterior direction, following the direction of the fibers. Work both muscles at the same time. Occasionally, as you get to the ends of the lengthened fibers, hold the stretch and keep your fingers in place. Check with the client to see if this relieves the tension. (See figure 14.5.)

Circular Friction on the Occipital Ridge

Place the client's head in the palms of your hands. With the pads of your fingers, perform circular friction all along the muscles of the occipital ridge. Pay particular attention to the levels of tension here. In the medial area where the trapezius attaches, note whether it is tight or relaxed and if it is tight deep to the trapezius. Think about the muscles you are treating. (See figure 14.6.)

Alternating-Hands Neck Stretch

The alternating-hands neck stretch should help loosen the superficial layers of tissue. Start at the base of the neck, cupping the cervical spine with one hand, and stroke with pressure in a superior direction up to the atlas-axis area. The other hand will replace the superior hand at the cervical base and repeat the

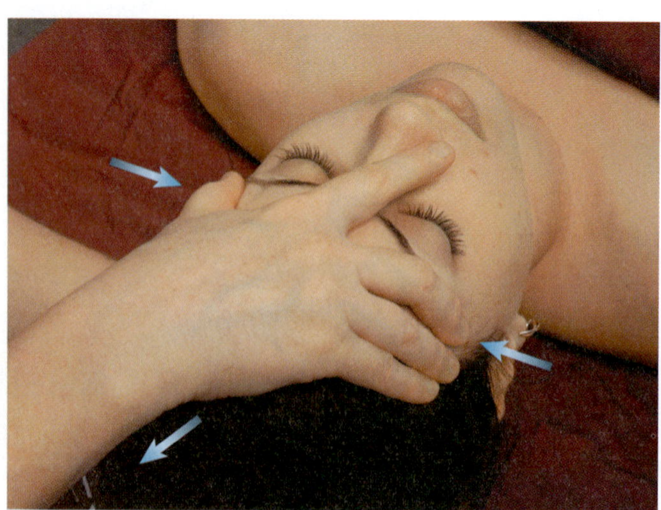

FIGURE 14.4 Temple lift

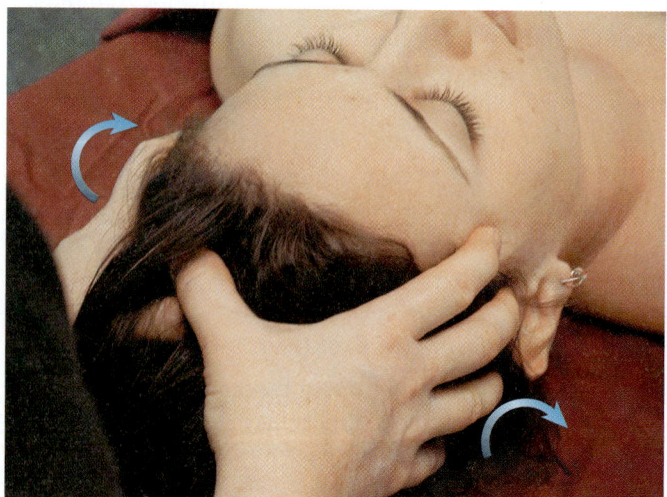

FIGURE 14.5 Circular friction on the scalp muscles

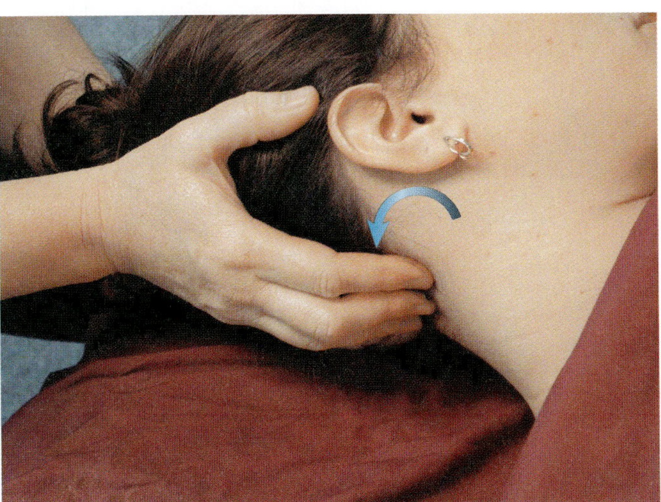

FIGURE 14.6 Circular friction on the occipital ridge

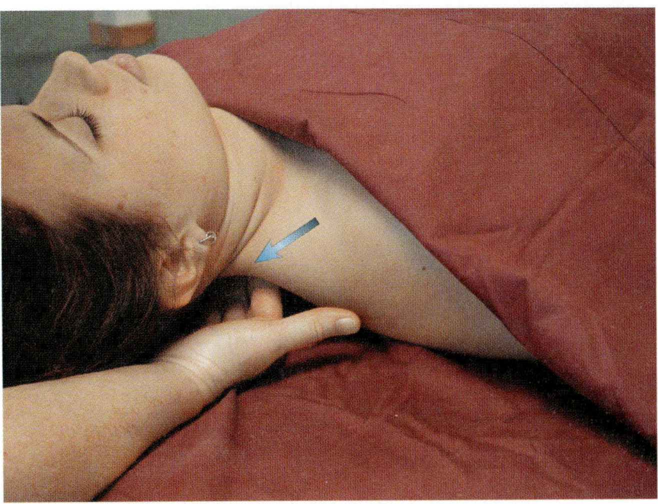

FIGURE 14.8 Hands under the back

directional stroke. Keep your hands under the client's neck, and repeat the alternating strokes a few times. When this stretch is done correctly, the cervical spine will slightly arch as the hands are alternately drawn toward the head. (See figure 14.7.)

Hands under the Back—Connecting the Trapezius

This technique connects the lower trapezius with the upper trapezius and lengthens fibers of the erectors. Place your hands under the back, and push down on your forearms to slide down to the lower thoracic spine. Stroke superiorly using any combination of effleurage, vibration, and circular friction. End with a little traction on the occipital ridge. For extra pressure, keep your fingers stiff. Repeat several times. *Note:* Do not try to lift the client, and do not do this technique if the client is physically too large. Never sacrifice yourself to a technique. (See figures 14.8 and 14.9.)

Edging the Upper Trapezius

Place one hand under the client's neck at a right angle to the spine, and locate the superior edge of the upper trapezius with your fingers. Slide the other hand under the trapezius so that your thumb rests on the anterior edge of the upper trapezius, making a slight pincer palpation. At the same time, draw the thumb and fingers together to hold the muscle mass. Edge the thumb toward the clavicle while drawing your fingers in a superior direction. The two hands will be going in opposite directions that will stretch this edge of the upper trapezius. (See figure 14.10.)

Effleurage around the Shoulders

Effleurage around the shoulders and up the posterior neck. Start with the fingers of both hands pointing toward each other in the flat area inferior to the

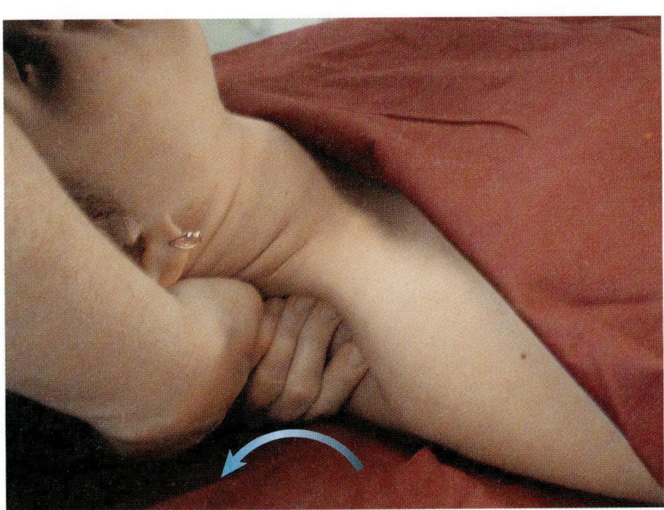

FIGURE 14.7 Alternating-hands neck stretch

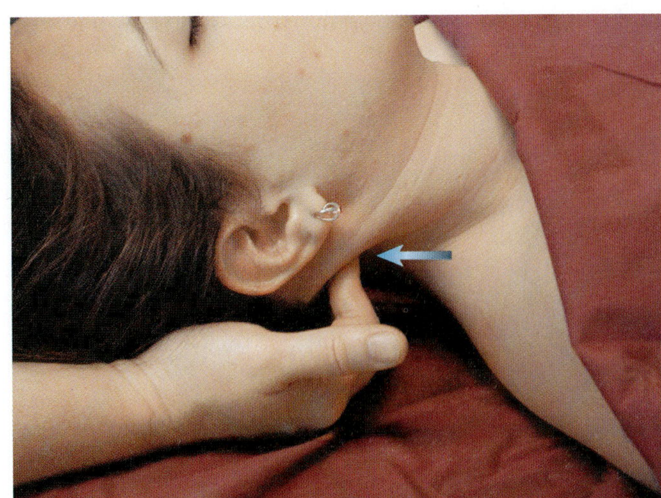

FIGURE 14.9 Traction on the occipital ridge

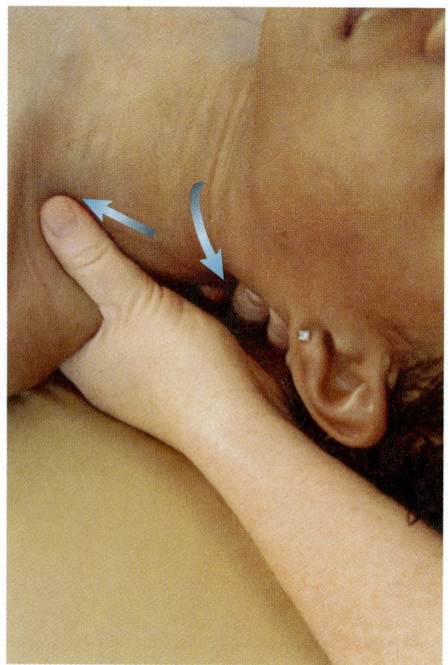

FIGURE 14.10 Edging the upper trapezius

clavicle bilaterally. Stroke with a smooth glide, and complete contact around the deltoids and up the sides of the trapezius to the occipital ridge. At the end of the stroke, give a little traction to the ridge. Use this stroke frequently during the routine to connect the shoulders to the head. It is easier to stand to do this technique effectively. Stand with one leg behind you for balance and stability, and use your body's momentum for strength. (See figure 14.11.)

Petrissage of the Trapezius

Turn the head to the side *slightly*. Petrissage the trapezius with one hand, while bracing the head with the forearm and grasping the trapezius with the other hand. You might have to bend the client's elbow to relax the trapezius a bit more. This will make it easier to release the fibers if the muscle is

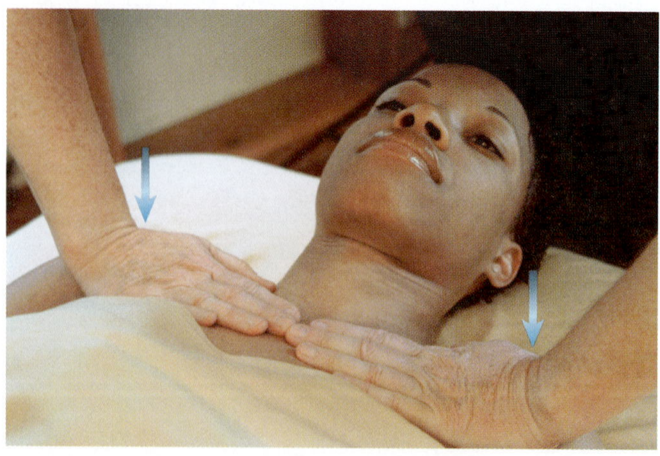

FIGURE 14.11 Effleurage around the shoulder

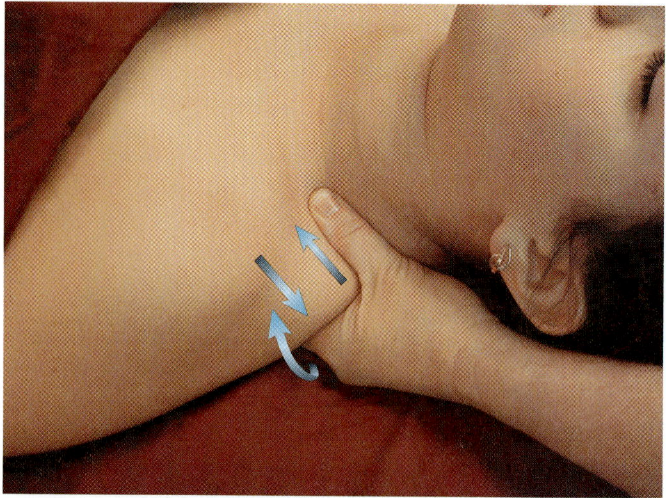

FIGURE 14.12 Petrissage of the trapezius

not lengthened. Next, petrissage the trapezius bilaterally, either at the same time or in an alternating side-to-side motion. Keep the strokes flowing from one action to the next without losing contact or flow. (See figure 14.12.)

Opposite-Side Petrissage of the Trapezius—Combing the Trapezius

Place your inferior hand under the client's head, and grasp the opposite trapezius. Use your fingers to "comb" and pull on the trapezius while your thumb completes a circular friction between the spine and the scapula. Use your superior hand to brace the head while you complete the technique. Repeat on the opposite side. (See figure 14.13.)

Closed-Palm Shaping

Make a relaxed, *loose fist* with the dorsal side of your hand, and while you support the other side of the

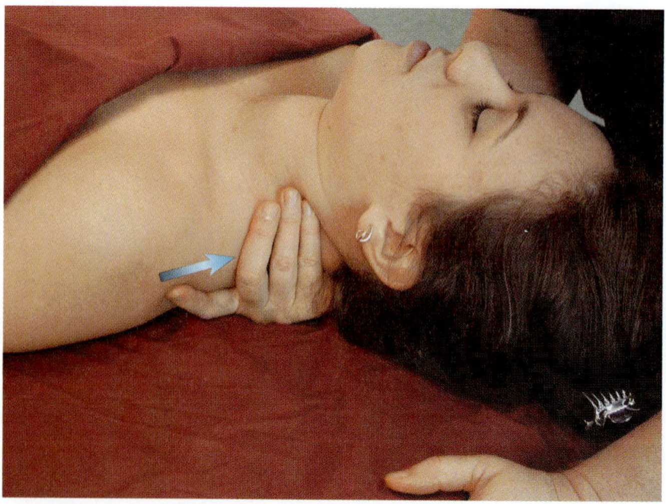

FIGURE 14.13 Opposite-side petrissage of the trapezius

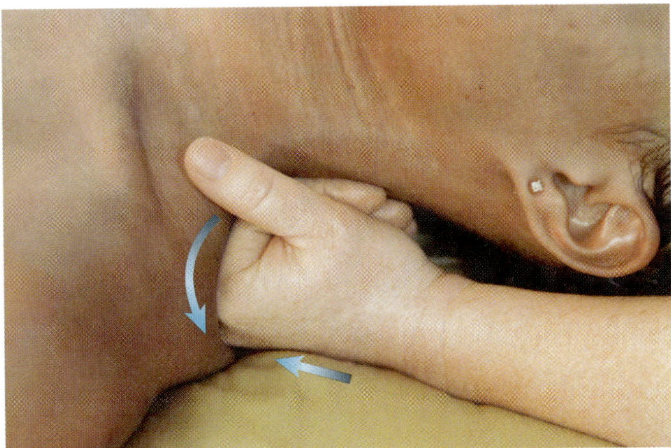

FIGURE 14.14 Closed-palm shaping of the trapezius

client's head with your forearm, stroke posterior to the sternocleidomastoid back and forth in a superior and inferior direction. Pay careful attention to shaping your hand to the client's structure. Lean into the stroke rather than using hand force, and use care, as always, to engage the tissues with an appropriate pressure. (See figure 14.14.)

Knuckling

With loose fists, move your hands in a circular motion on the trapezius bilaterally close to, but not on, the spine and away from the shoulder bones. Make sure that the client's upper arms are in a relaxed bent-elbow position to release tension in the trapezius as much as possible. Conform your hands to the shape of the structure, and lean into your strokes. Never use a tight, tense fist or press into the tissues.

Cervical Work

While holding the client's head with one hand above the cervical spine, strip the muscles parallel to the spinous processes from the atlas to C7. Repeat on the opposite side of the head, exchanging your hands to hold the head. You can use your thumb in this stroke, or you can straddle the spine and use your thumb on one side and your curled index finger on the other side. Apply some circular friction on as much soft tissue as possible all along the cervical spine. Your fingers should be between the spinous processes and the transverse processes. (See figure 14.15.)

Neck Stretch to the Side

First, gently rotate the client's head laterally. Position yourself just to the side of the table at the head. Place one hand on the shoulder and one hand on the back of the head. Slide the hand from the shoulder to the head. Take the other hand off the head and place it on the shoulder, and stretch, glide, and stretch again

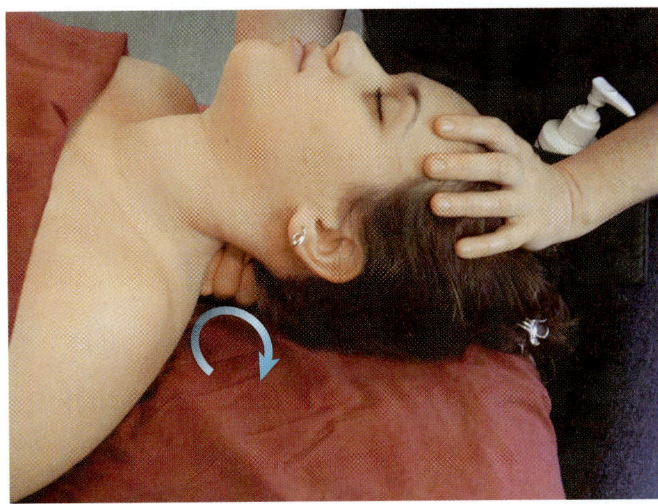

FIGURE 14.15 Cervical work

as you stroke alternately while stretching. Move your lower body with this stroke for better body mechanics. (See figure 14.16.)

Repeat either the alternating-hands neck stretch or effleurage of the client's shoulders.

The Neck Rock

Support the client's head in the palms of your hands, and place your finger pads under the occipital ridge. In an alternating motion, push up with your fingers and stretch the head back, pulling on the ridge with the fingers. The client must not try to help you accomplish this technique; it is successful only if the head remains passive. (See figure 14.17.)

Treating the Sternocleidomastoid

Assess how tight the sternocleidomastoid is bilaterally. Laterally tilt the client's head toward the shoulder, and slightly flex the head forward. On the side closest to the shoulder, repeatedly strip the fibers of the

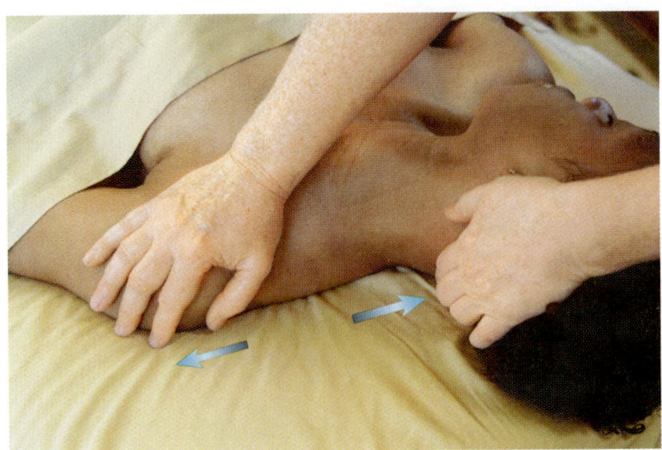

FIGURE 14.16 Neck stretch to the side

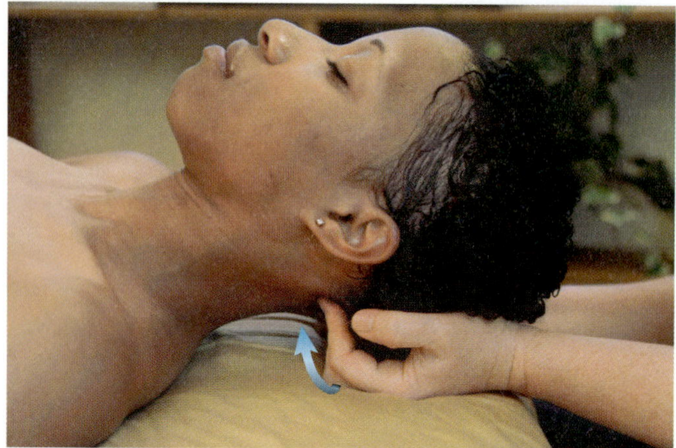

FIGURE 14.17 Neck rock

sternocleidomastoid from the mastoid process for a couple of inches toward the clavicle and sternum. Apply deep transverse friction or apply circular friction at the origins of the muscle on the sternum and clavicle. Jostle the length of the muscle, and work the muscle fibers between your thumb and index finger. Apply a pincer palpation to the trigger points in the muscles. Check with the client for the appropriate pressure; these trigger points can be exquisitely painful, and some might refer pain to the head. Remember to stretch the muscle after you treat the trigger points. Repeat the routine on the opposite sternocleidomastoid. (See figure 14.18.)

Scalenes

Lift the back of the client's head with one hand. Laterally flex the head toward the shoulder that you are working. Place your thumb behind the sternocleidomastoid on the same side, and glide inferiorly toward the 1st and/or 2nd rib as you continue to flex the head forward. Repeat several times. This technique can be omitted for treatment of a tension headache. (See figure 14.19.) *Note:* In a classroom, any work on the scalenes should be supervised by an experienced instructor.

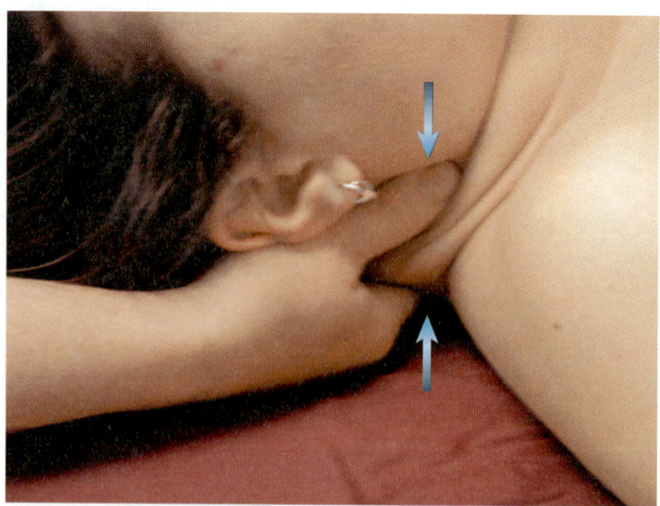

FIGURE 14.18 Treating the sternocleidomastoid

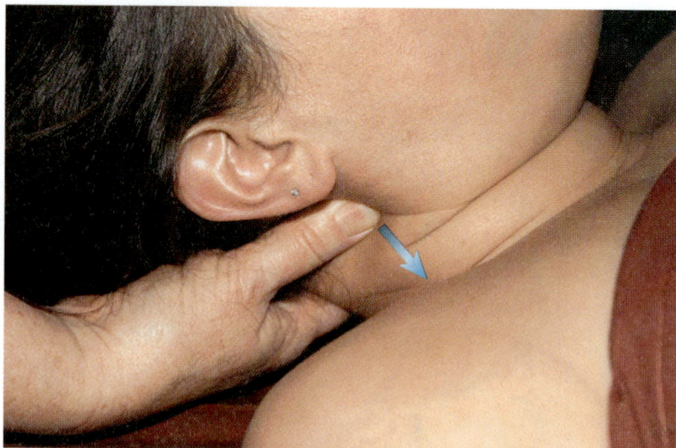

(a) Starting position

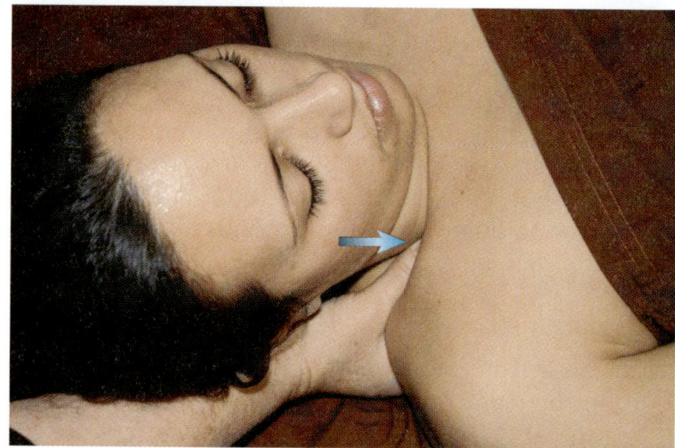

(b) End stroke

FIGURE 14.19 Stripping the scalenes

Now that all the superficial and some deeper-layer muscles have been treated and relaxed, the deeper posterior cervical muscles should be next to unwind if the client does not have a headache. If the client does have a headache, and the routine thus far has helped the headache to subside, the routine is over. Working deeply on these muscles might make the headache return with a vengeance, so check with the client and proceed with caution.

Treating the Deeper Posterior Cervical Muscles

The mastoid process is a hotbed of attachments. The sternocleidomastoid has already been treated. The splenius capitis and the longissimus lie underneath and posterior to the sternocleidomastoid. Angle the client's head so that these muscles are somewhat relaxed, and strip away from the mastoid process in the long fibers of the muscles. Apply circular friction

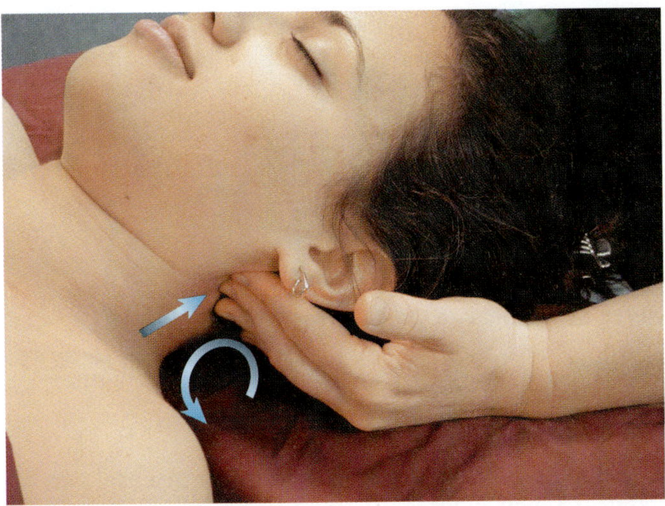

FIGURE 14.20 Treating the deeper posterior cervical muscles

and deep transverse friction to the attachments of the fibers on the mastoid process and the occiput. Treat the opposite side of the head. (See figure 14.20.)

Treating the Rectus Capitis Posterior Minor and Major

With the client's head nestled in the palm of your hands, curl your fingers under the occiput and apply circular friction all along the ridge. In the center of the occipital region, connecting to the spinous process of the atlas, is the rectus capitis posterior minor. Locate the superior attachment of this tiny muscle. With one or two fingers, deeply strip toward the atlas in the direction of the fibers. The muscle dips in at an angle, and you will not be able to palpate the C1 spinous process. The first spinous process you feel will be C2. Remember that you are pressing through the trapezius and semispinalis capitis, so be pressure-specific. Check with the client, as the rectus could have a horrific pain pattern. Apply deep transverse friction or use just circular friction on the rectus capitis posterior minor. Immediately lateral to the minor is the rectus capitis posterior major. Strip this muscle, and apply deep transverse friction or use circular friction on the attachments. The major extends to the spinous process of the axis (C2).

Other Suboccipitals

Locate the transverse processes of the atlas. Often headache sufferers may have an unbalanced atlas when one side or the other is held tighter by the muscles attaching to it. The culprits may be the obliquus capitis superior and obliquus capitis inferior. These two muscles form the sides and peak of the upside-down house of the suboccipitals. If you tilt the client's head and work on the shortened side, you can strip the obliquus capitis superior (side of the house) and apply deep transverse friction to the fibers. While the head is still tilted, locate the peak of the house, the obliquus capitis inferior, which connects the transverse process of the atlas to the spinous process of the axis. Strip and apply deep transverse friction to the obliquus capitis inferior. Repeat on the opposite side, starting with tilting the head in the opposite direction. Often, treating these muscles will allow the atlas to gently rotate back into place by itself. Remember that there is no adjustment involved with this technique. The relaxed muscles will do their own "adjusting" of the area, so let nature take its course. Physical adjustments must be administered by qualified professionals. Refer the client to an appropriate practitioner when necessary.

Finishing Strokes

Finish with an effleurage around the client's shoulders. Rest your hands on the shoulders for a few moments to signal your finish. Make sure the client rests on the table after the treatment. Place a cold cloth over the eyes, if necessary, and a cervical roll under the neck. Do not apply heat to the face or follow with a sauna or hot tub. Too much stimulation may cause the headache to return. Do not place a client with a headache prone on the table, even if it appears that you have helped the headache subside in the supine position. The prone position is an invitation for the headache to return, probably due to the pressure of the face in the face cradle.

Cervical Roll

Take a regular hand towel and fold it lengthwise toward the center. Allow about an inch gap for the cervical spine. Start at one end and roll the towel. It should be only large enough to support the cervical spine in a natural curve and not large enough to lift the head off the table. Place the cervical roll under the neck in a supine position. (See figure 14.21.)

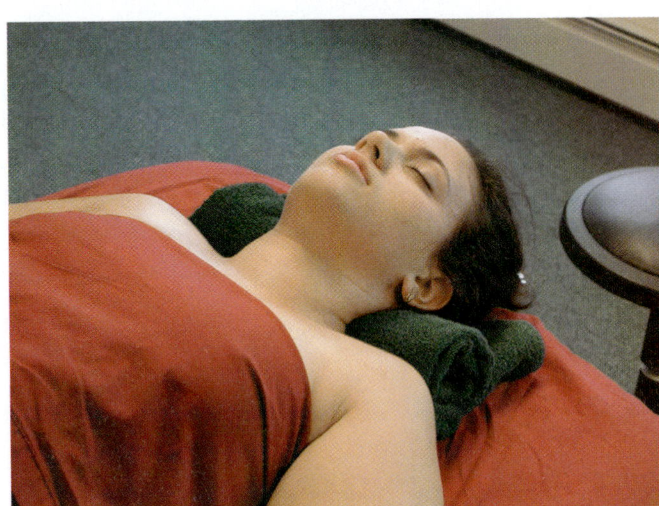

FIGURE 14.21 Cervical roll

CHAPTER summary

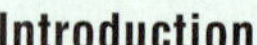

Introduction

- ✔ The head and neck are a harmony of balance and movement.
- ✔ Structure, positions of the head, and repetitive action are at fault for overuse syndromes and soft-tissue dysfunctions.
- ✔ Physical trauma also causes problems for the head and neck.
- ✔ Massage therapy can provide a great deal of relief for soft-tissue dysfunctions of the head and neck.

Structural Perspectives of the Head and Neck

- ✔ The head performs a balancing act on seven cervical vertebrae and disks that depends on the muscles, tendons, and ligaments of the head and neck for additional support.
- ✔ The thoracic and lumbar spines support the head, and the trunk supplies a base.
- ✔ Rounded shoulders can lead to a head-forward posture.
- ✔ Head-forward posture causes excessive stress on the posterior cervical muscles.

The Muscles

- ✔ Individual muscles that should be treated for various soft-tissue problems include the trapezius, levator scapulae, rhomboids, splenius capitis and cervicis, longissimus capitis, semispinalis capitis and cervicis, rotatores, multifidi, suboccipitals, occipitofrontalis, temporalis, and sternocleidomastoid.

Injuries and Overuse Syndromes

- ✔ Whiplash is an injury resulting from a violent impact.
- ✔ Torticollis is a spasmodic condition of the neck that can prevent movement and cause pain and discomfort.
- ✔ Tension headaches can be caused by posture and repetitive action of the head and neck.
- ✔ Massage therapy can help relieve discomfort from tension-type headaches.

Other Soft-Tissue Issues

- ✔ Massage therapy techniques can help the "everyday" stiff neck.

Nerve Complaints

- ✔ The greater occipital nerve can be entrapped by the trapezius and semispinalis capitis.
- ✔ The scalenes can entrap the brachial plexus.

Arthritis, Osteoarthritis, Degenerative Disk Disease, and Cervical Subluxations

- ✔ Arthritis, osteoarthritis, degenerative disk disease, and cervical subluxations can contribute to nerve complaints.

Unwinding the Muscles of the Head and Neck

- ✔ Massage therapy is a good choice for relieving tension in the head, neck, and shoulders.
- ✔ Follow a dimensional approach, and critically think about the involved joints and muscles.
- ✔ Always use treatment protocols to determine the sequence of a therapeutic session.
- ✔ Refer clients to appropriate professionals when necessary.

Sequence for a Tension Headache

- ✔ Prepare the environment well to work with a client with a tension headache.
- ✔ Approach techniques methodically, unwinding soft tissue superficially to deep.
- ✔ Allow time for rest following a treatment for a tension headache.

Dimensional Massage Therapy for the Muscles of the Head and Neck

- ✔ The techniques can be used as a complete sequence for a tension headache or be incorporated into other treatment sequences.
- ✔ Always practice good centering and grounding techniques.

CHAPTER *review*

True or False

Write true *or* false *after each statement.*

1. The rhomboids have no effect on posture.
2. The rotatores and multifidi are superficial muscles.
3. The sternocleidomastoid rotates to the same side.
4. The scalenes can entrap the brachial plexus.
5. Tension headaches can be caused by posture and hypertonic muscles.
6. Gravity assists the posterior cervical muscles in extension.
7. The levator scapulae and splenius cervicis both attach to transverse processes of the upper cervical vertebrae.
8. The accessory nerve innervates all the posterior cervical muscles.
9. The longissimus capitis is an erector spinae muscle.
10. The rotatores and multifidi are deep paraspinal muscles.

Short Answers

Write your answers on the lines provided.

1. Name the suboccipitals.

____

____

____

2. What three muscles are on or quite near the mastoid process?

____

____

____

3. What tiny muscle is a posterior muscle but is really not designed for extension of the head?

____

____

____

4. Explain why a head-forward posture applies pressure to the posterior cervical muscles.

____

____

____

5. What nerve innervates the sternocleidomastoid?

____

____

____

6. The rectus capitis posterior major attaches to what bones?

____

____

____

7. What is the definition of a headache?

____

____

____

8. What muscles might entrap the brachial plexus?

____

____

____

9. What muscles might entrap the greater occipital nerve?

____

____

____

10. Why is it important to work on the shoulder girdle muscles first?

____

____

____

11. Why would a therapist take a medical history of an individual who is presenting with a headache?

____

____

____

12. Should a therapist refer a client who has a headache and high blood pressure?

____

____

____

Multiple Choice

Circle the correct answers.

1. The splenius capitis and cervicis have the unique ability to:
   a. flex the head
   b. rotate the head and extend the head from opposite sides of the muscle
   c. extend the head only
   d. none of the above
2. The suboccipitals include:
   a. rectus capitis superior minor and major and obliquus capitis superior and inferior
   b. sternocleidomastoid, splenius capitis, and cervicis
   c. semispinalis
   d. all of the above
3. The trapezius could entrap:
   a. the accessory nerve
   b. the ulnar nerve
   c. the greater occipital nerve
   d. none of the above
4. Temporomandibular joint syndrome is:
   a. a problem with the jaw in closing or opening the mouth
   b. lack of movement in the upper cervicals
   c. not a problem at all
   d. a disease of the oral cavity
5. Whiplash victims need to be:
   a. massaged right away
   b. examined first by a physician
   c. given elaborate range-of-motion stretches
   d. none of the above
6. Muscles involved in whiplash might include:
   a. rectus femoris, biceps femoris, and quadratus lumborum
   b. sternocleidomastoid, splenius capitis and cervicis, and scalenes
   c. sternocleidomastoid only
   d. none of the above
7. Treatment protocol for working on the head and neck is to:
   a. start prone and work only on the back muscles
   b. start in a supine position and work superficial to deep
   c. work on the lower extremity first
   d. go as deep as you can right away
8. Posterior cervical muscles:
   a. flex the head
   b. extend the head and neck bilaterally
   c. do nothing to the head and neck
   d. none of the above
9. Regular massage for a person who suffers from headaches could:
   a. reduce the number of headaches, reduce pain levels, increase seratonin levels, and reduce stress hormones
   b. increase stress hormones and increase headaches
   c. do nothing for the client
   d. none of the above
10. If a client presented with an undiagnosed pain in the neck and had just had an accident, you would:
    a. massage the client and make repeated appointments
    b. make an appropriate referral
    c. examine the neck by having the client do complete range of motion
    d. do nothing

EXPLORE & practice

1. Locate the bony landmarks of the cervical vertebrae on a partner.
2. Locate on a partner the origins and insertions of the muscles discussed in this chapter and in Chapter 13.
3. Demonstrate how to passively shorten the flexors and extensors of the head and neck on a partner.
4. Demonstrate passive range of motion of the head and neck with a partner.
5. Demonstrate active range of motion of the head and neck with a partner.
6. List which muscles are agonists and synergists for flexion of the head and neck.
7. List which muscles are agonists and synergists for extension of the head and neck.
8. Describe how you would work on a client who has a tension headache.
9. Practice dimensional techniques individually and in a sequence on a partner.
10. Explain the precautions you would take if a client presents with a headache.

part 4

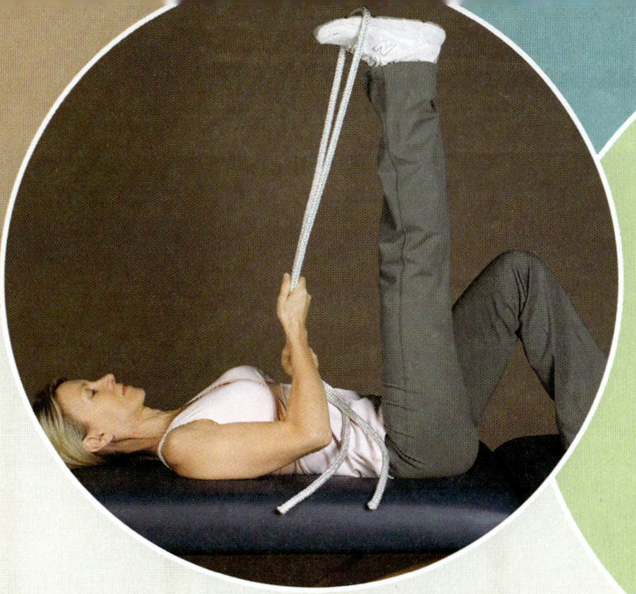

LOWER EXTREMITIES

chapter 15

The Hip Joint and Pelvic Girdle

LEARNING OUTCOMES

After completing this chapter, you should be able to:

15-1 Define key terms.

15-2 Identify on a human skeleton selected bony features of the hip joint and pelvic girdle.

15-3 Label on a skeletal chart selected bony features of the hip joint and pelvic girdle.

15-4 Draw on a skeletal chart the individual muscles of the hip joint, including origins and insertions.

15-5 Demonstrate all the active and passive movements of the hip joint and pelvic girdle with a partner.

15-6 Palpate the muscles of the hip joint and pelvic girdle, including attachments, on a partner.

15-7 Organize and list the agonists, antagonists, and synergists that produce movement of the hip joint and pelvic girdle.

15-8 Practice flexibility and strengthening exercises for each muscle group.

KEY TERMS

Acetabular femoral joint
Acetabulum
Adductor brevis
Adductor longus
Adductor magnus
Femoral nerve
Gemellus inferior
Gemellus superior
Gerdy's tubercle
Gluteus maximus
Gluteus medius
Gluteus minimus
Gracilis
Greater trochanter
Hamstrings
Iliacus
Iliopsoas
Iliotibial tract
Ilium
Ischial tuberosity
Ischium
Lesser trochanter
Linea aspera
Lumbosacral plexus
Obturator externus
Obturator internus
Obturator nerve
Pectineus
Pelvic bones
Peroneal nerve
Piriformis
Psoas major
Psoas minor
Pubis
Quadratus femoris
Rectus femoris
Sacroiliac joints
Sacrum
Sartorius
Sciatic nerve
Symphysis pubis
Tensor fasciae latae
Tibial nerve

Introduction

In the anatomical puzzle that is the human body, the pelvic girdle provides a sturdy foundation for the trunk and spine. The sacrum fits between the two sides of the ilium and creates a wide base for the larger lumbar vertebrae. Muscles span, like guy wires, from the ribs and vertebrae to the hip and pelvic bones. The structure of the trunk, spine, and pelvic girdle lends stability to the weight of the trunk. As the body ages, the weight of the trunk wears down the quality of the disks between the vertebrae, especially in the L4, L5, and S1 areas, making this region susceptible to dysfunction. Poor body mechanics, weak core muscles, trauma, and improper lifting postures make this area the weakest link in the mechanical musculoskeletal chain.

The vertebrae and the pelvic girdle provide attachments for muscles that have action on the hip joint. For the lower extremities to be involved in locomotion, muscles must attach to the trunk and pelvic girdle and extend to the femur. Similar to the ball-and-socket joint of the shoulder, the hip joint, or **acetabular femoral joint,** enjoys the entire free range of movements that the shoulder does. The difference between the two joints is that the distal end of the lower extremity is constantly concussing with the ground or floor, whereas the upper extremity often has an open kinetic chain. Gravity anchors the lower extremity in movement, and it gives the feet more stability and provides balance to the body's structure. Because of its bony architecture, strong ligaments, and large, supportive muscles, the lower extremity depends on the hip joint to be relatively stable.

Bones

The hip joint is a ball-and-socket joint that consists of the head of the femur connecting with the cup-shaped **acetabulum** of the pelvic girdle (figure 15.1). The femur (figure 15.2) projects out laterally from its head toward the **greater trochanter** and then angles back toward the midline as it runs inferiorly to form the proximal bone of the knee. It is the longest bone in the body. The pelvic girdle consists of a right and left pelvic bone joined together posteriorly by the sacrum. The **sacrum** can be considered an extension of the spinal column with its five fused vertebrae. Extending inferior to the sacrum is the coccyx. The **pelvic bones** consist of three bones: the **ilium,** the **ischium,** and the **pubis** (figure 15.3). At birth and during growth and development, these are three distinct bones. At maturity, they fuse to form one pelvic bone.

The pelvic bone can be divided roughly into three areas, starting from the acetabulum:

- Upper two-fifths = ilium
- Posterior and lower two-fifths = ischium
- Anterior and lower one-fifth = pubis

In studying the muscles of the hip and thigh, it is helpful to focus on the important bony landmarks, keeping in mind their purpose as key attachment points for the muscles. The anterior pelvis provides points of origin for the muscles generally involved in flexing the hip. Specifically, the tensor fasciae latae arises from the anterior iliac crest, the sartorius originates on the anterior superior iliac spine, and the rectus femoris originates on the anterior inferior iliac spine. Laterally, the gluteus medius and gluteus minimus, which abduct the hip, originate just below the iliac crest. Posteriorly, the gluteus maximus originates on the posterior

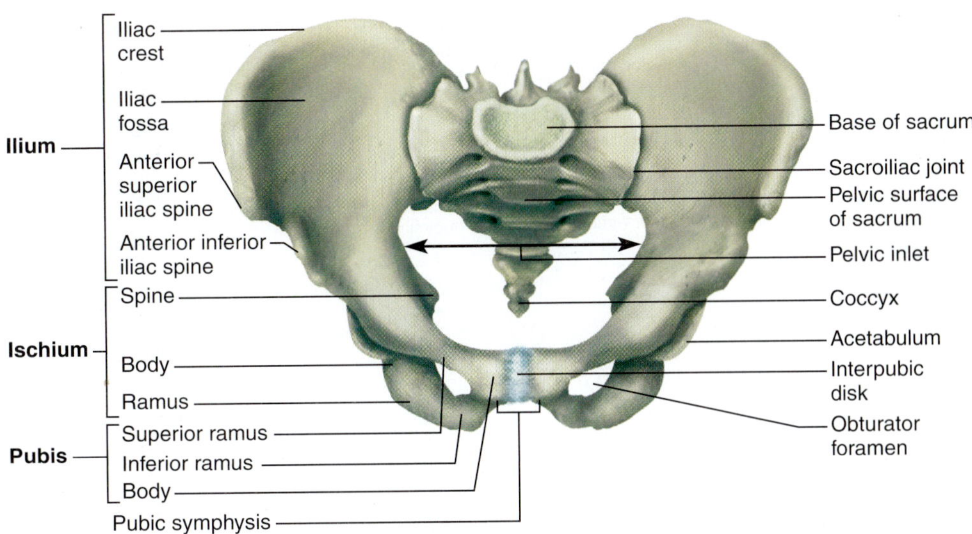

FIGURE 15.1 The pelvis, anterosuperior view

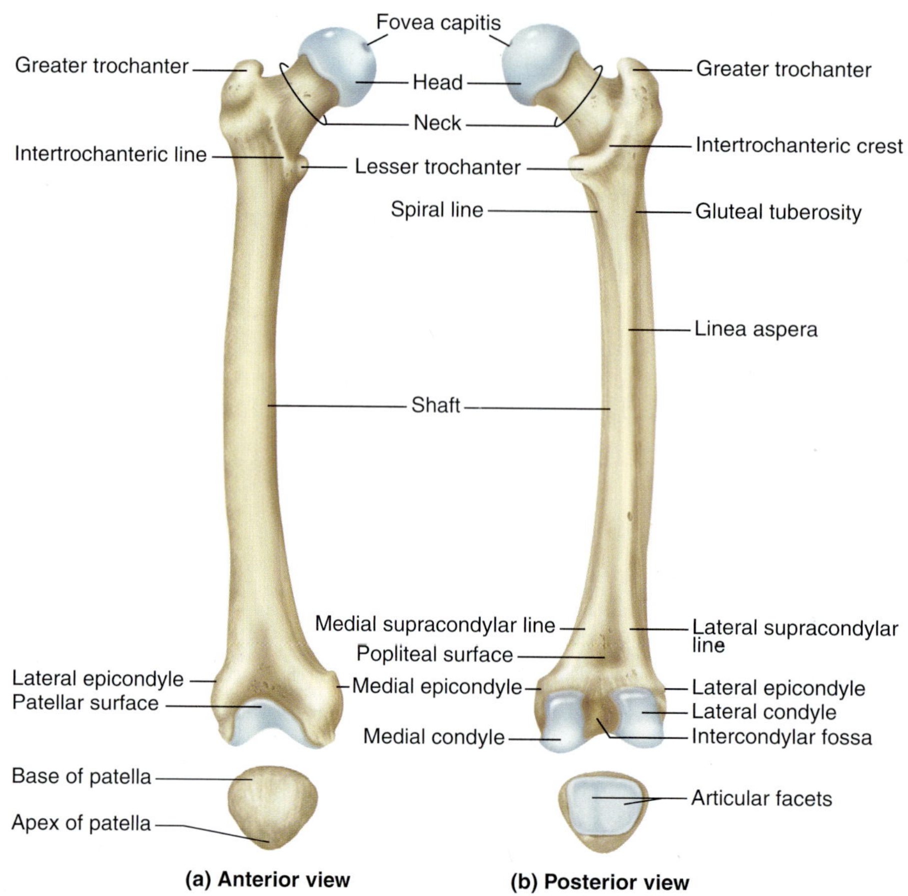

FIGURE 15.2 The right femur and patella

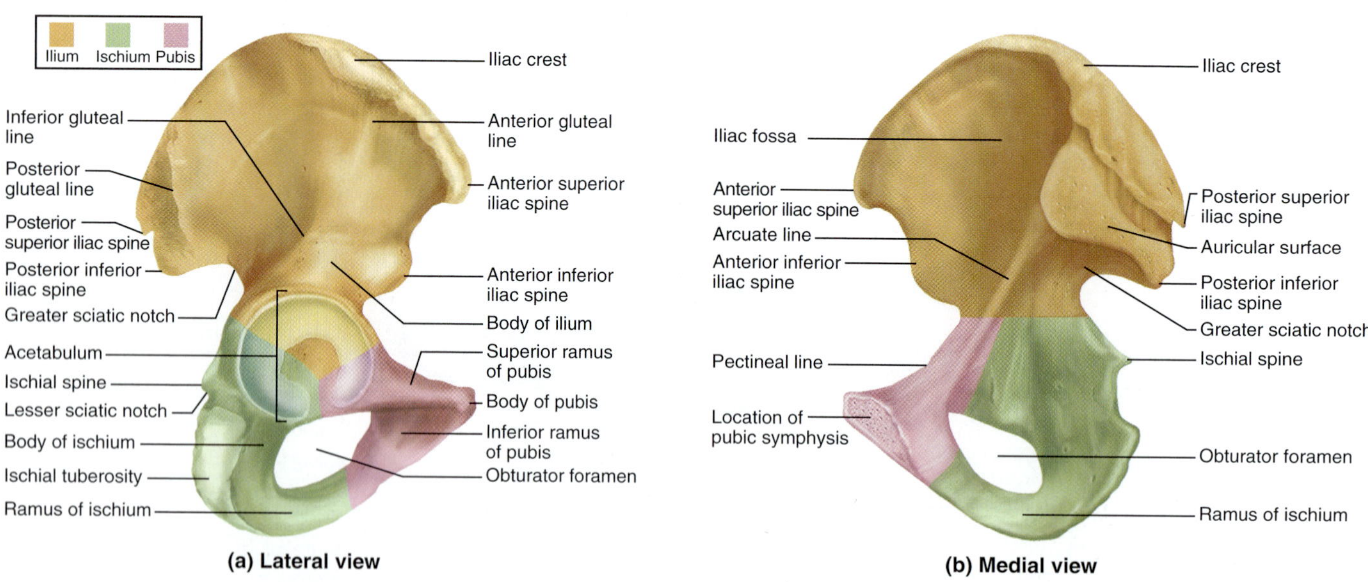

FIGURE 15.3 The ilium, ischium, and pubis

iliac crest, as well as the posterior sacrum and coccyx. Posteroinferiorly, the **ischial tuberosity** serves as the point of origin for the hamstrings, which extend the hip. Medially, the pubis and its inferior ramus serve as the point of origin for the hip adductors, which include the adductor magnus, adductor longus, adductor brevis, pectineus, and gracilis.

The proximal thigh generally serves as a point of insertion for some of the short muscles of the hip and as the origin for three of the knee extensors. Most notably, the greater trochanter is the point of insertion for all the gluteal muscles and most of the six deep external rotators. Although not palpable, the **lesser trochanter** serves as the bony landmark on which the iliopsoas inserts. Anteriorly, the three vasti muscles of the quadriceps originate proximally. Posteriorly, the **linea aspera** serves as the insertion for the hip adductors.

Distally, the patella serves as a major bony landmark, attaching all four quadriceps muscles by the patellar tendon and inferiorly inserting on the tibial tuberosity. The remaining hip muscles insert on the proximal tibia or fibula. The sartorius, gracilis, and semitendinosus insert on the upper anteromedial surface of the tibia just below the medial condyle, after crossing the knee posteromedially. The semimembranosus inserts posteromedially on the medial tibial condyle. Laterally, the biceps femoris inserts primarily on the head of the fibula, with some fibers attaching on the lateral tibial condyle. Anterolaterally, **Gerdy's tubercle** provides the insertion point for the **iliotibial tract** of the tensor fasciae latae.

Joints

In the anterior area, the pelvic bones join to form the **symphysis pubis,** an amphiarthrodial joint. In the posterior area, the sacrum is located between the two pelvic bones and forms the **sacroiliac joints.** Strong ligaments unite these bones to form rigid, slightly movable joints. The bones are large and heavy, and for the most part they are covered by thick, heavy muscles. Very minimal oscillating-type movements can occur in these joints, such as those in walking or in hip flexion when lying on one's back; however, movements usually involve the entire pelvic girdle and hip joints. In walking, there is hip flexion and extension with rotation of the pelvic girdle, forward in hip flexion and backward in hip extension. Jogging and running result in faster movements and in a greater range of movement.

Sports skills such as kicking a football or soccer ball provide other good examples of hip and pelvic movements. Pelvic rotation helps increase the length of the stride in running; in kicking, it can result in a greater range of motion, which translates to a greater distance or more speed to the kick.

Except for the glenohumeral joint, the hip is one of the most mobile joints of the body, largely because of its multiaxial arrangement. Unlike the glenohumeral, the hip joint's bony architecture provides a great deal of stability, resulting in relatively few hip joint subluxations and dislocations.

The hip joint is classified as an enarthrodial-type joint and is formed by the femoral head inserting into the socket provided by the acetabulum of the pelvis (figure 15.4). Its extremely strong and dense ligamentous capsule reinforces the joint, especially anteriorly.

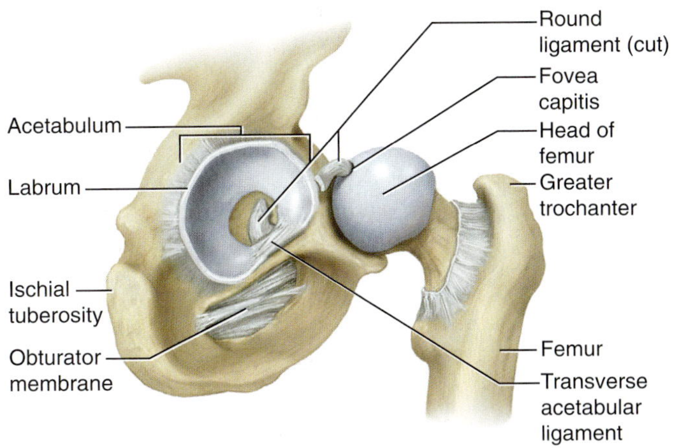

(a) Lateral view, femur retracted

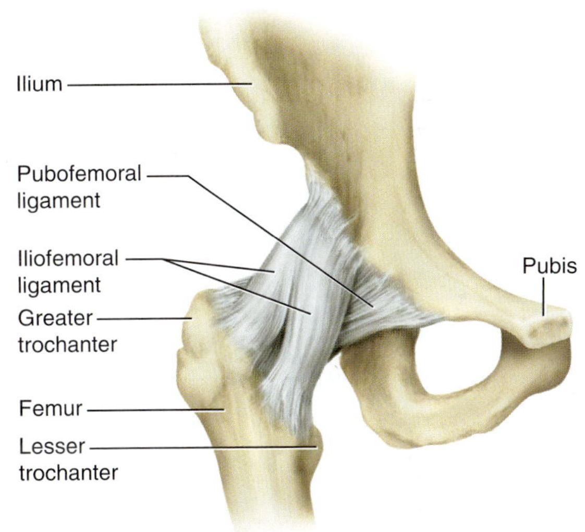

(b) Anterior view

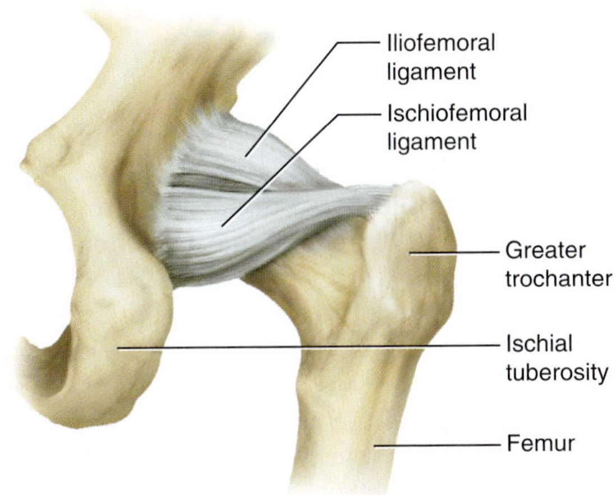

(c) Posterior view

FIGURE 15.4 Hip joint

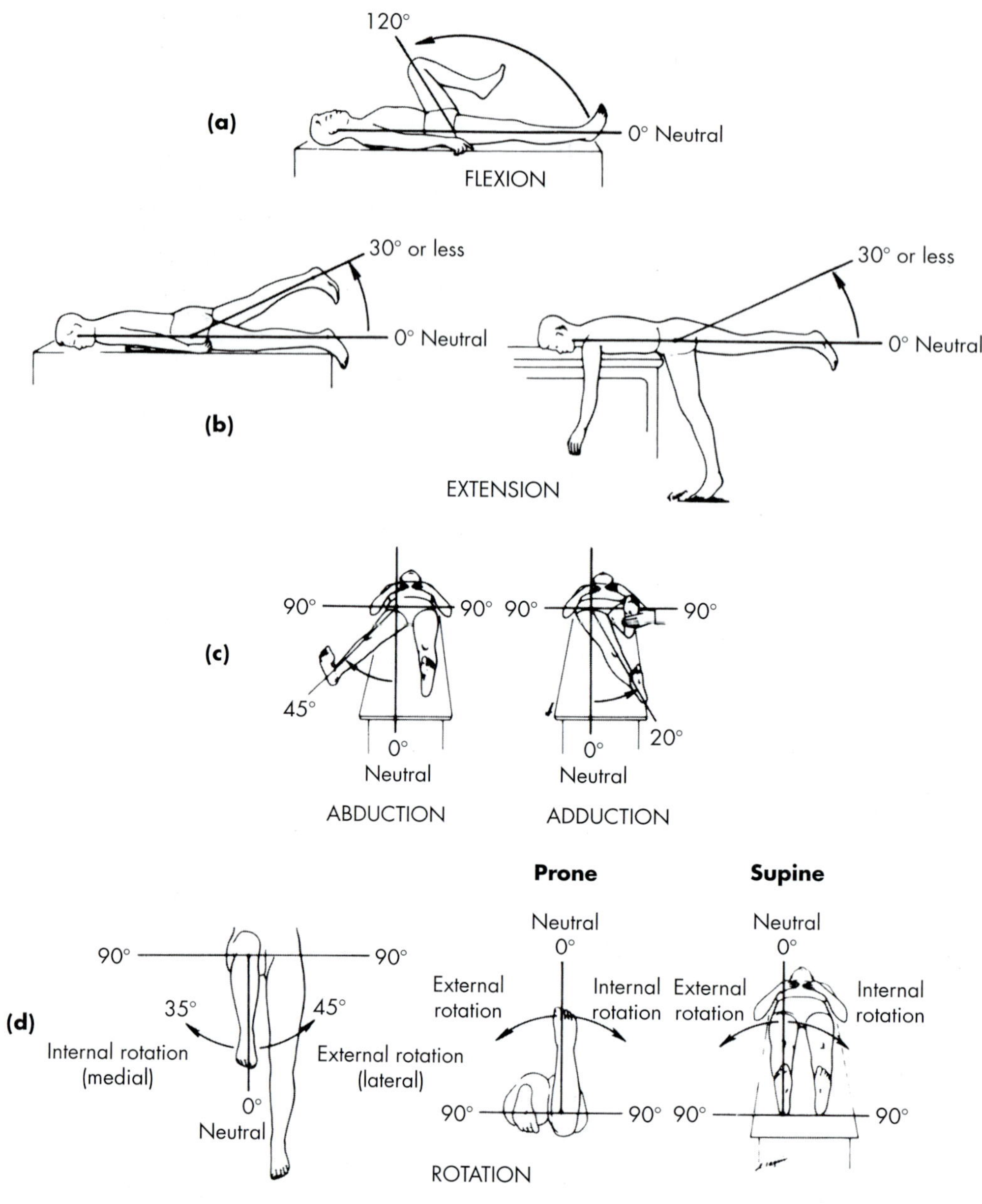

FIGURE 15.5 Active motions of the hip

Anteriorly, the iliofemoral, or Y ligament, prevents hip hyperextension. The teres ligament attaches from deep in the acetabulum to a depression in the head of the femur; it slightly limits adduction. The pubofemoral ligament is located anteromedially and inferiorly and limits excessive extension and abduction. Posteriorly, the triangular ischiofemoral ligament extends from the ischium below to the trochanteric fossa of the femur; it limits internal rotation.

Although there is some disagreement about the exact possible range of each movement in the hip joint, the ranges are generally 0 to 130 degrees of flexion, 0 to 30 degrees of extension, 0 to 35 degrees of abduction, 0 to 30 degrees of adduction, 0 to 45 degrees of internal rotation, and 0 to 50 degrees of external rotation (figure 15.5).

The pelvic girdle moves back and forth within three planes for a total of six different movements. To avoid confusion, it is important to analyze the pelvic girdle activity to determine the exact location of the movement. All pelvic girdle rotation actually results from motion at one or more of the following locations: the right hip, the left hip, and/or the lumbar spine. Although it is not essential for movement to occur in all three of these areas, it must occur in at least one for the pelvis to rotate

TABLE 15.1 Motions Accompanying Pelvic Rotation

Pelvic rotation	Lumbar spine motion	Right-hip motion	Left-hip motion
Anterior rotation	Extension	Flexion	Flexion
Posterior rotation	Flexion	Extension	Extension
Right lateral rotation	Left lateral flexion	Abduction	Adduction
Left lateral rotation	Right lateral flexion	Adduction	Abduction
Right transverse rotation	Left lateral rotation	Internal rotation	External rotation
Left transverse rotation	Right lateral rotation	External rotation	Internal rotation

in any direction. Table 15.1 lists the motions at the hips and lumbar spine that can often accompany rotation of the pelvic girdle.

Movements

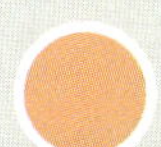

FLEXIBILITY & STRENGTH

Movements of the Hip and Pelvic Girdle

Anterior and posterior pelvic rotations occur in the sagittal or anteroposterior plane, whereas right and left lateral rotation occurs in the lateral or frontal plane. Right transverse (clockwise) rotation and left transverse (counterclockwise) rotation occur in the horizontal or transverse plane of motion. (See figures 15.6 and 15.7.)

Hip flexion
Movement of the femur straight anteriorly from any point in the sagittal plane toward the pelvis.

Hip extension
Movement of the femur straight posteriorly from any point in the sagittal plane away from the pelvis; sometimes referred to as *hyperextension*.

Hip abduction
Movement of the femur in the frontal plane laterally to the side away from the midline.

Hip adduction
Movement of the femur in the frontal plane medially toward the midline.

Hip external rotation
Lateral rotary movement of the femur in the transverse plane around its longitudinal axis away from the midline; lateral rotation.

Hip internal rotation
Medial rotary movement of the femur in the transverse plane around its longitudinal axis toward the midline; medial rotation.

Hip diagonal abduction
Movement of the femur in a diagonal plane away from the midline of the body.

Hip diagonal adduction
Movement of the femur in a diagonal plane toward the midline of the body.

Anterior pelvic rotation
Anterior movement of the upper pelvis in which the iliac crest tilts forward in a sagittal plane (anterior tilt); accomplished by hip flexion and/or lumbar extension.

Posterior pelvic rotation
Posterior movement of the upper pelvis in which the iliac crest tilts backward in a sagittal plane (posterior tilt); accomplished by hip extension and/or lumbar flexion.

Left lateral pelvic rotation
In the frontal plane, rotation in which the left pelvis moves inferiorly in relation to the right pelvis—either the left pelvis rotates downward or the right pelvis rotates upward (left lateral tilt); accomplished by left-hip abduction, right-hip adduction, and/or right lumbar lateral flexion.

Right lateral pelvic rotation
In the frontal plane, rotation in which the right pelvis moves inferiorly in relation to the left pelvis—either the right pelvis rotates downward or the left pelvis rotates upward (right lateral tilt); accomplished by right-hip abduction, left-hip adduction, and/or left lumbar lateral flexion.

Left transverse pelvic rotation
In a horizontal plane of motion, rotation of the pelvis to the body's left—the right iliac crest moves anteriorly in relation to the left iliac crest, which moves posteriorly; accomplished by right-hip external rotation, left-hip internal rotation, and/or right lumbar rotation.

Right transverse pelvic rotation
In a horizontal plane of motion, rotation of the pelvis to the body's right—the left iliac crest moves anteriorly in relation to the right iliac crest, which moves posteriorly; accomplished by left-hip external rotation, right-hip internal rotation, and/or left lumbar rotation.

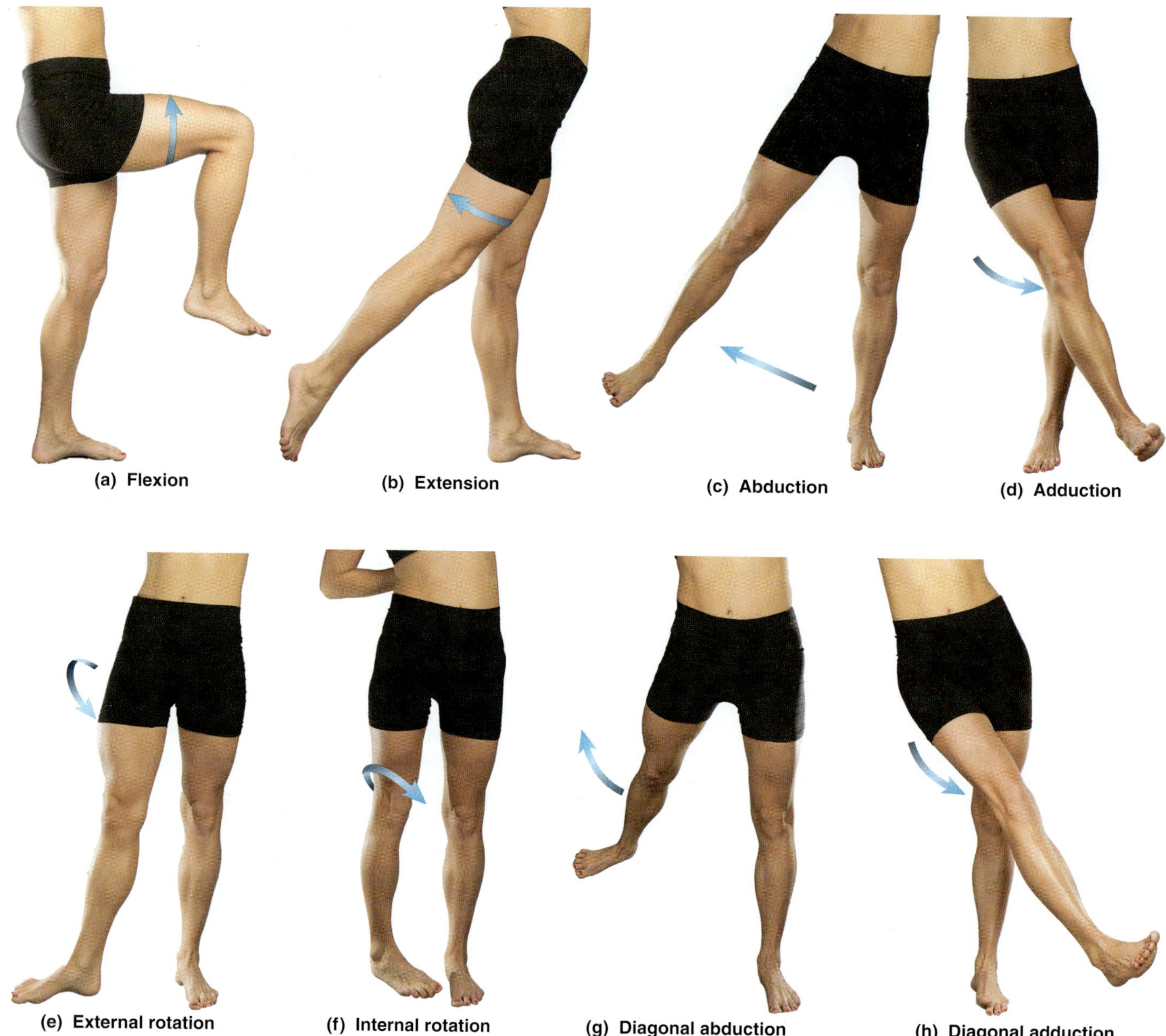

FIGURE 15.6 Movements of the hip

Muscles

At the hip joint, there are seven two-joint muscles that have one action at the hip and another at the knee. The muscles actually involved in hip and pelvic girdle motions depend largely on the direction of the movement and the position of the body in relation to the earth's gravitational forces. In addition, the body part that moves the most will be the part least stabilized. For example, when a person is standing on both feet and contracting the hip flexors, the trunk and pelvis will rotate anteriorly. When a person is lying supine and contracting the hip flexors, however, the thighs will move forward into flexion on the stable pelvis.

In another example, the hip flexor muscles are used to move the thighs toward the trunk. But the extensor muscles are used eccentrically when the pelvis and the trunk move downward slowly on the femur; they are used concentrically when the trunk is raised on the femur—this movement, of course, is rising to the standing position.

In the downward phase of the knee-bend exercise, the movement at the hips and knees is flexion. The muscles primarily involved are the hip and knee extensors in eccentric contraction.

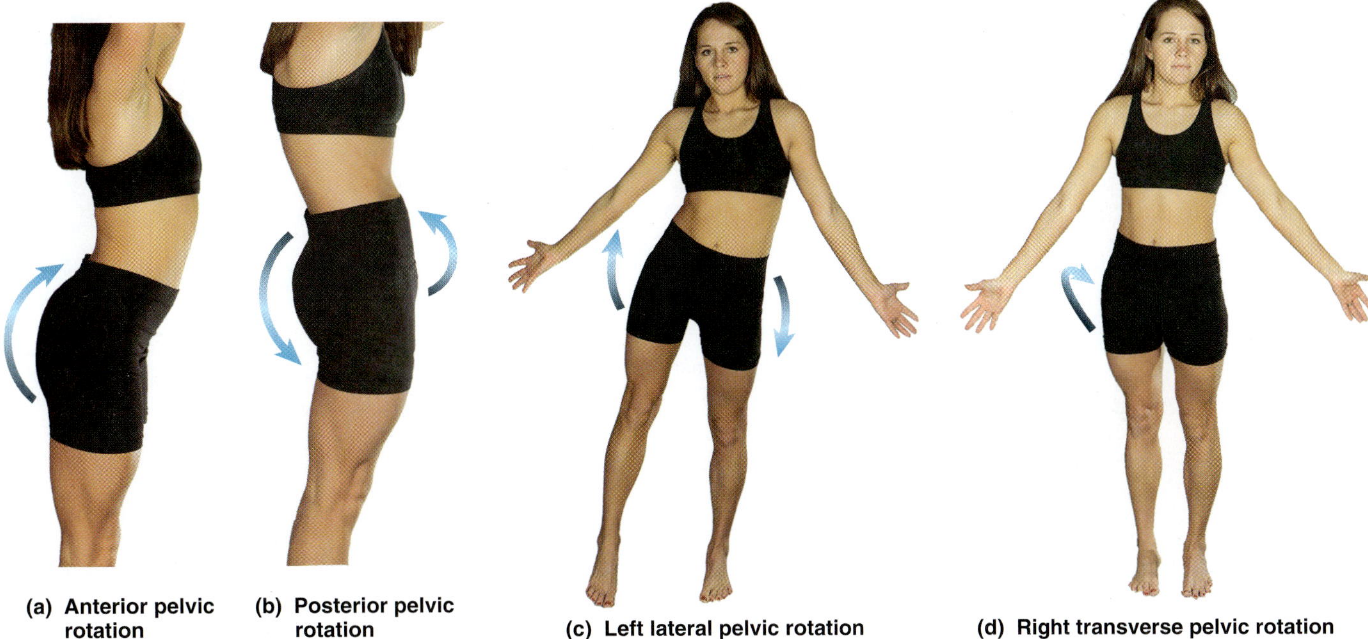

(a) Anterior pelvic rotation (b) Posterior pelvic rotation (c) Left lateral pelvic rotation (d) Right transverse pelvic rotation

FIGURE 15.7 Movements of the pelvic girdle

Hip joint and pelvic girdle muscles—location

MUSCLE SPECIFIC

Muscle location largely determines the muscle action. Seventeen or more muscles are found in the area (the six external rotators are counted as one muscle). Most hip joint and pelvic girdle muscles are large and strong.

Anterior—primarily hip flexion
- Iliopsoas (iliacus and psoas)
- Pectineus
- Rectus femoris
- Sartorius

Lateral—primarily hip abduction
- Gluteus medius
- Gluteus minimus
- Tensor fasciae latae

Posterior—primarily hip extension
- Gluteus maximus
- Biceps femoris
- Semitendinosus
- Semimembranosus
- Lateral rotators (six deep)

Medial—primarily hip adduction
- Adductor brevis
- Adductor longus
- Adductor magnus
- Gracilis

MUSCLE IDENTIFICATION

In developing a thorough and practical knowledge of the muscular system, it is essential for students to understand the functions of individual muscles. Figures 15.8, 15.9, and 15.10 illustrate groups of muscles that work together to produce joint movement. While viewing the muscles in these figures, correlate them with table 15.2.

The pelvis muscles that act on the hip joint may be divided into two regions—the iliac and gluteal regions. The iliac region contains the **iliopsoas** muscle (figure 15.8), which flexes the hip. The iliopsoas actually is composed of three different muscles—the **iliacus,** the **psoas major,** and the **psoas minor.** The 10 muscles of the gluteal region function primarily to extend and rotate the hip. Located in the gluteal region are the **gluteus maximus, gluteus medius, gluteus minimus,** and **tensor fasciae latae** and the six deep lateral rotators—**piriformis, obturator externus, obturator internus, gemellus superior, gemellus inferior,** and **quadratus femoris** (figures 15.9 and 15.10).

The thigh is divided into three compartments by the intermuscular septa (figure 15.11). The anterior compartment contains the **rectus femoris,** vastus medialis, vastus intermedius, vastus lateralis, and **sartorius** (see figure 15.8a). The **hamstring** muscle group, consisting of the biceps femoris, semitendinosus, and semimembranosus, is located in the posterior compartment. The medial compartment contains the thigh muscles primarily responsible for adduction of the hip; these are the **adductor brevis,**

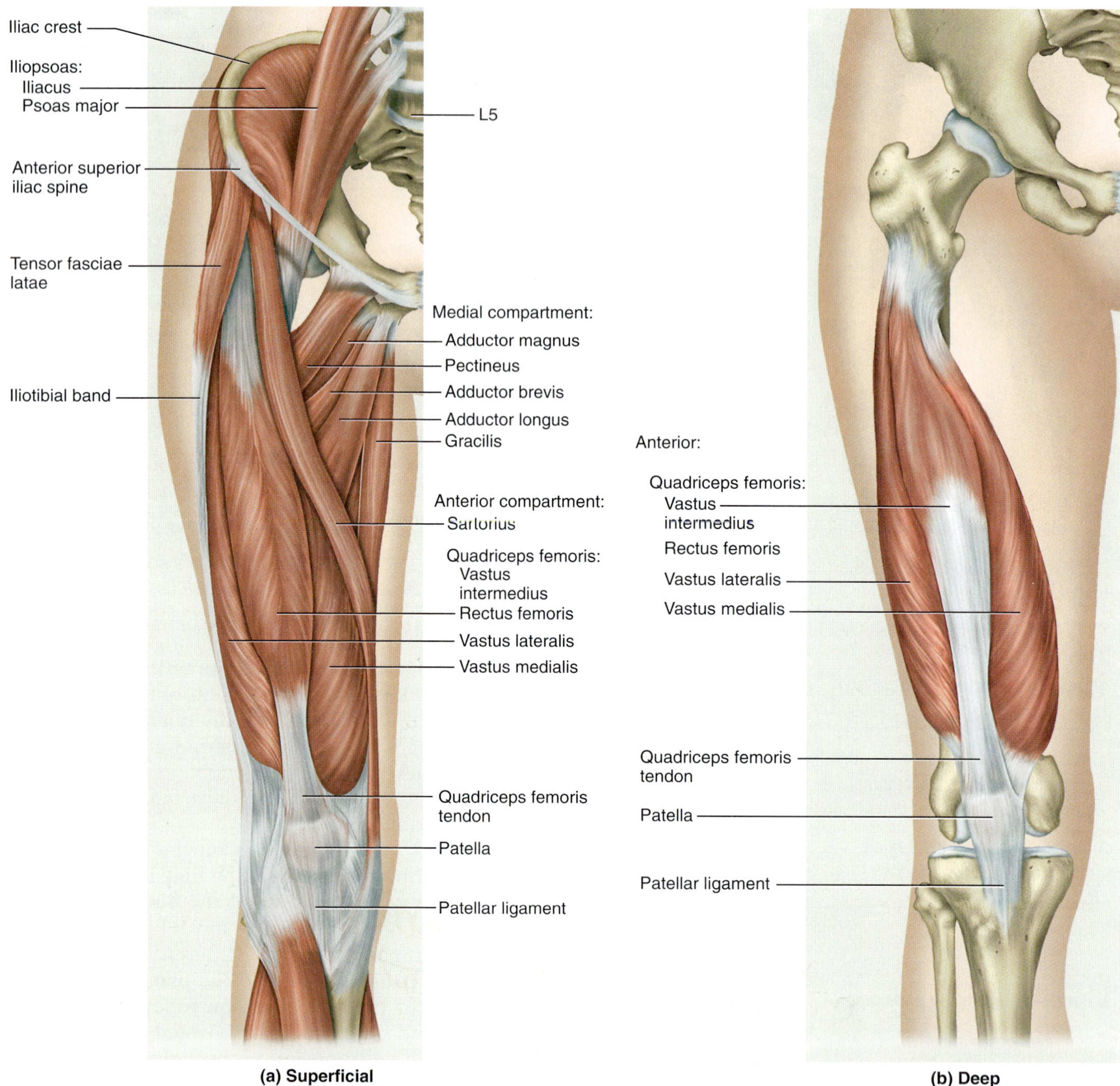

FIGURE 15.8 Anterior muscles of the thigh

adductor longus, adductor magnus, pectineus, and **gracilis** (see figures 15.8a, 15.8b, and 15.9).

Nerves

The hip and pelvic girdle muscles are all innervated from the *lumbar plexus* and *sacral plexus,* known collectively as the **lumbosacral plexus.** The lumbar plexus (figure 15.12) is formed by the anterior rami of spinal nerves L1 through L4 and some fibers from T12. The lower abdomen and the anterior and medial portions of the lower extremity are innervated by nerves arising from the lumbar plexus. The sacral plexus (figure 15.13) is formed by the anterior rami of L4, L5, and S1 through S4. The lower back, pelvis, perineum, posterior surface of the thigh and leg, and dorsal and plantar surfaces of the foot are innervated by nerves arising from the sacral plexus.

The major nerves of significance are the femoral and obturator nerves, which arise from the lumbar plexus

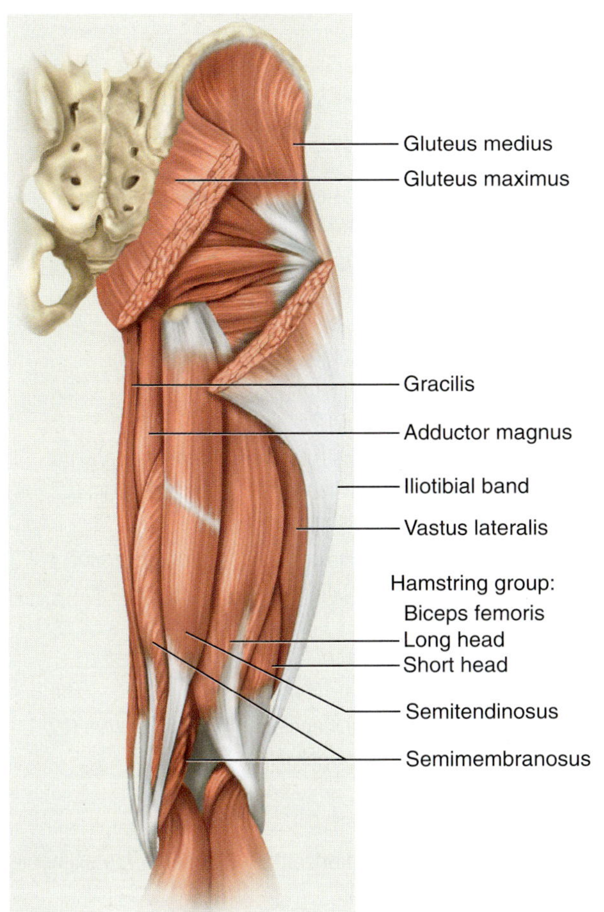

FIGURE 15.9 Superficial gluteal and thigh muscles, posterior view

to innervate the muscles of the hip. The **femoral nerve,** as shown in figure 15.12, arises from the posterior division of the lumbar plexus and innervates the anterior muscles of the thigh, including the iliopsoas, rectus femoris, vastus medialis, vastus intermedius, vastus lateralis, pectineus, and sartorius. It also provides sensation to the anterior and lateral thigh and the medial leg and foot. The **obturator nerve,** as shown in figure 15.12, arises from the anterior division of the lumbar plexus and provides innervation to the hip adductors, such as the adductor brevis, adductor longus, adductor magnus, and gracilis, as well as the obturator externus. The obturator nerve provides sensation to the medial thigh.

The nerves arising from the sacral plexus that innervate the muscles of the hip are the superior gluteal, inferior gluteal, sciatic, and branches from the sacral plexus. The superior gluteal nerve arises from L4, L5, and S1 to innervate the gluteus medius, gluteus minimus, and tensor fasciae latae. The inferior gluteal nerve arises from L5, S1, and S2 to supply the gluteus maximus. Branches from the sacral plexus innervate the piriformis (S1, S2), gemellus superior (L5, S1, S2), gemellus inferior and obturator internus (L4, L5, S1, S2), and quadratus femoris (L4, L5, S1).

The **sciatic nerve** is composed of the **tibial nerve** and common **peroneal** (fibular) **nerve,** which are

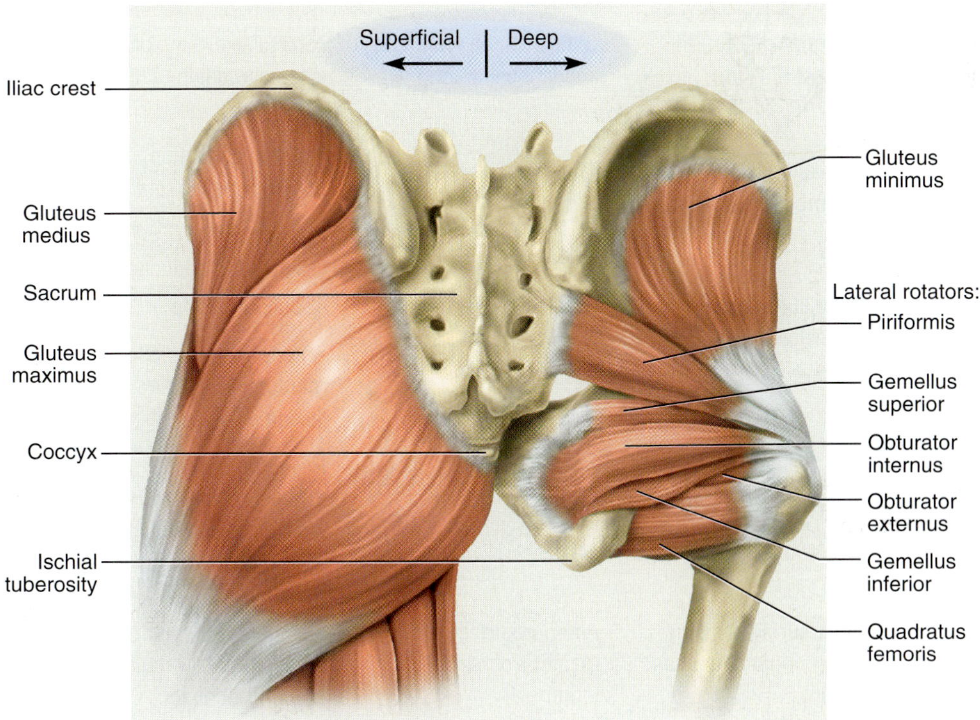

FIGURE 15.10 Deep gluteal muscles and lateral rotators, posterior view

TABLE 15.2 Agonist Muscles of the Hip Joint

Name of Muscle	Origins	Insertion	Actions	Innervations
Iliopsoas: psoas minor, psoas major, iliacus	Inner surface of ilium, base of sacrum and sides of bodies of last thoracic and all lumbar vertebrae, disks, transverse processes	Lesser trochanter of femur and shaft just below	Flexion of hip; lateral rotation of femur; when hip is fixed, iliopsoas muscle pulls on vertebrae and flexes spine and pelvis on thigh, as in rising to a sitting position from supine	Lumbar nerve and femoral nerve (L2–L4)
Psoas minor	Anterior aspect of 12 thoracic and 1 or 2 lumbar vertebrae	Pectineal line and iliopectineal eminence	Transverse pelvis rotation contralaterally when ipsilateral femur is stabilized	Lumbar nerve and femoral nerve (L2–L4)
Sartorius	Anterior superior iliac spine (ASIS) and notch just below spine	Anterior medial condyle of tibia just below condyle	Flexion of hip, flexion of knee, lateral rotation of thigh as it flexes hip and knee, abduction of hip, anterior pelvic rotation	Femoral nerve (L2–L3)
Rectus femoris	Anterior inferior iliac spine (AIIS) of ilium, groove (posterior) above acetabulum	Superior aspect of patella and patellar tendon to tibial tuberosity	Flexion of hip, extension of knee, anterior pelvic rotation	Femoral nerve (L2–L4)
Tensor fasciae latae	Anterior iliac crest and surface of ilium just below crest	Iliotibial tract on thigh one-fourth of way down (Iliotibial tract inserts into Gerdy's tubercle of anterolateral tibial condyle.)	Flexion of hip, horizontal abduction of hip, tendency to rotate hip internally as it flexes, anterior pelvic rotation	Superior gluteal nerve (L4–L5, S1)
Gluteus maximus	Posterior one-fourth of crest of ilium, posterior surface of sacrum near ilium and fascia of lumbar area, coccyx near ilium	Gluteal line of femur and iliotibial tract	Forceful extension of hip, external rotation of hip *Upper fibers:* assist in abduction, posterior pelvic rotation *Lower fibers:* assist in hip adduction	Inferior gluteal nerve (L5, S1–S2)
Gluteus medius	Outer surface of ilium just below crest	Greater trochanter of femur, posterior and middle surfaces	Abduction of hip *Anterior fibers:* medial rotation of thigh, weak flexion *Posterior fibers:* external rotation and weak extension of hip, lateral pelvic rotation to ipsilateral side	Superior gluteal nerve (L4–L5, S1)
Gluteus minimus	Outer surface of ilium below origin of gluteus medius	Anterior surface of greater trochanter of femur	Abduction of femur on pelvis, internal rotation as femur abducts, lateral pelvic rotation to ipsilateral side	Superior gluteal nerve (L4–L5, S1)

TABLE 15.2 (Continued)

Name of Muscle	Origins	Insertion	Actions	Innervations
Lateral rotators:				
Piriformis	Anterior sacrum	Superior aspect of posterior greater trochanter	External rotation	1st or 2nd sacral nerve (S1–S2)
Gemellus superior	Posterior portions of ischium	Posterior aspect of greater trochanter	External rotation	Sacral nerve (L5, S1–S2)
Gemellus inferior	Same	Posterior aspect of greater trochanter	External rotation	Branches from sacral plexus (L4–L5, S1–S2)
Obturator externus	Obturator foramen	Posterior aspect of greater trochanter	External rotation	Obturator nerve (L3–L4)
Obturator internus	Obturator foramen	Posterior aspect of greater trochanter	External rotation	Branches from sacral plexus (L4–L5, S1–S2)
Quadratus femoris	Anterolateral surface of ischium	Inferior aspect of greater trochanter	External rotation	Branches from sacral plexus (L4–L5, S1)
Adductor brevis	Front of inferior pubic ramus just below origin of longus	Upper portion of linea aspera between adductor longus and adductor magnus and posterior to pectineus	Adduction of hip, external rotation as it adducts the hip, assists in flexion of hip	Obturator nerve (L3–L4)
Adductor longus	Anterior pubis just below its crest	Middle third of linea aspera	Adduction of hip, assists in flexion of hip	Obturator nerve (L3–L4)
Adductor magnus	Pubic ramus, ischium, ischial tuberosity	Linea aspera of posterior femur and inner condyloid ridge, adductor tubercle of medial femur	Adduction of hip, external rotation as the hip adducts, extension of hip	*Anterior:* obturator nerve (L2–L4) *Posterior:* sciatic nerve (L4–L5, S1–S3)
Pectineus	Anterior pubis just above crest lateral to pubic tubercle	Between lesser trochanter and linea aspera of posterior femur	Flexion of hip, adduction of hip on pelvis, external rotation of hip	Femoral nerve (L2–L4)
Gracilis	Anteromedial edge of descending ramus of pubis	Medial proximal tibia just below condyle (pes anserinus)	Adduction of hip, internal rotation of flexed knee, flexion of knee from extension, weak flexion of hip, internal rotation of hip	Obturator nerve (L2–L4)

Anterior
Quadriceps
Rectus femoris
Vastus medialis
Medial
Sartorius
Vastus lateralis
Intermuscular septum
Vastus intermedius
Femur
Adductor longus
Adductor brevis
Gracilis
Biceps femoris short head
Adductor magnus
Semimembranosus
Biceps femoris long head
Semitendinosus
Lateral
Posterior

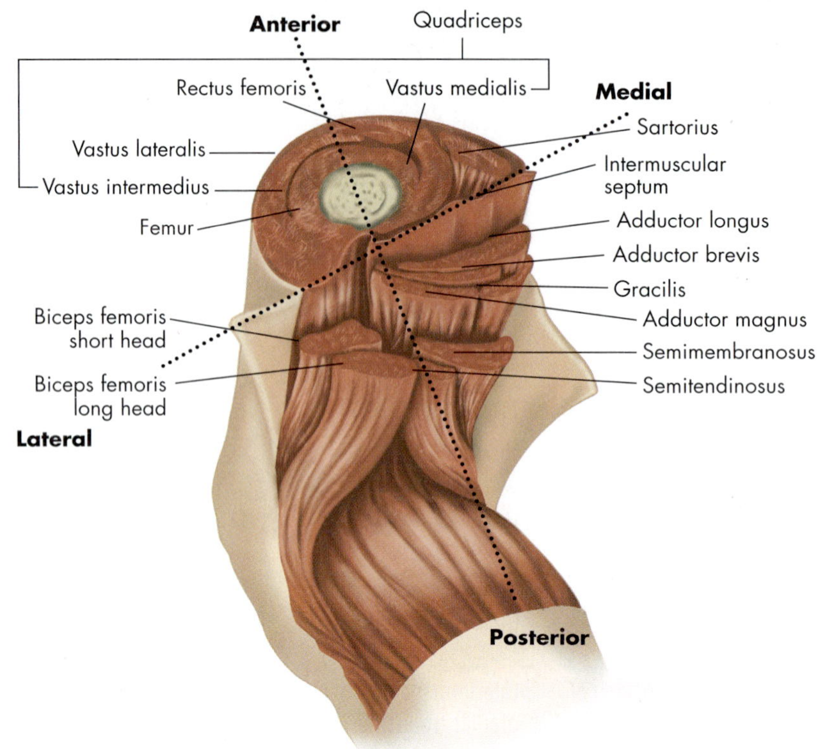

FIGURE 15.11 Cross section of midthigh at midsection

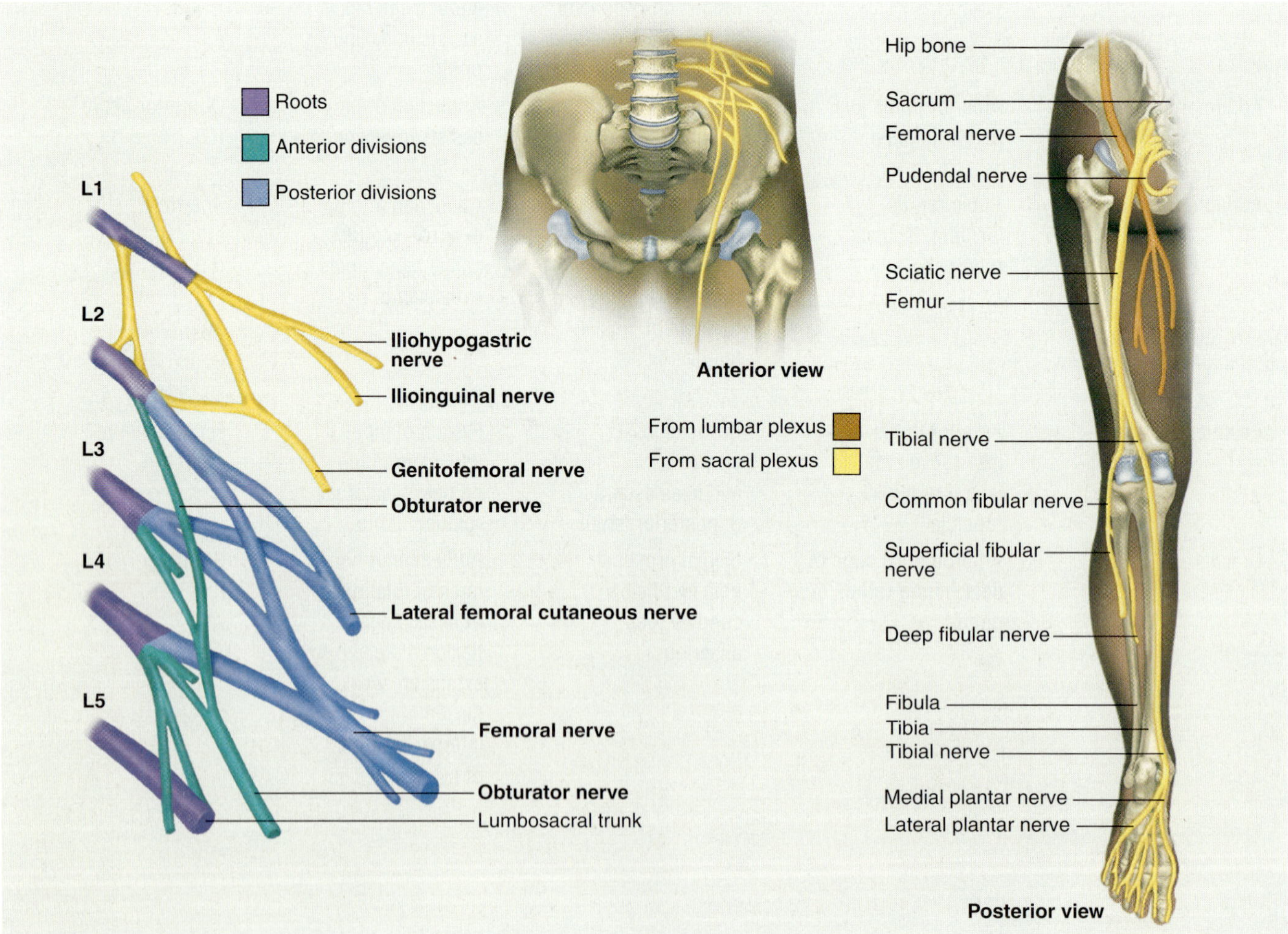

Roots
Anterior divisions
Posterior divisions
L1
L2
L3
L4
L5
Iliohypogastric nerve
Ilioinguinal nerve
Genitofemoral nerve
Obturator nerve
Lateral femoral cutaneous nerve
Femoral nerve
Obturator nerve
Lumbosacral trunk
Anterior view
From lumbar plexus
From sacral plexus
Hip bone
Sacrum
Femoral nerve
Pudendal nerve
Sciatic nerve
Femur
Tibial nerve
Common fibular nerve
Superficial fibular nerve
Deep fibular nerve
Fibula
Tibia
Tibial nerve
Medial plantar nerve
Lateral plantar nerve
Posterior view

FIGURE 15.12 The lumbar plexus

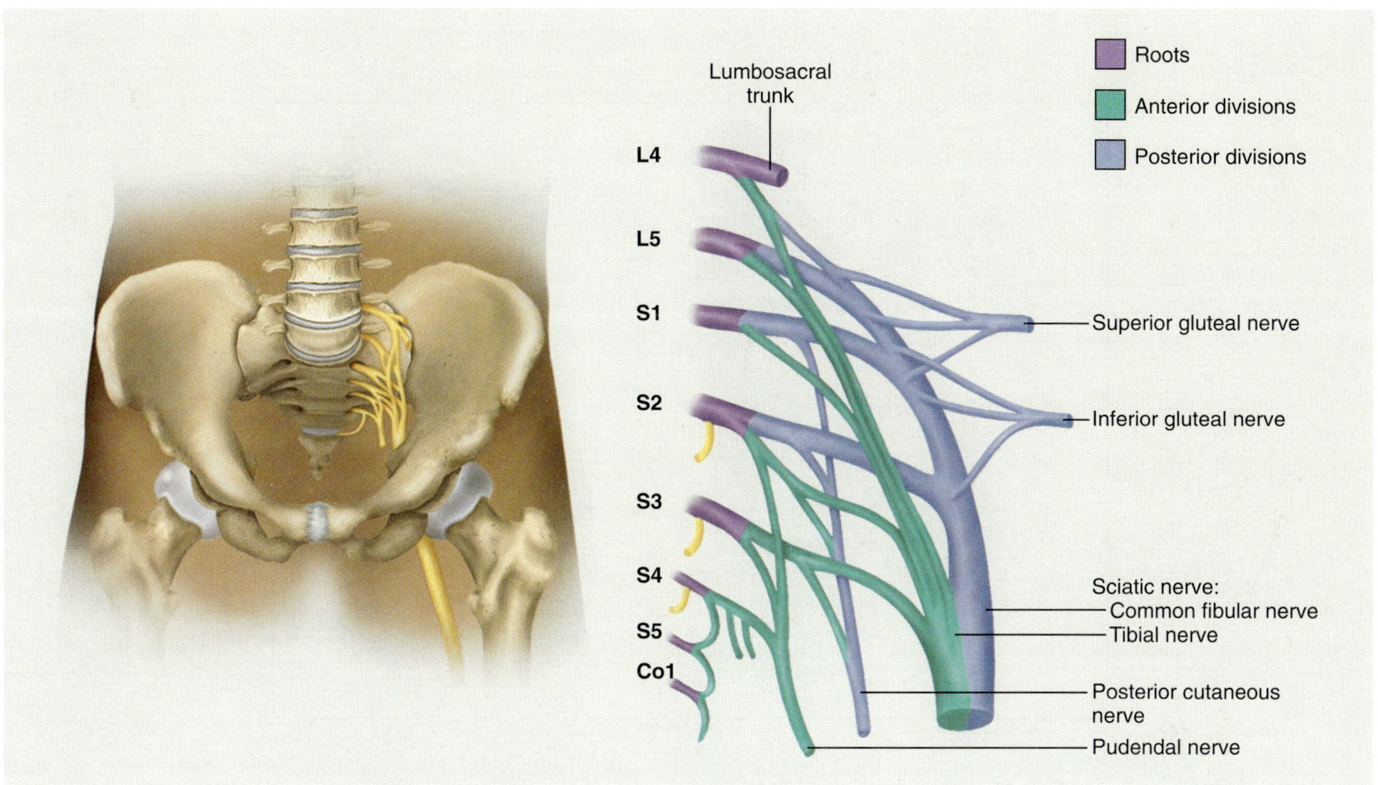

FIGURE 15.13 The sacral and coccygeal plexuses

wrapped together in a connective tissue sheath until the nerves reach approximately midway down the posterior thigh. The sciatic nerve tibial division (figure 15.13) innervates the semitendinosus, semimembranosus, biceps femoris (long head), and adductor magnus. The sciatic nerve supplies sensation to the anterolateral and posterolateral lower leg, as well as most of the dorsal and plantar aspects of the foot. The tibial division provides sensation for the posterolateral lower leg and the plantar aspect of the foot, while the peroneal division provides sensation to the anterolateral lower leg and dorsum of the foot. Both of these nerves continue down the lower extremity to provide motor and sensory function to the muscles of the lower leg; this is addressed in Chapters 17 and 19.

Individual Muscles of the Hip Joint and Pelvic Girdle—Anterior

ILIOPSOAS MUSCLE

Palpation

The iliopsoas is difficult to palpate as it is deep against the posterior abdominal wall. With the client seated and leaning slightly forward to relax the abdominal muscles, palpate the psoas major deeply between the iliac crest and the 12th rib, about halfway between the ASIS and the umbilicus, with active hip flexion. With the client supine, palpate the iliopsoas distal tendon on the anterior aspect of the hip approximately 1½ inches below the center of the inguinal ligament with active hip flexion and extension, immediately lateral to the pectineus and medial to the sartorius.

CLINICAL NOTES **Core Muscle**

The iliopsoas is considered a core muscle. Psoas major is very active when the abdominal muscles are weak; it assists in trunk flexion. The psoas major can cause painful low-back conditions because it is attached to the vertebrae. Tightness in this muscle pulls the lumbar vertebrae anteriorly into lordosis and can result in herniated L3–L4 disks. The psoas also can affect the body's posture if it is contracted on one side, can cause sore muscle responses up and down the back, and can hold the femur in a flexed position. Read the caution below in Muscle Specifics about exercising the iliopsoas.

OIAI MUSCLE CHART ILIOPSOAS (il´e-o-so´as) Major hip flexor

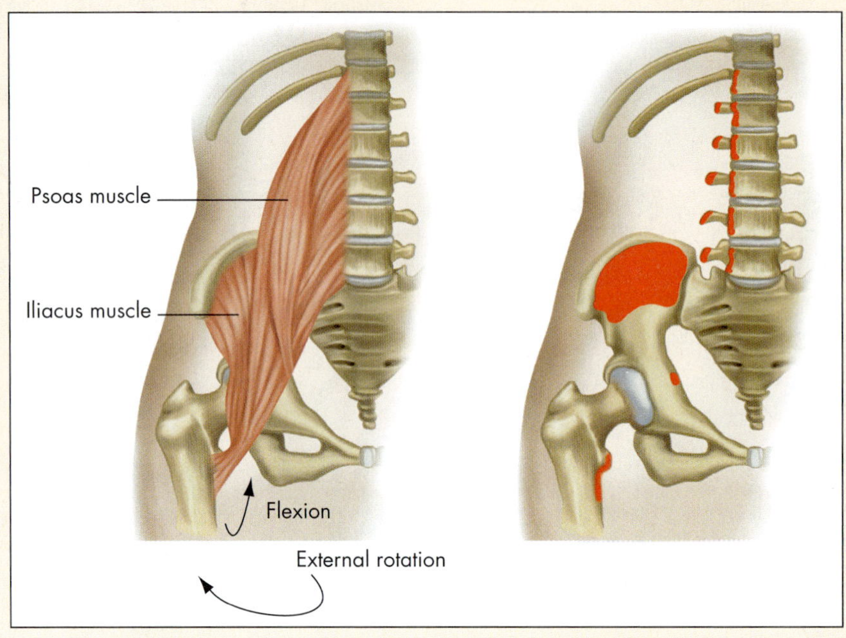

Name of Muscle	Origins	Insertion	Actions	Innervations
Iliopsoas: psoas minor, psoas major, iliacus	Inner surface of ilium, base of sacrum and sides of bodies of last thoracic and all lumbar vertebrae, disks, transverse processes	Lesser trochanter of femur and shaft just below	Flexion of hip; lateral rotation of femur; when hip is fixed, iliopsoas muscle pulls on vertebrae and flexes spine and pelvis on thigh, as in rising to a sitting position from supine	Lumbar nerve and femoral nerve (L2–L4)
Psoas minor*	Anterior aspect of 12 thoracic and 1 or 2 lumbar vertebrae	Pectineal line and iliopectineal eminence	Transverse pelvis rotation contralaterally when ipsilateral femur is stabilized	Lumbar nerve and femoral nerve (L2–L4)

*The psoas minor does not flex the hip because it inserts on the pelvis, but it does assist in posterior pelvic rotation.

Muscle Specifics

The iliopsoas is commonly referred to as if it were one muscle, but it is actually composed of the iliacus, the psoas major, and the psoas minor. Some anatomy texts make this distinction and list each muscle individually. The psoas minor is not always present; it is absent in 40 percent of individuals. The psoas minor does not flex the hip because it inserts on the pelvis, but it does assist in posterior pelvic rotation.

The iliopsoas muscle is powerful in performing some actions, such as raising the lower extremity from the floor while in a supine position. The psoas major's origin in the lower back tends to move the lower back anteriorly or, in the supine position, to pull the lower back up as it raises the legs. For this reason, lower-back problems are often aggravated by this activity, and bilateral leg raises are not usually recommended. Strong abdominal muscles can be used to prevent lower-back strain by pulling up on the front of the pelvis, thus flattening the back. Leg raising is primarily hip flexion and not abdominal action. Backs may be injured by strenuous and prolonged leg-raising exercises. The iliopsoas contracts strongly, both concentrically and eccentrically, in sit-ups, particularly if the hips are not flexed. The more flexed or abducted the hips are, the less the iliopsoas will be activated with abdominal strengthening exercises. Straight-leg sit-ups are extremely dangerous and should be avoided.

Clinical Flexibility

Stretching the psoas specifically can help reduce anterior forces on the lumbar disks and help herniated-disk issues. It also helps correct improper gait. To stretch the iliopsoas, which often becomes tight and contributes to anterior pelvic tilting, the hip must be hyperextended so that the femur is behind the plane of the body. Kneel on a towel or pad, with the leg bent at 90 degrees. Bring the other leg in front by flexing the hip in a lunge position. Tighten the abdominals and move the navel forward in a straight line. Feel for the stretch on the lower leg near the groin. You might also feel this at the lower back. Make certain that the forward leg is bent enough so that the foot is in front of the knee in the lunge position. *Contraindications:* Use caution if lumbar lesions are active. It is important to counteract the pull on the lumbar vertebrae by contracting the abdominals.

Strengthening

Hip flexion is an important movement in sports and normal activities. A weak and contracted psoas will distort gait by shortening stride, and it can cause the quadratus lumborum to spasm as it tries to resist the pull on the lumbar spine. The iliopsoas may be strengthened by lying on your back on a table (or bed). Shift your hip so that the involved side is even with the edge of the table. With ankle weights on and both legs bent, flex one leg up so that the femur is at a 90-degree angle. Leave the foot of the other leg on the table. The knee should remain flexed at 90 degrees throughout the movement. Lower the weight down and off the table slowly, keeping the abdominals contracted. Slowly lift the knee back toward the chest (hip flexion), and repeat. Be sure to use the stomach muscles on this exercise to protect the low back. *Contraindications:* It is important to keep the uninvolved leg bent during this movement to help protect the low back, especially if lumbar disk lesions exist. Begin with no weight if pain is present.

SARTORIUS MUSCLE

Palpation

The sartorius is located proximally just medial to the tensor fasciae latae and lateral to the iliopsoas. With the client in a supine position, palpate the sartorius superficially from the anterior superior iliac spine to the medial tibial condyle during combined resistance of hip flexion, external rotation, and abduction and knee flexion and internal rotation.

CLINICAL NOTES — **Strap Muscle**

The sartorius is considered a strap muscle, and it is the longest muscle in the body. It inserts on the most anterior position of the pes anserinus tendinous expansion (with the gracilis and semitendinosus) on the medial tibia. This muscle is not as large as the quadriceps, and although it is superficial, it may be virtually unseen on the thigh. Compressive effleurage in the direction of the fibers distal to proximal can help to release a tight sartorius. Stretching the anterior thigh (see Clinical Flexibility below) is also helpful. The therapist is encouraged to work on the gracilis and semitendinosus, as well as other hip and knee flexors, in addition to treating the pes anserinus area. See Chapter 18 for techniques and Chapter 21 for thigh muscle exercises.

Muscle Specifics

Pulling from the anterior superior iliac spine and the notch just below it, the sartorius tends to tilt the pelvis anteriorly (down in front) as the muscle contracts. The abdominal muscles must prevent this tendency by posteriorly rotating the pelvis (pulling up in front), thus flattening the lower back.

The sartorius, a two-joint muscle, is effective as a hip or knee flexor. It is weak when both actions take place at the same time. Overall, it is not a powerful muscle. Observe that, in attempting to cross the knees when in a sitting position, one customarily leans back, thus raising the origin to lengthen this muscle and make it more effective in flexing and crossing the knees. With the knees held extended, the sartorius becomes a more effective hip flexor.

Clinical Flexibility

The sartorius can be stretched using a quadriceps stretch. Although it is a thin muscle, the fibers may be isolated along with the quadriceps by taking the hip into hyperextension. From a side-lying position, tuck the bottom leg up into flexion, and hold it to your chest (or as high as possible). Grasp the ankle of the top leg, and, beginning from a flexed-hip position, contract the gluteals to move the hip back into hyperextension. Contract the abdominals to prevent the hip from rotating in the direction of the stretch. Gently pull on the ankle for 2 seconds, and repeat. Make certain that the hip stays down and in line with the shoulders; do not abduct the thigh during the movement. *Contraindications:* Use caution if lumbar disk lesions are present. The abdominals help protect the low back in this exercise.

Strengthening

The sartorius is strengthened by performing hip flexion activities in the manner described for developing the iliopsoas.

OIAI MUSCLE CHART SARTORIUS (sar-to´ri-us) The tailor cross-legged muscle

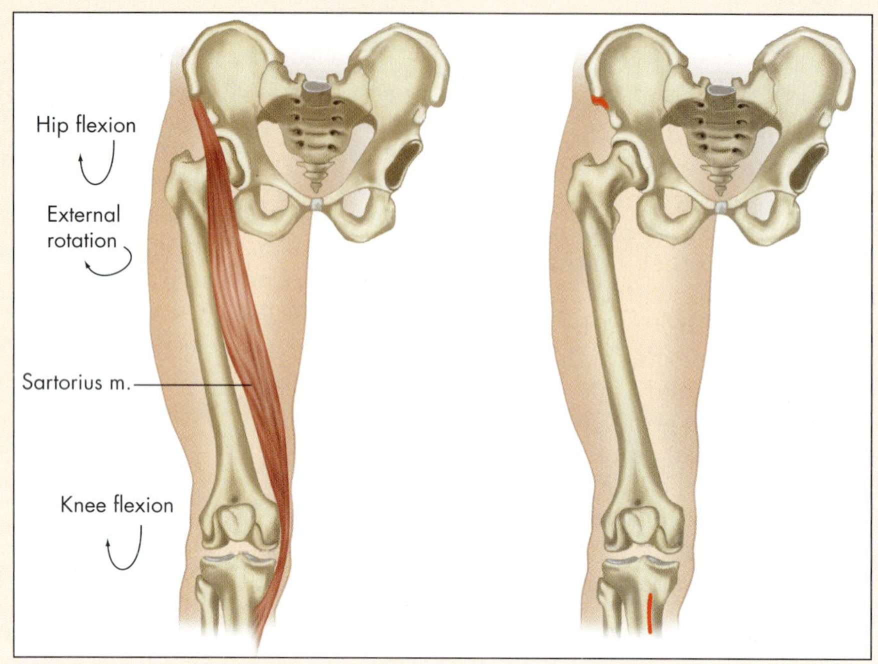

Name of Muscle	Origins	Insertion	Actions	Innervations
Sartorius	Anterior superior iliac spine (ASIS) and notch just below spine	Anterior medial surface of tibia just below condyle	Flexion of hip, flexion of knee, lateral rotation of thigh as it flexes hip and knee, abduction of hip, anterior pelvic rotation, medial rotation of knee	Femoral nerve (L2–L3)

RECTUS FEMORIS MUSCLE

Palpation

Palpate the rectus femoris straight down the anterior thigh from the anterior inferior iliac spine to the patella, with resisted knee extension and hip flexion.

CLINICAL NOTES **Two-Joint Muscle**

The rectus femoris sits on top of the vastus intermedius and inserts strongly into the patellar tendon. It is not as large as the vastus lateralis or vastus medialis, but it can be well developed as part of the whole quadriceps group. When fatigued, the rectus femoris and the other quadriceps tend to feel weak when one walks down stairs; this is especially true in individuals with arthritis. Because of its two-joint function, the therapist must remember how the muscle is used in its action. This muscle is an important "guide" for the patella; as it contracts, it pulls this bone along the trochlear groove of the femur. Rolling, elliptical movement, compression, and broadening are useful techniques for unwinding the quadriceps. Specifically stretching this muscle at both origin and insertion is extremely beneficial for knee-tracking issues and Osgood-Schlatter disease. See Chapter 18 for techniques and Chapter 21 for exercises for the thigh muscles.

Muscle Specifics

Pulling from the anterior inferior iliac spine of the ilium, the rectus femoris muscle, like the sartorius, has the tendency to anteriorly rotate the pelvis (down in front and up in back). Only the abdominal muscles can prevent

OIAI MUSCLE CHART RECTUS FEMORIS (rek´tus fem´or-is) Straight superficial quadricep

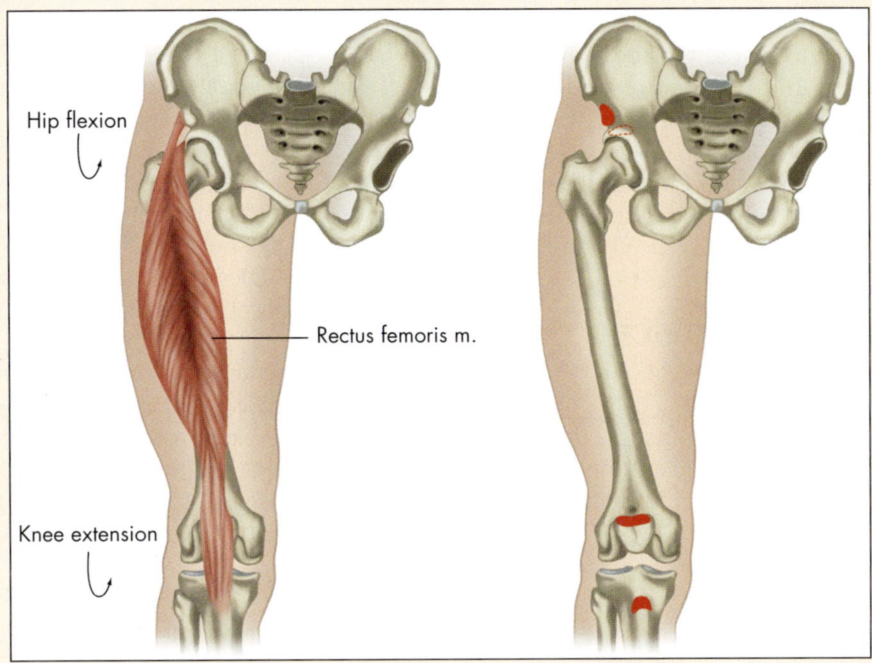

Name of Muscle	Origins	Insertions	Actions	Innervations
Rectus femoris	Anterior inferior iliac spine (AIIS) of ilium, groove (posterior) above acetabulum	Superior aspect of patella and patellar tendon to tibial tuberosity	Flexion of hip, extension of knee, anterior pelvic rotation	Femoral nerve (L2–L4)

this from occurring. Within the hip flexor group in general, many people develop an anteriorly tilted pelvis as they age. A weak abdominal wall does not help stabilize the pelvis and results in an increased lumbar curve.

Clinical Flexibility

Stretching this powerful muscle is important for everyday activities and sports. Knee-tracking issues, wherein the patella does not track the way it should along the trochlear groove, can lead to many painful conditions. The rectus femoris is a chronically tight muscle in many people. The shortened middle part, or belly, of its fibers must be released to take forces off the patella and improve knee biomechanics. Releasing this muscle also helps stabilize the pelvis in a more neutral position. The rectus femoris is best stretched as described for the sartorius. *Contraindications:* The psoas muscle should be stretched before the quadriceps, especially if there are low-back issues. The abdominals must be contracted during this stretch to help stabilize the pelvis and lumbar spine.

Strengthening

Generally, a muscle's ability to exert force decreases as it shortens. This explains why the rectus femoris muscle is a powerful extensor of the knee when the hip is extended but is weaker when the hip is flexed. This muscle is exercised, along with the vastus group, in running, jumping, hopping, and skipping. In these movements, the hips are extended powerfully by the gluteus maximus and the hamstring muscles, which counteract the tendency of the rectus femoris muscle to flex the hip while it extends the knee. The rectus femoris should be strengthened as a hip and knee flexor. To strengthen as a hip flexor, start supine, with the uninvolved leg bent. Using ankle weights, lift the extended leg up into flexion, and lower slowly to the starting position. Keep the foot dorsiflexed throughout the movement. Although psoas is brought into action in this exercise, the proximal end of the rectus femoris helps flex the weighted hip. To strengthen knee flexion, sit on a bench or therapy table with a pillow under the knees; this elevates the knees slightly above the hips. Contract the abdominals and lean the torso forward. Stay in this position throughout. Dorsiflex the ankle and slowly extend the leg; hold 3 to 4 seconds, and lower the weighted ankle slowly. *Contraindications:* Use caution if arthritis is present, and extend the knee only as far as is comfortable.

TENSOR FASCIAE LATAE MUSCLE

Palpation

Anterolaterally, palpate the tensor fasciae latae between the anterior iliac crest and the greater trochanter during internal rotation, flexion, and abduction.

CLINICAL NOTES **Contracted Iliotibial Tract**

The iliotibial tract (IT), or Maissiat's band, is not a muscle. It is an anatomical structure that braces the knee for walking or running, and it consists of a fibrous band that extends from the fasciae latae. The tensor fasciae latae (TFL) and the gluteus maximus are the two muscles that tug on it and provide tension and contracture. The TFL is an important muscle to release by stretching the entire iliotibial tract along with the muscle. Because the IT crosses the knee joint, the knee must stay extended to completely stretch this structure. Many dysfunctions of this region can snowball into chronic issues; therefore, restoring this structure's length is beneficial (see Clinical Flexibility below). To passively shorten the TFL, flex the knee and hip. Broad strip the muscle as the knee is passively drawn in horizontal adduction from the hip joint. Repeat. See Chapter 18 for thigh muscle techniques.

OIAI MUSCLE CHART TENSOR FASCIAE LATAE (ten´sor fas´i-e la´te) Pulls on the iliotibial tract

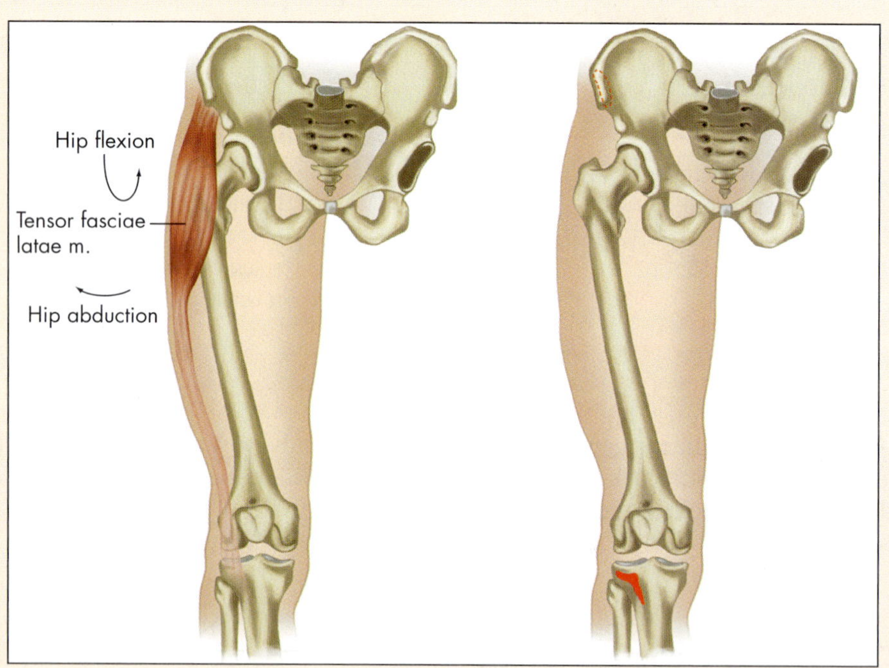

Name of Muscle	Origins	Insertion	Actions	Innervations
Tensor fasciae latae	Anterior iliac crest and surface of ilium just below crest	Iliotibial tract on thigh one-fourth of way down (Iliotibial tract inserts into Gerdy's tubercle of anterolateral tibial condyle.)	Flexion of hip, horizontal abduction of hip, tendency to rotate hip internally as it flexes, anterior pelvic rotation	Superior gluteal nerve (L4–L5, S1)

Muscle Specifics

The tensor fasciae latae muscle aids in preventing external rotation of the hip as it is flexed by other flexor muscles.

The tensor fasciae latae muscle is used when flexion and internal rotation take place. This is a weak movement, but it is important in helping direct the leg forward so that the foot is placed straight forward during walking and running. Thus, from the supine position, raising the leg with definite internal rotation of the femur will call the TFL into action.

Clinical Flexibility

Stretching the TFL effectively involves isolating the iliotibial tract along with it. The following gluteus maximus stretch is also beneficial. Runners and athletes will benefit from restoring this region because it has such a dramatic effect on gait and knee movement. While tensor fascia latae may be stretched with a flexed knee, the iliotibial tract must be isolated by locking the knee during the stretch. To do this, lie supine and bring the opposite leg across the midline, pointing the foot inward. This helps keep the hip stable on the side being stretched. Using an 8-foot rope, wrap the rope around the foot, and bring the rope around the lateral lower leg. Extend the knee with the quadriceps and laterally rotate the femur. Contracting the adductors, bring the leg just high enough to clear the other leg. Using the rope, gently stretch for 2 seconds. Repeat by locking the knee again and laterally rotating the thigh. *Contraindications:* Avoid using this exercise on hip arthroplasty clients.

Strengthening

Strengthening the TFL can greatly assist gait problems and improve lateral hip stability. To develop the tensor fasciae latae, perform hip abduction exercises against gravity and resistance while in a side-lying position. This is done simply by abducting the hip that is up and then slowly lowering it back to rest against the other leg, keeping the foot in dorsiflexion throughout. *Contraindications:* Strengthening is safe with controlled movement. If trochanteric bursitis is present, the leg may feel weak during the movement.

Individual Muscles of the Hip Joint and Pelvic Girdle—Posterior

GLUTEUS MAXIMUS MUSCLE

Palpation

Palpate gluteus maximus running downward and laterally between the posterior iliac crest superiorly, anal cleft medially, and gluteal fold inferiorly. Palpation of the muscle is emphasized with hip extension, external rotation, and abduction.

CLINICAL NOTES — Underdeveloped, Unused, and Padded

The gluteus maximus is the base on which people sit. Since it is activated by forceful extension, it tends to be more underdeveloped and heavily padded than other muscles. Many middle-aged people have difficulty getting out of chairs because of atrophy to this muscle. When it is overused for extreme sports such as marathon running, it will join the tensor fasciae latae to tighten the iliotibial tract. Since it has fibers that attach to the sacrum, it may be involved in sacroiliac dysfunctions and lower-back issues. See the techniques for releasing the gluteal muscles in Chapter 16 and the exercises in Chapter 21.

Muscle Specifics

The gluteus maximus muscle comes into action when movement between the pelvis and the femur approaches and moves beyond 15 degrees of extension. As a result, it is not used extensively in ordinary walking. It is important in extension of the thigh with external rotation.

Strong action of the gluteus maximus muscle is seen in hiking up an incline, running, hopping, skipping, and jumping. Powerful thigh extension is secured in the return to standing from a squatting position, especially if a barbell with weights is placed on the shoulders.

Clinical Flexibility

Since the sciatic nerve lies just beneath the large, powerful gluteus maximus, stretching this muscle can help relieve sciatic pain. While in the supine position, bring the opposite extended leg across the midline, pointing the foot laterally. Flex the stretched leg at the hip and knee, with one hand over the ankle and one just above the knee. Contract the adductors and bring the side of the knee to the opposite shoulder. Pull gently with both hands, and repeat. Pulling on the ankle creates a more intense stretch. This rotates the femur externally, placing force on the internal rotators of the hip. *Contraindications:* Sciatic patients may feel discomfort doing this stretch; it is safe with controlled movement.

Strengthening

Hip extension exercises from a forward-leaning or prone position may be used to develop the gluteus maximus. This muscle is most emphasized when the hip starts from a flexed position and moves to full extension and abduction, with the knee flexed 30 degrees or more to reduce the hamstrings' involvement in the action. A simple squat against a therapy ball without weight will strengthen the gluteus maximus. Stand with the back to the wall, with the feet shoulder-width apart, and place a therapy ball at the lower back for support. Slowly lower

OIAI MUSCLE CHART GLUTEUS MAXIMUS (glu´te-us maks´i-mus) Greek *(gloutos)* for "buttock"

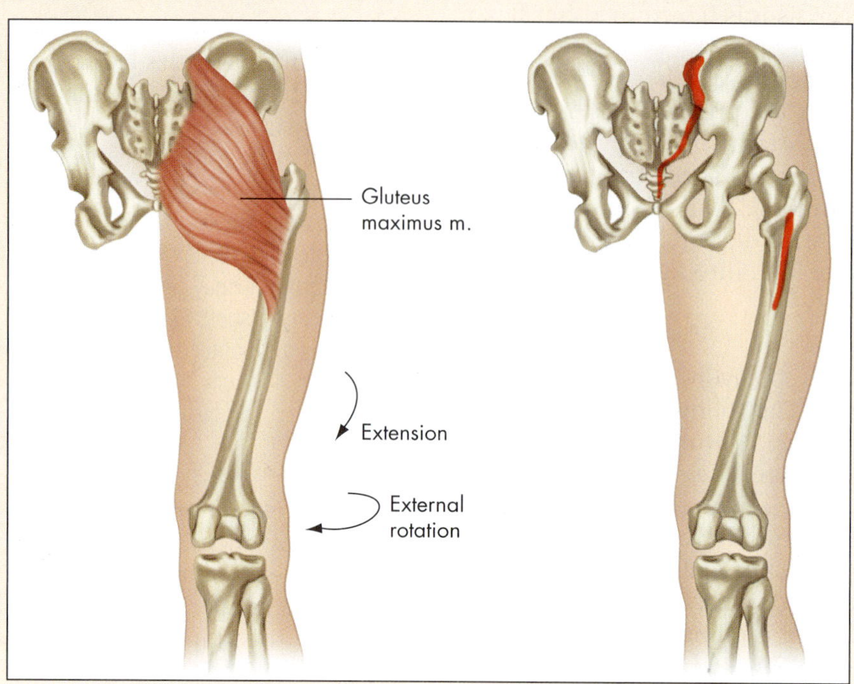

Name of Muscle	Origins	Insertion	Actions	Innervations
Gluteus maximus	Posterior one-fourth of crest of ilium, posterior surface of sacrum near ilium and fascia of lumbar area, coccyx near ilium	Gluteal line of femur and iliotibial tract	Forceful extension of hip, external rotation of hip *Upper fibers*: assist in abduction, posterior pelvic rotation *Lower fibers:* assist in hip adduction	Inferior gluteal nerve (L5, S1–S2)

the body by bending the knees, rolling the back against the ball. Repeat. Make sure to keep the abdominals contracted throughout the movement to protect the back. *Contraindications:* Individuals with knee issues should limit knee flexion to 50 to 60 degrees.

GLUTEUS MEDIUS MUSCLE

Palpation

Palpate the gluteus medius slightly in front of and a few inches above the greater trochanter with active elevation of the opposite pelvis when the client is in a standing position or with active abduction when the client is side-lying on the contralateral pelvis.

CLINICAL NOTES **Outer Thigh Muscle**

The outer thigh muscles shape the hips and are thus frequent targets of exercise for millions of women. The gluteus medius attaches to the posterior iliac crest and is in close quarters with the lower back. Because it is often one of the weakest muscles of the hip, it is directly involved with many soft-tissue problems that spill over into the hip area. When contracted, the gluteus medius tends to refer pain into the lower back. Stretching and strengthening this muscle will help improve pain patterns and gait issues. See Chapter 16 for techniques on the gluteals and Chapter 21 for exercises.

OIAI MUSCLE CHART GLUTEUS MEDIUS (glu´te-us me´di-us) Powerful abductor

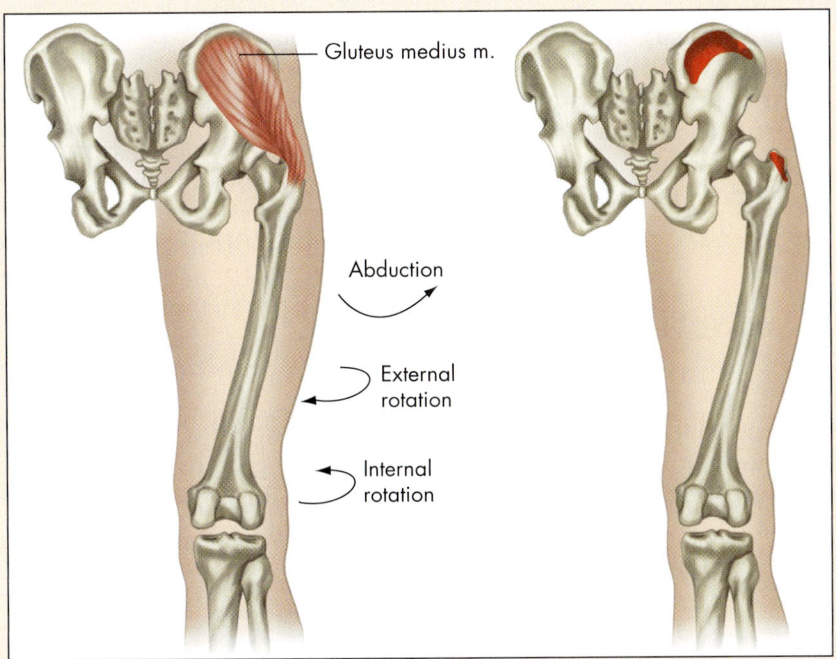

Name of Muscle	Origins	Insertion	Actions	Innervations
Gluteus medius	Outer surface of ilium just below crest	Greater trochanter of femur, posterior and middle surfaces	Abduction of hip *Anterior fibers:* internal rotation of thigh, weak flexion *Posterior fibers:* external rotation and weak extension of hip, lateral pelvic rotation to ipsilateral side	Superior gluteal nerve (L4–L5, S1)

Muscle Specifics

Typical action of the gluteus medius and gluteus minimus muscles is seen in walking. The gluteus medius moves the crest of the iliac toward the greater trochanter of the femur during gait. As the weight of the body is suspended on one leg, these muscles prevent the opposite pelvis from dropping. Weakness in the gluteus medius and gluteus minimus can result in a Trendelenburg gait. With this weakness, the individual's opposite pelvis will drop on weight bearing because the hip abductors cannot maintain proper alignment. As a result, the body will compensate to hike the hip, causing unnecessary force in other parts of the body.

Clinical Flexibility

Stretch the gluteus medius as a hip abductor by using the stretch for the gluteal. To stretch the gluteus medius as a rotator, stay supine and bend the involved leg at 90 degrees. Using the lateral rotators of the hip, rotate the thigh and use the rope to stretch at the end movement. You also can apply the same gluteal technique and perform this motion using just the hands during the gluteal stretch. *Contraindications:* These stretches are safe with controlled movement. Contracting the abdominals will help stabilize the low back.

Strengthening

The gluteus medius is often one of the weakest and most dysfunctional muscles in the hip. Strengthening it on a weekly basis will help gait, low-back pain, and posture. It is best strengthened by performing the side-lying leg raises or hip abduction exercises as described for the tensor fasciae latae. To isolate this muscle better, make certain that the hip remains pointed to the ceiling and not rotated forward or backward. Additionally, keep the foot in dorsiflexion throughout the exercise.

GLUTEUS MINIMUS MUSCLE

Palpation

Palpate gluteus minimus deep to the gluteus medius; it is covered by the tensor fasciae latae between the anterior iliac crest and the greater trochanter during internal rotation and abduction.

CLINICAL NOTES **An Outer Thigh Assister**

The gluteus minimus is closer to the greater trochanter, but it is under the gluteus medius. It supports the gluteus medius and tensor fasciae latae in abduction. The gluteus minimus develops soreness and can harbor trigger points that refer down the lower extremity. Runners can exhibit sore hips and painful referred patterns from the gluteus minimus. The gluteus minimus should be considered along with treatment for the gluteus medius and TFL. See Chapter 16 for techniques and Chapter 21 for exercises for the gluteals.

Muscle Specifics

Both the gluteus minimus and the gluteus medius are used in powerfully maintaining proper hip abduction during running. As a result, both of these

OIAI MUSCLE CHART GLUTEUS MINIMUS (glu´te-us min´i-mus) Small abductor

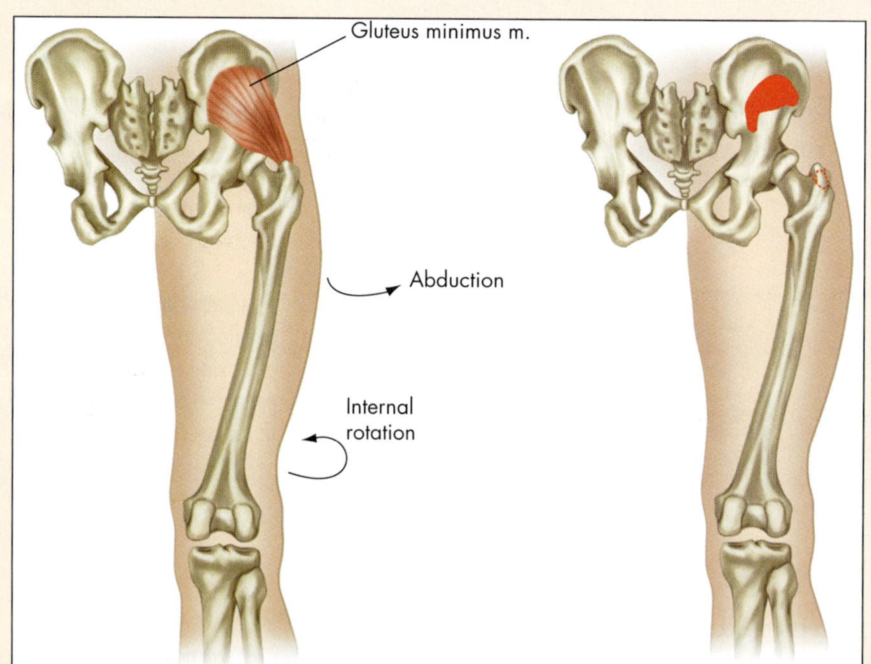

Name of Muscle	Origins	Insertion	Actions	Innervations
Gluteus minimus	Outer surface of ilium below origin of gluteus medius	Anterior surface of greater trochanter of femur	Abduction of femur on pelvis, internal rotation as femur abducts, lateral pelvic rotation to ipsilateral side	Superior gluteal nerve (L4–L5, S1)

muscles are exercised effectively in running, hopping, and skipping, actions in which weight is transferred forcefully from one foot to the other. Yet the gluteus minimus should be isolated and forced to work on its own to develop key muscular strength. As the body ages, the gluteus medius and gluteus minimus muscles tend to lose their effectiveness. It is common for these muscles to be weak in trained athletes. The spring of youth, as far as the hips are concerned, resides in these muscles. These muscles must be fully developed and maintained to have great drive in the legs and to support the hips in gravity.

Clinical Flexibility

The gluteus minimus is stretched in the same manner as that for the gluteus medius. To help isolate it better, bring the femur into adduction more during the stretch.

Strengthening

The gluteus minimus is best strengthened by performing hip abduction exercises similar to the ones described for the tensor fasciae latae and gluteus medius muscles. It also may be developed by performing hip internal rotation exercises against manual resistance. In the side-lying position with an ankle weight, flex the lower leg at the knee 90 degrees. Rotate the weight into internal rotation, and repeat.

THE SIX DEEP LATERAL ROTATOR MUSCLES

Palpation

Although the rotators are not directly palpable, deep palpation is possible between the posterior superior greater trochanter and the obturator foramen. With the client in the prone position, have the client keep the gluteus maximus relaxed. Passively flex the knee, and palpate the piriformis while internally and externally rotating the femur or alternating contracting and relaxing the lateral rotators slightly.

CLINICAL NOTES **Sciatic Nerve Entrapper**

Of special note, the sciatic nerve usually passes just underneath the piriformis muscle and—in rare occasions—through it. Should the piriformis become contracted, the sciatic nerve is then at risk for compression. Many people walk with the hips in external rotation. A constant gait in external rotation puts a postural torque on the deep lateral rotators and may place the sciatic nerve at risk. The therapist must exercise caution when working on the piriformis because of its close proximity to the sciatic nerve. Stretching is a very important component of unwinding any piriformis problem.

Muscle Specifics

The six lateral rotators are used powerfully in movements of femur external rotation, as in sports in which the individual takes off on one leg from preliminary internal rotation. Examples include throwing a baseball and swinging a baseball bat, both of which involve hip rotation.

Clinical Flexibility

The lateral rotator muscles are important to stretch for sciatic and hip problems. They can be stretched in the manner used for the gluteus medius, except that the femur is *internally* rotated with the rope assisting the stretch. The piriformis must be stretched as an abductor as well as a rotator. This is accomplished by lying supine, with the uninvolved extended leg angled into the midline. Bring the other leg into 90 degrees of hip flexion, with a slight flex in the knee. Wrap the rope around the foot; then, using the adductors, bring the leg across the body, almost horizontal, aiming just above the rib cage on the opposite side. Stretch gently for 2 seconds. *Contraindications:* Avoid using this exercise on hip arthroplasty clients.

Strengthening

The lateral rotator muscles are a little difficult to strengthen. While there are machines designed to specifically strengthen them, these small muscles also can be strengthened using ankle weights. In the side-lying position, flex the hip and bend both knees to 90 degrees. Rotate the ankle weight on the top leg into external rotation, and then slowly lower the weight. Make sure to keep the leg from abducting as you rotate. Repeat on each side. *Contraindications:* Use a pad between the knees to prevent bone on bone. Strengthening is safe with controlled movement.

HAMSTRINGS

The hamstring muscle group, consisting of the biceps femoris, semimembranosus, and semitendinosus, is covered in complete detail in Chapter 17, but additional discussion is included here because of the hamstrings' importance in hip extension.

Muscle strains involving the hamstrings are common in football and other sports that require explosive running. The hamstring muscle group is often referred to as the "running muscle" because of its function in acceleration. The hamstring muscles are antagonists to the quadriceps muscles at the knee and are named for their cordlike attachments at the knee. All the hamstring muscles originate on the ischial tuberosity of the pelvic bone, except the short head of the biceps femoris, which originates on the linea aspera of the femur. The semitendinosus and

OIAI MUSCLE CHART LATERAL ROTATORS

PIRIFORMIS (pi-ri-for´mis) Pear shaped

GEMELLUS SUPERIOR (je-mel´us su-pe´ri-or) Upper twin

GEMELLUS INFERIOR (je-mel´us in-fe´ri-or) Lower twin

OBTURATOR EXTERNUS (ob-tu-ra´tor eks-ter´nus) From the obturator

OBTURATOR INTERNUS (ob-tu-ra´tor in-ter´nus) From the obturator

QUADRATUS FEMORIS (kwad-ra´tus fem´or-is) Square muscle

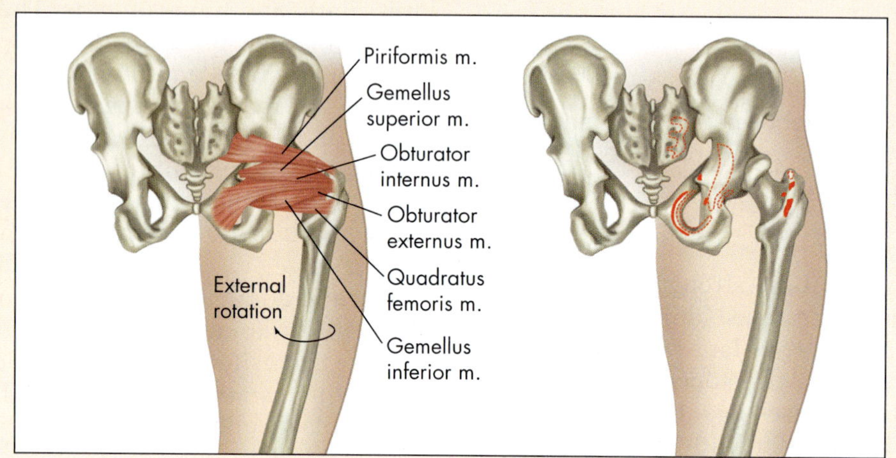

Name of Muscle	Origins	Insertion	Actions	Innervations
Piriformis	Anterior sacrum	Superior aspect of posterior greater trochanter	External rotation	1st or 2nd sacral nerve (S1–S2)
Gemellus superior	Posterior portions of ischium	Posterior aspect of greater trochanter	External rotation	Sacral nerve (L5, S1–S2)
Gemellus inferior	Same	Posterior aspect of greater trochanter	External rotation	Branches from the sacral plexus (L4–L5, S1–S2)
Obturator externus	Obturator foramen	Posterior aspect of greater trochanter	External rotation	Obturator nerve (L3–L4)
Obturator internus	Obturator foramen	Posterior aspect of greater trochanter	External rotation	Branches from sacral plexus (L4–L5, S1–S2)
Quadratus femoris	Anterolateral surface of ischium	Inferior aspect of greater trochanter	External rotation	Branches from sacral plexus (L4–L5, S1)

semimembranosus insert on the anteromedial and posteromedial side of the tibia, respectively. The biceps femoris inserts on the lateral tibial condyle and head of the fibula—hence the saying, "Two to the inside and one to the outside."

Specific exercises to improve the strength and flexibility of this muscle group are important in decreasing knee injuries. The hamstring muscles are also major culprits of low-back pain. Standing straight and touching one's toes is not a safe technique for assessing hamstring flexibility; this movement places great forces on the lumbar spine and can cause injury. A safer test is accomplished by taking the body out of gravity. From a supine position, the hip should flex to a 90-degree position with the knee extended; degrees less than this suggest a lack of hamstring flexibility. The hamstrings should be strengthened where they act on the hip and the knee. The main belly of the hamstring is developed by performing knee or hamstring curls on a knee table against resistance. Additional exercises are included in Chapters 17 and 21.

Individual Muscles of the Medial Thigh

ADDUCTOR BREVIS MUSCLE

Palpation

Palpate the adductor brevis deep to the adductor longus and superficial to the adductor magnus. The adductor brevis is very difficult to palpate and to differentiate from the adductor longus, which is immediately inferior; the proximal portion of the adductor brevis is just lateral to the adductor longus.

OIAI MUSCLE CHART ADDUCTOR BREVIS (ad-duk´tor bre´vis) Short adductor

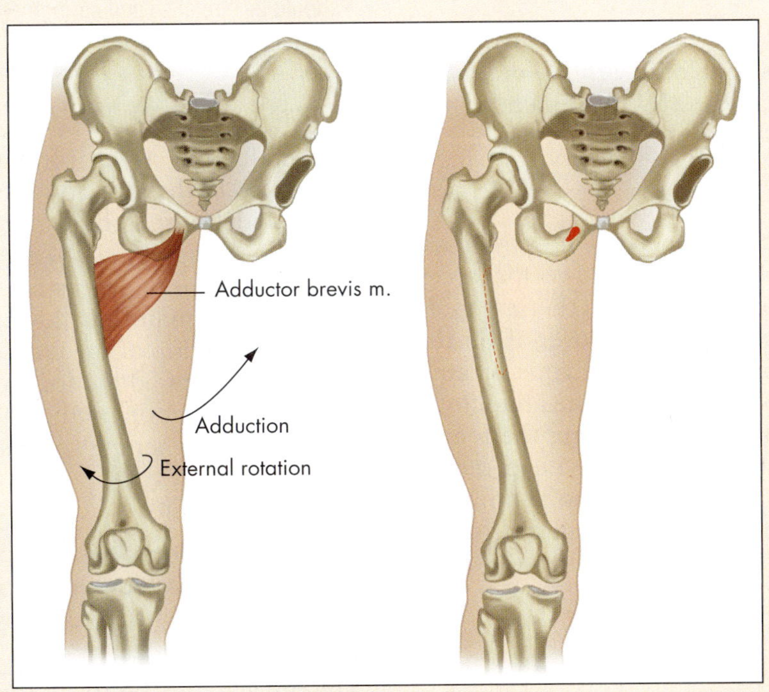

Name of Muscle	Origins	Insertion	Actions	Innervations
Adductor brevis	Front of inferior pubic ramus just below origin of longus	Upper portion of linea aspera between adductor longus and adductor magnus and posterior to pectineus	Adduction of hip, external rotation as it adducts the hip, assists in flexion of the hip	Obturator nerve (L3–L4)

> **CLINICAL NOTES — Hidden Adductor**
>
> The adductor brevis originates on the outer surface of the inferior ramus of the pubis, making it extremely difficult to palpate. Because of the larger and more powerful adductor muscles, adductor brevis is rarely injured. Specific tearing of this muscle can occur during a powerful eccentric contraction that exceeds the strength of the muscle-tendon units. Fatigue and previous strains to the muscle are also factors. Since the adductor magnus and longus are larger and more powerful muscles, it is important to stretch and strengthen the entire group to allow support for the smaller adductor brevis. Specific strengthening of the adductors is often overlooked in gyms and fitness-based programs, as more focus is placed on the hamstring and quadriceps group. A solid exercise program should involve every muscle that surrounds the femur, and the exercises should include specific isolation of each group.

Muscle Specifics

The adductor brevis muscle, along with the other adductor muscles, provides powerful movement of the thighs toward each other.

Clinical Flexibility

Stretching the adductors is beneficial for low-back and hip issues, because it helps eliminate vector forces acting on these areas. Lying supine on a therapy table or floor, bring the opposite leg off (or over, if on the floor), away from the midline. Wrap a rope around the foot on the involved side. Contract the abductors, and move the leg into abduction, keeping the femur down and along the table. Stretch at the end movement, and repeat. *Contraindications:* The abdominal muscles should remain contracted during this movement to help protect the back.

Strengthening

The adductors should be strengthened along with the abductors. Doing so helps support the knee joint as well as the hip, especially in forceful movements. In the side-lying position with an ankle weight on the bottom leg, extend the leg completely. Flex the top leg over the bottom leg so that it is not in the way. Bring the foot into dorsiflexion, and while contracting the adductors, lift the weight up, leading with the heel. Hold 2 seconds, and slowly lower the weight. Repeat. *Contraindications:* Strengthening is safe with controlled movement.

ADDUCTOR LONGUS MUSCLE

Palpation

Palpate the adductor longus, a most prominent muscle proximally on the anteromedial thigh, just inferior to the pubic bone, with resisted adduction.

> **CLINICAL NOTES — Prone to Injury**
>
> The adductor longus muscle is sometimes injured in sports like football or any activity requiring explosive lateral movements. The injury to this muscle is often misdiagnosed as a torn hamstring muscle, and it can be injured along with the biceps femoris. While a complete rupture of the adductor longus tendon is rare, it can occur, especially in movements with eccentric loading of the adductors in forced hyperabduction of the thigh. Pain is usually felt at the origin of the adductor longus, and externally rotating the femur often produces pain. It is important for the clinician to consider the adductor group, especially the adductor longus, with any injury to muscles on the thigh. Because the actions of this muscle include adduction, lateral rotation, and assisted hip flexion, it should be stretched and strengthened in all of these movements.

Muscle Specifics

The adductors as a group may be underdeveloped compared to the more powerful quadriceps and other more widely used thigh muscles. The adductor longus is more superficial than the adductor brevis and is therefore more accessible to treatment and can be stretched to maintain flexibility. While its main action is adduction of the femur, it contributes to lateral rotation during adduction and assisted flexion of the hip. See the section on the adductor brevis for stretching and strengthening suggestions.

Clinical Flexibility

The adductor longus is stretched in the same manner as that for the adductor brevis.

Strengthening

The muscle may be strengthened in the manner used for the adductor brevis.

ADDUCTOR MAGNUS MUSCLE

Palpation

Palpate the adductor magnus on the medial aspect of the thigh, between the gracilis and the medial hamstrings, from the ischial tuberosity to the adductor tubercle with resisted adduction from the abducted position.

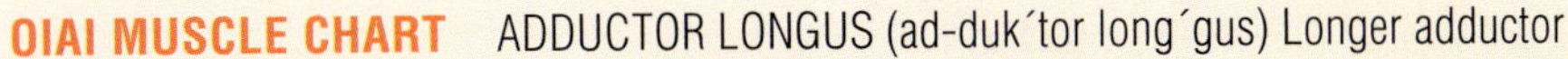

OIAI MUSCLE CHART ADDUCTOR LONGUS (ad-duk´tor long´gus) Longer adductor

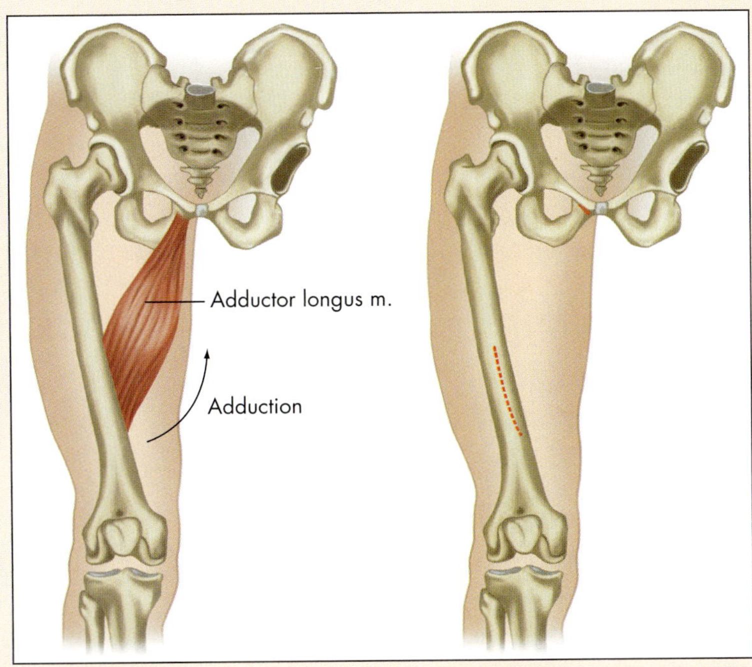

Name of Muscle	Origins	Insertion	Actions	Innervations
Adductor longus	Anterior pubis just below its crest	Middle third of linea aspera	Adduction of hip, assists in flexion of hip	Obturator nerve (L3–L4)

CLINICAL NOTES **The Day after Horseback Riding**

Those who have experienced horseback riding for the first time often wake the next day to discover pain or discomfort in muscles they did not know they possessed! The adductors are weaker as a group than the hip extensors or flexors and, as such, are often underdeveloped; however, the adductors are important muscles to consider in treatment when low-back pain is present because they can skew the pelvis and place pressure on the lumbar spine. For avid or competitive riders, sports massage techniques and stretching are essential for unwinding the adductors. See Chapter 18 for techniques and Chapter 21 for exercises for the thigh.

Muscle Specifics

The adductor magnus muscle is used in swimming (in the breaststroke kick) and in horseback riding. Since the adductor muscles (adductor magnus, adductor longus, adductor brevis, and gracilis muscles) are not heavily used in ordinary movement, some prescribed activity for them should be provided. This is especially true for athletes, who rely on powerful, forceful lateral movements.

Clinical Flexibility

Stretch the adductor magnus in the same manner as stretching the adductor brevis and adductor longus. It can be further isolated by externally rotating the femur 45 degrees and by bringing the femur down at the end movement.

Strengthening

Hip adduction exercises, such as those described for the adductor brevis and the adductor longus, may be used for strengthening the adductor magnus.

OIAI MUSCLE CHART ADDUCTOR MAGNUS (ad-duk´tor mag´nus) Largest adductor

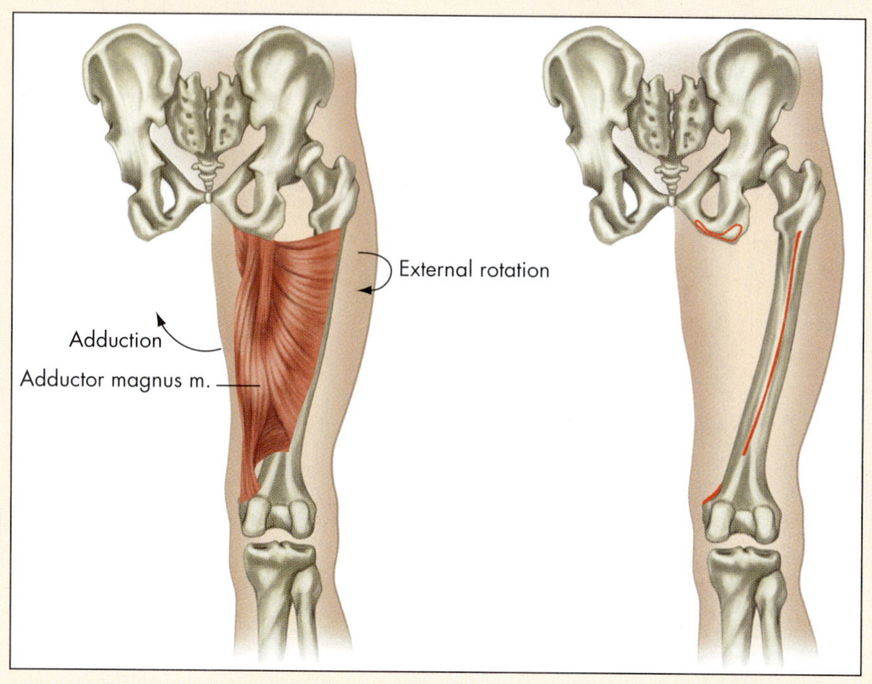

Name of Muscle	Origins	Insertion	Actions	Innervations
Adductor magnus	Pubic ramus, ischium, ischial tuberosity	Linea aspera of posterior femur and inner condyloid ridge, adductor tubercle of medial femur	Adduction of hip, external rotation as the hip adducts, extension of hip	*Anterior:* obturator nerve (L2–L4) *Posterior:* sciatic nerve (L4–L5, S1–S3)

PECTINEUS MUSCLE

Palpation

The pectineus is difficult to distinguish from other adductors. Palpate the pectineus on the anterior aspect of the hip approximately 1½ inches below the center of the inguinal ligament, just lateral and slightly proximal to the adductor longus and medial to the iliopsoas, during flexion and adduction of the supine client.

CLINICAL NOTES **Endangerment Zone**

Superficial to the pectineus runs the femoral artery, nerve, and vein. Because of the close proximity to vessels and nerve, this inguinal triangle area is considered an endangerment zone. The therapist has to be very careful working on the pectineus, passively shortening the muscle by bringing the thigh into flexion and palpating for the femoral artery and a pulse. Only experienced therapists should attempt to work on this muscle due to the endangerment zone and its close proximity to the genital region. Isolated stretching of this muscle is safe, as no direct hand pressure is placed on the danger zone. Athletes tend to strain this muscle in extreme sprinting or hurdling events. Massage and stretching can relieve a very painful pectineus.

Muscle Specifics

As the pectineus contracts, it tends to rotate the pelvis anteriorly. The abdominal muscles stabilizing the pelvis anteriorly prevent this tilting action. For this reason, the pectineus should be stretched along with the other adductors on a daily basis.

OIAI MUSCLE CHART PECTINEUS (pek-tin´e-us) Groin muscle

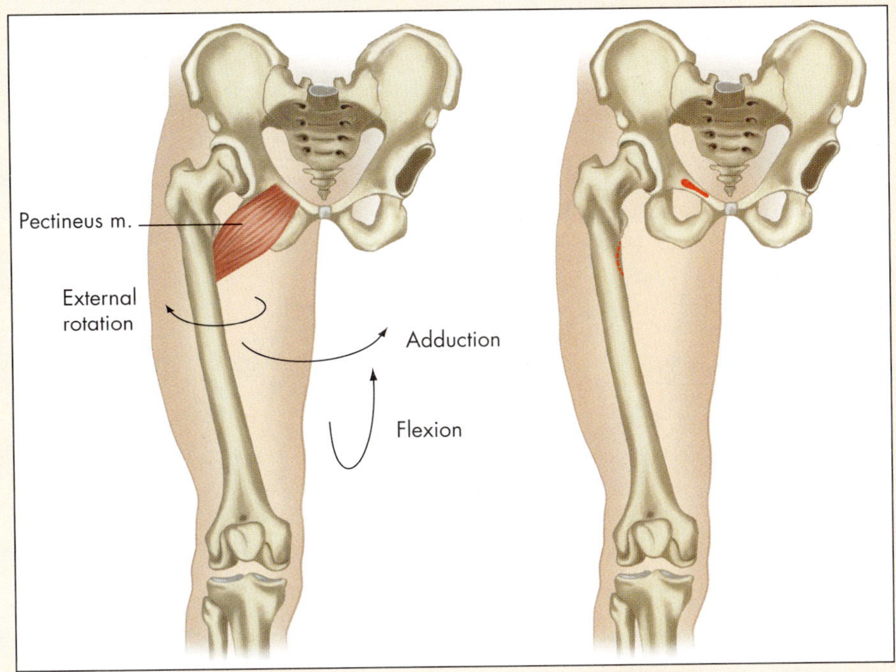

Name of Muscle	Origins	Insertion	Actions	Innervations
Pectineus	Anterior pubis just above crest lateral to pubic tubercle	Between lesser trochanter and linea aspera of posterior femur	Flexion of hip, adduction of hip on pelvis, external rotation of hip	Femoral nerve (L2–L4)

Clinical Flexibility

The pectineus is stretched in the same manner as that for the other adductors. Specific isolation occurs when the hip is externally rotated, flexed, and brought into abduction.

Strengthening

The pectineus muscle is exercised together with the iliopsoas muscle in leg raising and lowering from a table, as described above for the iliopsoas. It can also be strengthened using the side-lying leg raises described for the adductors.

GRACILIS MUSCLE

Palpation

Palpate the thin tendon of the gracilis on the anteromedial thigh with knee flexion and resisted adduction just posterior to the adductor longus and medial to the semitendinosus.

CLINICAL NOTES **Pes Anserinus**

The anatomical tripod is made up of three muscles: the sartorius, gracilis, and semitendinosus. They attach to a small slip of tissue on the medial tibia called the *pes anserinus,* located just below the condyle. Structurally these muscles support the knee from the different directions—anteriorly, medially, and posteriorly—of the pelvic girdle. For these reasons, the attachment area can be very sore on individuals and must be examined. Use circular friction on the attachment site, and make sure to treat all three muscles. The gracilis is stretched effectively with the adductors.

OIAI MUSCLE CHART GRACILIS (gras´-il-is) The second-longest muscle in the body

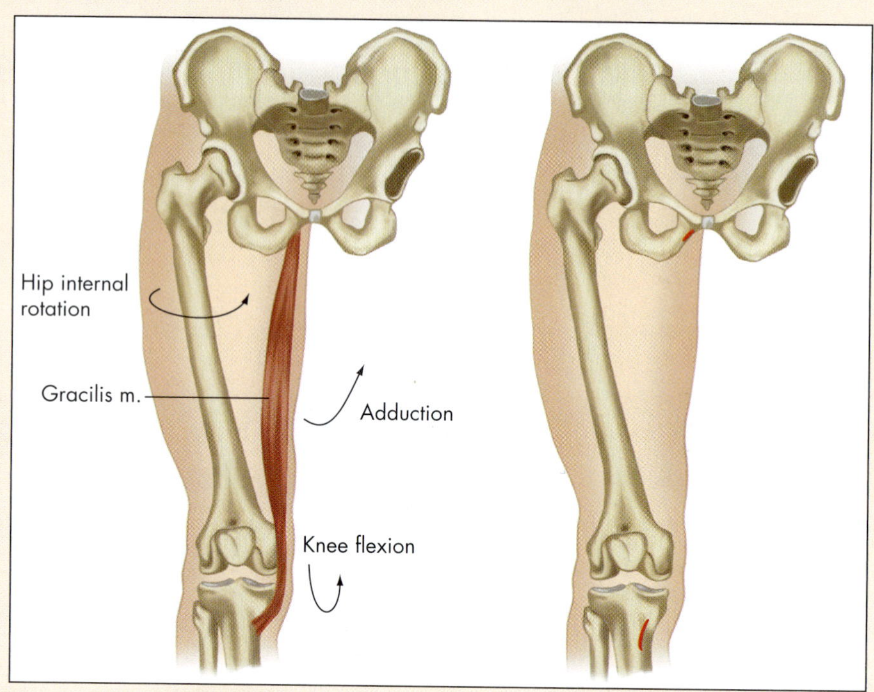

Name of Muscle	Origins	Insertion	Actions	Innervations
Gracilis	Anteromedial edge of descending ramus of pubis	Medial proximal tibia just below condyle (pes anserinus)	Adduction of hip, internal rotation of flexed knee, flexion of knee from extension, weak flexion of hip, internal rotation of hip	Obturator nerve (L2–L4)

Muscle Specifics

Also known as the *adductor gracilis,* the gracilis muscle performs the same function as that of the other adductors, but it adds some weak assistance to knee flexion.

The adductor muscles as a group (adductor magnus, adductor longus, adductor brevis, and gracilis) are called into action in horseback riding and in doing the breaststroke kick in swimming. Proper development of the adductor group prevents soreness after participation in these sports.

Clinical Flexibility

The gracilis may be stretched in the manner used for for the adductors.

Strengthening

The gracilis is strengthened using the exercise described for the other hip adductors.

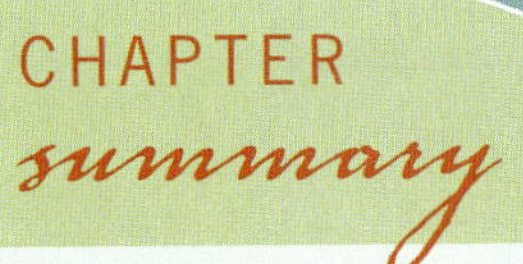

CHAPTER summary

Introduction

- In the anatomical puzzle that is the human body, the pelvic girdle provides a sturdy foundation for the trunk and spine. The sacrum fits between the two sides of the ilium and creates a wide base for the larger lumbar vertebrae. Muscles span, like guy wires, from the ribs and vertebrae to the hip and pelvic bones. The structure of the trunk, spine, and pelvic girdle lends stability to the weight of the trunk.

Bones

- The femur is the longest bone in the body.
- Bony landmarks for muscular attachments on the femur include the greater and lesser trochanters, the linea aspera, and the medial and lateral condyles.
- The pelvic girdle is divided into the ilium, ischium, and pubis.
- The sacrum and coccyx connect the posterior portions of the pelvic girdle.
- Landmarks for muscular attachments on the ilium include the iliac crest and portions thereof anteriorly and posteriorly.
- Muscles attach to the pubic bone, superior and inferior pubic ramus, and pubic crest.
- The ischial tuberosity of the ischium houses many muscular attachments.

Joints

- The hip joint is an enarthrodial ball-and-socket joint.
- The acetabulum and the femoral head form the joint called the acetabular femoral joint.
- The pelvic girdle is joined anteriorly by the symphysis pubis, which is an amphiarthrodial joint.
- The sacroiliac joint posteriorly is formed by ligaments and is slightly movable.
- Many ligaments give stability and strength to the joints.

Movements

- Movement of the hip joint permits flexion, extension, abduction, adduction, internal and external rotation, and diagonal movements of the hip.
- Movements of the pelvic girdle include anterior and posterior rotation, right and left lateral rotation, and right and left transverse rotation.

Muscles

- The iliopsoas is composed of three muscles: the iliacus, psoas major, and psoas minor. It is a primary hip flexor and is located deep in the anterior trunk.
- The sartorius runs from the anterior superior crest to the tibia medially.
- The rectus femoris is a superficial quadriceps that flexes the femur.
- The tensor fasciae latae is a flexor and abductor of the hip and is located anterior and lateral.
- The pectineus is considered a flexor and adductor of the hip; it spans from the pubic bone to the femur.
- The other adductors include the adductor brevis, adductor longus, adductor magnus, and gracilis. They are medial thigh muscles.
- The hamstrings include the biceps femoris, semitendinosus, and semimembranosus.
- The hamstrings extend the hip and are located posteriorly.
- Gluteal muscles include the gluteus maximus, gluteus medius, and gluteus minimus; they are located posteriorly.
- The deep-six lateral rotators are the piriformis, gemellus superior and inferior, obturator internus and externus, and quadratus femoris; they are located deep to the gluteals.

Nerves

- Nerves from the lumbar and sacral plexus innervate the muscles of the hip and pelvic girdle.
- Nerves of significance from the lumbar plexus include the femoral nerve and the obturator nerve.
- The largest nerve of significance of the sacral plexus is the sciatic nerve.
- The sciatic nerve is composed of the tibial and common peroneal nerves.

Individual Muscles of the Hip Joint and Pelvic Girdle—Anterior

- *Iliopsoas* is a combination of the psoas major, psoas minor, and the iliacus. The psoas major spans from the anterior vertebrae and joins the iliacus to insert on the lesser trochanter and the shaft just below. The iliopsoas is a primary hip flexor.
- *Sartorius* is the longest muscle in the body and runs from the anterior superior crest to the medial tibia, where it inserts along with the gracilis and the semitendinosus. It flexes the hip and externally rotates the hip as it flexes the knee.
- *Rectus femoris* is a biarticular muscle that acts on two joints. It spans from the anterior inferior iliac crest and inserts with the other quadriceps at the tibial tuberosity. The rectus femoris flexes the hip and extends the knee.
- *Tensor fasciae latae* spans from the anterior crest and inserts in the iliotibial tract. It flexes and abducts the hip.

Individual Muscles of the Hip Joint and Pelvic Girdle—Posterior

- ✔ *Gluteus maximus* is the largest of the gluteal muscles. It covers a greater portion of the posterior ilium and the edge of the sacrum and coccyx. It inserts on the femur and into the iliotibial tract. It causes forceful extension and external rotation, and it assists in abduction and adduction depending on the fiber attachments.
- ✔ *Gluteus medius* covers up the rest of the ilium and is a major abductor of the hip. It inserts on the greater trochanter.
- ✔ *Gluteus minimus* originates below the medius and inserts on the greater trochanter. It gives depth and support to the gluteus medius in abduction of the hip.
- ✔ *Deep-six lateral rotators—piriformis, gemellus superior, gemellus inferior, obturator externus, obturator internus, quadratus femoris*—all externally rotate the hip. The most notable, the piriformis, is the only muscle of the group that has an anterior sacrum origin. It inserts on the greater trochanter with the other lateral rotators. The piriformis is a possible entrapper of the sciatic nerve. The other lateral rotators originate on various parts of the ischium and obturator foramen.
- ✔ *Hamstrings—semitendinosus, semimembranosus, long head of the biceps femoris*—originate on the ischial tuberosity. The short head of the biceps femoris begins on the linea aspera and joins the long head to insert on the lateral side of the tibia and fibula. The semitendinosus and semimembranosus insert on the medial tibia. The hamstrings extend the hip and flex the knee. They are explained individually in Chapter 17.

Individual Muscles of the Medial Thigh

- ✔ *Adductor brevis* is the smallest of the adductor muscles and is sandwiched between the adductor longus and pectineus anteriorly and the adductor magnus posteriorly. Its primary action is adduction of the hip.
- ✔ *Adductor longus* originates on the anterior pubis and inserts on the middle of the linea aspera of the femur. It assists in hip flexion and has the primary function of adduction.
- ✔ *Adductor magnus* is the largest of the adductors and has a more posterior presentation because it begins on the ischial tuberosity and pubic ramus. It inserts into the entire length of the linea aspera and forms a great deal of the inner-thigh soft tissue. It is a major adductor of the hip, but it does assist in other actions.
- ✔ *Pectineus* originates on the anterior pubis and inserts between the lesser trochanter and the linea aspera. It is a hip flexor and adductor.
- ✔ *Gracilis* begins on the ramus of the pubis medially and inserts with the sartorius and semitendinosus on the pes anserinus of the medial tibia. Another two-joint muscle, it adducts the hip and weakly flexes the knee.

CHAPTER *review*

Worksheet Exercises

As an aid to learning, for in-class or out-of-class assignments, or for testing, tear-out worksheets are found at the end of the text, on pages 539–542.

True or False

Write true *or* false *after each statement.*

1. The rectus femoris is the only hip flexor.
2. The piriformis can entrap the sciatic nerve.
3. The gluteus maximus originates on the whole posterior crest of the ilium.
4. The sartorius is the longest muscle in the body.
5. The pectineus adducts and flexes the hip.
6. The adductor brevis is sandwiched between the tensor fasciae latae and the pectineus.
7. Gluteus medius and minimus both adduct the hip.
8. The sacroiliac joint is bound by ligaments.
9. The iliopsoas is made up of the iliacus, psoas minor, and psoas major.
10. The symphysis pubis connects the sacrum to the ischium.

Short Answers

Write your answers on the lines provided.

1. Distinguish between hip flexion and trunk flexion.

____

____

____

2. Name the bones of the hip joint. What is the hip joint called?

____

____

____

3. What is the cup of the hip joint called?

____

____

____

4. Name the hip joint's actions.

____

____

____

5. Which muscles flex the hip?

____

____

____

6. Which muscles extend the hip?

____

____

____

7. Which muscles adduct the hip?

____

____

____

8. Where on the femur do a lot of the hip adductors insert?

____

____

____

9. Which two muscles insert into the iliotibial tract?

____

____

____

10. Name the deep-six lateral rotators.

____

____

____

Multiple Choice

Circle the correct answers.

1. The nerve that comes from the lumbar plexus to innervate the quads is the:
   a. sciatic nerve
   b. femoral nerve
   c. tibial nerve
   d. median nerve
2. The bones that make up the pelvic girdle are:
   a. ilium, ischium, and pubis
   b. femur, iliac crest, and pubis
   c. iliac crest, anterior iliac crest, and pubis
   d. none of the above
3. The muscles that adduct the hip are:
   a. adductor magnus, biceps femoris, adductor brevis
   b. adductor magnus, adductor brevis, adductor longus
   c. adductor magnus, rectus femoris, adductor brevis
   d. none of the above
4. The iliopsoas inserts on the:
   a. linea aspera
   b. greater trochanter
   c. lesser trochanter and shaft just below
   d. tibia
5. The piriformis is the only one of the deep-six lateral rotators that originates on the:
   a. pubic bone
   b. iliac crest
   c. obturator foramen
   d. anterior sacrum
6. The hamstrings:
   a. flex the hip
   b. extend the hip
   c. extend the knee
   d. none of the above
7. The lateral rotators all insert on the:
   a. lesser trochanter
   b. iliotibial tract
   c. greater trochanter
   d. tibia
8. Gluteus medius originates on:
   a. the lateral surface of the ilium just below the crest
   b. the sacrum

c. the anterior superior iliac crest
d. none of the above

9. The muscle that was named for the tailor was the:
   a. tensor fasciae latae
   b. rectus femoris
   c. biceps femoris
   d. sartorius

10. The psoas major originates on the:
    a. anterior ilium
    b. posterior ilium
    c. bodies of the lumbar vertebrae
    d. femur

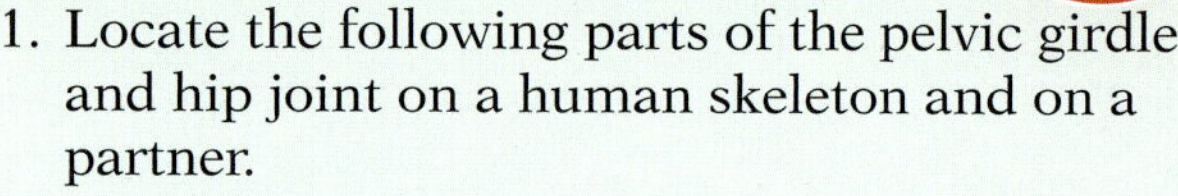

1. Locate the following parts of the pelvic girdle and hip joint on a human skeleton and on a partner.

   a. Skeleton:
   1. Ilium
   2. Ischium
   3. Pubis
   4. Symphysis pubis
   5. Acetabulum
   6. Rami (ascending and descending)
   7. Obturator foramen
   8. Ischial tuberosity
   9. Anterior superior iliac spine
   10. Greater trochanter
   11. Lesser trochanter

   b. Partner:
   1. Crest of the ilium
   2. Anterior superior iliac spine
   3. Ischial tuberosity
   4. Greater trochanter

2. How and where can the following muscles be palpated on a human?
   a. Gracilis
   b. Sartorius
   c. Gluteus maximus
   d. Gluteus medius
   e. Gluteus minimus
   f. Biceps femoris
   g. Rectus femoris
   h. Semimembranosus
   i. Semitendinosus
   j. Adductor magnus
   k. Adductor longus
   l. Adductor brevis

3. Be prepared to indicate on a human skeleton, using a long rubber band, where each muscle has its origin and insertion.

4. Demonstrate the movement and list the muscles primarily responsible for the following hip movements:
   a. Flexion
   b. Extension
   c. Adduction
   d. Abduction
   e. External rotation
   f. Internal rotation

5. How is walking different from running in relation to the use of the hip joint muscle actions and the range of motion?

6. How may the walking gait be affected by a weakness in the gluteus medius muscle? Have a partner demonstrate the gait pattern associated with gluteus medius weakness. What is the name of this dysfunctional gait?

7. How might bilateral iliopsoas tightness affect the posture and movement of the lumbar spine in the standing position? Demonstrate and discuss this effect with a partner.

8. How might bilateral hamstring tightness affect the posture and movement of the lumbar spine in the standing position? Demonstrate and discuss this effect with a partner.

9. *Muscle analysis chart:* Fill in the chart below by listing the muscles primarily involved in each movement.

Flexion	Extension
Abduction	**Adduction**
External rotation	**Internal rotation**

10. *Antagonistic muscle action chart:* Fill in the chart below by listing the muscle(s) or parts of muscles that are antagonistic in their actions to the muscles in the left column.

Agonist	Antagonist
Gluteus maximus	
Gluteus medius	
Gluteus minimus	
Biceps femoris	
Semimembranosus/Semitendinosus	
Adductor magnus/Adductor brevis	
Adductor longus	
Gracilis	
Lateral rotators	
Rectus femoris	
Sartorius	
Pectineus	
Iliopsoas	
Tensor fasciae latae	

chapter 16

Deep Tissue of the Low Back and Posterior Pelvis

LEARNING OUTCOMES

After completing this chapter, you should be able to:

16-1 Define key terms.

16-2 Locate on a human skeleton selected bony structures of the trunk, spine, and pelvic girdle.

16-3 Palpate bony landmarks and the muscles of the trunk, spine, and pelvic girdle on a partner.

16-4 Explore the origins and insertions of the muscles of the trunk and pelvic girdle on a partner.

16-5 Review general pathologies and conditions of the muscles of the trunk and pelvic girdle.

16-6 Discuss a treatment protocol for conditions of sciatica, back-pocket sciatica, and piriformis syndrome.

16-7 Demonstrate safe body mechanics.

16-8 Practice specific techniques on the low-back and pelvic girdle muscles.

16-9 Incorporate dimensional massage therapy techniques in a regular routine or use them when needed.

16-10 Determine safe treatment protocols and refer clients to other health professionals when necessary.

KEY TERMS

Axial pain	Foraminal stenosis	Myofascial pain	Referred pain
Back-pocket sciatica	Herniated disk	Piriformis syndrome	Sciatica
Cryotherapy	Laminectomy	Radicular pain	

Introduction

A back massage is similar to dessert after dinner. It often comes last in the massage sequence and may, therefore, be anticipated with the most excitement. Since it reduces regular tension and sore muscles, the back massage completes the treatment. There is also tremendous need for low-back massage, since millions of people complain of and endure chronic back pain. It is estimated that 80 percent of the general population will, at some time, experience back pain. Since 50 percent of people generally feel relief from low-back pain within 2 weeks and 90 percent usually recover fully within 3 months, one can assume that some of the problem encompasses soft-tissue dysfunction. Sources of pain include muscles, tendons, ligaments, bones, disks, and facet joints. Unfortunately, once the back has sustained an injury, there is every likelihood of a recurrence within the same year. Lifting, repetitive action, posture, and trauma cause recurrences with alarming frequency.

Helping people through chronic back pain requires a team approach. Conservative care beyond diagnosis can include rest, physical therapy, ergonomic evaluation of the work site, postural awareness and body mechanics training, a home exercise and stretching program, **cryotherapy** (the safe use of ice and exercise to reduce inflammation and acute responses), chiropractic or manipulative osteopathic care, acupuncture, and medication. Massage therapy is an integral part of this team effort.

Structural Perspectives of the Low Back and Pelvic Girdle

The low back includes the last thoracic vertebra, all the lumbar vertebrae, and soft tissue of the posterior pelvic girdle. The sacrum completes the spine and connects the pelvic girdle to the low back. Erector spinae fibers connect the sacrum to the occiput in a network of trunk muscles. There is a large aponeurosis that provides attachment for the latissimus dorsi and lumbar fasciae to the pelvic girdle and spine. Attachments at and around the sacrum connect lumbar fasciae to gluteal muscles, providing more communication between the low back and the pelvic girdle. The sides of the abdomen are the sides of the back; the obliques tuck into the posterior pelvic girdle and interdigitate with low-back fasciae and the musculature. All of this information provides sound reasoning for including the low-back, sacral area, and pelvic girdle soft tissue in a treatment scenario.

The movement of the pelvic girdle can have a dramatic effect on the low back, spinal curvature, and its soft tissue, depending on its position. An anteriorly rotated pelvis will enhance the lumbar curve in a lordosis. The low back needs the abdominal muscles to help control anterior rotation. A posterior rotation of the hips can cause a reduced curve in the low back and possibly tighten the psoas major and the abdominals.

Contracted muscles in the lower extremities contribute to the position of the hips and subsequently affect the lower back in a domino effect. Quadriceps and anterior thigh muscles affect anterior rotation of the pelvis and give cause to treat the thigh musculature. Tight hamstrings pull on the pelvis from the posterior direction.

These structural perspectives provide the massage therapist reason enough to design treatments based on each individual, medical history, postural observations, and palpation of associated hypertonic soft tissue. A dimensional approach to treatment will encompass areas that, in turn, affect the low back.

Injuries and Overuse Syndromes

Back pain is debilitating and frustrating, and it can deny a person freedom to live a full life. Trauma and inappropriate lifting causing back sprains and strains are some of the foremost causes of back injuries. **Axial pain** can be sharp or dull, constant or intermittent, and mild or severe and can be confined to the low back. It gets worse with certain activities and position changes, and it is often relieved by rest. Since it is usually mechanical in origin, different treatment approaches, including rest, massage therapy, physical therapy, chiropractic care, and medication assist recovery 90 percent of the time in 6 weeks to 3 months.

Back pain, however, is not always caused by soft-tissue injury. Kidney stones, bladder infections, tumors, and internal injury can all be causative factors of back pain. Diagnosis is the premise of the physician. Should a client present with any of the following, it is appropriate to refer the client to a medical professional.

TREATMENT PROTOCOL

Reasons for Referral

- Fever and/or chills
- History of cancer with recent weight loss
- Severe trauma
- Significant leg weakness
- Sudden bowel and/or bladder incontinence
- Severe continuous abdominal and back pain
- Nausea and/or vomiting

SOFT-TISSUE ISSUES

Lifting a heavy item in an unbalanced position is a recipe for low-back injury, especially if the object is a moving target, such as a child. Children can change the balance differential by throwing their weight in another direction, which causes them to weigh more. If a person lifts a child who is positioned directly in front of him, and he lifts with the back instead of using the lower extremities, the erector spinae and latissimus dorsi will be at considerable risk. Lifting a heavy object off to the side might call the quadratus lumborum, erector spinae, and gluteus medius into action or possibly into too much eccentric lengthening and/or braking. The opposing stabilizers of the spine can be strained in the activity of inappropriate lifting. Clients can suffer from considerable low-back pain as the result of lifting accidents. They may find it difficult to move or even take a deep breath. It would not be unusual to hear that a client had crawled on hands and knees to the bathroom and/or was having trouble standing from a seated position. Aside from the diagnosis, a conservative team approach can help resolve most soft-tissue lifting injuries.

Nerve Complaints

SCIATICA

Pain from the sciatic nerve radiates down the thigh to the calf and may spread to the foot. **Radicular pain** is unilateral, deep, steady, and reproducible with certain activities (walking or sitting), and it follows the involved dermatome. It can include numbness and tingling, muscle weakness, and loss of specific reflexes. **Sciatica** can be defined as an inflammation of the sciatic nerve, but since the sciatic nerve traverses through the pelvic girdle and down the lower extremity, it is at risk at several different locations. Sciatica really should not be a diagnosis unless the cause is included in the statement. Impingement can result from a herniated disk, **foraminal stenosis** (narrowing of the intervertebral space through which the spinal nerve exits, due to bone spurs or arthritis), diabetes, nerve root injuries, or scarring from a previous spinal surgery.

A **herniated disk** occurs when the gelatinous nucleus pulposus protrudes into or through the annulus fibrosus. This herniation produces a "bulging" of the disk tissue posteriorly into the vertebral canal and pinches the spinal cord and/or spinal nerves branching off the spinal cord. Lumbar herniated disks (commonly from L4 and L5) frequently cause low-back pain and may be a cause of sciatica. Herniated disks are treated conservatively first before moving to more drastic, surgical solutions. Often, rest, physical therapy, and specific lumbar exercises help to resolve the injury. Massage therapy is helpful to relieve soft-tissue discomfort and referred pain patterns. It should be included in a conservative team approach. Caution should be used around the injured-disk site.

Entrapment of the sciatic nerve can take place by the piriformis in a prolonged state of external rotation or by different structural scenarios of the nerve actually passing around or through the piriformis itself. This is often called **piriformis syndrome.** (See Chapter 15 for the piriformis and appropriate stretches.) The sciatic nerve also runs between the adductor magnus and the biceps femoris. Runners might experience entrapment from contracted posterior thigh muscles. (See Chapter 17 for clinical notes on the biceps femoris and for appropriate stretches.) Another, more peculiar, cause of sciatic pain can be a lumpy wallet kept on only one side in the back pocket. The wallet adds a lift to one side of the pelvis and compresses the piriformis area. If the problem is many years in the making, it may take a considerable amount of time for the pelvis to readapt itself to a normal position, if at all. A conservative team approach is useful in treating **back-pocket sciatica.** Whatever the cause, sciatica is a painful condition and a common complaint. Diagnosis for cause is essential, but even an MRI is not always accurate.

Massage can help release soft tissue entrapping the sciatic nerve and can calm tissue fibers that have a referred pain pattern passing through them. **Referred pain** can be achy, dull, migratory, and intermittent with varied intensity. It can radiate from the low back to groin, buttock, and upper thigh. This type of pain may be different from the referred pain of myofascial pain and trigger points. **Myofascial pain** is associated with soft tissue; it may or may not hurt at the location of the trigger point; and it is not linked with the distribution of a nerve. When the myofascial discomfort is located somewhere other than on the offending trigger point, it is called *referred pain.* In this case, the pain may not be a very reliable indicator of its source, as it may hurt in a completely different location than the soft-tissue cause. Injury, disease, repetitive action, posture, and surgery can cause myofascial pain. Myofascial pain is often treatable with conservative care, including massage therapy.

Arthritis, Osteoarthritis, Degenerative Disk Disease, and Lumbar and Sacroiliac Subluxations

The low back is particularly vulnerable to degenerative disk disease and osteoarthritis. The weight alone wears down the disks in time. Osteoarthritis exacerbates old injuries and aging, and it adds its own spin to the development of bony growth on the vertebrae. Stenosis, a narrowing of the vertebral foramen, which limits room for the spinal cord and spinal nerves, can result in predictable pain patterns to distal regions. To reduce stenosis, orthopedic methods might include a surgery called a **laminectomy,** wherein the posterior arch and the spinous processes of the midline of the vertebrae are removed, giving the spinal cord room. Should the massage therapist suspect involvement and/or nerve compression, it is appropriate to refer the client to a medical professional. Suspected lumbar and/or sacroiliac subluxations are reasons to refer the client for further evaluation and possible manual therapy. After diagnosis, massage therapy, manual therapy, postural correction, and specific rehabilitation exercises are a good combination of conservative care for low-back and sacral subluxations.

Unwinding the Muscles of the Low Back: Prone or Supine?

Sometimes, a client may tell her massage therapist, "I want only my back done." Much as the therapist may want to fulfill the client's wish, the therapist must consider if doing so really best serves the client's needs and if the sequence will give the anticipated result. The treatment also depends on the client's medical history, the mechanism of injury (if any), and which muscles are involved in any soft-tissue dysfunction. It is much easier and more efficient to work on the neck and shoulders in a supine position first than to try and unwind the shoulder girdle muscles only from a prone position. In the prone position, the head cannot be used to passively shorten the muscles as easily, nor is it possible to work on any anterior muscles of the head, neck, and shoulder girdle. Positioning should be part of the expertise that the therapist lends to the client, thereby aiming to make the treatment more successful. It is up to the therapist to communicate and educate the client about the appropriate options that will be most advantageous to the session.

COMFORT, SUPPORT, AND SEQUENCE

Once you have softened the head, neck, and shoulder muscles in a supine position, position the client face-down or prone on the table. Make sure the client is thoroughly comfortable on the table. For a female client, use a table with breast recesses, if possible. Then place the pads from the recess holes under the anterior part of the shoulders. This supports the shoulders and shortens lengthened fibers. Rolled towels can provide similar support. Place a bolster under the anterior feet. The bolster will relax the hamstrings that are connected to the pelvic girdle via the ischial lower back. A small pillow or folded towel placed under the client's abdominal region could relieve some of the anterior pelvic rotation.

When the client is comfortable on the table, proceed with unwinding the layers of the back muscles. Release the soft tissue in the posterior shoulder girdle region first. Remember that the erector spinae muscles are under the trapezius, rhomboids, and latissimus dorsi and are all connected from the neck to the sacrum. Unwind the back from top to bottom. Work superficial to deep, warming up the tissues sufficiently before sinking into underlying layers. Methodically, make sure you address the soft tissue necessary to achieve a successful treatment goal. See the section below on dimensional massage therapy for techniques to unwind the low-back muscles.

Dimensional Massage Therapy for the Muscles of the Low Back and Pelvic Girdle

DEEP-TISSUE TECHNIQUES FOR LOW-BACK PAIN AND TENSION

The following techniques can be used as a complete sequence for the low back and posterior pelvic girdle muscles. Remember to adequately prepare the entire back with introductory strokes of effleurage,

TREATMENT PROTOCOL

How do you unwind the back muscles in a sequence?

- Take a careful medical history, appropriate for the client; look for contraindications; and refer the client to an appropriate professional when necessary.
- Always use treatment protocols to determine the sequence of a therapeutic session; assess active and passive ranges of motion of the neck and trunk.
- Position the client on the table with appropriate support.
- Palpate tissues.
- Follow a dimensional approach, and critically think about the involved joints and muscles.
- Determine pressure intelligently; ask for feedback from the client.
- Work superficial to deep.
- Visit all the muscles possibly involved in the problem.
- Visit all the attachments of the involved muscles.
- Passively shorten muscles whenever possible with your techniques to decrease tension.
- Do not overwork sore areas.
- Intersperse compressive effleurage after applying deep, detailed techniques.
- Practice shoulder girdle, head, and neck routines in a supine position before using the prone techniques.
- See the techniques below for additional suggestions.

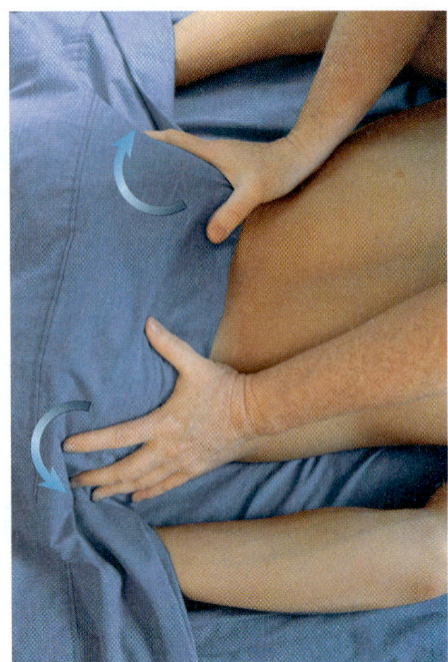

FIGURE 16.1 Elliptical movement of the hips

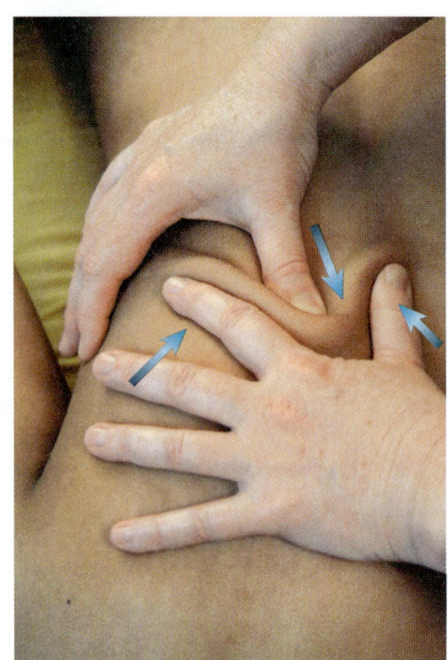

FIGURE 16.2 Myofascial warm-up

compression, skin rolling, petrissage, and rocking, along with myofascial strokes and stretches, elliptical movements, parallel thumbs, and so on, before using specific deep-tissue techniques.

PRONE BODY POSITION

Elliptical Movement of the Hips

Stand to the side of the face cradle. Place your hands on either side of the client's hips at or below the posterior crest on either side of the sacrum. Mobilize the hips in an elliptical manner, alternating clockwise and counterclockwise directions with each hand. Move your hands around the posterior pelvic area to compress and access different areas of the hips. Be gentle and slow, and use a rhythmic pace. Repeat several times during the sequence of the massage. (See figure 16.1.)

Myofascial Stretches and Techniques

Picking up the fasciae and releasing it from underlying structures provides a unique opportunity for deep-tissue work. One simple technique involves pushing the fasciae in a clockwise manner with one thumb into the opposite hand that is also gathering tissue between a thumb and a forefinger. Use all fingers of that hand to help with the momentum of the stroke. (See figure 16.2.) Another myofascial stroke involves picking up the tissue with the fingers of both hands in a slight half-moon and drawing it over the thumbs as the thumbs press forward toward the fingers. Apply both strokes repetitively over a region. (See figure 16.3.)

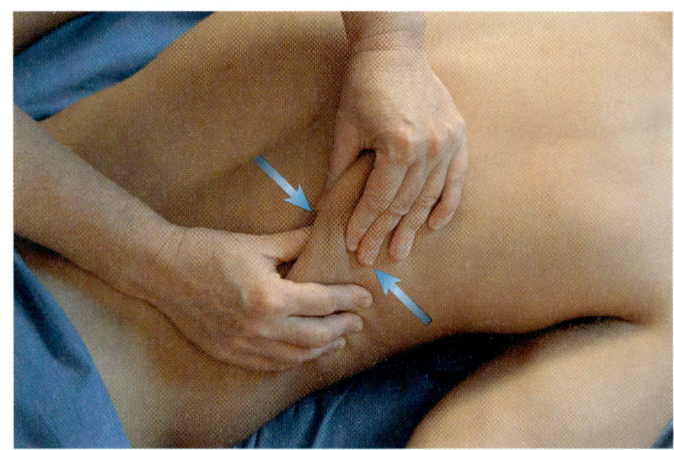

FIGURE 16.3 Half-moon warm-up

Elliptical Movement for Lower-Back Muscles

Facing the client's body, engage the external oblique and lower-back muscles on the opposite side of the body in an elliptical manner, moving the hands in opposing clockwise and counterclockwise directions. (See figure 16.4.)

Alternating Effleurage

With a small amount of lubrication, apply a sweeping alternating effleurage on the lumbar section of the erector spinae group and quadratus lumborum. Remain on one side of the table, and reach across to the opposite side of the low back. Keeping your fingers together, move your hands away from each other in an alternating effleurage movement. Sweep

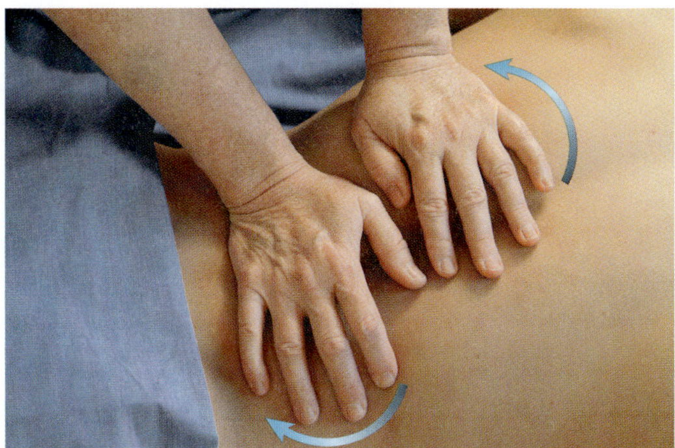

FIGURE 16.4 Elliptical movement for lower-back muscles

from the 12th-rib area to the hip with the inferior hand and from the last lumbar vertebra and sacrum to the end of the 12th rib with the superior hand. Start the secondary movement before you let go of the initial stroke to sustain the pressure and stretch. Move to the opposide side of the table, and repeat the action. *Note:* One side of the back can be treated at a time to layer the techniques listed below. When finished, move to the opposite side and start over with the sequence. (See figure 16.5.)

Figure Eight of the Low Back

Face the table at the low back. Place one hand on one side of the low back between the posterior crest and the 12th rib and the other hand on the side closest to you. Keep your hands in a straight line with your forearms and in the direction you are facing. Make large circles on the low back with both hands on each side: The hand on the opposite side of the table goes clockwise; the hand closest to you goes counterclockwise. After you have completed one circle, glide your hands over the spine and repeat the stroke. Keep alternating to opposite sides of the back several times for a fluid effect. Use enough pressure. Move your body along with the stroke. (See figure 16.6.)

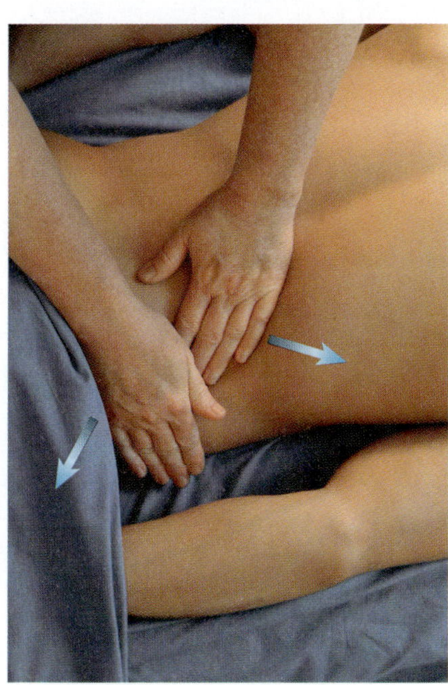

FIGURE 16.5 Alternating effleurage

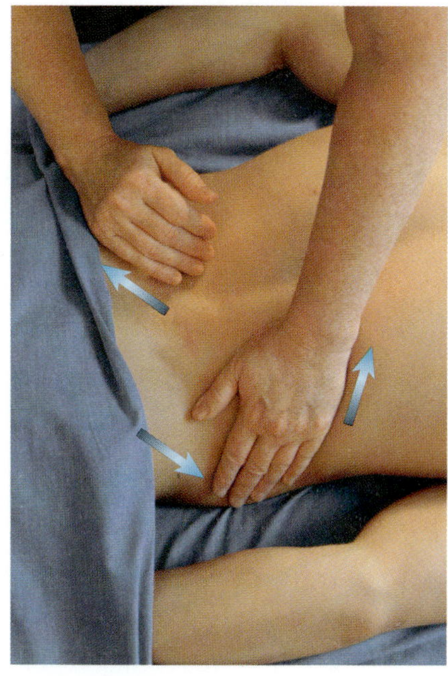

FIGURE 16.6 Figure eight of the low back

Petrissage of the External Oblique

Facing the client's back, petrissage the external oblique on the opposite side of the body from hip to ribs. (See figure 16.7.)

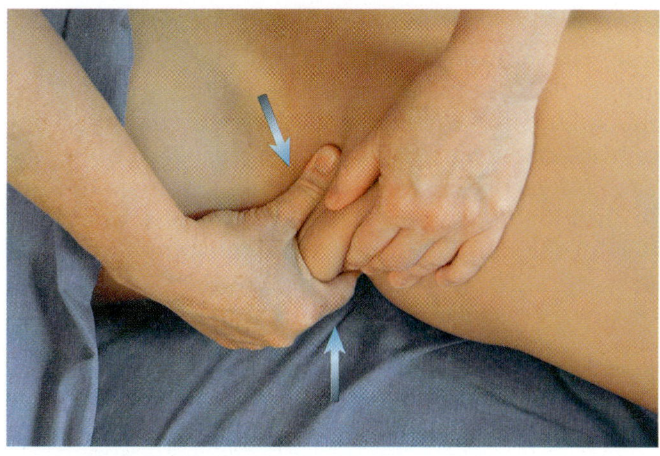

FIGURE 16.7 Petrissage of the external oblique

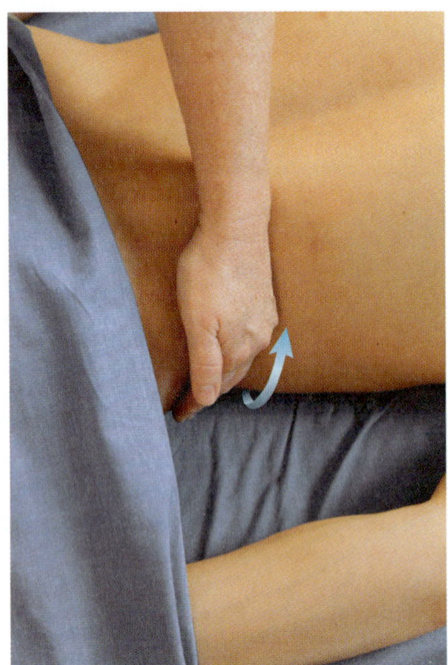

FIGURE 16.8 Edging the hip

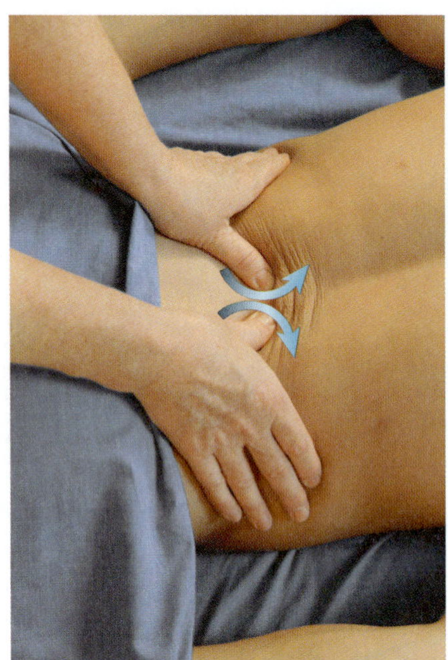

FIGURE 16.9 Thumb friction

Edging the Hip

Face the client's back. On the opposite side of the body, place the ulnar side of your superior hand on the outside lateral edge of the iliac crest. Draw your hand medially, conforming to the shape of the iliac crest and pinning the muscles against the ilium as you engage the tissues. Repeat a few times. Remember to use a soft hand, and use your body weight and momentum to bring you backward. (See figure 16.8.)

Thumb Friction

Apply thumb friction with half circles on either side of the spinous processes, beginning just above the sacrum and ending at the 12th thoracic vertebra. Use appropriate thumb pressure to sink into the structure of soft tissue around the vertebrae. (See figure 16.9.)

Deep Transverse Friction to the Erectors

Apply deep transverse friction on the lumbar erector group. Start at the base of the lumbar spine. From the side of the table where you are standing, work on the opposite erectors. Place your hands on top of each other. Using straight fingertips, apply a to-and-fro motion 90 degrees to the spine, and cross the fibers of the muscle group with a constant downward pressure. Change sides and repeat the stroke on the other erector group. (See figure 16.10.)

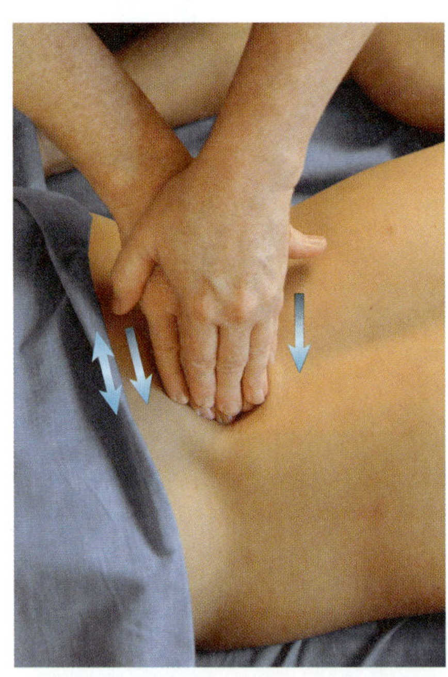

FIGURE 16.10 Deep transverse friction to the erectors

Forearm Effleurage to the Erector Spinae

Using your forearm closest to the body, apply the ulnar edge to the lower erector spinae group. Glide superiorly over the muscle group until the muscles change diameter. At this point, you can release your pressure and glide back down to your original position or continue up between the scapula and glide around laterally and back down to your original position. Check with the client for feedback about pressure. Be careful of the position of your olecranon process and your proximity to the spinous processes. (See figure 16.11.)

Trigger Points for Quadratus Lumborum

Locate trigger points on the quadratus lumborum and erectors, two to four points if any. On the same

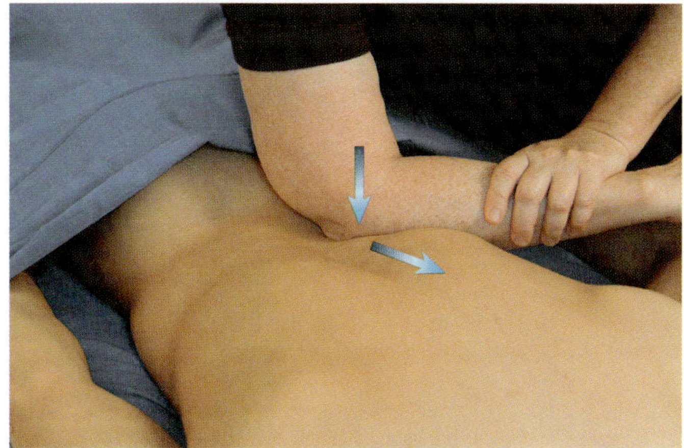

FIGURE 16.11 Forearm effleurage to the erector spinae

side of the table, facing the client's head, press thumb on top of thumb, under the end of the 12th rib. Have the client inhale, and on exhalation sink into the trigger point. Apply pressure for 7 to 10 seconds. Ease out gently. Stretch the tissue. Repeat where necessary. Use intelligent pressure. (See figure 16.12.)

Quadratus Lumborum and Erectors Stretch

Stretch all fiber lengths of the muscles. Reach across to the opposite side of the client. For the first stretch, use your inferior hand to grasp the anterior iliac crest. Place your superior hand on the ribs. Lift the pelvis and push the ribs to provide a stretch. (See figure 16.13.) Let the pelvis down gently, and place your

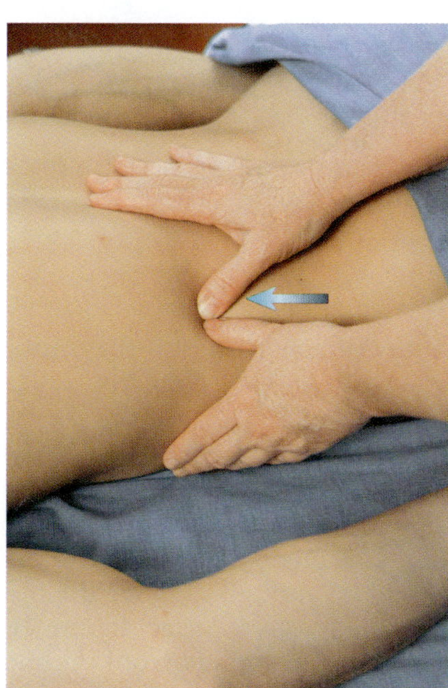

FIGURE 16.12 Trigger points

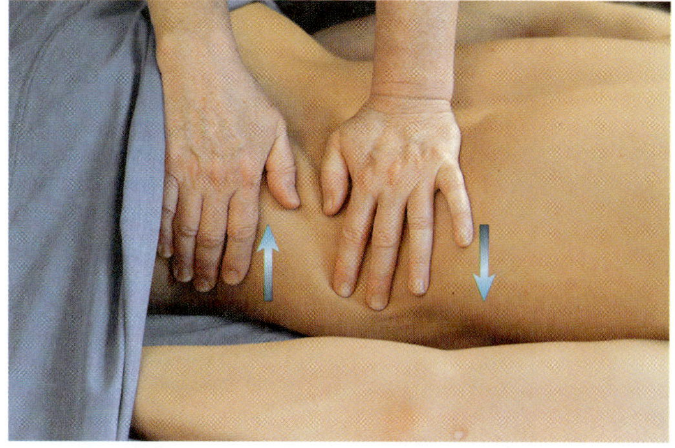

FIGURE 16.13 Quadratus lumborum stretch, lifting pelvis

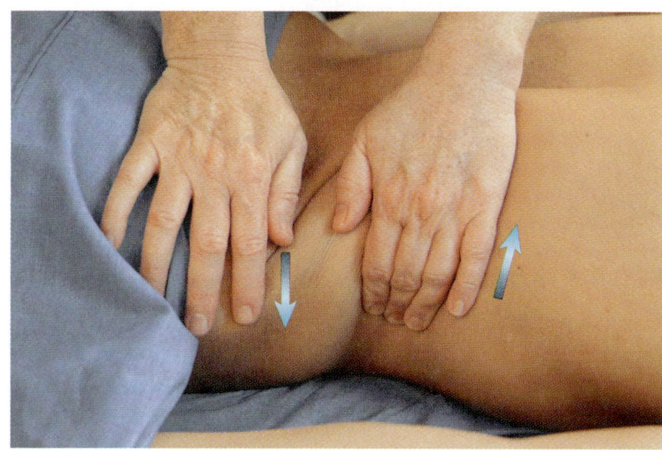

FIGURE 16.14 Quadratus lumborum stretch, pushing pelvis

hands so that you can push on the pelvis and lift the ribs. (See figure 16.14.) For the erectors and fibers of the quadratus lumborum that run from the 12th rib to the crest, cross your hands, and pin and stretch the fibers. (See figure 16.15.)

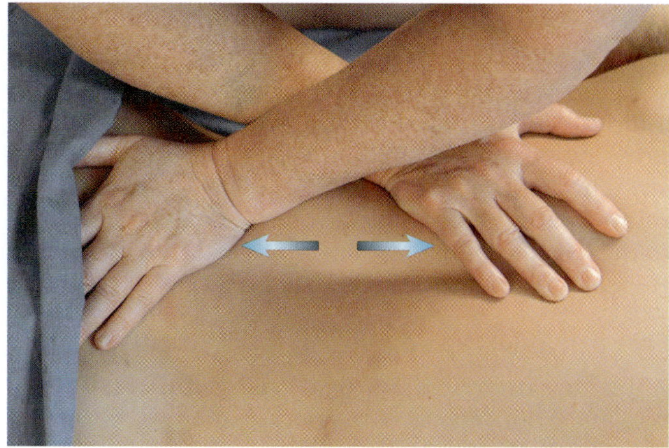

FIGURE 16.15 Erectors stretch

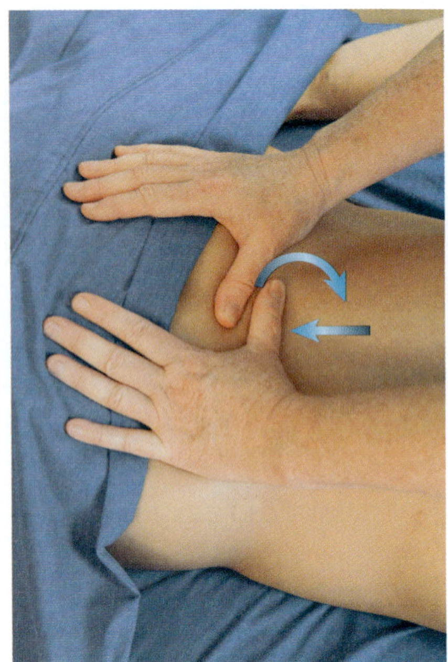

FIGURE 16.16 Parallel thumbs

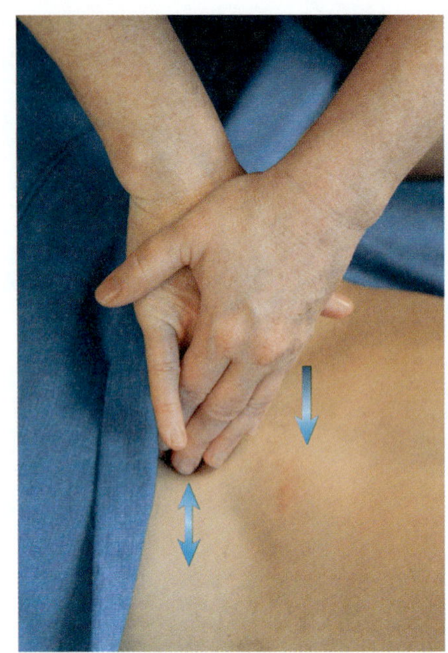

FIGURE 16.17 Deep transverse friction to the sacrum

SACRUM

Parallel Thumbs

Facing the client's feet, line your thumbs up in a parallel line. As you press into the tissue, place one thumb over the next, moving down the length of the sacrum. Stroke the fibers first on one side of the sacrum and then on the other side. (See figure 16.16.)

Deep Transverse Friction to the Sacrum

Apply deep transverse friction across the iliac crest using your middle finger over your index finger from the same side of the table; switch sides to repeat on the opposite crest. Edge across the crest lateral to medial with the side of your hand. (See figure 16.17.)

Trigger Points on the Sacrum and Crest of Ilium

Locate trigger points on the sacrum and the crest of the ilium. Use care to position yourself on the sacrum and not in the sacroiliac joint. As the client exhales, press down with your thumbs on top of each other straight into the surface. Hold for 7 to 10 seconds to 2 minutes. Roll under the iliac crest, and apply pressure to the trigger point. Ease out gently. Stretch the tissue. Repeat where necessary.

Forearm Effleurage on the Posterior Crest

Apply forearm effleurage on the posterior crest twice, moving from inferior to superior; change sides and repeat. (See figure 16.18.)

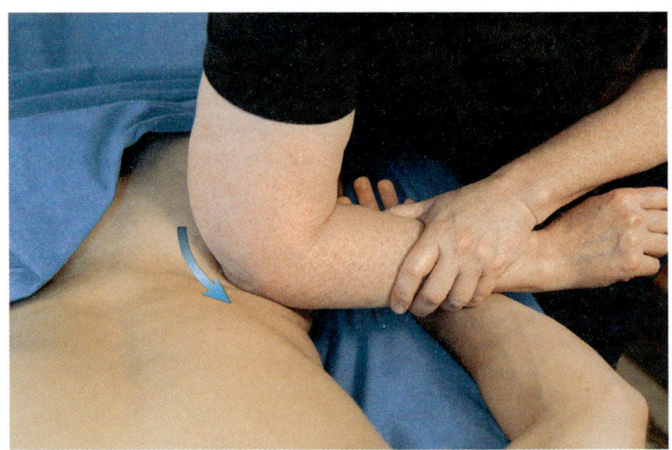

FIGURE 16.18 Forearm effleurage on the posterior crest

GLUTEALS

Repeat elliptical movement of the hips. (See figure 16.1.)

Elliptical Movement on the Gluteals

From the opposite side of the table, place your hands on the gluteal muscles. Apply a clockwise and counterclockwise movement alternately to the gluteals. Pressure should be enough to move the muscle mass rather than glide over it. (See figure 16.19.) The technique also can be applied from the same side of the table. (See figure 16.20.)

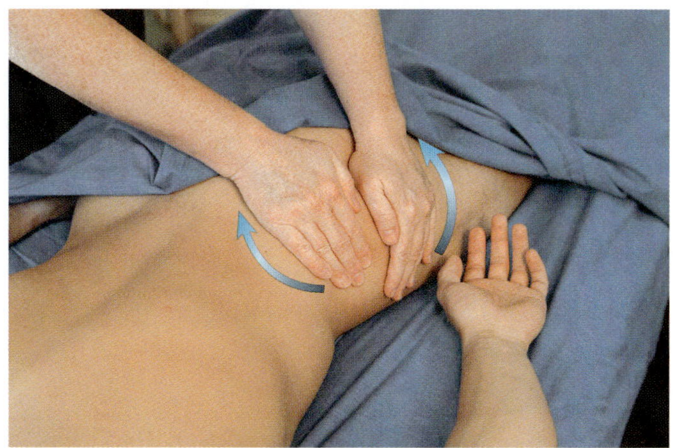

FIGURE 16.19 Elliptical movement on the gluteals, from opposite side of the table

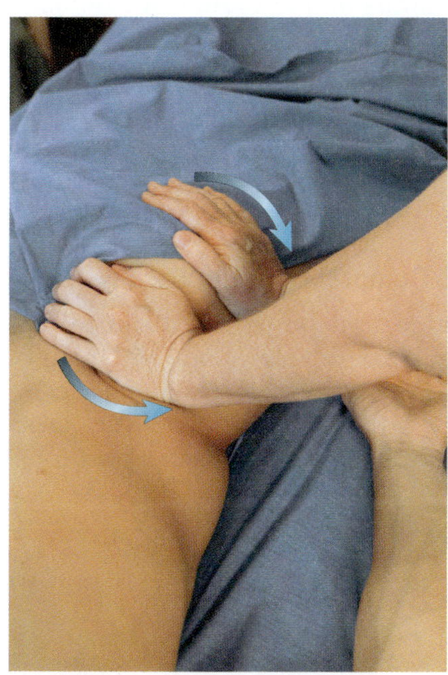

FIGURE 16.20 Elliptical movement on the gluteals, from same side of the table

Circular Effleurage on the Gluteals

Work on the same side of the table, facing the client's head. With one hand over the other, press and effleurage in a circular direction toward the sacrum. (See figure 16.21.)

Anchor Hip and Separate Fibers

Stand on the opposite side of the table, facing the client's low back and gluteal region. Place your superior hand above the crest on the opposite side of the spine of the low back. While you brace the low back with your superior hand, draw your inferior hand medially over the fibers of the gluteal muscles. Reposition the inferior hand, and repeat. (See figure 16.22.)

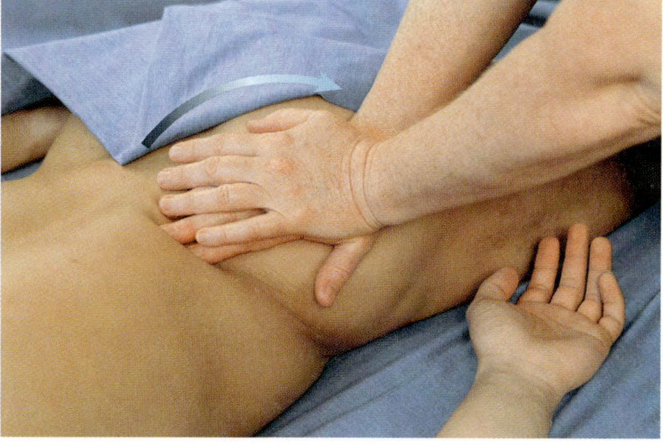

FIGURE 16.21 Circular effleurage on the gluteals

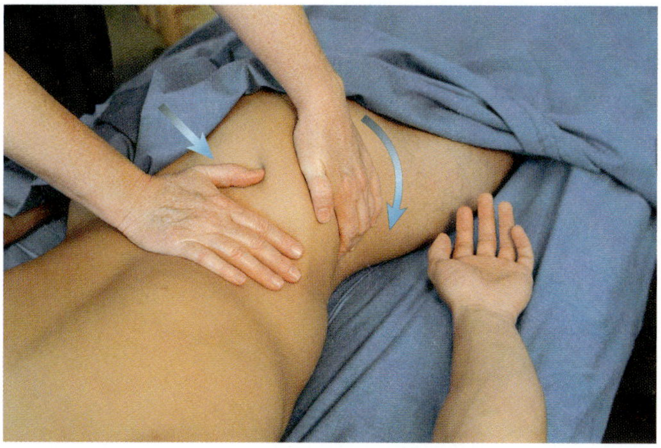

FIGURE 16.22 Anchoring the hip and separating the fibers

Palm Compressive Effleurage to the Gluteus Medius

Face the client's head. Place your inside hand on the sacrum. With your outside hand, use a soft palm compressive effleurage to the gluteus medius in a circular direction from the sacrum to the lateral crest. Repeat several times. (See figure 16.23.)

Closed-Fist Stripping of the Gluteus Medius

In a lunge position, stand to the side of the table, facing the feet. With your outside hand, apply a relaxed closed fist to the gluteus medius at the crest. Stroke in the direction of the fibers, toward the greater trochanter. Repeat the stroke, starting again at the crest in a slightly different position on the muscle. (See figure 16.24.)

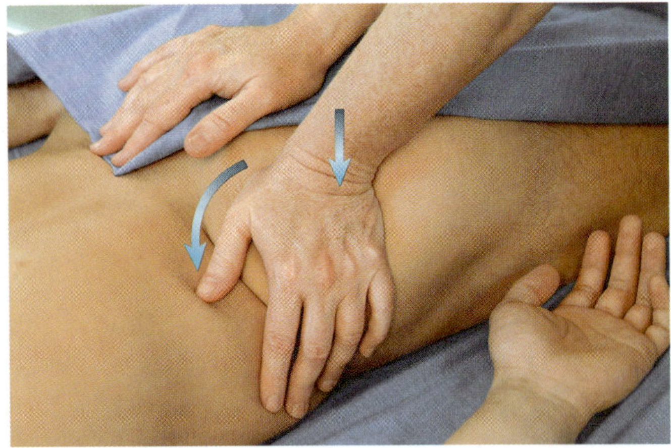

FIGURE 16.23 Palm compressive effleurage to the gluteus medius

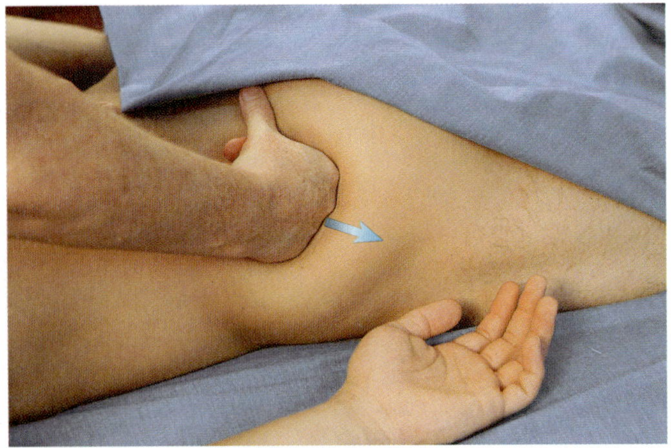

FIGURE 16.24 Closed-fist stripping of the gluteus medius

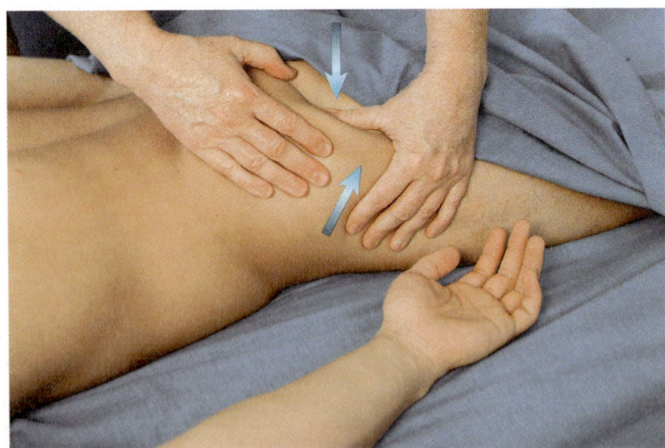

FIGURE 16.25 Deep petrissage of the gluteals

Deep Petrissage of the Gluteals

Standing on the opposite side of the table, facing the client, petrissage the gluteals. (See figure 16.25.)

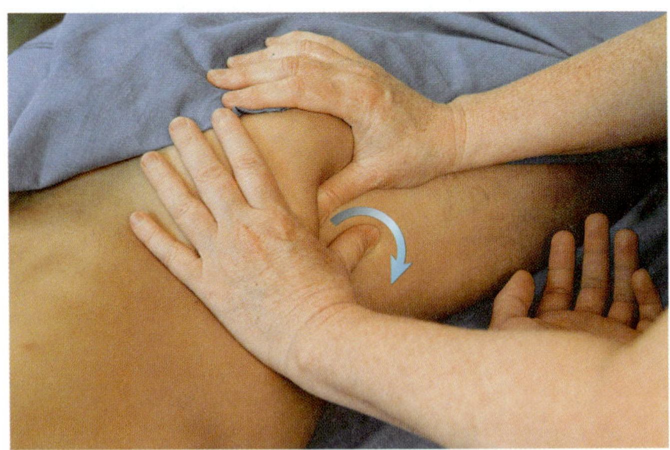

FIGURE 16.26 Parallel thumbs on the gluteus maximus

Parallel Thumbs on the Gluteus Maximus

On the same side of the table, place your hands close to the greater trochanter. Apply even pressure, and roll the thumbs over each other one at a time in a strip toward the sacrum. Repeat as you move in the shape of a fan with each strip toward the sacrum. (See figure 16.26.)

Bent-Knee Compression with Passive Movement

Face the table, and flex the client's knee closest to you. Hold the ankle with your hand. With your other hand, palpate the lateral hip rotators and gluteals, and compress them with a relaxed fist as you passively move the leg in external and internal positions. (See figure 16.27.)

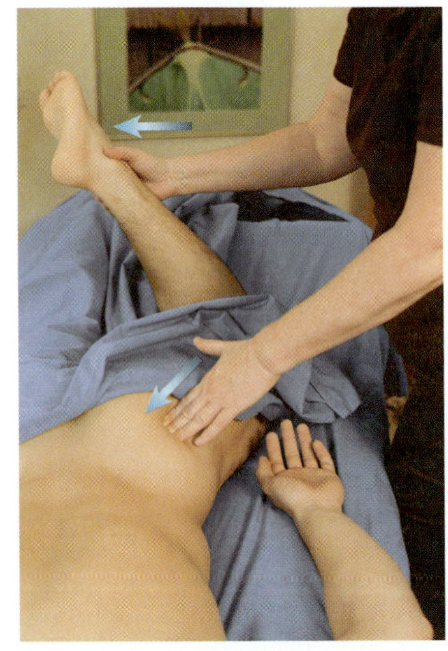

FIGURE 16.27 Bent-knee compression with passive movement

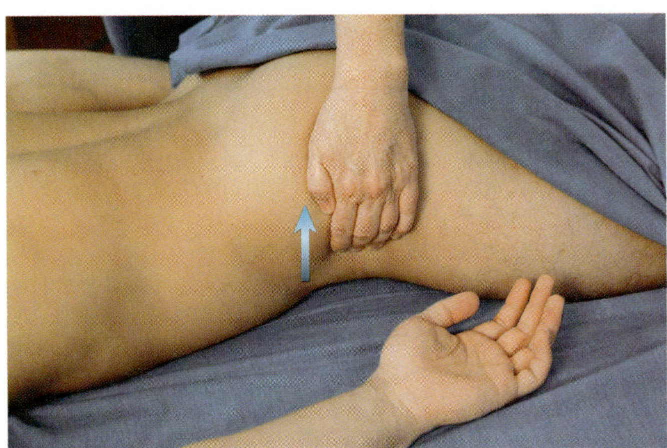

FIGURE 16.28 Deep transverse friction of the tensor fasciae latae

Deep Transverse Friction of the Tensor Fasciae Latae

Reaching across the table, locate the tensor fasciae latae just inferior to the iliac crest. Apply deep transverse friction in a hand-over-hand position to the medial side of the tensor fasciae latae. Allow the body to do the work for you. As you draw your fingers over the fibers, the weight of the body will assist you in the technique. (See figure 16.28.)

Deep Transverse Friction of the Anterior and Posterior Crest

Facing the client's feet, apply deep transverse friction from the ASIS to the PIIS using hand over hand in a to-and-fro motion. (See figure 16.29.)

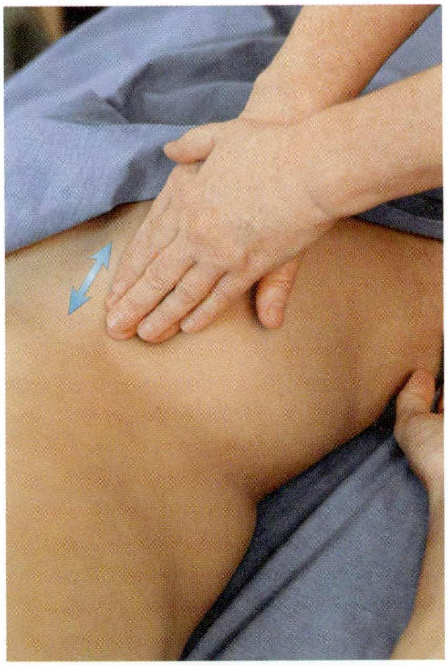

FIGURE 16.29 Deep transverse friction of the crest

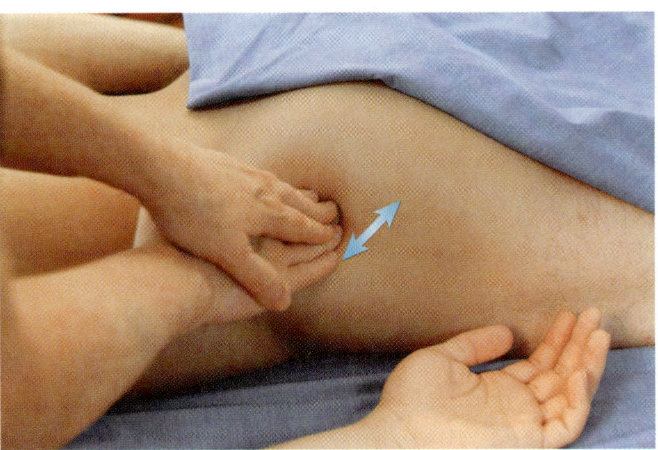

FIGURE 16.30 Deep transverse friction to the piriformis and lateral rotators

Deep Transverse Friction to the Piriformis

Facing the client's head, apply deep transverse friction to the piriformis and the lateral rotator using hand over hand in a to-and-fro motion. (See figure 16.30.)

Trigger Points in the Lateral Rotators

Locate trigger points in the piriformis and lateral rotators. As the client exhales, press into the trigger points. Be cautious to avoid the sciatic nerve when you are locating the trigger points. This may be a very painful area. Release as before, usually within 7 to 10 seconds. Ease out slowly and stretch the tissue. (See figure 16.31.)

Forearm Effleurage of the Sacrum and Crest

Facing the client's head, place the inside forearm on or near the PIIS. Stroke toward the ASIS of the crest. Repeat 2 times. (See figure 16.32.)

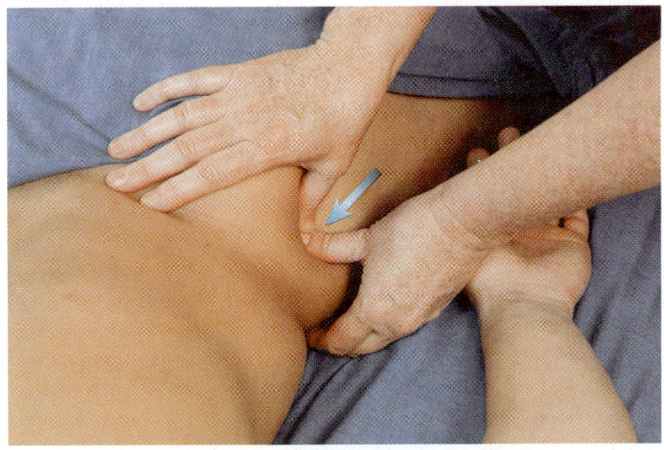

FIGURE 16.31 Trigger points in the lateral rotators

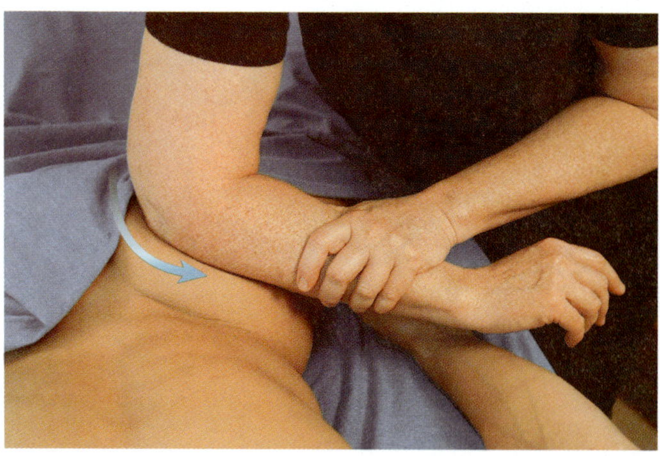

FIGURE 16.32 Forearm effleurage of the sacrum and crest

Repeat the above techniques to the other gluteal region.

Assess the success of the treatment by the release of the soft tissue, decrease in pain, and increase in the client's mobility. Remember, Rome was not built in a day. If the client has been in pain for a period of time, resolution of soft-tissue dysfunction may take more than one or two treatments. Chart the progress, and work with a conservative team approach for the client's benefit.

Complete the sequence with full-back effleurage and any ending strokes.

CHAPTER *summary*

Introduction

- ✔ Chronic low-back pain affects millions of people.
- ✔ Sources of pain include muscles, tendons, ligaments, bones, disks, and facet joints.
- ✔ Physical trauma, repetitive action, posture, and improper lifting cause problems for the low back and pelvic girdle.
- ✔ Massage therapy is part of a conservative approach to relieving chronic back pain.

Structural Perspectives of the Low Back and Pelvic Girdle

- ✔ The abdomen is the front and sides of the low back.
- ✔ The movement of the pelvic girdle can affect the low back.
- ✔ Contracted muscles in the low back, hips, and lower extremities can contribute to the position of the hips.
- ✔ Structural perspectives give massage therapists a reason for approaching massage treatments dimensionally.
- ✔ Different positions in lifting inappropriately might involve a variety of lower-back muscles.

Injuries and Overuse Syndromes

- ✔ Trauma and inappropriate lifting contribute to back injuries.
- ✔ Diagnosis is reserved for the physician.
- ✔ Massage therapists should refer undiagnosed clients to a medical professional when they present with pain and fever or chills, a history of cancer with recent weight loss, severe trauma, significant leg weakness, sudden bowel and/or bladder incontinence, severe continuous abdominal and back pain, and nausea and/or vomiting.

Nerve Complaints

- ✔ Sciatica can be defined as an inflammation of the sciatic nerve.
- ✔ Sciatica can be caused by a herniated disk, foraminal stenosis, and/or soft-tissue entrapment.
- ✔ Massage therapy can help release nerve entrapment and relieve soft-tissue discomfort.

Arthritis, Osteoarthritis, Degenerative Disk Disease, and Lumbar and Sacroiliac Subluxations

- ✔ Arthritis, osteoarthritis, degenerative disk disease, and lumbar subluxations can contribute to nerve complaints.
- ✔ A laminectomy is a surgical procedure that removes the posterior arch and spinous processes of the midline of the vertebrae to reduce stenosis in the spinal canal and give the spinal cord more room.

Unwinding the Muscles of the Low Back: Prone or Supine?

- ✔ Positioning the client is important to the success of the treatment.
- ✔ Support the client with pillows, pads, or rolled towels to passively shorten muscles and provide comfort.
- ✔ Follow a dimensional approach, and critically think about the involved joints and muscles.
- ✔ Always use treatment protocols to determine the sequence of a therapeutic session.
- ✔ Refer clients to an appropriate professional when necessary.

Dimensional Massage Therapy for the Muscles of the Low Back and Pelvic Girdle

- ✔ Apply appropriate warm-up techniques to soften tissue.
- ✔ Approach techniques methodically, unwinding soft tissue superficially to deep.
- ✔ Practice techniques, and incorporate them into a sequence.

CHAPTER *review*

True or False

Write true *or* false *after each statement.*

1. Sciatica is inflammation of the sciatic notch.
2. A conservative team approach for back pain would require surgery.
3. Always put heat on painful new injuries.
4. Erector spinae fibers stop at lumbar vertebra 1.
5. It is important to exert caution with clients with a herniated disk.
6. The muscles of the lower extremities have no effect on the movement and position of the pelvic girdle.
7. Abdominal muscles can affect the position of the pelvic girdle.
8. It is all right to massage an undiagnosed client who has nausea, vomiting, and severe continuous abdominal and back pain.
9. Bone spurs and/or arthritis can cause foraminal stenosis.
10. The sciatic nerve can go through the piriformis muscle in some cases.
11. Removing a wallet out of a person's back pocket will automatically fix any sciatic compression.

Short Answers

Write your answers on the lines provided.

1. Name the superficial muscle of the low back that is attached to a large aponeurosis.

____

____

____

2. Define *foraminal stenosis.*

____

____

____

3. Name the muscles of the posterior thigh that the sciatic nerve passes between.

____

____

____

4. Define *myofascial pain.*

____

____

____

5. Which lateral rotator may have an effect on the sciatic nerve?

____

____

____

6. What can cause sciatica?

____

____

____

7. Define *radicular pain.*

____

____

____

8. What contributes to the degeneration of disks in the low back?

____

____

____

9. What is a laminectomy?

____

____

____

10. Define *herniated disk.*

____

____

____

11. What is cryotherapy?

____

____

____

12. Give five reasons for referring an undiagnosed client with back pain to a medical professional.

____

____

____

Multiple Choice

Circle the correct answers.

1. A conservative approach to chronic back pain would include:
   a. surgery
   b. massage, chiropractic, exercise, and physical therapy
   c. a laminectomy
   d. none of the above
2. Axial pain can be:
   a. sharp or dull, constant or intermittent, mild or severe
   b. found in the lower extremities
   c. only sharp
   d. all of the above
3. The piriformis can entrap:
   a. the accessory nerve
   b. the femoral nerve
   c. the sciatic nerve
   d. none of the above
4. Myofascial pain can be caused by:
   a. injury, trauma, lifting, surgery, posture
   b. only injury
   c. only repetitive action
   d. the client's imagination
5. Trauma victims experiencing back pain need to be:
   a. massaged right away
   b. examined first by a physician
   c. given elaborate range-of-motion stretches
   d. none of the above
6. Myofascial pain is:
   a. caused by the distribution of a nerve
   b. not associated with the distribution of a nerve
   c. linked to the spinal nerves
   d. none of the above
7. Treatment protocol for working on the low back is to:
   a. start prone and work only on the back muscles
   b. start in a supine position and work superficial to deep
   c. work on the lower extremity first
   d. go as deep as you can right away
8. Abdominal muscles:
   a. posteriorly rotate the hips
   b. anteriorly rotate the hips
   c. do not support the back at all
   d. none of the above
9. Regular massage for a person who suffers from chronic back pain could:
   a. assist the release of entrapped nerves and help relieve discomfort
   b. relieve all pain immediately
   c. do nothing for the client
   d. none of the above
10. Fifty percent of people with back pain from mechanical origin have some relief in:
    a. 2 days
    b. 2 weeks
    c. 10 days
    d. 2 years

EXPLORE & *practice*

1. Locate bony landmarks of the lumbar vertebrae on a partner.
2. Locate on a partner the origins and insertions of the muscles discussed in this chapter and in Chapter 15.
3. List conservative approaches that might be possible for a client with back pain.
4. List which muscles are agonists and synergists for flexion of the trunk.

5. List which muscles are agonists and synergists for extension of the trunk.
6. Describe how to interview a client who has back pain.
7. Practice dimensional techniques individually and in a sequence on another student.
8. What precautions might you take should a client present with acute back pain?
9. What precautions might you take should a client present with chronic back pain?

chapter 17

The Knee Joint

LEARNING OUTCOMES

After completing this chapter, you should be able to:

17-1 Define key terms.

17-2 Identify on a human skeleton selected bony features of the knee joint.

17-3 Describe the cartilaginous and ligamentous structures of the knee joint.

17-4 Draw and label on a skeletal chart the muscles, including origins and insertions, and ligaments of the knee joint.

17-5 Palpate the superficial knee joint structures and muscles, including origins and insertions, on a partner.

17-6 Demonstrate all the active and passive movements of the knee joint with a partner.

17-7 Name and explain the actions and importance of the quadriceps and hamstring muscles.

17-8 List and organize the muscles that produce the movements of the knee joint and list their antagonists.

17-9 Practice flexibility and strengthening exercises for each muscle group.

KEY TERMS

Anterior cruciate ligament (ACL)
Biceps femoris
Chondromalacia
Femoral nerve
Fibula
Fibular (lateral) collateral ligament (LCL)
Hamstrings
Lateral meniscus
Medial and lateral femoral condyles
Medial collateral ligament (MCL)
Medial meniscus
Medial tibial condyle
Patella
Pes anserinus
Plica
Popliteus
Posterior cruciate ligament (PCL)
Q angle
Rectus femoris
Semimembranosus
Semitendinosus
Sesamoid
Tibia
Tibial plateau
Tibial tuberosity
Tibiofemoral joint
Vastus intermedius
Vastus lateralis
Vastus medialis

Introduction

Skiing down a slope is only one of the many sports that are possible because of the knee's ability to flex, extend, and internally and externally rotate, with its dynamic stability provided by its muscles balancing the forces from the hip and the lower extremity. Similar in function, in many respects, to the elbow joint in the upper extremity, the knee joint is the largest, most complex joint in the body; it divides the hip and the foot by providing the mechanism of movement and the attachments for powerful knee extensor and flexor muscles. These muscles enable the body to utilize the mobile hip joints to their maximum capacities in skiing, jumping, dancing, and other similar activities. Weight bearing and locomotion are the primary functions of the knee joint. The knee joint also has an effect on the position of the hips. When the knees are locked in extension, the hips rotate anteriorly. Observe, for example, the gymnast's final stance in a landing or a woman's posture in her last trimester of pregnancy. A locked-knee position forces the individual's lower back to have an accentuated lordosis, thereby pulling on the lower-back muscles. To find balance, the body often leans over, causing the back extensors to oppose trunk flexion and sometimes producing a head-forward posture position. The domino effect caused by the position of the knee joint can result in many imbalances in the body.

The powerful and movable knee joint is vulnerable to many injuries. It is often injured in sports and other activities that require a great amount of mobility, yet a simple turn of the body in the wrong position can also cause damage. The articular surfaces of both the femur and the tibia are common areas for knee fractures, especially in athletics. Age, regular wear and tear, and torque break the joint down over time. Each time the body takes a step, its weight concusses through the joint structures to the tibia, placing major stress on the menisci. Guy wire, or tension, ligaments connect the sides and insides of the knee joint to provide static stability. Trauma and continual torque affect ligament stability. It is no wonder that this joint is one of the most replaced joints in the body. The bones' structures are designed to provide the mobility and weight bearing that is necessary from this powerful joint.

Bones

The enlarged femoral condyles articulate on the matching condyles of the tibia, in a somewhat horizontal line. Since the femur projects downward at an oblique angle toward the midline, its medial condyle is slightly larger than the lateral condyle.

The tops of the medial and lateral tibial condyles, known as the medial and lateral **tibial plateaus,** serve as receptacles for the femoral condyles. The **tibia** is the medial bone in the leg; it bears much more of the body's weight than does the **fibula.** The fibula serves as the attachment for important knee joint structures, although it does not articulate with the femur or patella. It is connected to the femur through the fibular collateral ligament.

The **patella** is a **sesamoid** (floating) bone contained within the quadriceps muscle group and patellar tendon. Its location allows it to serve the quadriceps in a manner similar to the work of a pulley by creating an improved angle of pull. This results in a greater mechanical advantage during knee extension.

Key bony landmarks of the knee include the superior and inferior poles of the patella, the **tibial tuberosity,** Gerdy's tubercle, the **medial and lateral femoral condyles,** the upper anterior medial surface of the tibia, and the head of the fibula. The three vasti muscles of the quadriceps originate on the proximal femur and insert, along with the rectus femoris, on the superior pole of the patella (figures 17.1 and 17.2). Their specific insertion into the patella varies in that the vastus medialis and the vastus lateralis insert into the patella from a superomedial and superolateral angle, respectively. The superficial rectus femoris and the vastus intermedius, which lies directly beneath it, both attach to the patella from a superior direction. From there, their insertion is ultimately on the tibial tuberosity by way of the large patellar tendon, which runs from the inferior patellar pole to the tibial tuberosity. Because this structure comes from bone to bone, it is often distinguished as a ligament. Gerdy's tubercle, located on the anterolateral aspect of the lateral tibial condyle, is the insertion point for the iliotibial tract of the tensor fasciae latae.

The upper anteromedial surface of the tibia just below the medial condyle serves as the insertion for the sartorius, gracilis, and semitendinosus. The semimembranosus inserts posteromedially on the **medial tibial condyle.** The head of the fibula is the primary location of the biceps femoris insertion, although some of its fibers insert on the lateral tibial condyle. The popliteus origin is located on the lateral aspect of the lateral femoral condyle.

Additionally, the tibial collateral ligament originates on the medial aspect of the upper medial femoral condyle and inserts on the medial surface of the tibia. Laterally, the shorter fibular collateral ligament originates on the lateral femoral condyle very close to the popliteus origin and inserts on the head of the fibula.

Joints

The knee joint proper, or **tibiofemoral joint** (figures 17.2 and 17.3), is classified as a ginglymus joint because it functions like a hinge. It moves between flexion and extension without side-to-side movement into abduction or adduction. However, it is sometimes referred to as a *trochoginglymus* joint because of the internal and external rotation movements that can

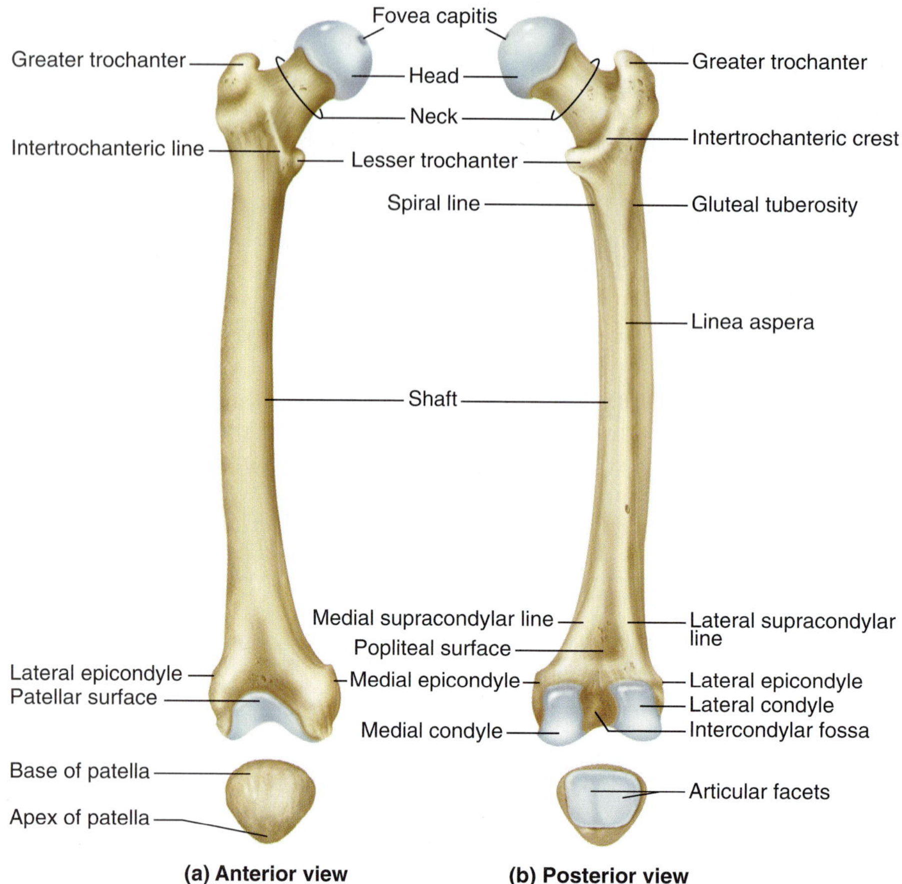

FIGURE 17.1 The femur and patella

occur during flexion. Some authorities even suggest that it should be classified as a condyloid or "double-condyloid" joint due to its bicondylar structure. The patellofemoral joint is classified as an arthrodial joint due to the gliding nature of the patella on the femoral condyles.

The ligaments provide static stability to the knee joint, and contractions of the quadriceps and hamstrings produce dynamic stability. Articular cartilage protects the surfaces between the femur and the tibia, as is true of all diarthrodial joints. In addition to the articular cartilage that covers the ends of the bones, specialized cartilages known as the *menisci* (figure 17.3) form cushions between the bones. The menisci are attached to the tibia and deepen the tibial plateaus, thereby enhancing stability.

The medial semilunar cartilage or, more technically, the **medial meniscus,** is located on the medial tibial plateau to form a receptacle for the medial femoral condyle. The lateral semilunar cartilage **(lateral meniscus)** sits on the lateral tibial plateau to receive the lateral femoral condyle. Both of these menisci are thicker on the outside border and taper down, becoming thinner on the inside border. They can slip about slightly and are held in place by various small ligaments. The medial meniscus is the larger of the two and has a more open C appearance than the rather closed C configuration of the lateral meniscus. Either or both of the menisci may be torn in several different areas from a variety of mechanisms, resulting in varying degrees of severity and problems. These injuries often occur because of the significant compression and shear forces that develop as the knee rotates while flexing or extending during quick directional changes, such as those in running.

Ligaments of the Knee Joint

Two very important knee ligaments are the **anterior cruciate ligament (ACL)** and **posterior cruciate ligament (PCL),** so named because they cross within the knee between the tibia and the femur. These ligaments are vital to maintaining the anterior and posterior stability of the knee joint, respectively, as well as the rotary stability. (See figure 17.3.)

An anterior cruciate ligament tear is one of the most common and serious injuries to the knee. It is significantly more common in females than in males

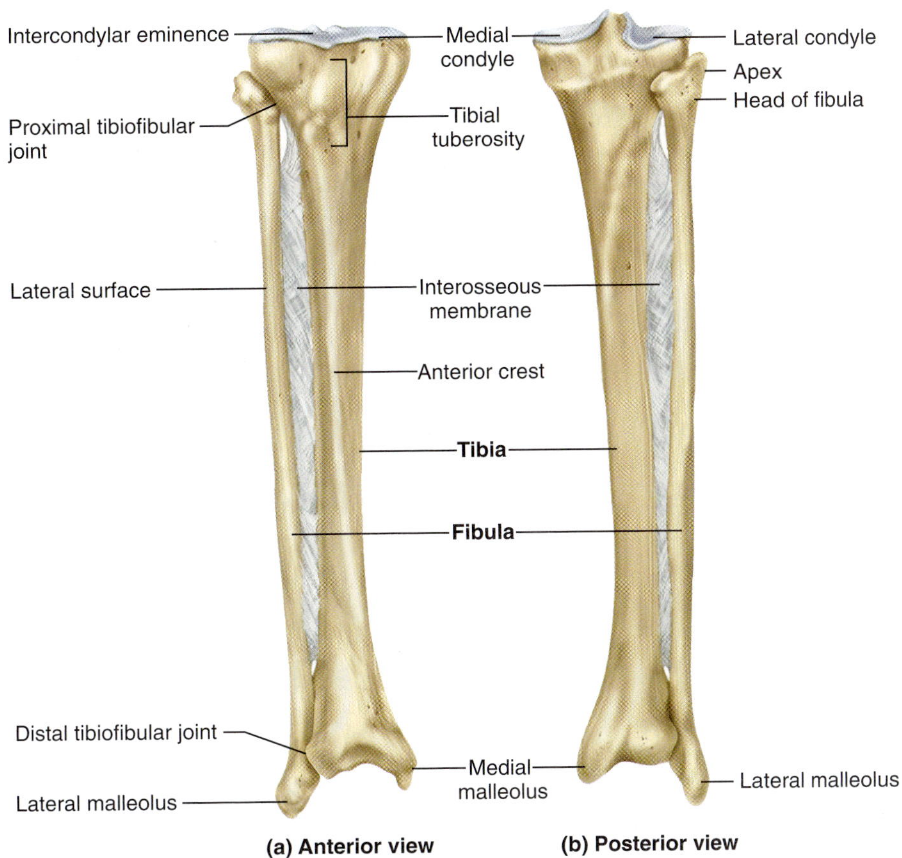

FIGURE 17.2 The right tibia and fibula

during the performance of sports, such as basketball or soccer. The mechanism of this injury often involves noncontact rotary forces associated with planting and cutting. Studies have shown that the ACL may also be disrupted in a hyperextension mechanism or solely by a violent contraction of the quadriceps that pulls the tibia forward on the femur. Recent studies suggest that ACL injury-prevention programs may be effective in reducing the likelihood of injury when the programs incorporate detailed conditioning exercises and techniques that are designed to improve neuromuscular coordination and control among the hamstrings and quadriceps, maintain proper knee alignment, and utilize proper landing techniques.

Fortunately, the posterior cruciate ligament is not often injured. Injuries of the posterior cruciate usually occur through direct contact with an opponent or the playing surface. Many PCL injuries are partial tears with minimal involvement of other knee structures. In many cases, even with complete tears, athletes may remain fairly competitive at a high level after a brief nonsurgical treatment and rehabilitation program.

On the medial side of the knee is the tibial **medial collateral ligament (MCL)** (figure 17.3), which maintains medial stability by resisting valgus forces or preventing the knee joint from being abducted. Injuries to the tibial collateral occur quite commonly, particularly in contact or collision sports in which a teammate or an opponent falls against the lateral aspect of the knee or leg, causing a medial opening of the knee joint and stress to the medial ligamentous structures. The tibial collateral's deeper fibers are attached to the medial meniscus, which may be affected by injuries to the ligament.

On the lateral side of the knee, the **fibular (lateral) collateral ligament (LCL)** joins the fibula and the femur. Injuries to this ligament are infrequent; however, it is subject to postural issues and problems with the knee.

In addition to the intraarticular ligaments detailed in figure 17.3, there are numerous other ligaments not shown that are contiguous with the joint capsule.

CLINICAL NOTE — **Prepatellar Bursitis**

The knee joint, as shown in figure 17.3, is well supplied with synovial fluid from the synovial cavity, which lies under the patella and between the surfaces of the tibia and the femur. This

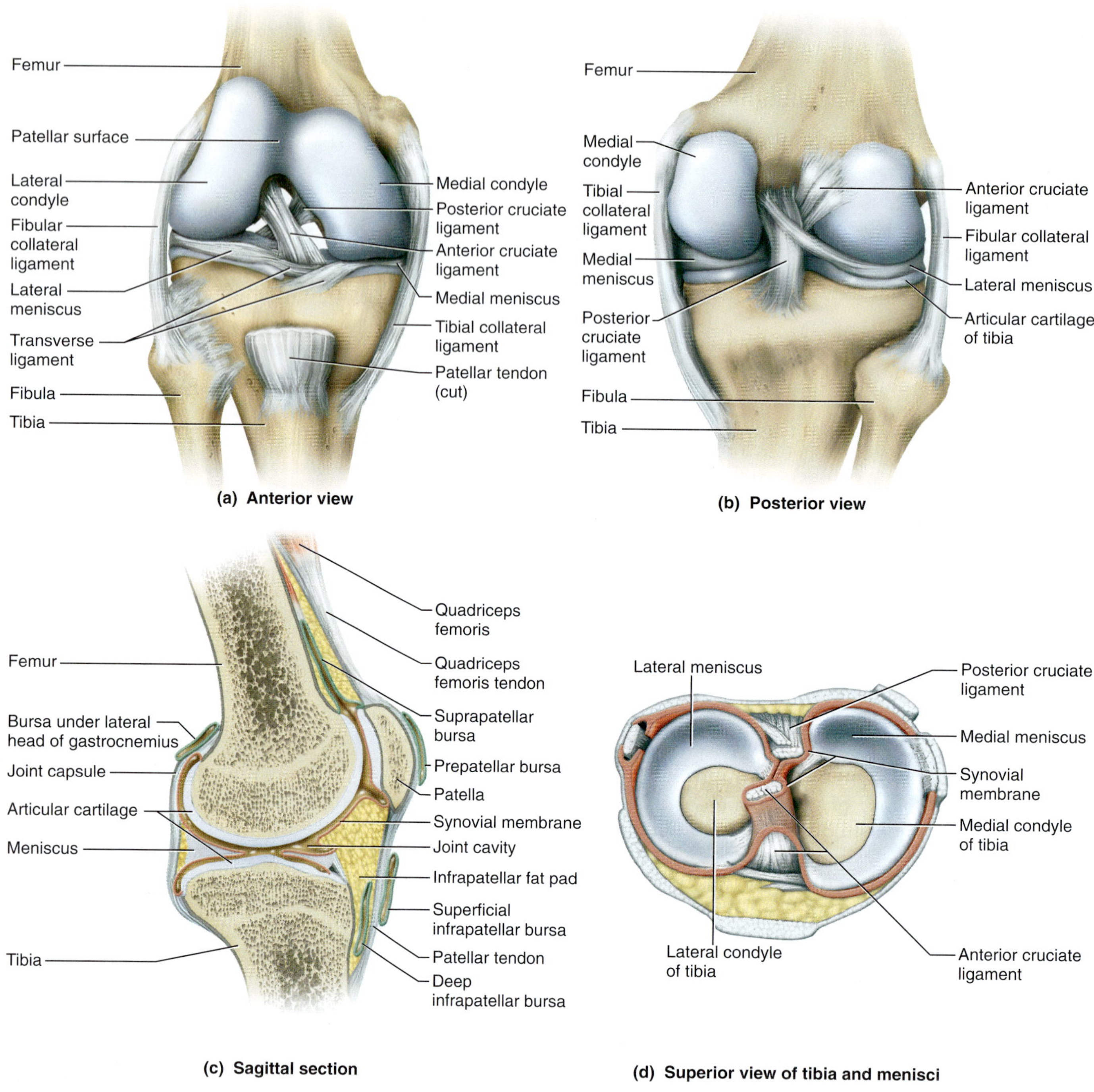

FIGURE 17.3 Knee joint

synovial cavity is also called the *knee capsule*. Just posterior to the patellar tendon is the infrapatellar fat pad, which is often an insertion point for synovial folds of tissue known as *plicae*. A **plica** is an anatomical variant among some individuals that may be irritated or inflamed with injuries or overuse of the knee. More than 10 bursae are located in the knee, some of which are connected to the synovial cavity. Bursae are located in areas where they can absorb shock or prevent friction. The prepatellar bursa often is irritated by kneeling and develops "water on the knee," or "housemaid's knee," which are common names for prepatellar bursitis. Stretching the quadriceps can help release pressure on the bursae.

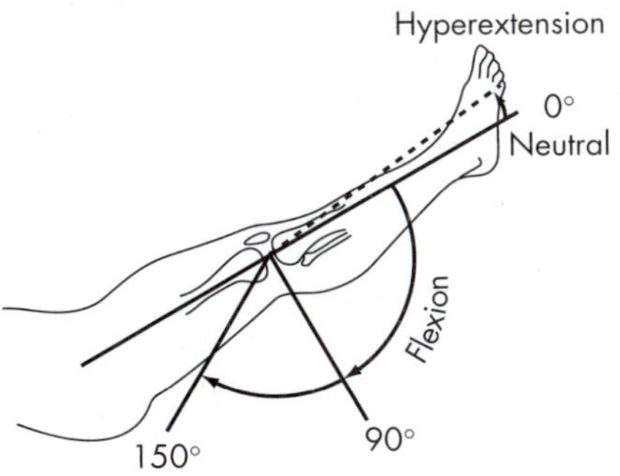

FIGURE 17.4 Active motion of the knee

The knee can usually extend to 180 degrees, or a straight line, although it is not uncommon for some knees to hyperextend up to 10 degrees or more. When the knee is in full extension, it can move from there to about 140 degrees of flexion. With the knee flexed 30 degrees or more, approximately 30 degrees of internal rotation and 45 degrees of external rotation can occur (figure 17.4).

Due to the shape of the medial femoral condyle, the knee must externally rotate to fully extend. As the knee approaches full extension, the tibia must externally rotate approximately 10 degrees to achieve proper alignment of the tibial and femoral condyles. In full extension, due to the close congruency of the articular surfaces, there is no appreciable rotation of the knee. During initial flexion from a fully extended position, the knee "unlocks" by the tibia rotating internally, to a degree, from its externally rotated position to achieve flexion.

Movements

FLEXIBILITY & STRENGTH

Movements of the Knee

Flexion and extension of the knee occur in the sagittal plane, whereas internal and external rotation occur in the horizontal plane. The knee will not allow rotation unless it is flexed 20 to 30 degrees or more (figure 17.5).

Flexion

Bending or decreasing the angle between the femur and lower leg; characterized by the heel moving toward the buttock.

Extension

Straightening or increasing the angle between the femur and the lower leg.

External rotation

Rotary movement of the lower leg laterally away from the midline.

Internal rotation

Rotary movement of the lower leg medially toward the midline.

Muscles

Chapter 15 discussed some of the muscles involved in knee joint movements because of their biarticular arrangement with both the hip joint and the knee joint; they are not covered again fully in this chapter. The knee joint muscles that have already been addressed are the rectus femoris (knee extensor) and the sartorius and gracilis (knee flexors). The gastrocnemius, discussed in Chapter 19, also assists minimally with knee flexion.

The quadriceps muscle group extends the knee and is located in the anterior compartment of the thigh. It consists of the rectus femoris, vastus lateralis, vastus intermedius, and vastus medialis. All four of these muscles work together to pull the patella superiorly; this, in turn, pulls the leg into extension at the knee by its attachment to the tibial tuberosity via the patellar tendon.

The central line of pull for the entire quadriceps runs from the anterior superior iliac spine (ASIS) to the center of the patella. The line of pull of the patellar tendon runs from the center of the patella to the center of the tibial tuberosity. The angle formed by the intersection of these two lines at the patella is known as the **Q angle,** or quadriceps angle (figure 17.6). Normally, this angle is 15 degrees or less in males and 20 degrees or less in females. Generally, females have higher angles due to having wider pelvises. Higher Q angles generally predispose people, in varying degrees, to a variety of potential knee problems, including patellar subluxation or dislocation, patellar compression syndrome, chondromalacia, and ligamentous injuries. Young athletic women in jumping sports have suffered an increase in knee injuries over the last few years, attributed to the biomechanics of the structure of the wider pelvis. Additionally, females injure their ACL up to six times more than do males.

The hamstring muscle group is located in the posterior compartment of the thigh and is responsible for knee flexion. The **hamstrings** consist of three muscles: the **semitendinosus,** the **semimembranosus,** and the **biceps femoris.** The semimembranosus and semitendinosus muscles (medial hamstrings) are assisted by the **popliteus** in internally rotating the knee, whereas the biceps femoris (lateral hamstring) is responsible for knee external rotation.

Two-joint muscles are most effective when either the origin or the insertion is stabilized to prevent movement in the direction of the muscle when it contracts. Additionally, muscles are able to exert greater force when lengthened than when shortened. All the hamstring muscles, as well as the rectus femoris, sartorius, and gracilis, are biarticular (two-joint) muscles.

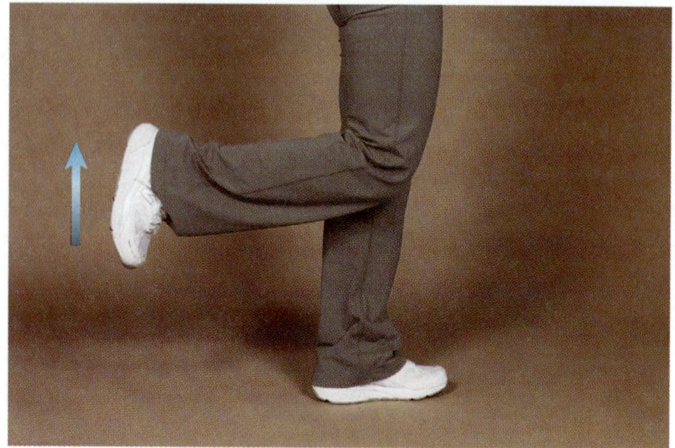
Flexion

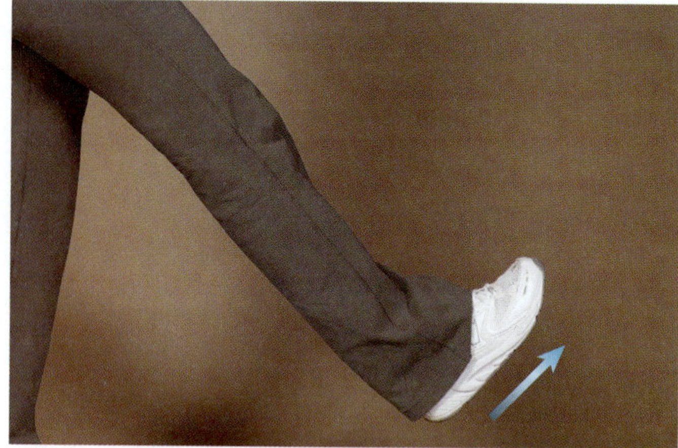
Extension

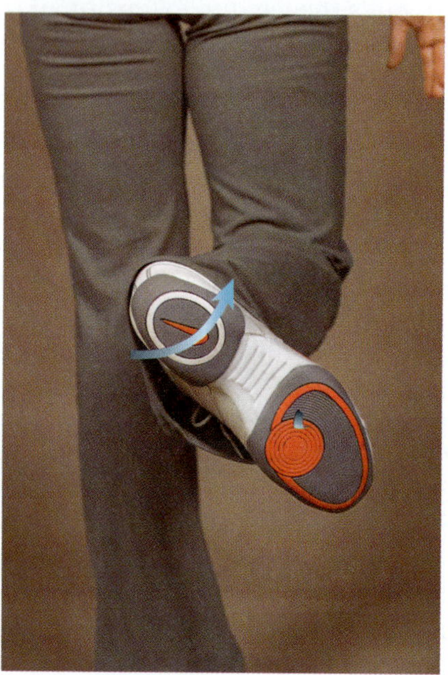
External rotation

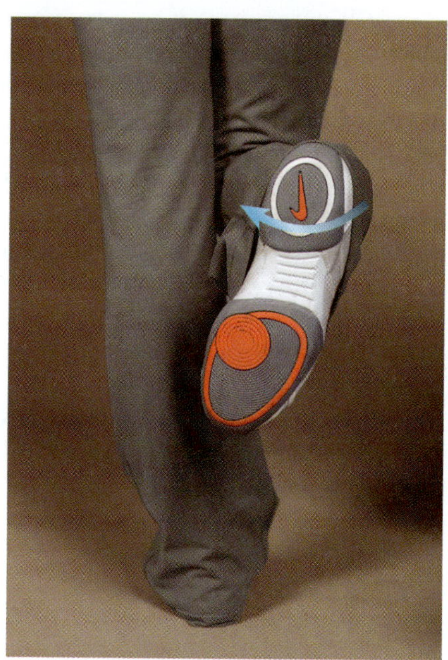
Internal rotation

FIGURE 17.5 Movements of the knee

For example, the sartorius muscle becomes a better flexor at the knee when the pelvis is rotated posteriorly and stabilized by the abdominal muscles, thus increasing its total length by moving its origin farther from its insertion. This is exemplified by trying to flex the knee and cross the legs in the sitting position. One usually leans backward to flex the legs at the knees. Again, this is illustrated by kicking a football. The kicker invariably leans backward to raise and fix the origin of the rectus femoris muscle to make it more effective as a leg and knee extensor. When children hang by the knees, they flex the hips to fix or raise the origin of the hamstrings to make the latter more effective knee flexors.

The sartorius, gracilis, and semitendinosus—the muscles of the anatomical tripod—all join together distally to form a tendinous expansion known as the **pes anserinus,** which attaches to the anteromedial aspect of the proximal tibia below the level of the tibial tuberosity. This attachment and the line of pull these muscles have posteromedially to the knee enable them to assist with knee flexion, particularly once the knee is flexed and the hip is externally rotated. The medial and lateral heads of the gastrocnemius attach posteriorly on the medial and lateral femoral condyles, respectively. This relationship to the knee provides the gastrocnemius a line of pull to assist with knee flexion. (See table 17.1.)

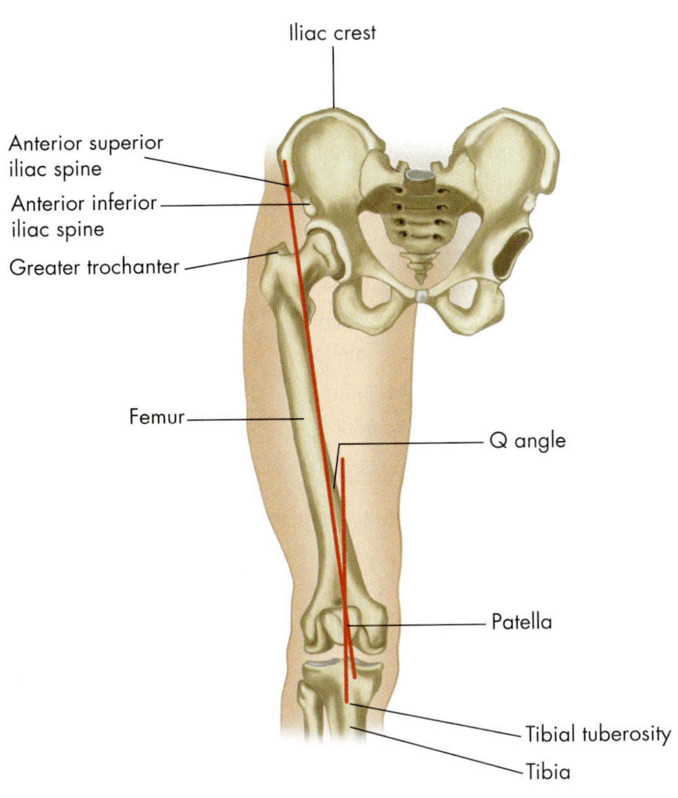

FIGURE 17.6 Q angle

Muscles that move the knee—location

MUSCLE SPECIFIC

Muscle location closely relates to muscle function with the knee.

Anterior—primarily knee extension

Rectus femoris	Vastus intermedius
Vastus medialis	Vastus lateralis

Posterior—primarily knee flexion

Biceps femoris	Sartorius	Gastrocnemius
Semimembranosus	Gracilis	
Semitendinosus	Popliteus	

Nerves

The **femoral nerve** (see figure 15.12 on page 324), innervates the knee extensors—rectus femoris, vastus medialis, vastus intermedius, and vastus lateralis. The knee flexors, consisting of the semitendinosus, semimembranosus, biceps femoris (long head), and popliteus are innervated by the tibial division of the sciatic nerve. The biceps femoris short head is supplied by the peroneal nerve.

TABLE 17.1 Agonist Muscles of the Knee Joint

Name of Muscle	Origins	Insertion	Actions	Innervations
Vastus lateralis	Lateral surface of femur, below greater trochanter and upper half of linea aspera	Lateral border of patella and via patellar tendon to tibial tuberosity	Extension of knee	Femoral nerve (L2–L4)
Vastus intermedius	Upper two-thirds of anterior femoral shaft	Upper border of patella and via patellar tendon to tibial tuberosity	Extension of knee	Femoral nerve (L2–L4)
Vastus medialis	Linea aspera on posterior femur and medial condyloid ridge	Medial half of upper border of patella and via patellar tendon to tibial tuberosity	Extension of knee	Femoral nerve (L2–L4)
Semitendinosus	Ischial tuberosity	Upper anterior medial of tibia just below condyle	Extension of hip, flexion of knee, internal rotation of flexed knee, internal rotation of hip, posterior pelvic rotation	Sciatic nerve—tibial division (L5, S1–S2)
Semimembranosus	Ischial tuberosity	Posterior surface of medial condyle of tibia	Extension of hip, flexion of knee, internal rotation of flexed knee, internal rotation of hip, posterior pelvic rotation	Sciatic nerve—tibial division (L5, S1–S2)

(Continued)

TABLE 17.1 (Continued)

Name of Muscle	Origins	Insertion	Actions	Innervations
Biceps femoris	*Long head:* ischial tuberosity	Lateral condyle of tibia and head of fibula	*Long head:* extension of hip	*Long head:* sciatic nerve—tibial division (S1–S3)
	Short head: lower half of linea aspera, and outer condyloid ridge		*Both heads:* flexion of knee, external rotation of hip and flexed knee, posterior pelvic rotation	*Short head:* sciatic nerve—peroneal division (L5, S1–S2)
Popliteus	Posterior surface of lateral condyle of femur	Upper posteromedial surface of tibia	Flexion of knee, internal rotation of knee as it flexes	Tibial nerve (L5, S1)

Individual Muscles of the Knee Joint—Anterior

QUADRICEPS GROUP: FOUR POWERFUL KNEE EXTENSORS

The ability to jump is essential in nearly all sports. Individuals who have good jumping ability always have strong quadriceps muscles that extend the leg at the knee. The quadriceps (kwod´ri-seps) functions as a decelerator when it is necessary to decrease speed in order to change direction or to prevent falling when landing. This deceleration function is also evident in stopping the body when it is coming down from a jump. The contraction that occurs in the quadriceps during braking or decelerating actions is eccentric. This eccentric action of the quadriceps controls the slowing of movements initiated in previous phases of the sports skill.

The quadriceps muscles are the **rectus femoris** (the only two-joint muscle of the group), **vastus lateralis** (the largest muscle of the group), **vastus intermedius,** and **vastus medialis.** All attach to the patella and by the patellar tendon to the tuberosity of the tibia. All are superficial and palpable, except the vastus intermedius, which is under the rectus femoris. The vertical jump is a simple test that may be used to indicate the strength or power of the quadriceps. This muscle group is generally desired to be 25 to 33 percent stronger than the hamstring muscle group (knee flexors).

Development of strength and flexibility of the quadriceps, or "quads," is essential for maintenance of patellofemoral stability, which is often a problem in many physically active individuals. This problem is further perpetuated due to the quadriceps being particularly prone to atrophy when injuries occur. Muscles should be released through stretching before attempting resistance. This better prepares them to contract and work.

RECTUS FEMORIS MUSCLE

Palpation

Palpate the rectus femoris straight down the anterior thigh from the anterior inferior iliac spine to the patella, with resisted knee extension and hip flexion.

CLINICAL NOTES — **Two-Joint Muscle**

The rectus femoris sits on top of the vastus intermedius and inserts strongly into the patellar tendon. It is not as large as the vastus lateralis or vastus medialis, but it can be well developed as part of the whole quadriceps group. When fatigued, the rectus femoris and the other quadriceps tend to feel weak going down stairs. Because of its two-joint function, the therapist must keep in mind how the muscle is used in its action. Rolling, elliptical movement, compression, and broadening are useful techniques for unwinding the quadriceps. Specifically stretching this muscle at both origin and insertion is extremely beneficial for knee-tracking issues and Osgood-Schlatter dysfunction. See Chapter 18 for techniques and Chapter 21 for exercises for the thigh muscles.

Muscle Specifics

When the hip is flexed, the rectus femoris becomes shorter, and this reduces its effectiveness as an extensor of the knee. The work is then done primarily by the three vasti muscles. Also see the rectus femoris discussion in Chapter 15, page 328.

OIAI MUSCLE CHART RECTUS FEMORIS (rek´tus fem´o-ris) Two-joint muscle

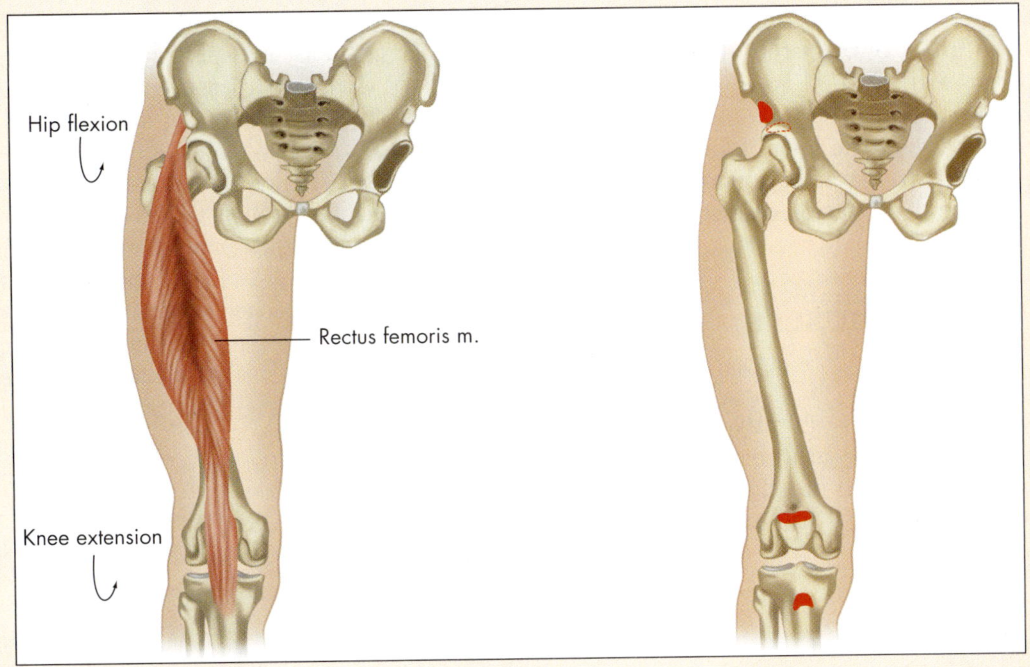

Name of Muscle	Origins	Insertion	Actions	Innervations
Rectus femoris	Anterior inferior iliac spine (AIIS) of ilium and superior margin of acetabulum	Superior aspect of patella and patellar tendon to tibial tuberosity	Flexion of hip, extension of knee, anterior pelvic rotation	Femoral nerve (L2–L4)

Clinical Flexibility

Stretching this powerful muscle is important for everyday activities and sports. Knee-tracking issues, wherein the patella does not track the way it should along the tibia, can lead to many painful conditions. The rectus femoris is a chronically tight muscle in many people. The shortened middle part of its fibers must be lengthened to take forces off the patella and improve knee biomechanics. Releasing this muscle also helps stabilize the pelvis in a more neutral position. From a side-lying position, tuck the bottom leg up into flexion, and hold it to your chest (or as high as possible). Grasp the ankle of the top leg, and beginning from a flexed-hip position, contract the gluteals to move the hip back into hyperextension. The abdominals are contracted. Gently pull on the ankle for a gentle 2-second stretch, and repeat. Be certain the hip stays down and in line with the shoulders; do not abduct the thigh during the movement. *Contraindications:* The psoas muscle should be released (lengthened) before attempting this stretch. The abdominals help prevent strain to the low back during this movement. Knee arthroplasty patients should use caution when performing this stretch.

Strengthening

The rectus femoris should be strengthened as a hip flexor and knee extender. Overall, the quadriceps may be developed by resisted knee extension activities from a seated position. Seated positions take the place of exercises such as lunges, which many people cannot perform due to arthritic or painful knees. It is safer, especially for those with current or past injuries, to keep the pelvis fixed while extending the knees with the quadriceps.

To strengthen as a hip flexor, start supine, with the uninvolved leg bent. Using ankle weights, lift the extended leg up into flexion, and lower slowly to the start position. Keep the foot dorsiflexed throughout the movement. Although the psoas is brought into action in this exercise, the proximal end of the rectus femoris helps flex the weighted hip. To strengthen knee extension, sit on a bench or therapy table with a pillow under the knees. This elevates the knees slightly above the hip. Contract the abdominals and lean the torso forward. Hold this position throughout. Dorsiflex the foot and slowly extend the leg; hold 3 to 4 seconds, and lower the weighted ankle slowly. *Contraindications:* During knee extension, there may be tenderness if knee dysfunction exists. If so, do not completely extend the knee.

VASTUS LATERALIS MUSCLE

Palpation

Palpate the vastus lateralis slightly distal to the greater trochanter down the anterolateral aspect of the thigh to the superolateral patella, with extension of the knee, particularly with full extension against resistance.

CLINICAL NOTES **Connection to Iliotibial Tract**

The largest muscle of the quadriceps group is the vastus lateralis. Connective tissue from the vastus lateralis binds the iliotibial tract enough to make it necessary to release the lateralis fibers when there is a contracted IT band. The vastus lateralis braces the lateral side of the knee, as does the iliotibial tract. A tight vastus lateralis can pull on the lateral side of the patella and make it difficult for the patella to track appropriately. Strengthening the vastus medialis muscle can help balance the pull of an overcompensating vastus lateralis. The vastus lateralis should be stretched along with the tensor fasciae latae and iliotibial tract. See Chapter 18 for techniques to release quadriceps muscles and Chapter 21 for exercises.

OIAI MUSCLE CHART VASTUS LATERALIS (vas´tus lat-er-a´lis) Lateral quadriceps

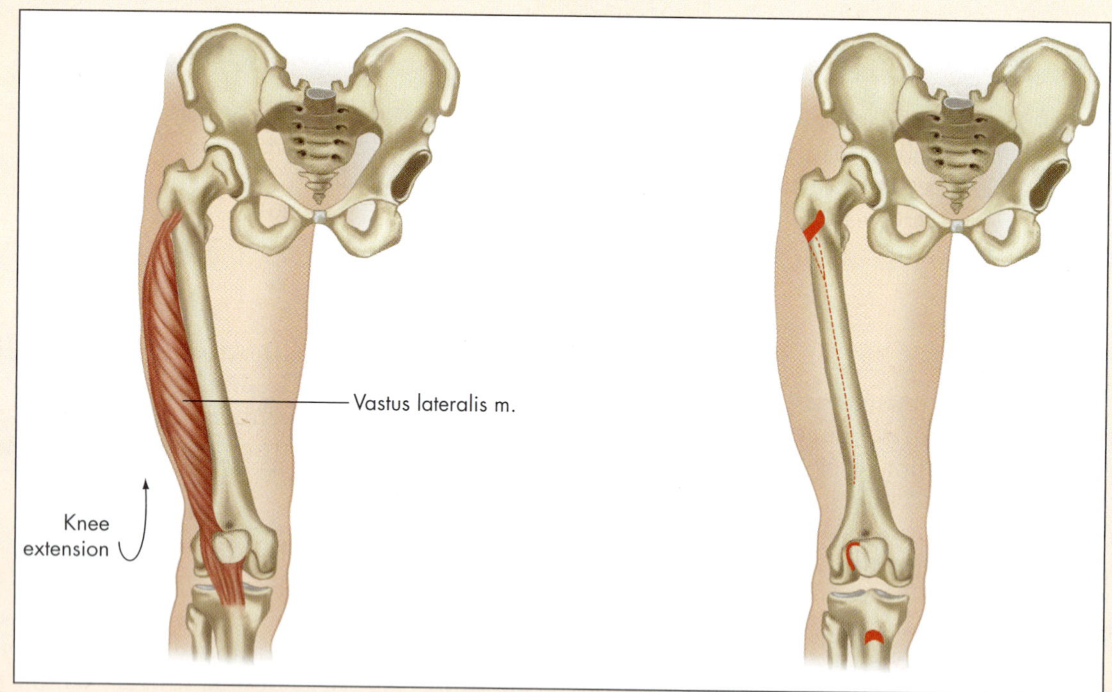

Name of Muscle	Origins	Insertion	Actions	Innervations
Vastus lateralis	Lateral surface of femur, below greater trochanter and upper half of linea aspera	Lateral border of patella and via patellar tendon to tibial tuberosity	Extension of knee	Femoral nerve (L2–L4)

Muscle Specifics

All three of the vasti muscles function with the rectus femoris in knee extension. They are typically used in walking and running and must be used to keep the knees straight, as in standing. The vastus lateralis has a slightly superolateral pull on the patella and, as a result, is occasionally blamed in part for common lateral patellar subluxation and dislocation problems.

Clinical Flexibility

Releasing the vastus lateralis muscle can help with lateral tracking issues of the patella. Stretch this muscle the same way as stretching the rectus femoris.

Strengthening

The vastus lateralis often pulls the patella laterally, especially in cyclists. The vastus lateralis is strengthened through knee extension activities against resistance.

VASTUS INTERMEDIUS MUSCLE

Palpation

Palpate the vastus intermedius on the anteromedial distal one-third of the thigh just above the superomedial patella and deep to the rectus femoris, with extension of the knee, particularly with full extension against resistance.

CLINICAL NOTES **Invisible Quadriceps**

The vastus intermedius develops problems only after the rectus femoris does. Buried under the rectus femoris, it is difficult to treat as it is virtually inaccessible. However, the techniques for the quadriceps will help unwrap any problems of the vastus intermedius. It is stretched along with the other quadriceps. See Chapters 18 to 21 for quadriceps techniques.

OIAI MUSCLE CHART VASTUS INTERMEDIUS (vas´tus in´ter-me´di-us) Hidden quadriceps

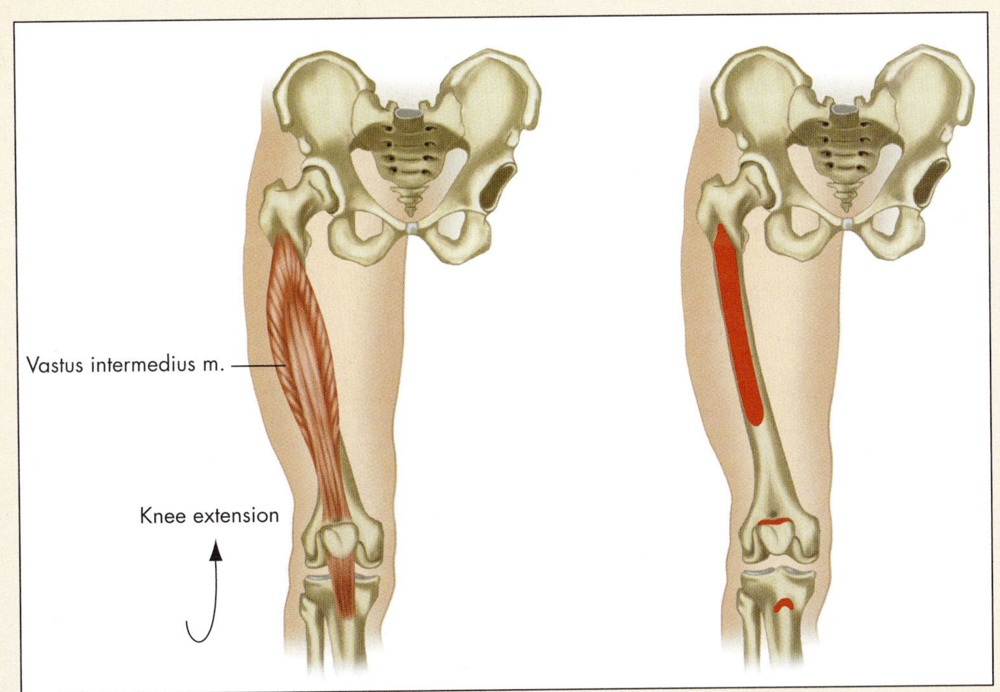

Name of Muscle	Origins	Insertion	Actions	Innervations
Vastus intermedius	Upper two-thirds of anterior femoral shaft	Upper border of patella and via patellar tendon to tibial tuberosity	Extension of knee	Femoral nerve (L2–L4)

Muscle Specifics

The three vasti muscles all contract in knee extension. They are used together with the rectus femoris in running, jumping, hopping, skipping, and walking. The vasti muscles are primarily responsible for extending the knee while the hip is flexed or being flexed. Thus, in doing a knee bend with the trunk bent forward at the hip, the vasti are exercised with little involvement of the rectus femoris. The natural activities mentioned here develop the quadriceps.

Clinical Flexibility

The quadriceps stretches apply for this muscle.

Strengthening

The knee extension exercises for the vastus lateralis apply here.

VASTUS MEDIALIS MUSCLE

Palpation

Palpate the vastus medialis on the anteromedial side of the thigh just above the superomedial patella, with extension of the knee, and particularly with full extension against resistance.

CLINICAL NOTES **Chondromalacia**

The vastus medialis is an important muscle to consider in helping alleviate patellar tracking issues. **Chondromalacia,** or wear and tear of the cartilage on the underside of the patella, is often caused by the lateral movement of the patella, which may not "track" smoothly in the patellar groove as it moves. The vastus

OIAI MUSCLE CHART VASTUS MEDIALIS (vas´tus me-di-a´lis) Medial quadriceps

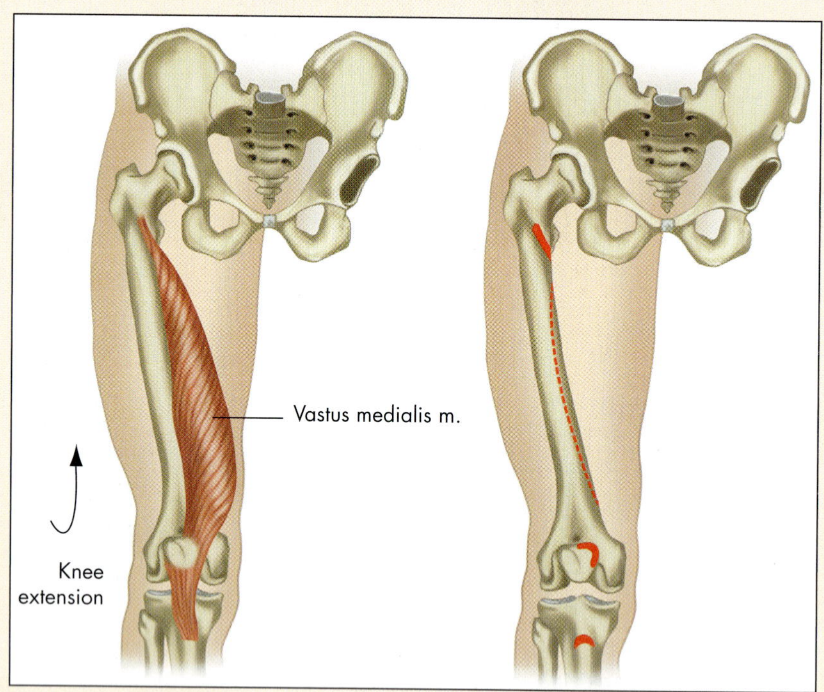

Name of Muscle	Origins	Insertion	Actions	Innervations
Vastus medialis	Linea aspera on posterior femur and medial condyloid ridge	Medial half of upper border of patella and via patellar tendon to tibial tuberosity	Extension of knee	Femoral nerve (L2–L4)

lateralis and the iliotibial tract work together to laterally pull the patella, causing friction to the joint. The iliotibial tract can develop tendonitis at its attachment as well. Stretching the quadriceps and IT band, as well as the tensor fasciae latae, can help balance this pull of the quadriceps, but vastus medialis should also be isolated in resistance exercises to better strengthen its pull. See the exercises in this chapter and in Chapter 21.

Muscle Specifics

The vastus medialis is very important in maintaining patellofemoral stability because of the oblique attachment of its distal fibers to the superior medial patella. This portion of the vastus medialis is referred to as the *vastus medialis obliquus (VMO)*.

Clinical Flexibility

Full knee flexion for the rectus femoris stretches all the quadriceps muscles.

Strengthening

The vastus medialis is strengthened by knee extensions, but the VMO is not really emphasized until the last 10 to 20 degrees of knee extension. To help isolate the medialis and correct lateral tracking of the patella, rotate the tibia internally during extension with resistance. The foot is dorsiflexed throughout the movement.

Individual Muscles of the Knee Joint—Posterior

HAMSTRING MUSCLES

The hamstrings are primarily knee flexors in addition to serving as hip extensors. Knee rotation can occur when the knee is in a flexed position. Knee rotation is brought about by the hamstring muscles (figure 17.7). The biceps femoris externally rotates the lower leg at the knee. The semitendinosus and semimembranosus perform internal rotation. Knee rotation permits pivoting movements and change in body direction. This rotation of the knee is vital in accommodating to forces developing at the hip or ankle during directional changes in order to make the total movement more functional as well as more fluid in appearance.

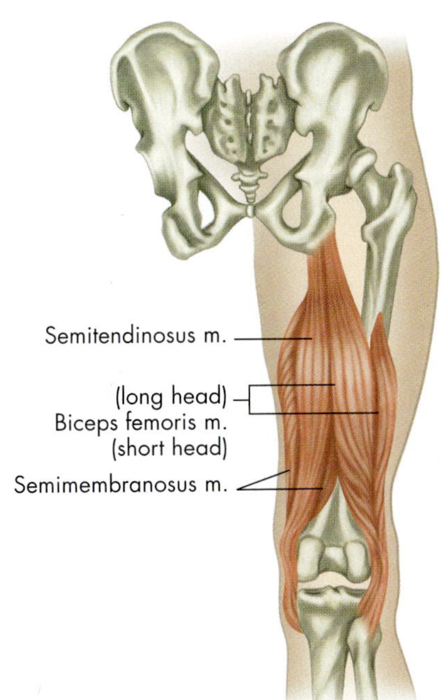

FIGURE 17.7 Hamstring muscles

SEMITENDINOSUS MUSCLE

Palpation

Palpate the semitendinosus on the posteromedial aspect of the distal thigh with combined knee flexion and internal rotation against resistance and just distal to the ischial tuberosity, in a prone position, with the hip internally rotated during active knee flexion.

CLINICAL NOTES **Anatomical Tripod**

The third guy wire from the hip that connects to the pes anserinus is the semitendinosus. Together, the semitendinosus, sartorius, and gracilis form an anatomical tripod that supports the structure and function of the medial knee. Therapists must keep these muscles and attachments in mind as they treat the thigh and knee region. Should any of these muscles be contracted, the pes anserinus area may cause painful knee problems and gait issues. See Chapter 18 for techniques for the hamstrings and Chapter 21 for exercises.

Muscle Specifics

This two-joint muscle is most effective when contracting to either extend the hip or flex the knee. When there is extension of the hip and flexion of the knee at the same time, both movements are weak. When the trunk is flexed forward with the knees straight, the hamstring muscles have a powerful pull on the rear pelvis and tilt it down in back by full contraction. If the knees are flexed when this movement takes place, one can observe that the work is done chiefly by the gluteus maximus muscle.

OIAI MUSCLE CHART SEMITENDINOSUS (sem´i-ten-di-no´sus) Long tendon

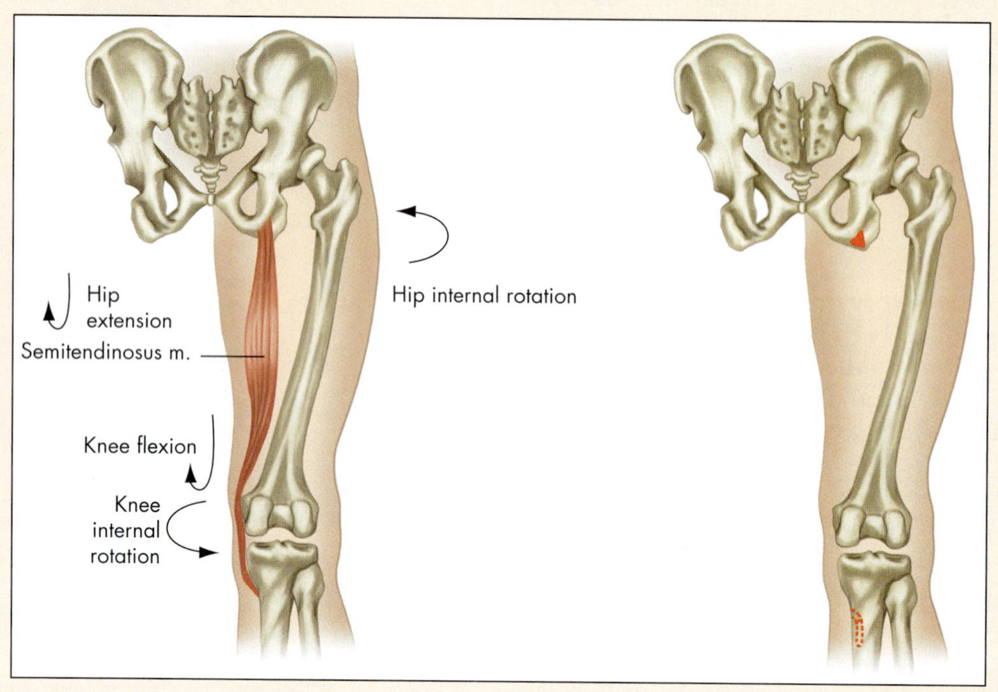

Name of Muscle	Origins	Insertion	Actions	Innervations
Semitendinosus	Ischial tuberosity	Upper anterior medial of tibia just below condyle	Extension of hip, flexion of knee, internal rotation of flexed knee, internal rotation of hip, posterior pelvic rotation	Sciatic nerve—tibial division (L5, S1–S2)

In contrast, when the muscles are used in powerful flexion of the knees, as in hanging by the knees from a bar, the hip flexors come into play to raise the origin of these muscles and make them more effective as knee flexors. Through full extension of the hips in this movement, the knee flexion movement is weakened. These muscles are used in ordinary walking as extensors of the hip and allow the gluteus maximus to relax in the movement.

Clinical Flexibility

Since the hamstring muscles act on the hip and knee, stretching should be performed for both areas. To stretch the semitendinosus as it crosses the knee, lie supine with a rope wrapped around the foot. Bend the involved leg to 90 degrees. Extend the knee, and use the rope for a gentle 2-second stretch that should be felt behind the knee. Keep the other hand planted on the anterior thigh to prevent the femur from moving forward. To stretch the semitendinosus at the hip, begin the same way, except extend the involved leg. Keep the knee extended throughout the movement. Lift with the psoas and rectus femoris into hip flexion, walking up the rope with both hands. Stretch 2 seconds at the end movement, feeling for a stretch at the ischial tuberosity. To further isolate this muscle, try wrapping the rope on the inside of the leg, effectively rotating the femur internally as you stretch. See Chapter 21 for photographs showing this stretch. *Contraindications:* Make certain that the uninvolved leg stays flexed to help protect the lower back. Use caution if disk herniations are present.

Strengthening

The semitendinosus is best developed through knee flexion exercises against resistance. Commonly known as *hamstring curls* or *leg curls,* they may be performed in a prone position on a knee flexion machine or in a standing position with ankle weights attached. This muscle is emphasized when a person is performing hamstring curls while attempting to maintain the knee joint in internal rotation. This internally rotated position brings its insertion into alignment with its origin. The hamstrings are typically weak at the hip insertion, as resistance exercises for this area are not normally part of a fitness program. To strengthen the proximal hip attachment, use ankle weights. Stand with the anterior pelvis against a table. Turn the involved leg internally, and keep it rotated throughout. Extend the knee and hyperextend the thigh, lifting without abducting. Hold at the top, and slowly lower. See Chapter 21 for photographs of this exercise. *Contraindications:* This is beneficial for low-back pain, but use caution if lumbar dysfunction exists.

SEMIMEMBRANOSUS MUSCLE

Palpation

Largely covered by other muscles, the tendon of the semimembranosus can be felt at the posteromedial aspect of the knee just deep to the semitendinosus tendon with combined knee flexion and internal rotation against resistance.

OIAI MUSCLE CHART SEMIMEMBRANOSUS (sem´i-mem´bra-no´sus) Meniscus protector

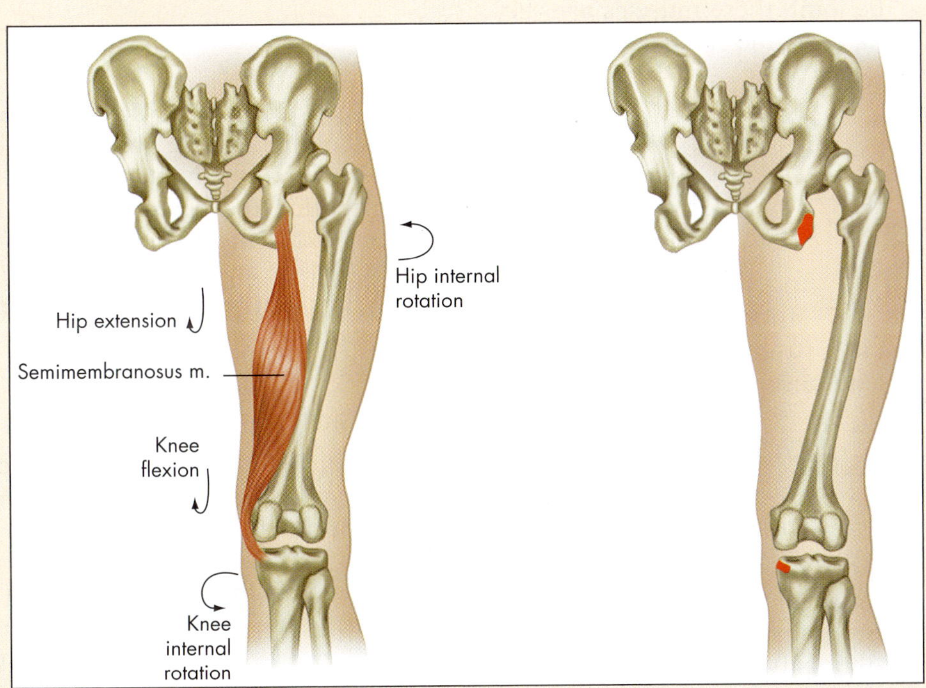

Name of Muscle	Origins	Insertion	Actions	Innervations
Semimembranosus	Ischial tuberosity	Posterior surface of medial condyle of tibia	Extension of hip, flexion of knee, internal rotation of flexed knee, internal rotation of hip, posterior pelvic rotation	Sciatic nerve—tibial division (L5, S1–S2)

CLINICAL NOTES **Semimembranosus: Meniscus Protector**

The semimembranosus can be injured along with the adductor longus or magnus because of its medial insertion on the ischial tuberosity. While this muscle helps to medially rotate the knee, it also serves another supportive function. Its insertion on the posterior surface of the medial condyle of the tibia has a tendinous branch that supports the medial meniscus during knee flexion. In some people, this branch may also support and pull on the lateral meniscus as well. The semimembranosus should be stretched and strengthened at the knee as well as at the hip. See Chapter 18 for techniques and Chapter 21 for exercises.

Muscle Specifics

Both the semitendinosus and the semimembranosus, along with the popliteus muscle, are responsible for internal rotation of the knee. Because of the manner in which they cross the joint, these muscles are very important in providing dynamic medial stability to the knee joint.

Clinical Flexibility

The semimembranosus is stretched in the same manner as the semitendinosus is.

Strengthening

The semimembranosus is strengthened in the manner used for the semitendinosus.

BICEPS FEMORIS MUSCLE

Palpation

Palpate the biceps femoris on the posterolateral aspect of the distal thigh with combined knee flexion and external rotation against resistance and just distal to the ischial tuberosity, in a prone position, with the hip internally rotated during active knee flexion.

CLINICAL NOTES **Possible Sciatic Nerve Entrapper**

The sciatic nerve passes between the adductor magnus and the biceps femoris in the posterior thigh musculature. Runners sometimes experience referred pain from contracted muscles entrapping the sciatic nerve. Releasing the thigh muscles can help relieve painful conditions such as sciatica and low-back pain. The tendon of origin of the long head of the biceps femoris is directly continuous with the fibers of the sacrotuberous ligament, so releasing the thigh muscles helps stabilize the sacrum as well. See Chapter 18 for techniques to release the hamstrings and Chapter 21 for exercises.

Muscle Specifics

The semitendinosus, semimembranosus, and biceps femoris muscles are known as the *hamstrings*. These muscles, together with the gluteus maximus muscle, are used in extension of the hip when the knees are straight or nearly so. Thus, these muscles are used together in running, jumping, skipping, and hopping. The gluteus maximus is used without the aid of the hamstrings when the knees are flexed while the hips are being extended. This occurs when rising from a seated to a standing position.

Clinical Flexibility

The biceps femoris is stretched in the manner described earlier for the hamstrings, except that the leg is externally rotated. Lift the leg to the opposite shoulder, isolating the biceps femoris on the lateral hip. *Contraindications:* Use caution if lumbar dysfunction exists. This is an extremely beneficial stretch for sciatic issues, but tenderness may be present during the movement.

Strengthening

The biceps femoris is best developed through hamstring curls, as described for the semitendinosus, but it is emphasized more if the knee is maintained in external rotation throughout the range of motion, thus bringing the origin and insertion more in line with each other. The hip portion can be strengthened using the exercise used for the other hamstrings, except that the thigh is held in the externally rotated position.

POPLITEUS MUSCLE

Palpation

With the client sitting and the knee flexed 90 degrees, palpate the popliteus deep to the gastrocnemius medially on the posterior proximal tibia; proceed superolaterally toward the lateral epicondyle of the tibia, just deep to the fibular collateral ligament, while the client internally rotates the knee.

OIAI MUSCLE CHART BICEPS FEMORIS (bi´seps fem´or-is) Two-headed hamstring

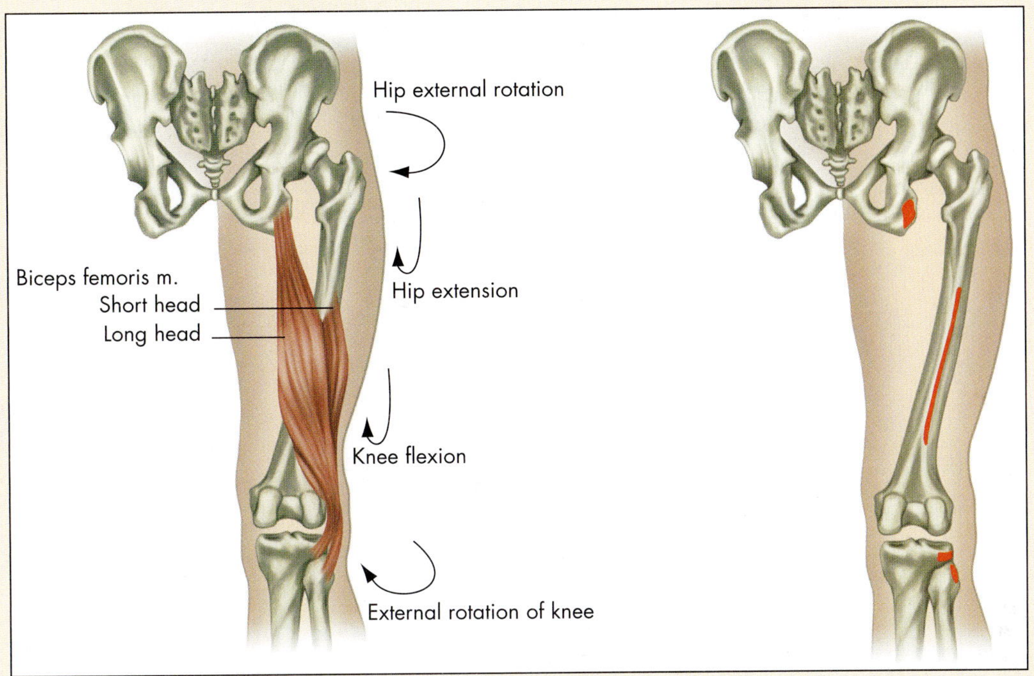

Name of Muscle	Origins	Insertion	Actions	Innervations
Biceps femoris	*Long head:* ischial tuberosity *Short head:* lower half of linea aspera, and outer condyloid ridge	Lateral condyle of tibia and head of fibula	*Long head:* extension of hip *Both heads:* flexion of knee, external rotation of hip and flexed knee, posterior pelvic rotation	*Long head:* sciatic nerve—tibial division (S1–S3) *Short head:* sciatic nerve—peroneal division (L5, S1–S2)

CLINICAL NOTES **Unlocks the Knee**

The popliteus attaches to the lateral meniscus in the knee; it shifts the meniscus posteriorly during knee flexion to prevent pinching the meniscus between the tibia and the femur. The popliteus assists in flexing the leg; when the leg is flexed, it will rotate the tibia inward. It is used at the start of knee flexion, as it produces slight internal rotation of the tibia in the first stages of flexion. The posterior compartment of the knee often needs increased circulation because of its pocketed shape; scar tissue often forms in this area after arthroscopy procedures.

Muscle Specifics

The popliteus muscle is the only true flexor of the leg at the knee. All other flexors are two-joint muscles. The popliteus is vital in providing posterolateral stability to the knee. It assists the medial hamstrings in internal rotation of the lower leg at the knee, and it is crucial in internally rotating the knee to unlock it from the full extension position.

Clinical Flexibility

Stretching the popliteus is accomplished using the bent-knee hamstring stretch described earlier.

Strengthening

This muscle is strengthened using the bent-knee hamstring exercises with ankle weights.

OIAI MUSCLE CHART POPLITEUS (pop´li-te´us) Knee unlocker

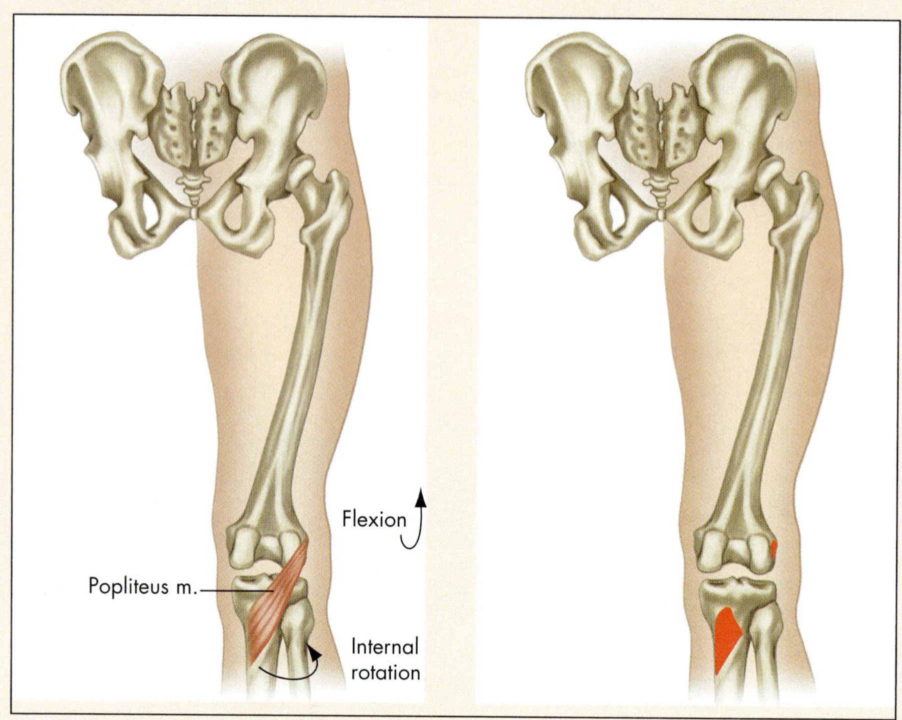

Name of Muscle	Origins	Insertion	Actions	Innervations
Popliteus	Posterior surface of lateral condyle of femur	Upper posteromedial surface of tibia	Flexion of knee, internal rotation of knee as it flexes	Tibial nerve (L5, S1)

CHAPTER *summary*

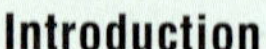

Introduction

- Similar in many respects to the elbow joint in the upper extremity, the knee joint is the largest, most complex joint in the body. It serves to divide the hip and foot by providing the mechanism of movement and attachments for powerful knee extensor and flexor muscles. These muscles give the body the ability to utilize the mobile hip joints to their maximum capacities in skiing, jumping, and dancing.

Bones

- The bones of the knee joint include the femur, patella, tibia, and fibula.
- The medial and lateral condyles of the femur are attachment sites for muscles.
- The tibial tuberosity is the attachment site for the quadriceps.
- The medial condyle area of the tibia is an attachment site for many muscles.
- The head of the fibula and Gerdy's tubercle on the tibia are attachment sites for muscles and the iliotibial tract.

Joints

- The tibiofemoral joint is classified as a ginglymus joint because it functions as a hinge.
- The patellofemoral joint is classified as an arthrodial joint.
- The superior tibiofibular joint is held together by ligaments.

- The menisci are cartilages that cushion the knee joint; they are the medial and lateral meniscus, respectively.
- Strong ligaments called collateral ligaments attach the fibula to the femur and the tibia to the femur.
- Many ligaments inside the knee joint add stability to the knee.
- There are many bursae in the knee joint; the prepatellar bursa is most frequently inflamed.
- The anterior cruciate ligament (ACL) and posterior cruciate ligament (PCL) cross within the knee joint.
- Medial and lateral collateral ligaments maintain stability on both sides of the knee joint.

Movements

- The movements of the knee joint permit flexion, extension, and internal and external rotation.
- The ball-and-socket hip joint allows better positioning of the knee regardless of the limited movement ability of the knee joint.

Muscles

- The quadriceps are located anteriorly and extend the knee.
- Knee flexors include the sartorius, gracilis, hamstrings, popliteus, and gastrocnemius.
- The sartorius, gracilis, and semitendinosus share a tendinous expansion known as the pes anserinus at the anteromedial aspect of the proximal tibia below the level of the tibial tuberosity.
- The biceps femoris accomplishes minimal external rotation of the knee joint.
- The semitendinosus, semimembranosus, and popliteus work together to do internal rotation of the knee joint.

Nerves

- The femoral nerve innervates the knee extensors.
- The sciatic nerve's tibial division innervates the popliteus and the hamstrings, except the biceps femoris short head, which is innervated by the peroneal nerve.

Individual Muscles of the Knee Joint—Anterior

- *Rectus femoris* is named for its fibers and location. It flexes the hip and extends the knee. It is the only member of the quadriceps that has action on the hip. The quadriceps has a common attachment at the tibial tuberosity.
- *Vastus lateralis* is the largest of the quadriceps; it is located laterally and posteriorly around the femur and extends the knee.
- *Vastus intermedius* is located beneath the rectus femoris on the anterior femur and assists in extending the knee.
- *Vastus medialis* is located medially and posteriorly and extends the knee.
- *Sartorius* flexes the knee because it externally rotates and flexes the hip. It is covered in Chapter 15.
- *Gracilis* is a primary adductor but also flexes the knee. It is covered in Chapter 15.

Individual Muscles of the Knee Joint—Posterior

- *Semitendinosus,* a hamstring muscle, originates on the ischial tuberosity and attaches to the inside of the tibia. It flexes and internally rotates the knee. (The hamstrings consist of the semitendinosus, semimembranosus, and biceps femoris.)
- *Semimembranosus,* a hamstring muscle, originates on the ischial tuberosity and inserts on the medial tibia. It flexes and internally rotates the knee.
- *Biceps femoris,* a hamstring muscle, has two heads; the long head originates at the ischial tuberosity, and the short head begins on the linea aspera. The heads come together and split on the tibia and fibula. Together they flex the knee and externally rotate it.
- *Popliteus* is a triangular-shaped muscle that spans from the lateral posterior femur to the medial posterior tibia. It flexes the knee and internally rotates the knee as it flexes.
- *Gastrocnemius* is one of the most superficial calf muscles. It can flex the knee or plantar flex the foot but not at the same time. It is covered in Chapter 19.

CHAPTER *review*

Worksheet Exercises

As an aid to learning, for in-class or out-of-class assignments, or for testing, tear-out worksheets are found at the end of the text, on pages 543–546.

True or False

Write true *or* false *after each statement.*

1. The vastus lateralis is the quadriceps that flexes the hip and extends the knee.
2. The hamstrings all insert on Gerdy's tubercle.
3. The hamstrings all flex the knee.
4. The vastus medialis originates on the whole length of the linea aspera and the medial condyloid ridge.
5. The knee joint is a true ball-and-socket joint.
6. The ligament of Wrisberg is a ligament in the back of the knee.
7. The tibial division of the sciatic nerve innervates the quadriceps.

8. The ischial tuberosity is the origin for the rectus femoris.
9. The popliteus originates on the posterior surface of the lateral condyle of the femur.
10. The short head of the biceps femoris originates on the adductor tubercle.
11. The hamstrings are twice as strong as the quadriceps.

Short Answers

Write your answers on the lines provided.

1. What bones articulate at the knee joint?

2. The knee joint is what type of joint?

3. What are the structures inside the knee joint that cushion shock? What are their names?

4. Name the ligaments on the medial and lateral side of the knee joints.

5. What is the bursa on the front of the patella called?

6. Name the muscles that extend the knee.

7. List the muscles that flex the knee.

8. What is the structure that attaches to Gerdy's tubercle?

9. Name the nerve that innervates the quadriceps.

10. List the muscles that internally rotate the knee.

Multiple Choice

Circle the correct answers.

1. The quadriceps consists of:
   a. rectus femoris, vastus lateralis, vastus medialis, and vastus intermedius
   b. biceps femoris, vastus lateralis, vastus medialis, and vastus intermedius
   c. rectus femoris, biceps femoris, vastus lateralis, and vastus intermedius
   d. none of the above
2. The pes anserinus area has which three muscles attached to it?
   a. gracilis, vastus lateralis, and sartorius
   b. sartorius, gracilis, and semimembranosus
   c. sartorius, gracilis, and semitendinosus
   d. none of the above
3. The hamstrings consist of:
   a. semitendinosus, biceps femoris, and gracilis
   b. sartorius, gracilis, and semimembranosus
   c. biceps femoris, semitendinosus, and semimembranosus
   d. none of the above

4. The primary knee flexors are:
   a. hamstrings, sartorius, gracilis, popliteus, and gastrocnemius
   b. hamstrings, quadriceps, gracilis, popliteus, and gastrocnemius
   c. biceps femoris, quadriceps, gracilis, popliteus, and gastrocnemius
   d. none of the above
5. The vastus intermedius originates on:
   a. the posterior surface of the femur
   b. the anterior surface of the femur
   c. Gerdy's tubercle
   d. none of the above
6. The two ligaments that cross inside the joint are:
   a. ligament of Wrisberg and the medial meniscus
   b. anterior and posterior cruciate ligaments
   c. medial and lateral collateral ligaments
   d. none of the above
7. The joint between the fibula and the tibia is called:
   a. Gerdy's tubercle
   b. superior tibiofibular joint
   c. tibiofemoral joint
   d. hip joint
8. The flat area on the superior tibia that has cartilage on it is often called:
   a. the tibial plateau
   b. the landing
   c. the tibial tuberosity
   d. none of the above
9. The bony landmark on the posterior femur that runs the length of the bone and is an attachment site for some quadriceps and hamstrings is called the:
   a. medial and lateral condyles
   b. linea aspera
   c. adductor tubercle
   d. ischial tuberosity
10. The Q angle is the angle between the line from:
    a. the anterior superior iliac spine to the central patella and the line from the central patella to the tibial tuberosity
    b. the anterior superior iliac spine to the ischial tuberosity and the line from the central patella to the tibial tuberosity
    c. the anterior inferior iliac spine to the central patella and the line from the central patella to the tibial tuberosity
    d. none of the above

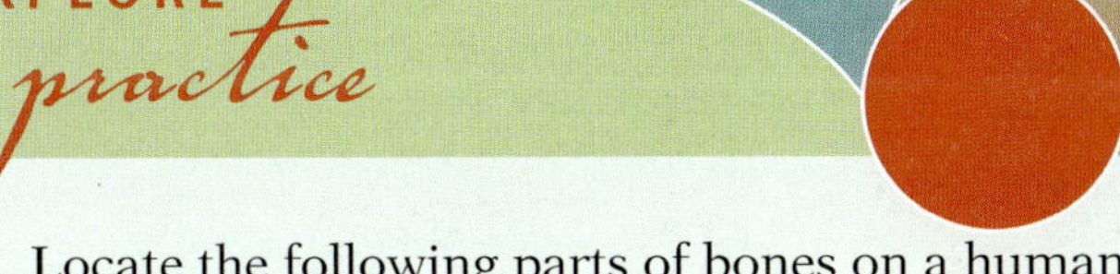

1. Locate the following parts of bones on a human skeleton and on a partner.

   a. Skeleton:
   1. Head and neck of femur
   2. Greater trochanter
   3. Shaft of femur
   4. Lesser trochanter
   5. Linea aspera
   6. Adductor tubercle
   7. Medial femoral condyle
   8. Lateral femoral condyle
   9. Patella
   10. Fibula head
   11. Medial tibial condyle
   12. Lateral tibial condyle
   13. Tibial tuberosity
   14. Gerdy's tubercle

   b. Partner:
   1. Greater trochanter
   2. Adductor tubercle
   3. Medial femoral condyle
   4. Lateral femoral condyle
   5. Patella
   6. Fibula head
   7. Medial tibial condyle
   8. Lateral tibial condyle
   9. Tibial tuberosity
   10. Gerdy's tubercle

2. How and where can the following muscles be palpated on a human? (*Note:* Palpate the previously studied hip joint muscles while they are performing actions at the knee.)
   a. Gracilis
   b. Sartorius
   c. Biceps femoris
   d. Semitendinosus
   e. Semimembranosus
   f. Rectus femoris
   g. Vastus lateralis
   h. Vastus intermedius
   i. Vastus medialis
   j. Popliteus

3. Be prepared to indicate on a human skeleton, by using a long rubber band, the origin and insertion of the muscles just listed.
4. Demonstrate the following movements, and list the muscles primarily responsible for each:
   a. Extension of the leg at the knee
   b. Flexion of the leg at the knee
   c. Internal rotation of the leg at the knee
   d. External rotation of the leg at the knee
5. With a laboratory partner, determine how and why maintaining the position of full knee extension limits the ability to maximally flex the hip both actively and passively. Does maintaining excessive hip flexion limit your ability to accomplish full knee extension?
6. With a laboratory partner, determine how and why maintaining the position of full knee flexion limits the ability to maximally extend the hip both actively and passively. Does maintaining excessive hip extension limit your ability to accomplish full knee flexion?
7. Compare and contrast the bony, ligamentous, articular, and cartilaginous aspects of the medial knee joint to those of the lateral knee joint.
8. Research preventive and rehabilitative exercises to strengthen the knee joint, and report your findings in class.
9. Which muscle group at the knee would be most important to develop for an athlete with a torn anterior cruciate ligament, and why? A torn posterior cruciate ligament? Why?
10. *Muscle analysis chart:* Fill in the chart below by listing the muscles primarily involved in each joint movement.

Flexion	Extension
Internal rotation	External rotation

11. *Antagonistic muscle action chart:* Fill in the chart below by listing the muscle(s) or parts of muscles that are antagonistic in their actions to the muscles in the left column.

Agonist	Antagonist
Biceps femoris	
Semitendinosus	
Semimembranosus	
Popliteus	
Rectus femoris	
Vastus lateralis	
Vastus intermedius	
Vastus medialis	

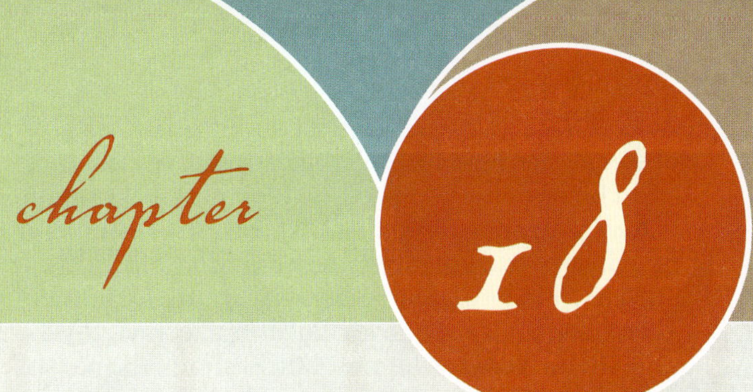

Dimensional Massage Techniques for the Muscles of the Thigh and Knee Joint

LEARNING OUTCOMES

After completing this chapter, you should be able to:

- **18-1** Define key terms.
- **18-2** Locate on a human skeleton bony structures of the hip and knee joints.
- **18-3** Palpate bony landmarks of the hip joint and knee joint on a partner.
- **18-4** Explore the origins and insertions of the muscles of the knee joint on a partner.
- **18-5** Review general pathologies and conditions of the muscles and soft-tissue structures of the knee joint.
- **18-6** Discuss a treatment protocol for working on muscles of the thigh for the hip and knee joints.
- **18-7** Demonstrate safe body mechanics.
- **18-8** Practice specific techniques on the knee joint muscles.
- **18-9** Incorporate dimensional massage therapy techniques in a regular routine or use them when needed.
- **18-10** Determine safe treatment protocols and refer the client to other health professionals when necessary.

KEY TERMS

Contracted iliotibial tract
Genu valgum
Genu varum
Hematoma
Knee replacement
Meralgia paresthetica
Ober's test
Osgood-Schlatter disease
Patellar tracking
Prosthesis

Introduction

With appropriate training and practice, the thigh muscles have the ability to provide the strength and power to complete amazing athletic accomplishments. The size of the thigh should be directly related to the amount of power and strength needed for a particular sport. For example, sprinters and hurdlers have massive thigh muscles, whereas marathon runners, who need to maintain endurance, require less mass to go the distance. The strength of the thigh muscles provides a supportive structure for the pelvic girdle, hip, and knee joint. Strong, flexible thigh muscles help guide the knees to the positions that the hip joint allows. Like guy wires, the muscles connect from the pelvic girdle to both sides of the knee to provide a line of pull and supportive mechanism for movement. The thigh carries the largest bone in the body and has the longest muscles. The knee joint, the largest joint in the body, provides attachments for the massive thigh muscles, mobility, and structural components that try to ward off wear and tear, injury, and disease throughout one's life.

Massage therapy for the muscles of the thigh and knee joint can help facilitate rehabilitation from injury or surgery, prevent atrophy, relieve back pain, provide relaxation, or be included as part of a sports training or event program for athletes, dancers, and others. A conservative team effort might also include stretching and flexibility exercises, physical therapy for rehabilitation, acupuncture, and chiropractic for back involvement. While this is by no means a complete list, it is an example of modalities working together for common goals. Surgery, a more dramatic therapy, might be necessary for injury repair or knee replacement. Massage therapy and other modalities should be part of the rehabilitation process.

Structural Perspectives of the Knee Joint

The pelvic girdle supports the femur and supplies a base for the muscles of the thigh. The thigh is the first part of the lower extremity and needs to be in the best shape for power and support. Many people do not have a perfect stance and gait. When the thigh muscles are not able to support the knee joint or when the body has too much weight or an individual walks with hips in externally or internally rotated positions, the trunk and pelvic girdle muscles might shorten, eventually leading to lower-leg length deformities and abnormal gait patterns. Foot problems and/or structure may affect the position of the feet as they strike the ground. The mechanism of walking spirals up the kinetic chain, thereby affecting the position of the knees and hips as the body moves. Several other structural problems might occur.

Genu valgum, or knock-knees, is a walking pattern marked by a lateral angulation of the leg in relation to the thigh. The thigh responds by medially rotating, thus putting strain on the hip muscles and torque on the medial knee and resulting in probable patellar-tracking issues and an apparent corrective foot pattern. This can be a congenital condition, but the cause is not always known. **Genu varum,** or bowlegs, is a walking pattern marked by a medial angulation of the leg in relation to the thigh. This variation puts strain on the lateral side of the knee and often presents with walking on the lateral side of the foot. It is important to determine the cause of the above knee positions and gait issues. Podiatrists, exercise physiologists, and experts in gait and foot problems are best at diagnosing walking patterns and thigh-leg relationships.

Patellar tracking is often the result of unusual gait problems that prevent the patella from riding normally over the knee in a superior and inferior direction during extension and flexion, respectively. When the knee is torqued in a more medial or lateral position, it may lead to proper, normal tracking of the patella during movement, causing pain in and around the knee. Releasing the tight muscles used to prevent the patella from tracking erratically will help, but the structural cause of the gait problem needs to be addressed.

The iliotibial tract braces the knee for walking and for running. The tract or band becomes contracted from overuse as the muscles that lead into it shorten. The tensor fasciae latae and the gluteus maximus are the primary culprits of hypertonicity and can contribute to a **contracted iliotibial tract.** The tract itself has no properties of contractility, but when palpated on a marathon runner, it can feel like a taut guitar string. This problem can lead to knee issues and gait dysfunctions. **Ober's test** is an orthopedic test for a contracted iliotibial tract. Position the client side-lying with the presenting extremity on top of the uninvolved limb. Support the bent knee. If the tract is contracted, the knee will not be able to stretch medially to close the gap between the two extremities. Massage, exercise, and stretching will assist in resolving a contracted iliotibial tract resulting from tight muscles, but problems with gait, foot structure, and so on, should be approached with a conservative team and appropriate diagnosis.

As mentioned in Chapter 17, the thigh muscles and knee joint can have a direct effect on the position of the pelvic girdle and its rotation. An external rotation of the hip can throw off gait, cause discomfort in the lower back, and create an imbalance in the muscular group relationships. The thigh muscles serve as communication links between the hip and the knee.

Muscles

The thigh muscles between the pelvic girdle and the knee house several two-jointed muscles that service both major joints. The muscles are located in their line of pull and in groups. The hip flexors and knee extensors are anterior and oppose the posterior hip extensors and knee flexors. Adductors of the thigh and internal knee rotators are located medially, and outer thigh muscles abduct the thigh. (See Chapter 17 for a review of the muscles, their locations, and groups of action.)

Balancing the muscles of the thigh requires appropriate stretching, strengthening, and training. The quadriceps are stronger than the hamstrings; only one of the quadriceps, the rectus femoris, is a two-joint muscle, whereas the hamstrings are all multiarticular with the exception of the short head of the biceps femoris. Hamstring strains are more common in track-and-field events than are quadriceps strains or injuries. With hamstring strains and injuries, it is not unusual to see a large **hematoma** with extensive ecchymosis or bruising on the posterior thigh. Athletes recover from hamstring injuries, but recovery requires a conservative team approach that includes massage therapy.

Injuries and Overuse Syndromes

Though not specifically designed for anything but flexion and extension, the knee joint can wear out over time. The tibial plateau receives the brunt of the body's weight, and this compromises the structures inside the knee. Traumatic falls (including motorcycle accidents, for example), excessive weight, aging, and arthritis can all lead to knee surgeries that include knee replacements and repair of torn cartilage and/or ligaments. Ligament injury can involve the anterior and/or posterior cruciate ligaments inside the knee or the collateral ligaments that bind the medial and lateral sides of the knee. Knee sprains involving ligaments may be resolved though physical therapy, exercise, and appropriate stretching. Some ligament tears have to be surgically repaired. The knee cartilage, known as the *medial and lateral menisci,* can become torn, particularly from torsional and compressive forces. The menisci are necessary to reduce friction between the femur and the tibia, and they help stabilize the knee joint. Problems with injured menisci cause much knee pain and probable development of arthritis. There are many interim steps to take in the management of arthritic knee pain, including exercise, weight loss, orthotics, therapeutic injections, and possible arthroscopic surgery. Ultimately, if enough deterioration occurs and conservative measures fail, a knee replacement might be inevitable.

Structural changes in the knee joint, abnormal gait patterns, or imbalanced muscular development in the thigh can cause a trigger point in the fibular collateral ligament. Trigger points are not necessarily limited to the muscles and/or tendons. Structural torque to the fibular collateral ligament can provoke the development of pain in the lateral side of the knee from an irritated trigger point. Therapists should take care to rule out iliotibial band issues. Strengthening, stretching, correcting gait patterns and structural problems, and massage therapy can help reduce and sometimes resolve the lateral knee pain from a trigger point in the fibular collateral ligament.

Osgood-Schlatter disease is a dysfunction with the growth plate of the tibial tuberosity that causes pain in the superior anterior tibial region, probable tracking issues, and tendonitis of the patella. It may be genetic and most problematic in active adolescent boys, but most often trauma to the front of the knee is involved. Although the massage therapist can do nothing about the growth plate, ice massage may help the patellar tendon at its attachment at the tibia. A conservative approach includes stretching and exercise, as well as massage to the soft tissue of the thigh muscles.

There are many more injuries and problems in relation to the knee joint. As discussed in Chapter 17, prepatellar bursitis, or "water on the knee," can be painful for anyone who spends time kneeling. A swollen patellar tendon may be tendonitis. Patellar subluxations or even dislocations can occur and may require management by an orthopedist, followed by rehabilitation by an athletic trainer or physical therapist. See Chapter 17 for a discussion of the Q angle. Many patellofemoral conditions are partially due to a weak vastus medialis. Additionally, nerve complaints can be a painful complication.

Nerve Complaints

FEMORAL NERVE AND SCIATIC NERVE

As discussed in Chapter 17, it is possible for thigh soft tissue to entrap either the femoral nerve or the sciatic nerve. Pain in the anterior thigh, or **meralgia paresthetica,** can be attributed to branches of the femoral nerve being compromised at some location, often from soft tissue. Since it can be a bit of a mystery, an experienced diagnostician should be consulted, but massage therapy can release the soft tissues of this troublesome condition.

The sciatic nerve passes between the biceps femoris and the adductor magnus in the posterior thigh. Hypertonic tissues, and sometimes compressed tissues from sitting, can cause pain in the posterior thigh muscles. Remember that the sciatic nerve can be compromised in a variety of ways in the lower-back and pelvic girdle region. Since the sciatic nerve traverses through the lower extremity in its divisions, it should not be assumed that problems with the nerve come only from the lower back and pelvic girdle. See Chapter 16 for more information on the involvement of the piriformis with the sciatic nerve (piriformis syndrome).

Arthritis, Osteoarthritis, and Surgical Intervention

In addition to trauma, osteoarthritis in the knee joint can lead to friction, meniscal wear, and eventual knee replacement. If the patella does not track appropriately, arthritic changes can develop in the articular surfaces of the patellofemoral joint, causing increased friction. Age and obesity hasten arthritic changes in the knee joint.

Knee replacement is a common solution for a painful hinge joint that no longer functions properly. Replacing the existing hinge joint requires a complete substitute hinge, or **prosthesis.** The patellar tendon may be partially or completely severed, and the femur and tibia are cut to fit the new hinge joint. Very soon after surgery, the patient is fitted with a passive motion machine that starts the rehabilitation process with a repetitive flexing of the knee joint, passively exercising the thigh muscles. Knee replacements are one of the most successful prostheses for the human body. Massage therapy, stretching, and additional physical therapy will assist the recovery and aid in compensatory changes in the back and other areas. A regular exercise program will be necessary for keeping the thigh muscles fit and is an important part of the success and maintenance of the new joint.

KNEE REPLACEMENT

Consider this scenario: A 48-year-old male hit a rock in his driveway with a motorcyle doing about 15 mph. Unfortunately, he stuck his right foot out to brace his fall. The momentum of the accident forced his femur to split his tibia as he tumbled over and landed on his back, fracturing his left scapula. The first surgery's focus was on saving his tibia by screwing the bone together. The second surgery removed the screws, especially the one that had worked its way up into the joint and was making a groove in the femur as he walked. The third surgery was an arthroscopy to see what was left, if anything, of the meniscal cartilage. The fourth and final surgery replaced the knee with a prosthesis. The knee joint could not be replaced in the first surgery, as the tibia was too damaged for replacement. The tibia had to repair enough to accept the eventual prosthesis.

This true story briefly outlines the possibilities with extreme trauma and surgical intervention. Generally, a healthy knee joint, without trauma or problematic gait issues, just needs exercise, stretching, and massage to provide maintenance for regular function.

Unwinding the Muscles of the Thigh and Knee Joint: Where to Start?

Ordinary soft tissue can be manipulated with regular Swedish techniques, but athletic thighs that are designed like tree trunks have to be approached with techniques that will compress, lengthen, and broaden fibers successfully. Techniques listed in the dimensional massage section will help to unwind the thigh muscles systematically, superficial to deep. Add the techniques to your tool belt, and choose the appropriate strokes for the desired outcome and individual needs of the client.

More than the specific sequence, the questions to consider are what soft-tissue problem affects which joints and what is the purpose of the massage treatment. Since so many thigh muscles are two-joint activators, it makes sense to approach the knee joint first from the hip and anterior thigh. Unwind the quadriceps first, as they are stronger and stacked together logistically with the hip flexors. Addressing the hip flexors helps relieve any restraints on the hip joint in flexion. Treat the sartorius, gracilis, and semitendinosus as a "group," as they insert on the medial knee at the pes anserinus. This medial knee area is often sore because of the functional connection of these guy wires.

Adductors have a tendency to be weak, but if you are working with an equestrian, these muscles are going to be primary targets. Adductor muscles fill in the gaps of the middle and posterior thigh. If the lateral thigh is very dense and is pulling on the iliotibial tract, work on the quadriceps first, paying particular attention to the vastus lateralis. Connective tissue from the vastus lateralis connects to the iliotibial tract. Make sure to address the tensor fasciae latae and the gluteus maximus, as they both insert into the iliotibial tract. Do not ignore the fibular collateral ligament and the lateral knee.

A dimensional approach to the posterior thigh must include work on the muscles of the posterior pelvic girdle. Remember that the hamstrings, which are posterior thigh muscles, are multiarticular muscles and affect the pelvic girdle position, the hip joint, and the knee joint. Apply techniques to all the attachments of the hamstrings. Soreness can develop at the attachment areas. The hamstrings and posterior muscles may be the last stronghold of back dysfunction, since you have already addressed the overpowering quadriceps and hip flexors. They must be included when treating the lower-back and pelvic girdle musculature. See Chapter 16 for low-back techniques. Naturally, you would not ignore the leg muscles. See techniques for the leg, ankle, and foot in Chapter 20.

Dimensional Massage Therapy on the Muscles of the Thigh and Knee Joint

The following techniques can be used as a complete sequence for the thigh muscles and knee joint issues or can be incorporated into other treatment sequences. To make smooth transitions between strokes, use effleurage or compressive effleurage liberally.

TREATMENT PROTOCOL

How do you unwind the thigh muscles and knee joint in a sequence?

- Take a careful medical history appropriate for the client; look for gait issues, patellar tracking, and foot structure problems.
- Always use treatment protocols to determine the sequence of a therapeutic session; assess active and passive ranges of motion of the hip and knee.
- Palpate tissues.
- Follow a dimensional approach, and critically think about the involved joints and muscles; work the muscles in groups and in paired opposition.
- Determine pressure intelligently; ask for feedback from the client.
- Work superficial to deep.
- Visit all the muscles possibly involved in the problem.
- Visit all the attachments of the involved muscles.
- Passively shorten muscles whenever possible with your techniques to decrease tension.
- Do not overwork sore areas.
- Begin supine, and try the techniques below for a dimensional approach.

SUPINE BODY POSITION

Rock and Roll

This technique is a great choice for initial contact, especially for thighs that have a lot of density. For the quadriceps and femoral muscles, stand to the side of the table and place both hands on either side of the lateral and medial thigh. Alternately pass the large muscle masses from hand to hand, lateral to medial and back, as you roll the muscles around the femur vigorously. Start as superior as possible, and work toward the knee. Use this technique at any time again throughout the routine. (See figure 18.1.)

Elliptical Movement of the Quadriceps

Stand to the side of the table, and place your hands in position for the rock-and-roll technique on the medial and lateral quadriceps. Grasp and mobilize the tissue in alternating clockwise and counterclockwise directions. Reposition your hands more toward the knee, and repeat the alternating directions. Keep repositioning your hands until you are right above the knee on the patellar tendon area. (See figure 18.2.)

Jostling the Quadriceps

Jostle all four muscles by tossing the quadriceps back and forth between both hands, starting superiorly

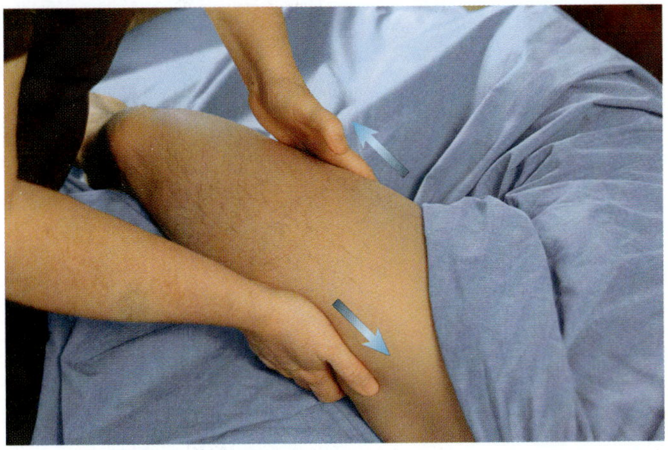

FIGURE 18.1 Rock and roll

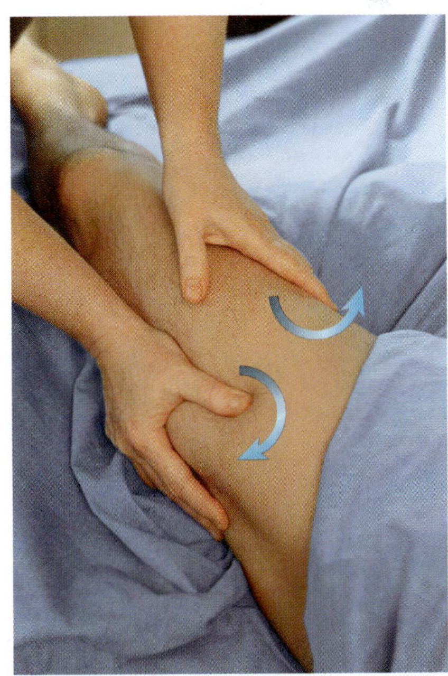

FIGURE 18.2 Elliptical movement of the quadriceps

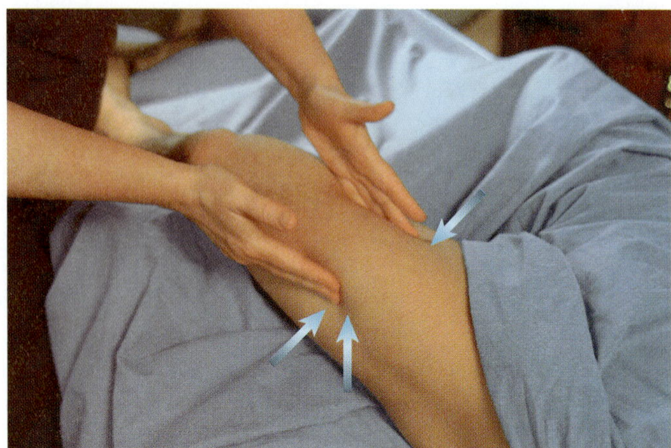

FIGURE 18.3 Jostling the quadriceps

and moving toward the knee. (See figure 18.3.) To isolate the rectus femoris, pick it up with one hand and jostle the muscle from origin to insertion. (See figure 18.4.)

Compression Using Thigh Rotation

For regular compression, apply one or two hands to the quadriceps and compress the tissue, moving from origin to insertion. Be careful not to "roll" off the muscles as you compress. For compression using medial thigh rotation, place one hand on the medial thigh. Place your other hand on the lateral thigh close to the knee. As you compress into the medial thigh musculature, roll the thigh in a medial direction. For the lateral thigh muscles, reposition the hand on the lateral thigh, and repeat compression toward the knee as you roll the thigh laterally. (See figure 18.5.)

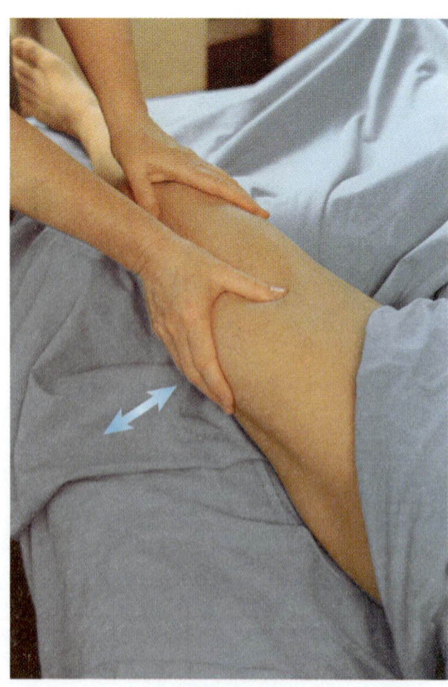

FIGURE 18.4 Jostling the rectus femoris

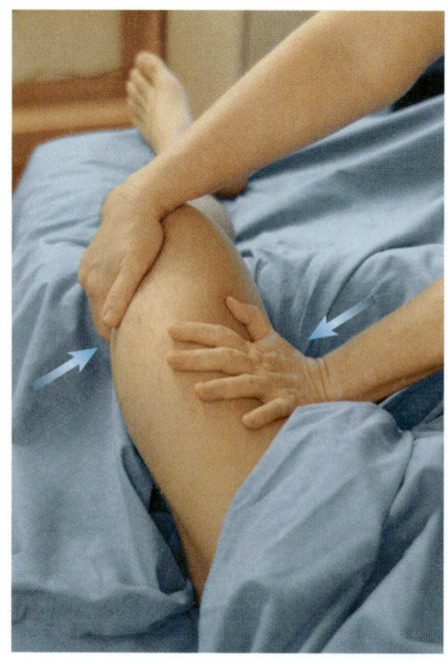

FIGURE 18.5 Compression using medial thigh rotation

Myofascial Techniques for the Quadriceps

Face the client's thigh at the side of the table. Place your hands side by side on the quadriceps. Place your thumbs on the lateral side of the quadriceps, and draw the muscle over your thumbs with your fingers. Repeat superiorly to inferiorly. The same technique can be utilized from the opposite side of the table for the vastus medialis. (See figure 18.6.)

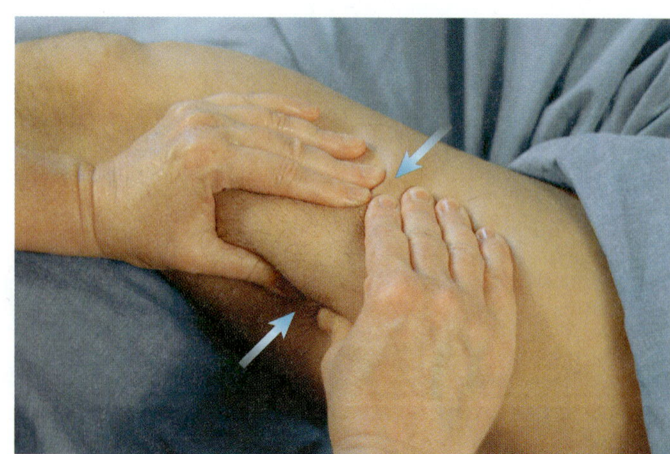

FIGURE 18.6 Myofascial techniques for the quadriceps

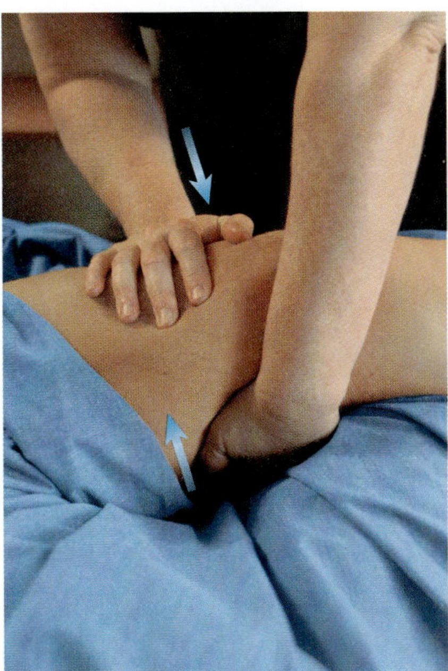

FIGURE 18.7 Wringing the thigh muscles

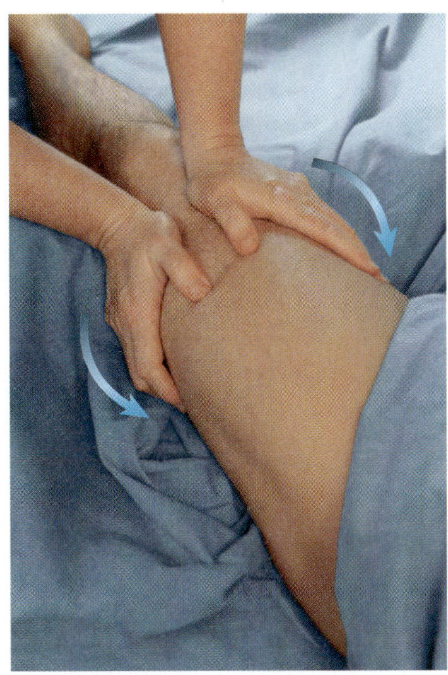

FIGURE 18.8 Broadening the quadriceps

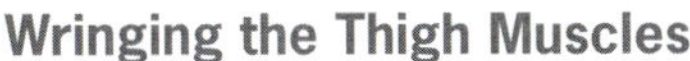

Wringing the Thigh Muscles

Place your hands on the client's lateral and medial thigh muscles. Compress, and as you let go of the pressure, lightly wring, and switch your hand positions. From the superior thigh, move toward the knee, compressing, lightly wringing, and switching hand positions. You also can place one hand on the rectus femoris and the other on the posterior thigh muscles, compress, lightly wring, and switch hand positions. (See figure 18.7.)

Broadening the Quadriceps

Place your hands next to each other on top of the client's thigh. Compress and spread the tissues laterally. Start superiorly and work toward the knee. Some therapists slightly lift the tissues before they broaden them. Use a small amount of lubrication. (See figure 18.8.)

Compressive Effleurage

Effleurage the client's entire lower extremity, but use a deeper penetrable pressure that literally compresses the tissues as you stroke toward the hip. Isolate the quadriceps and anterior thigh muscles, and stroke toward the hip. Repeat liberally throughout the routine. (See figure 18.9.)

Palmar Circular Friction Superior to the Knee

Apply your palms above and to the medial and lateral sides of the client's knee. Make compressive circles on the insertions of the vastus lateralis and medialis.

Tensor Fasciae Latae Technique with Flexed Hip and Knee

To passively shorten the tensor fasciae latae, flex the hip and knee. With your superior hand, grasp the tensor fasciae latae and draw your fingers across the fibers as you rotate the hip internally. Repeat. (See figure 18.10.)

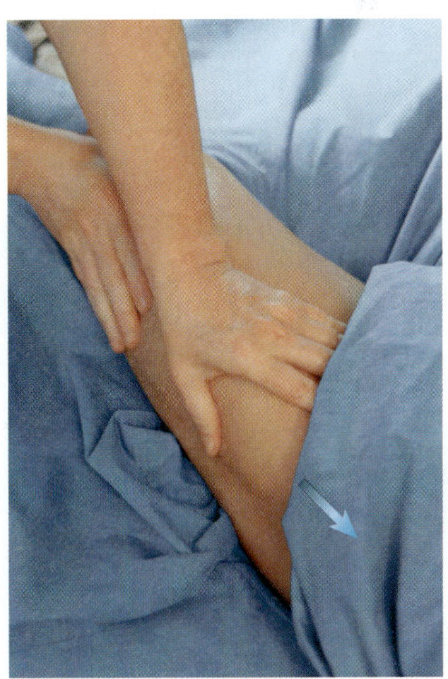

FIGURE 18.9 Compressive effleurage

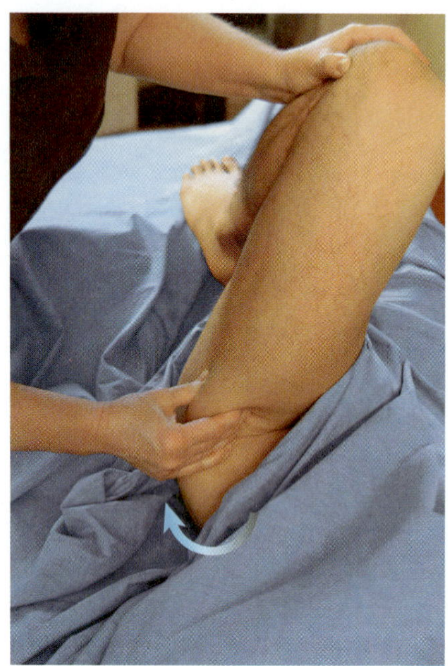

FIGURE 18.10 Tensor fasciae latae technique

Parallel Thumbs to the Vastus Lateralis

Isolate the vastus lateralis. Place your thumbs underneath the muscle close to its origin laterally. Move in an inferior fashion with the parallel thumbs technique, ending just above the knee. (See figure 18.11.)

Bent Fingers to the Iliotibial Tract and Vastus Lateralis

Place your inferior hand on the client's knee. Roll the thigh internally from the hip with your hand at the knee. With your superior hand, press your fingers, bending at the metacarpophalangeal joints, against the lateral knee on the iliotibial tract and vastus lateralis. Move your hand in a superior direction toward the hip. Your hand should be relaxed as it collapses

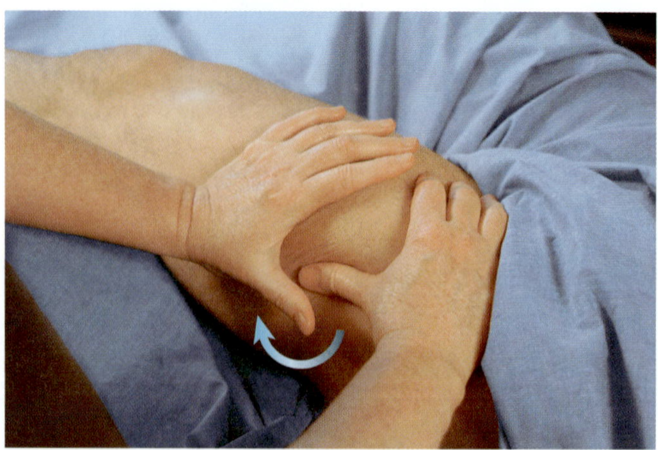

FIGURE 18.11 Parallel thumbs to the vastus lateralis

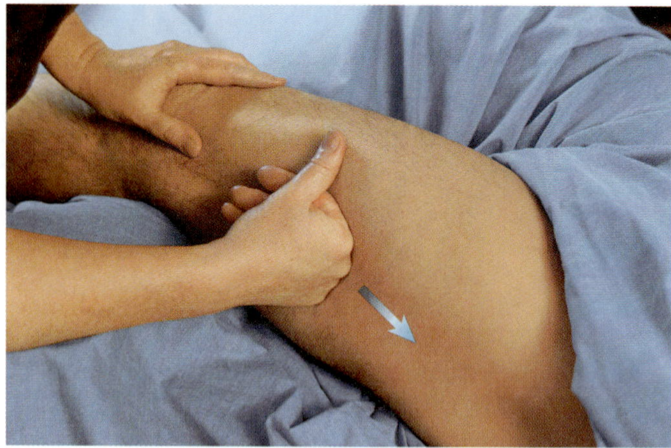

FIGURE 18.12 Bent fingers to the iliotibial tract and vastus lateralis

into the soft tissue. Do not use a fist. Use caution with your pressure. (See figure 18.12.)

Vibrate the Iliotibial Tract and Vastus lateralis

With your inferior hand, roll the client's hip internally. With your superior hand, start at the tensor fasciae latae and vibrate toward the tibia. Repeat several times. (See figure 18.13.)

Petrissage and Friction

Apply alternating petrissage and circular friction to the client's thigh muscles.

Deep Transverse Friction for Attachments of the Rectus Femoris

Flex the client's knee and hip. Locate the origin of the rectus femoris. Slide across the origin with your thumb to separate the fibers. Return the thigh to the table. Locate the patellar tendon above the knee. Apply deep transverse friction to the tendon with both thumbs simultaneously going in lateral and medial directions.

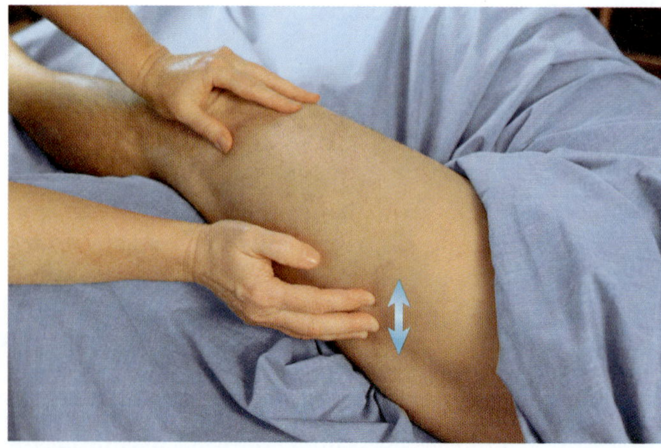

FIGURE 18.13 Vibrating the iliotibial tract and vastus lateralis

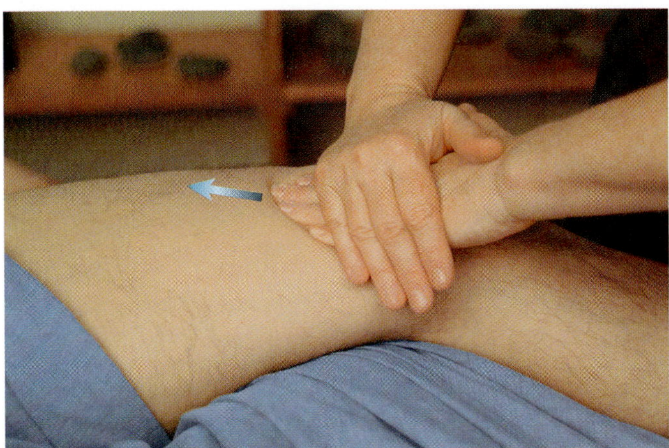

FIGURE 18.14 Stripping the sartorius

Stripping the Sartorius

The sartorius can be successfully stripped, as it is a superficial muscle. Locate the insertion and strip toward its origin. Place one hand on top of your fingers at a right angle and strip toward the origin, using the pressure of both hands. (See figure 18.14.)

Forearm Stroking

Forearms can stroke the quadriceps in three sections: lateral-, middle-, and inner-thigh areas. Angle your forearm, and secure the tissues before compressing the muscles and gliding from knee to hip area. (See figure 18.15.)

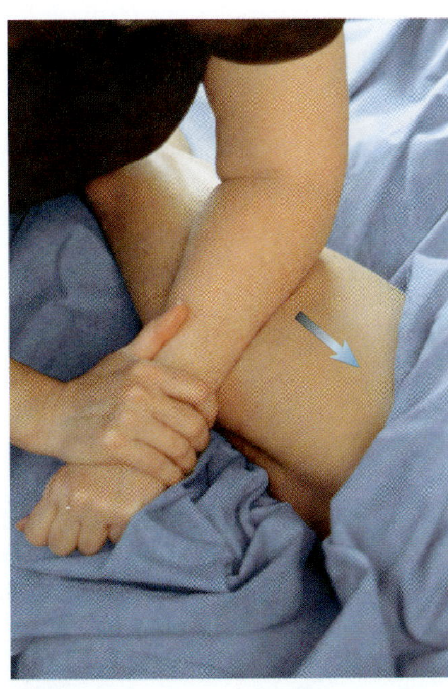

FIGURE 18.15 Forearm stroking

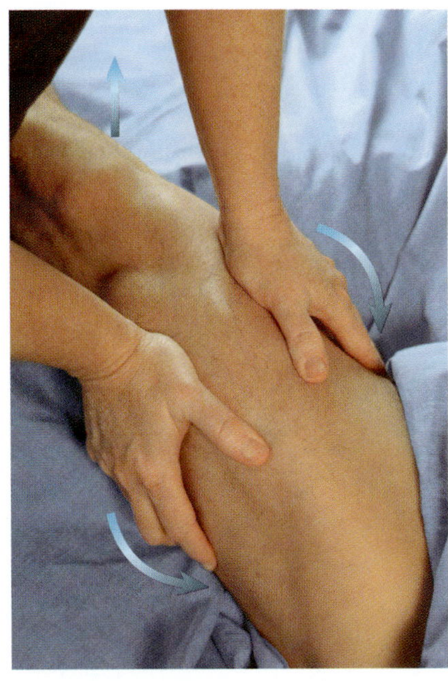

FIGURE 18.16 Broadening the quadriceps with active shortening

Broadening the Quadriceps with Active Shortening

The whole lower extremity can be off the table or over a bolster, as pictured. Start just above the client's knee. As the client actively and slowly begins to raise the leg in knee extension, broaden the quadriceps fibers. Have the client repeat knee extension as you move in a superior position, broadening the fibers. (See figure 18.16.)

Lengthening the Rectus Femoris with Active Engagement

Have the client flex the hip. Position your collapsed fingers just above the knee. As the client slowly brings the lower extremity to the table, strip superiorly with your collapsed fingers. Repeat the procedure again until you reach the hip. (See figure 18.17.)

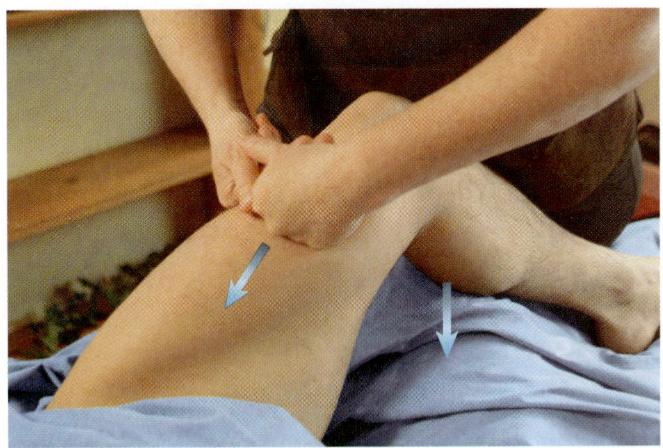

FIGURE 18.17 Lengthening the rectus femoris with active engagement

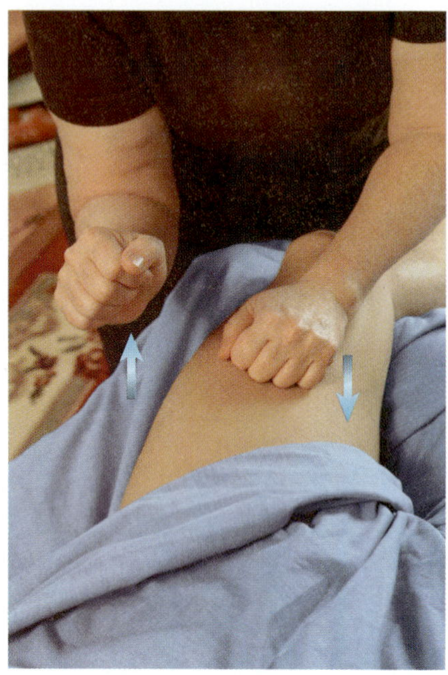

FIGURE 18.18 Loose-fist percussion

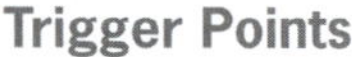

Trigger Points

Locate and apply digital pressure to trigger points in taut bands of tissue. Follow with stretches of the tissue.

Loose-Fist Percussion

Practice a variety of tapotement on these large anterior thigh muscles. (See figure 18.18.)

PRONE

Elliptical Movement of the Posterior Thigh Muscles

Passively shorten the hamstrings by flexing the knee. Place your hands on the medial and lateral sides of the posterior thigh muscles. Alternately move the musculature in clockwise and counterclockwise directions. Move your hands, grasp the soft tissue in different positions, and repeat the technique. (See figure 18.19.)

Compression of the Posterior Thigh

In the same position as above, instead of applying elliptical movement, apply compression to the posterior thigh muscles.

Myofascial Hamstrings and Posterior Thigh Muscles

Face the client's thigh at the side of the table. Place your hands side by side on the posterior thigh muscles. Place your thumbs on the lateral side of the

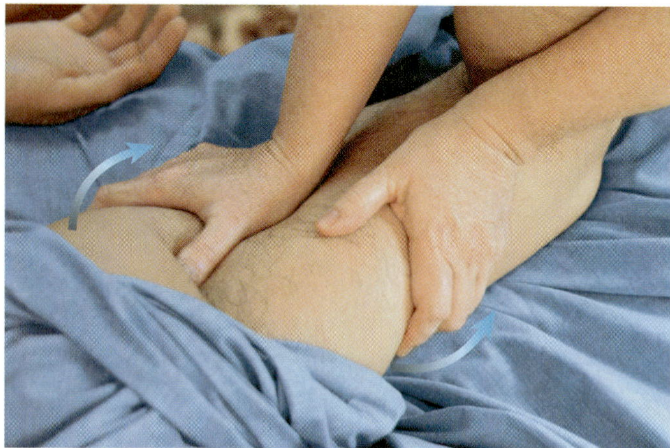

FIGURE 18.19 Elliptical movement of the posterior thigh muscles

thigh, and draw the muscle over your thumbs with your fingers. Repeat superiorly to inferiorly. The same technique can be utilized from the opposite side of the table for the medial side of the posterior thigh. (See figure 18.20.)

Broaden the Hamstrings and Posterior Thigh Muscles

Place your hands next to each other on top of the client's thigh. Compress and spread the tissues laterally. Start superiorly and work toward the knee. Some therapists slightly lift the tissues before they

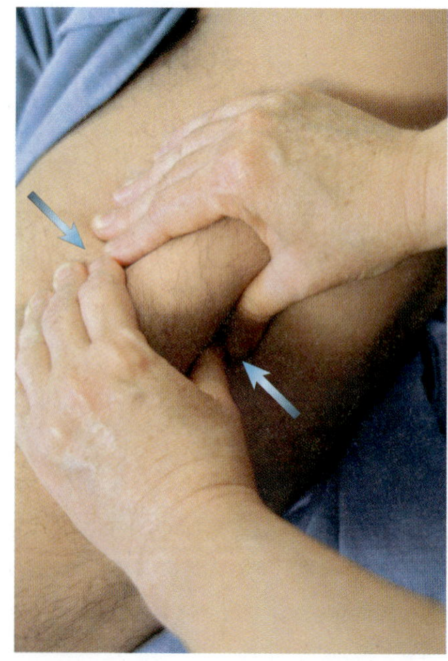

FIGURE 18.20 Myofascial hamstrings and posterior thigh muscles

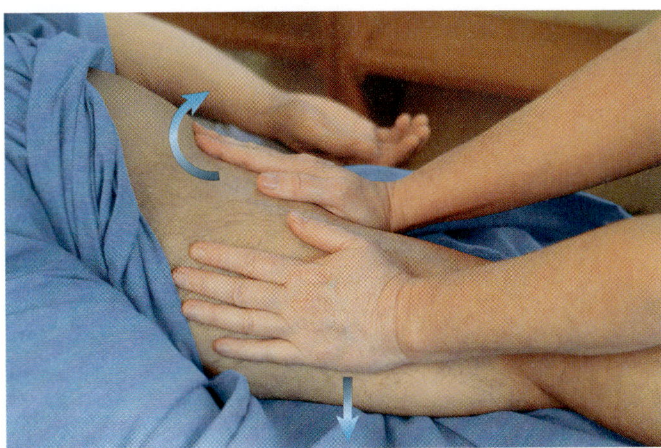

FIGURE 18.21 Broadening the hamstrings and posterior thigh muscles

broaden them. Use a small amount of lubrication. (See figure 18.21.)

Stripping with Collapsed Fingers and Flexed Knee

Passively shorten the client's hamstrings by flexing the knee. Surround the flexed knee, and place your collapsed fingers next to each other on the posterior thigh muscles. Sink into the tissue, and glide toward the hip. (See figure 18.22.)

Olympic Hamstring Tendon Stretch

This technique, among others, was designed for athletes with massive thighs at the sports medicine clinic in the Olympic Village for the 1996 Olympic Games in Atlanta, Georgia. For the biceps femoris, flex the client's knee, and wrap your inside arm around the posterior

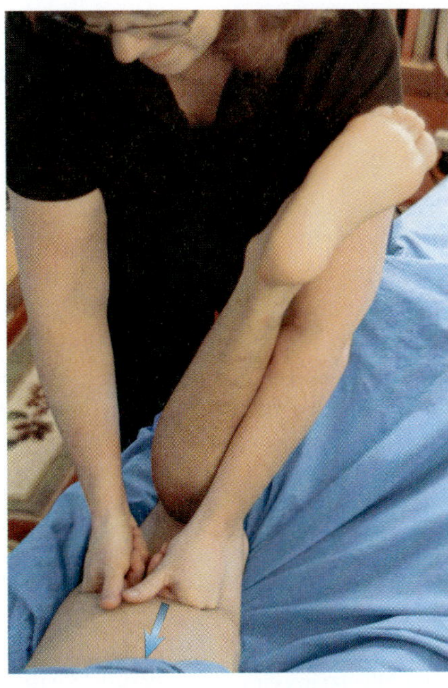

FIGURE 18.22 Stripping with collapsed fingers and flexed knee

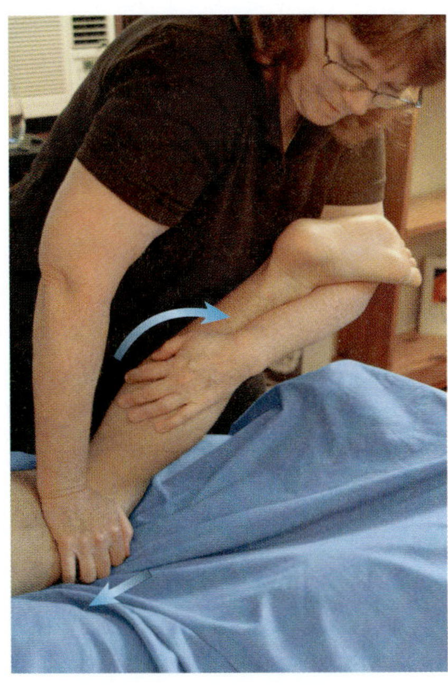

FIGURE 18.23 Olympic hamstring tendon stretch

leg muscles. Hold the gastrocnemius with your inside hand. Place your outside hand on the biceps femoris tendon, starting at the insertion. As you stroke toward the hip, extend the knee on a slight inward rotation. For the semitendinosus and semimembranosus, reverse the process so that your outside hand is on the medial tendons and you move the knee in an external knee rotation as you stroke the tendons. This could easily be called *palmar stripping* of the hamstrings. (See figure 18.23.)

Petrissage the Medial Hamstrings and Adductors with Flexed Knee

Passively shorten the client's hamstrings by flexing the knee. Bring your inferior arm around the front of the leg, and join your superior hand to petrissage the medial hamstrings and adductors. (See figure 18.24.)

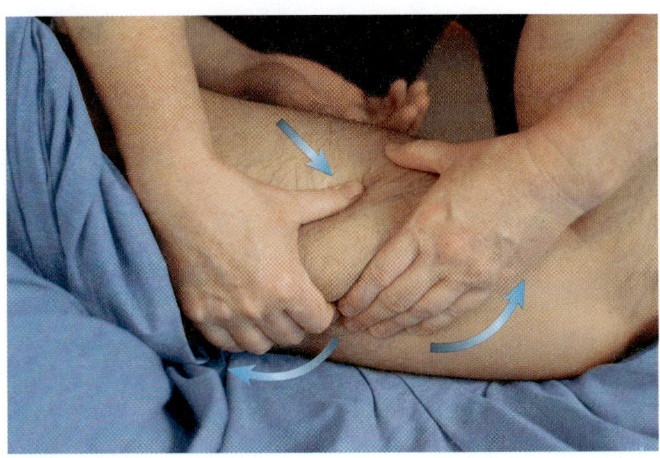

FIGURE 18.24 Petrissage of the medial hamstrings and adductors with flexed knee

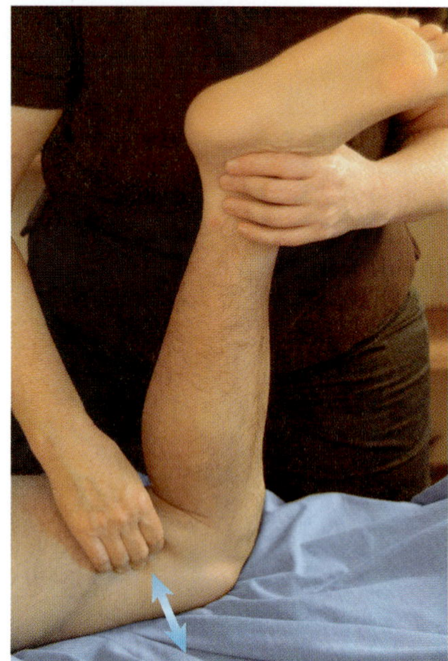

FIGURE 18.25 Vibrating the hamstrings

Vibrate the Hamstrings

Vibrate the tendons from each of the bellies of the muscles to the insertions. (See figure 18.25.)

Palmar Circular Friction of the Hamstrings

Using the soft palms of your hands, apply compressive circular strokes above the client's knee on the tendons.

Deep Transverse Friction for Hamstring Attachments

Apply deep transverse friction to the hamstring origin at the ischial tuberosity. (See figure 18.26.) Locate and apply deep transverse friction to the insertions of the biceps femoris and medial hamstring tendons.

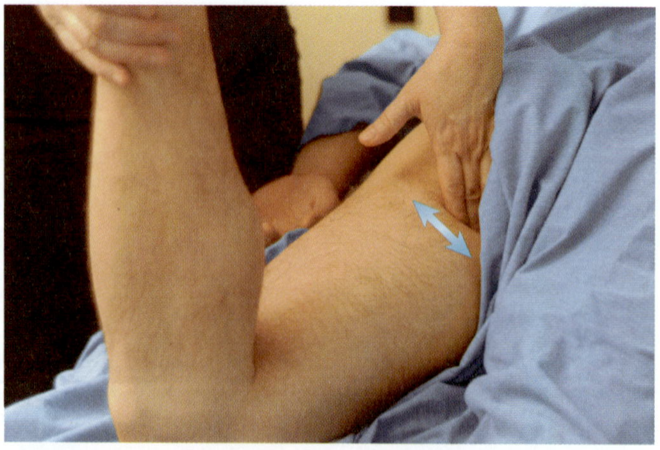

FIGURE 18.26 Deep transverse friction at the ischial tuberosity

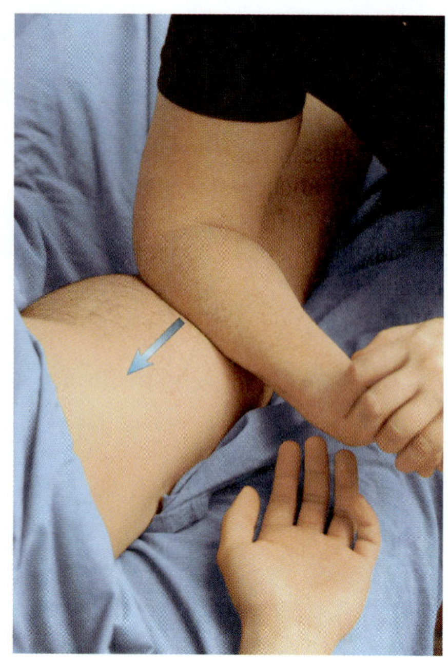

FIGURE 18.27 Forearm stroking on the posterior thigh

Intersperse with Compressive Effleurage

Utilize effleurage between your other strokes and techniques for maximum benefit.

Forearm Stroking

Use forearm stroking on the client's posterior thigh. (See figure 18.27.)

Trigger Points

Locate and apply digital pressure or a pincer palpation to trigger points. Follow with stretches to the muscle tissue.

Tapotement

Practice a variety of tapotement on the client's large posterior muscles. See figure 18.18 for loose-fist percussion.

Stretches

Place one hand on the ischial tuberosity and the other on the calcaneus. Lean over and stretch. Stretch the quadriceps by flexing the knee and bringing the calcaneus to the gluteals. Some individuals are so limber that you may have to lift the knee off the table to give an adequate stretch. Flex the knee, and lift it off the table with the ankle. Grasp the foot, and shake the ankle and leg muscles.

Ending

Finishing an area is as important as beginning it. Remember to use some finishing strokes such as effleurage and to apply nerve strokes last. Leave the area with a slight pressure or stroke from one to another for fluidity.

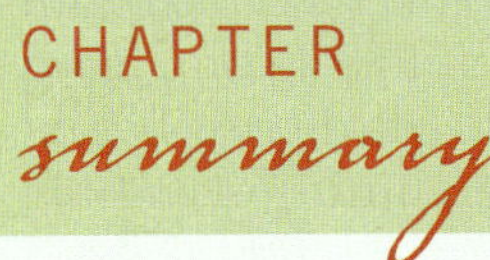

CHAPTER summary

Introduction

- ✔ The thigh muscles provide the strength and support to guide the knees in movement.
- ✔ Physical trauma causes problems for the knee joint.
- ✔ Massage therapy can provide a great deal of relief for soft-tissue dysfunction of the thigh muscles and knee joint.

Structural Perspectives of the Knee Joint

- ✔ The pelvic girdle supports the femur and supplies a base for the muscles of the thigh.
- ✔ The thigh muscles must be in good shape to support the knee in movement and stability.
- ✔ Structural problems might include genu valgum, genu varum, patellar tracking, contracted iliotibial tract, and hip alignment variances.

The Muscles

- ✔ The thigh muscles are the connecting links between the hip and the knee.
- ✔ The muscles are located logically within a line of pull to the knee joint.
- ✔ Balancing the thigh muscles requires a conservative team approach, including stretching, strengthening, training, and massage therapy.

Injuries and Overuse Syndromes

- ✔ The knee can fall victim to trauma, excessive weight, aging, and arthritis.
- ✔ Ligament injury is common to the knee joint.
- ✔ Meniscal tears are painful and may lead to eventual knee replacement.
- ✔ The fibular collateral ligament can have a trigger point develop from structural issues.
- ✔ Osgood-Schlatter disease is a dysfunction of the tibial tuberosity growth plate that causes pain and other knee issues.

Nerve Complaints

- ✔ Meralgia paresthetica is pain in the anterior thigh from entrapment of branches of the femoral nerve.
- ✔ Sciatic nerve pain in the posterior thigh can come from compression in the lower back, entrapment from soft tissue in the pelvic girdle, or by entrapment from the biceps femoris and adductor magnus in the posterior thigh.

Arthritis, Osteoarthritis, and Surgical Intervention

- ✔ Arthritis and osteoarthritis can contribute to friction or meniscal wear in the knee joint.
- ✔ A knee replacement is a prosthesis or substitute hinge joint fitted to the femur and tibia.
- ✔ Healthy knees need exercise, stretching, and massage to provide maintenance for regular function.

Unwinding the Muscles of the Thigh and Knee Joint: Where to Start?

- ✔ Massage therapy is a good choice for relieving hypertonicity in the thigh muscles.
- ✔ Follow a dimensional approach, and critically think about the involved joints and muscles.
- ✔ Always use treatment protocols to determine the sequence of a therapeutic session.

Dimensional Massage Therapy on the Muscles of the Thigh and Knee Joint

- ✔ Start with the anterior thigh muscles first.
- ✔ Approach techniques methodically, unwinding soft tissue superficially to deep.
- ✔ Passively shorten muscles when possible.
- ✔ Work the muscles in groups.

CHAPTER review

True or False

Write true *or* false *after each statement.*

1. Osgood-Schlatter affects old men only.
2. The gluteus medius and the sartorius feed the iliotibial tract.
3. Multiarticular muscles never have any problems, as they completely support all joints equally.
4. Patellar tracking can be affected by gait.
5. The knee joint is the largest joint in the body.
6. There are no two-joint muscles among the thigh muscles.

7. The weight of the body rests on the tibial plateau.
8. The medial meniscus is the only part of the cartilage that can be injured by trauma.
9. Compressive forces might injure ligaments inside the knee.
10. Massage therapy for the muscles of the thigh and knee joint can be part of a sports training or event program.

Short Answers

Write your answers on the lines provided.

1. What condition requires Ober's test?

2. Which muscles extend the knee?

3. Which muscles flex the knee?

4. Which muscles might make the iliotibial tract contract?

5. Name the hamstrings.

6. What is the difference between genu valgum and genu varum?

7. List three things that might contribute to knee replacement.

8. Which muscles are stronger, the quadriceps or the hamstrings?

9. What disease can develop inside the knee if the cartilage is worn?

10. Why might the medial knee often be sore to the touch?

Multiple Choice

Circle the correct answers.

1. A large bruise is called:
   a. a bump
   b. a hematoma
   c. an edema
   d. none of the above
2. Healthy knees just need:
   a. stretching, strengthening, and massage for the thigh muscles
   b. regular visits to the physician
   c. to be ignored
   d. all of the above
3. Meralgia paresthetica is pain:
   a. in the pelvic girdle
   b. in the posterior thigh
   c. presenting on the anterior thigh
   d. none of the above

4. A knee replacement requires:
   a. a prosthesis fit into the femur and tibia
   b. an arthroscopy
   c. a lot of exercise first
   d. none of the above
5. Genu valgum is:
   a. never a problem
   b. often called knock-knees
   c. a bowleg
   d. none of the above
6. The anterior cruciate ligament is on:
   a. the lateral side of the knee
   b. the inside of the knee
   c. the medial side of the knee
   d. none of the above
7. When the patella tracks correctly, it:
   a. moves side to side
   b. rides over the knee in a superior and inferior direction during flexion and extension
   c. does not move at all
   d. none of the above
8. Prepatellar bursitis is located:
   a. in back of the knee
   b. anterior to the patella
   c. on the lateral side of the knee
   d. none of the above
9. The sciatic nerve passes between:
   a. biceps femoris and adductor magnus
   b. semitendinosus and biceps femoris
   c. rectus femoris and biceps femoris
   d. none of the above
10. The quadriceps all insert into portions of:
    a. the femur
    b. the patellar tendon
    c. the fibula
    d. none of the above

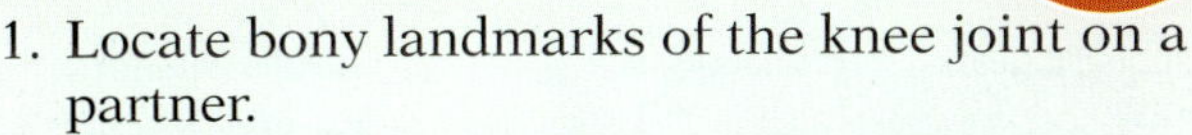

EXPLORE & *practice*

1. Locate bony landmarks of the knee joint on a partner.
2. Locate on a partner the origins and insertions of the muscles discussed in Chapters 15 and 17 associated with the knee joint.
3. Demonstrate how to passively shorten the flexors and extensors of the knee joint.
4. Demonstrate passive range of motion of the knee joint with a partner.
5. Demonstrate active range of motion of the knee joint with a partner.
6. List which muscles are agonists and synergists for flexion of the knee joint.
7. List which muscles are agonists and synergists for extension of the knee joint.
8. Which muscles insert on the pes anserinus?
9. Practice dimensional techniques individually and in a sequence on a willing individual.
10. Describe the effect the hamstrings might have on the pelvic girdle.

chapter 19

The Ankle and Foot Joints

LEARNING OUTCOMES

After completing this chapter, you should be able to:

19-1 Define key terms.

19-2 Identify on a human skeleton the most important bony features, ligaments, and arches of the ankle and foot.

19-3 Draw and label on a skeletal chart the muscles, including the origins and insertions, of the ankle and foot.

19-4 Demonstrate the active and passive movements of the ankle and foot with a partner.

19-5 Explore on a partner the superficial joint structures and muscles, including origins and insertions, of the ankle and foot.

19-6 List and organize the muscles that produce movement of the ankle and foot and list their antagonists.

19-7 Practice flexibility and strengthening exercises for each muscle group.

KEY TERMS

Achilles tendon
Anterior compartment
Calcaneus
Cuboid
Cuneiforms
Extensor digitorum longus
Extensor hallucis longus
Flexor digitorum longus
Flexor hallucis longus
Gastrocnemius
Heel-strike
Lateral compartment
Lateral longitudinal arch
Malleoli
Medial longitudinal arch
Metatarsals
Metatarsophalangeal (MP) joints
Midstance
Navicular
Peroneus brevis
Peroneus longus
Peroneus tertius
Phalanges
Plantaris
Posterior compartment
Pronation
Soleus
Stance
Subtalar and transverse tarsal joints
Supination
Swing
Talocrural joint
Talus
Tarsals
Tibialis anterior
Tibialis posterior
Tibiofibular joint
Toe extension
Toe flexion
Toe-off
Transverse arch
Trendelenburg test
Triceps surae

Introduction

The foot is one of the most abused structures in the human body because many individuals tend to sacrifice comfort for fashion by wearing high heels, pointed-toe shoes, and other types of footwear that do not properly support the feet. The continued use of improper shoes frequently leads to shortened muscles, poor foot mechanics, and deformed foot structure; it also interferes with the body's ability to balance and walk safely, resulting in gait abnormalities. Poor foot mechanics early in life inevitably lead to foot discomfort in later years, and it is not unusual for individuals to complain of knee, hip, back, and neck pain that stems from the use of improper shoes. At the end of the distal lower-extremity kinetic chain, the feet are often dismissed until it has been clearly established that they are the source of pain. Fortunately, today's wide selection of footwear made specifically for running, walking, cross-training, hiking, and other activities has helped support proper foot mechanics; however, massage therapy, strength training, and appropriate stretching should also be part of a conservative approach in supporting healthy feet.

CLINICAL NOTES **Walking Gait Cycle**

Walking and running consist of stance and swing phases (figure 19.1). The **stance** phase contains three components: heel-strike, midstance, and toe-off. Midstance is further separated into loading response and terminal stance. A normal **heel-strike** is characterized by the foot landing on the heel, with the foot in supination and the leg in external rotation; this is followed immediately by pronation and internal rotation of the foot and leg, respectively, during **midstance.** The foot returns to supination and the leg returns to external rotation immediately before and during **toe-off,** the movement in the gait cycle when the toe (primarily the first metatarsal) pushes off the ground to advance that particular foot forward. The **swing** phase occurs when the foot leaves the ground and the leg moves forward to another point of contact. The swing phase consists of initial swing, midswing, and terminal swing. Problems often arise when the foot is too rigid and does not pronate adequately or when the foot remains in pronation past midstance. When the foot remains too rigid and does not pronate adequately, impact forces are not absorbed through the gait; this results in shock being transmitted up the kinetic chain. If the foot overpronates, or remains in pronation too much past midstance, propulsive forces are diminished and additional stresses are placed on the kinetic chain. In walking, one foot is always in contact with the ground, and there is a point at which both feet are in contact with the ground. In running, both feet are never in contact with the ground at the same time, and there is a point when neither foot is in contact with the ground.

GAIT ASSESSMENT FOR MUSCLE WEAKNESS

Gait assessment is complicated, and there are many different tests available that help evaluate gait issues. Briefly, it is helpful to understand basic muscle weakness and how it affects gait. Weakness of the abductor area of the hip is a common area of muscle weakness and one that causes dysfunction in the gait cycle in addition to low-back pain. The gluteus medius muscle is often weak, as discussed in Chapter 21. During gait, this muscle acts to support the hip and moves the crest of the iliac spine toward the greater trochanter; it should provide pain-free movement as one walks. When it is weak, however, an individual will exhibit a lurch as he attempts to counteract the imbalance caused by the weakness. This lurch, or hiking, can be minimal or extreme, depending on the severity of muscle dysfunction. If left untreated, continued activity and normal walking can cause low-back pain, as well as possible bursitis and tendonitis. While a skilled kinesiologist can assess for gluteus medius weakness by observing gait, the **Trendelenburg test** is an easy and effective way to assess gluteus medius weakness. The therapist stands behind the patient and asks her to stand on one leg. If the muscle is strong, the gluteus medius muscle on the involved side should contract when the other leg leaves the ground. This elevates the pelvis on the unsupported side, giving support and causing a straight line across both sides of the pelvis. A positive test occurs when the pelvis on the unsupported side drops or remains in a skewed position. Assessing this muscle for weakness is one of the most powerful tools for addressing gait and low-back issues. See Chapter 21 for techniques that stretch and strengthen the gluteus medius.

The complex structure of the foot contains 26 bones, not including the tibia and fibula; 19 large muscles; many small (intrinsic) muscles; and more than 100 ligaments that connect the bones. This chapter reviews the bones, joints, muscles, movements, and nerves of the leg, ankle, and foot. Clinical Notes boxes throughout address common leg and foot ailments. Each prime mover is discussed in detail to illustrate the roles the muscles play in working together and in paired opposition. For ease of comprehension, the posterior leg muscles are presented first, superficial to deep, followed by the lateral leg and anterior leg muscles. The intrinsic foot muscles are briefly discussed at the end of the chapter.

Bones

Each foot has 26 bones, which collectively form the shape of an arch. They connect with the thigh and the remainder of the body through the fibula and tibia (figure 19.2). Body weight is transferred from the tibia to the **talus** and the **calcaneus.**

In addition to the talus and calcaneus, there are five other bones in the rear foot and midfoot known as the **tarsals.** Between the talus and the three **cuneiform** bones lies the **navicular.** The **cuboid** is located between the calcaneus and the 4th and 5th **metatarsals.** Distal to the tarsals are the five metatarsals, which in turn correspond to each of the five toes. The toes are known as the **phalanges.** (See figure 19.3.) There are three individual bones in each phalange, except

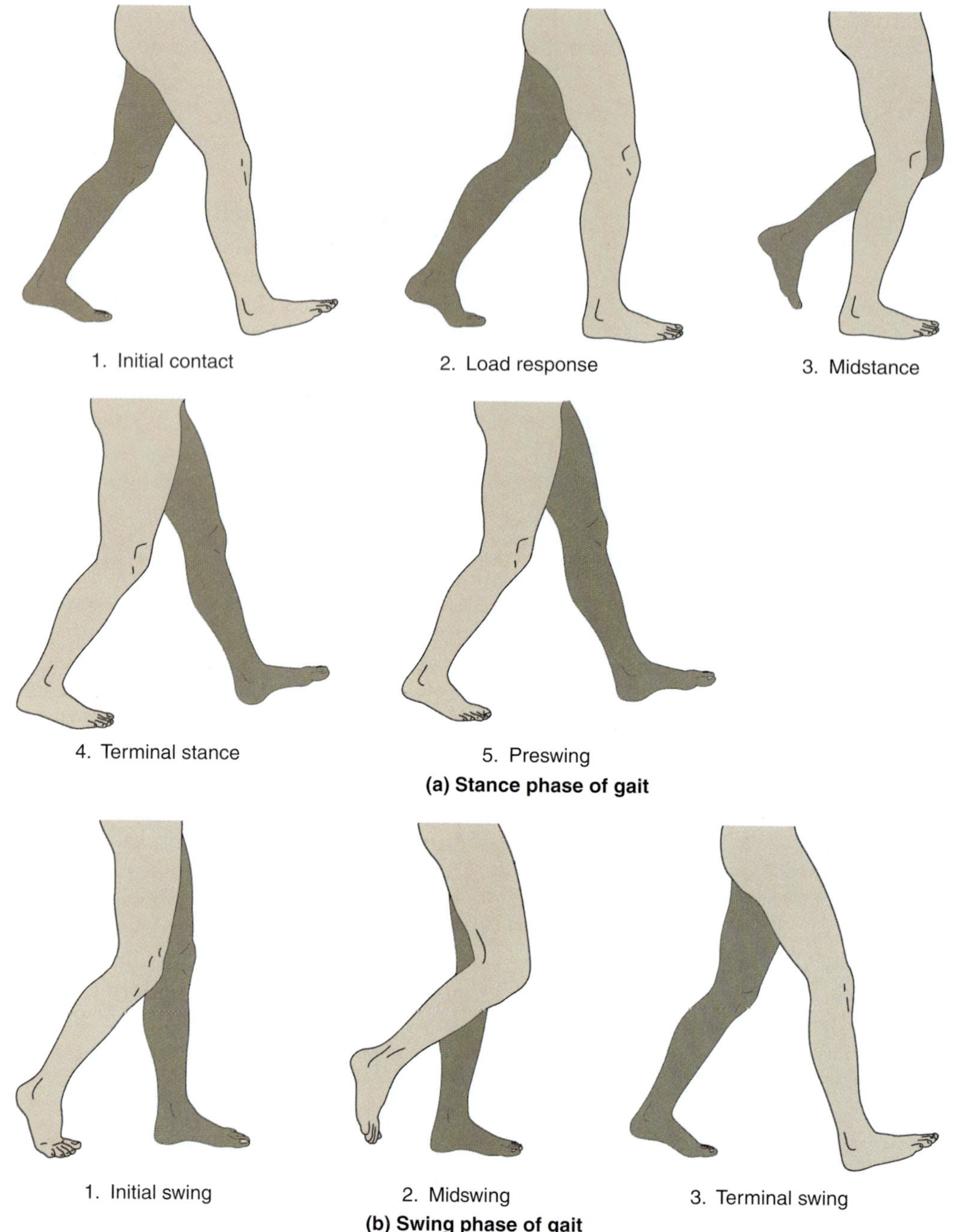

FIGURE 19.1 Gait

for the great toe, or hallux, which has only two. Each of these bones is known as a *phalanx*. Finally, there are two sesamoid bones located beneath the 1st metatarsophalangeal joint and contained within the flexor hallucis longus tendons.

The distal ends of the tibia and fibula are enlarged and protrude horizontally and inferiorly. These bony protrusions, known as **malleoli,** serve as a pulley of sorts for the tendons of the muscles that run directly posterior to them. Specifically, the peroneus brevis and peroneus longus are immediately behind the lateral malleolus. The muscles immediately posterior to the medial malleolus may be remembered by the phrase "Tom, Dick, and Harry," with the "T" for the tibialis posterior, the "D" for the flexor digitorum longus, and the "H" for the flexor hallucis longus. This bony arrangement increases the mechanical advantage of these muscles in performing their actions of inversion and eversion. The base of the 5th metatarsal is enlarged and prominent to serve as an attachment point for the peroneus brevis and tertius.

The inner surface of the medial cuneiform and the base of the 1st metatarsal provide insertion points for the tibialis anterior, while the undersurface of the same bones serves as the insertion for the peroneus longus. The tibialis posterior has multiple insertions on the lower inner surfaces of the navicular, cuneiform, and

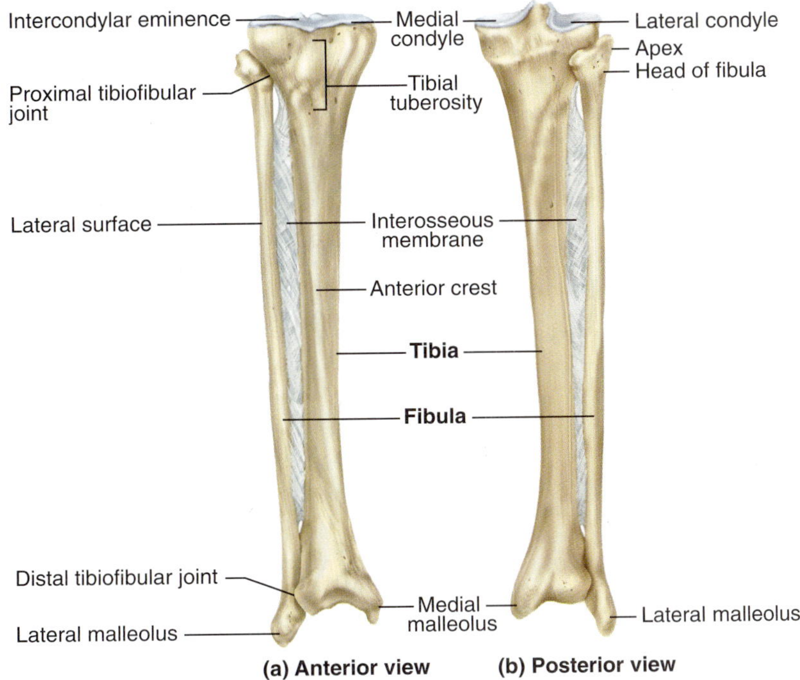

FIGURE 19.2 Tibia and fibula

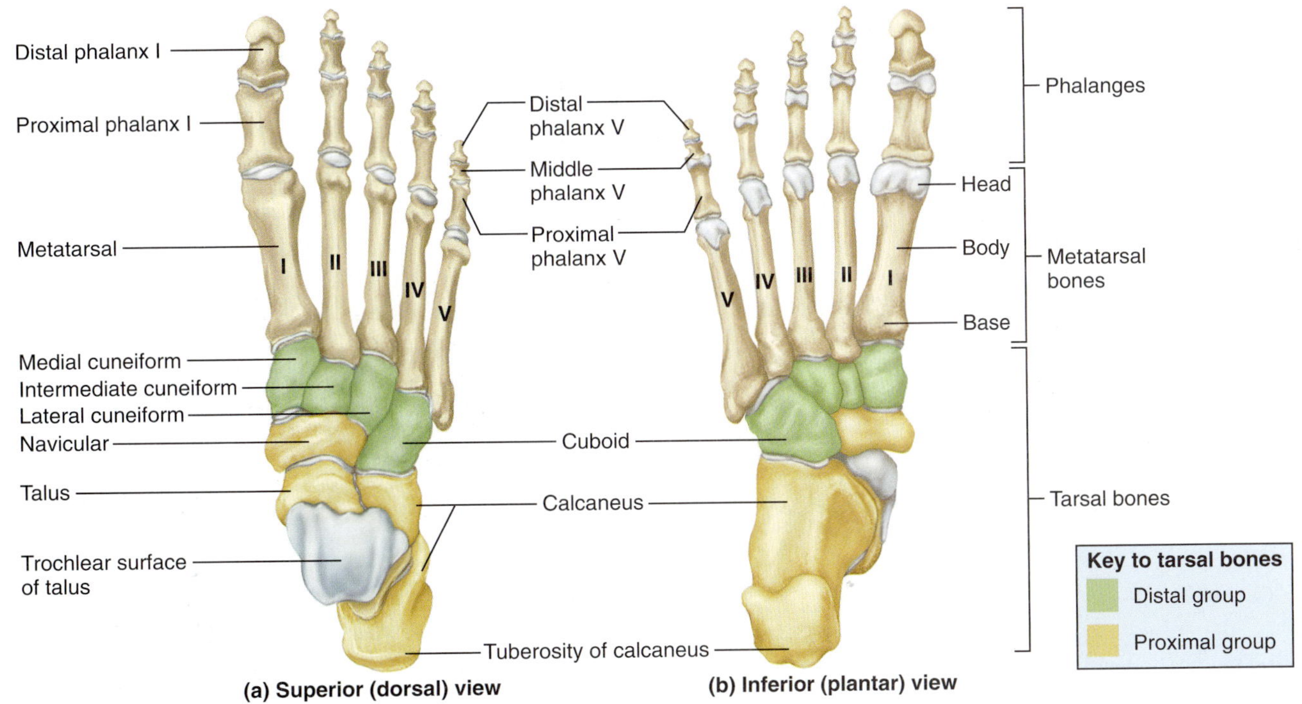

FIGURE 19.3 Bones of the feet

2nd through 5th metatarsal bases. The tops and undersurfaces of the bases of the 2nd through 5th distal phalanxes are the insertion points for the extensor digitorum longus and the flexor digitorum longus, respectively. Similarly, the top and undersurface of the base of the 1st distal phalanx provide insertions for the extensor hallucis longus and flexor hallucis longus, respectively.

The posterior surface of the calcaneus is very prominent and serves as the attachment point for the Achilles tendon of the gastrocnemius-soleus complex.

Joints

The tibia and fibula form the **tibiofibular joint,** a syndesmotic amphiarthrodial joint (figure 19.4). The bones are joined at both the proximal and distal tibiofibular joints. In addition to the ligaments supporting both of

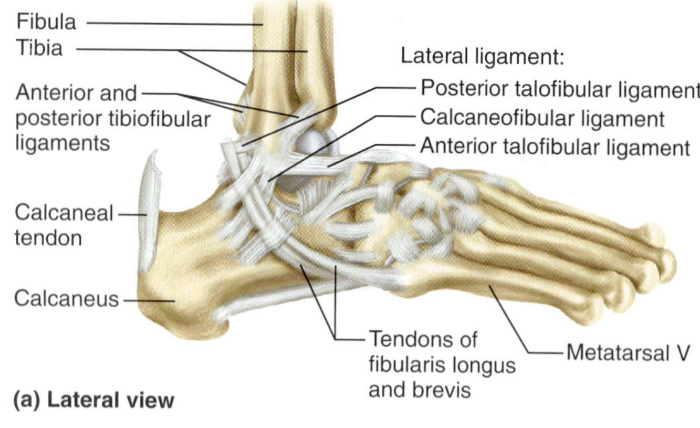

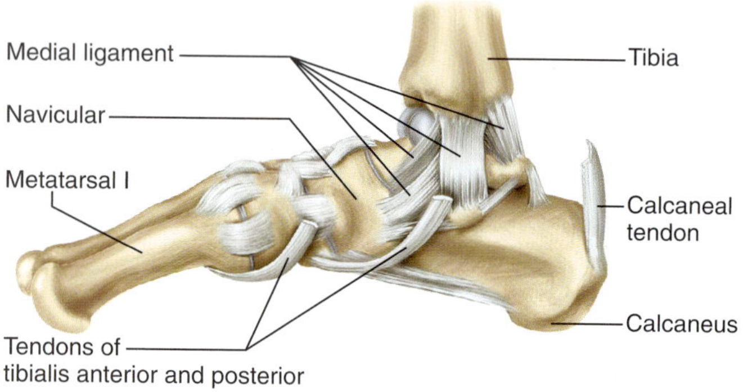

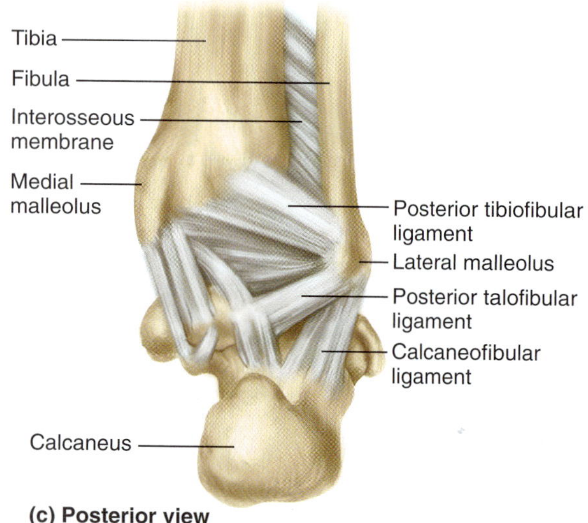

FIGURE 19.4 Right ankle joint views

these joints, there is a strong, dense interosseous membrane between the shafts of these two bones. Although only minimal movement is possible between these bones, the distal joint becomes sprained occasionally during heavy contact sports such as football. A sprain of the syndesmosis joint is commonly referred to as a *high ankle sprain* and primarily involves the anterior inferior tibiofibular ligament. With more severe injuries, the posterior tibiofibular ligament, interosseous ligament, and interosseous membrane may be secondarily involved.

The ankle joint, technically known as the **talocrural joint,** is a hinge or ginglymus-type joint (figure 19.4). Specifically, it is the joint made up of the talus, the distal tibia, and the distal fibula. The ankle joint allows approximately 50 degrees of plantar flexion and 15 to 20 degrees of dorsiflexion (figure 19.5). A greater range of dorsiflexion, particularly in weight bearing, is possible when the knee is flexed, as this reduces the tension of the biarticular gastrocnemius muscle. The fibula rotates on its axis 3 to 5 degrees externally with dorsiflexion of the ankle and 3 to 5 degrees internally during plantar flexion. The syndesmosis joint widens by approximately 1 to 2 millimeters during full dorsiflexion.

Inversion and eversion, although commonly thought to be ankle joint movements, technically occur in the **subtalar and transverse tarsal joints.** These joints, classified as gliding or arthrodial, combine to allow approximately 20 to 30 degrees of inversion and 5 to 15 degrees of eversion. There is minimal movement within the remainder of the intertarsal and tarsometatarsal arthrodial joints.

The phalanges join the metatarsals to form the **metatarsophalangeal (MP) joints,** which are classified as condyloid-type joints. The metatarsophalangeal joint of the great toe flexes 45 degrees and extends 70 degrees, whereas the interphalangeal (IP) joint can flex from 0 degrees of full extension to 90 degrees of flexion. The MP joints of the four lesser toes allow approximately 40 degrees of flexion and 40 degrees of extension. The MP joints also abduct and adduct minimally. The proximal interphalangeal (PIP) joints in the lesser toes flex from 0 degrees of extension to 35 degrees of flexion. The distal interphalangeal (DIP) joints flex 60 degrees and extend 30 degrees. There is much variation from joint to joint and from person to person in all of these joints.

CLINICAL NOTES

Ankle Sprain

Ankle sprains are one of the most common injuries among physically active people. Sprains involve the stretching or tearing of one or more ligaments. There are far too many ligaments in the foot and ankle to discuss in this text, but a few of the more important ankle ligaments are shown in figure 19.4. Ninety-five percent of all ankle sprains result from excessive inversion, which causes damage to the lateral ligamentous structures, primarily the anterior talofibular ligament and the calcaneofibular ligament. Although the fibula prevents most eversion sprains, excessive eversion forces can occur, causing injury to the deltoid ligament on the medial aspect of the ankle. Ankle sprains can be avoided by keeping the entire ankle strong and flexible. See Chapter 20 for more specific ligament and inversion sprain information.

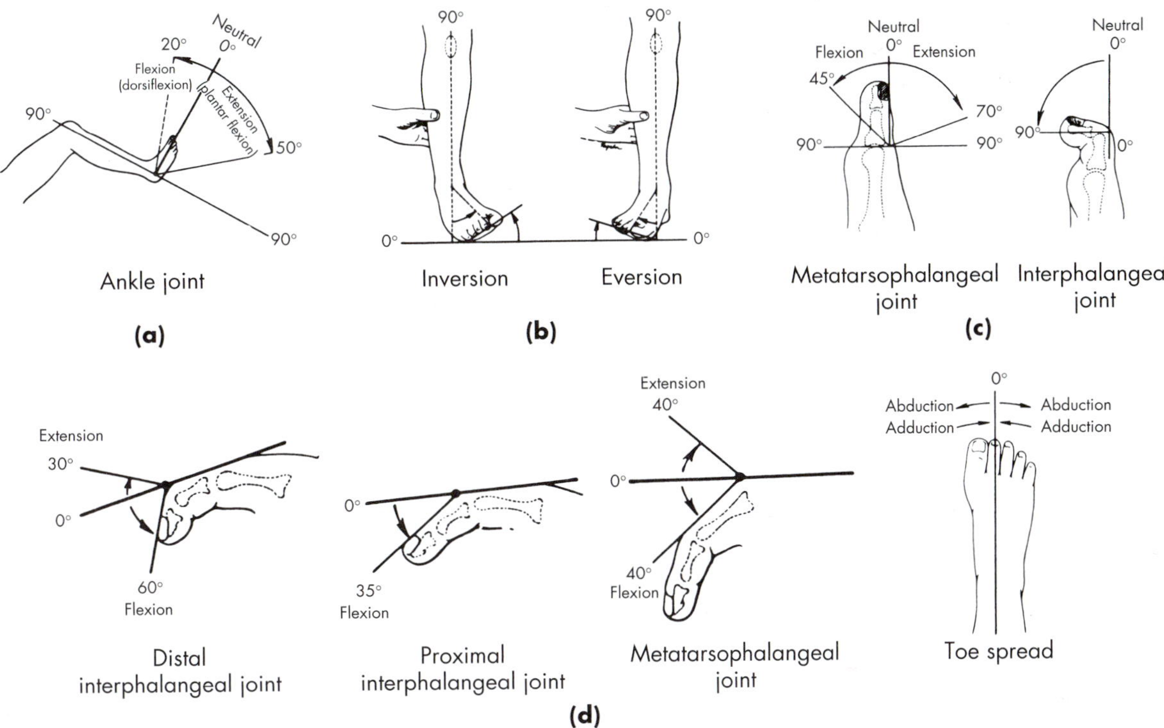

FIGURE 19.5 Active motion of the ankle, foot, and toes

Ligaments in the foot and the ankle maintain the position of an arch, which is also supported by the plantar fascia. All 26 bones in the foot are connected with ligaments. This brief discussion is focused on the longitudinal and transverse arches.

There are two longitudinal arches (figure 19.6). The **medial longitudinal arch** is located on the medial side of the foot and extends from the calcaneus bone to the talus, the navicular, the three cuneiforms, and the distal ends of the three medial metatarsals. The

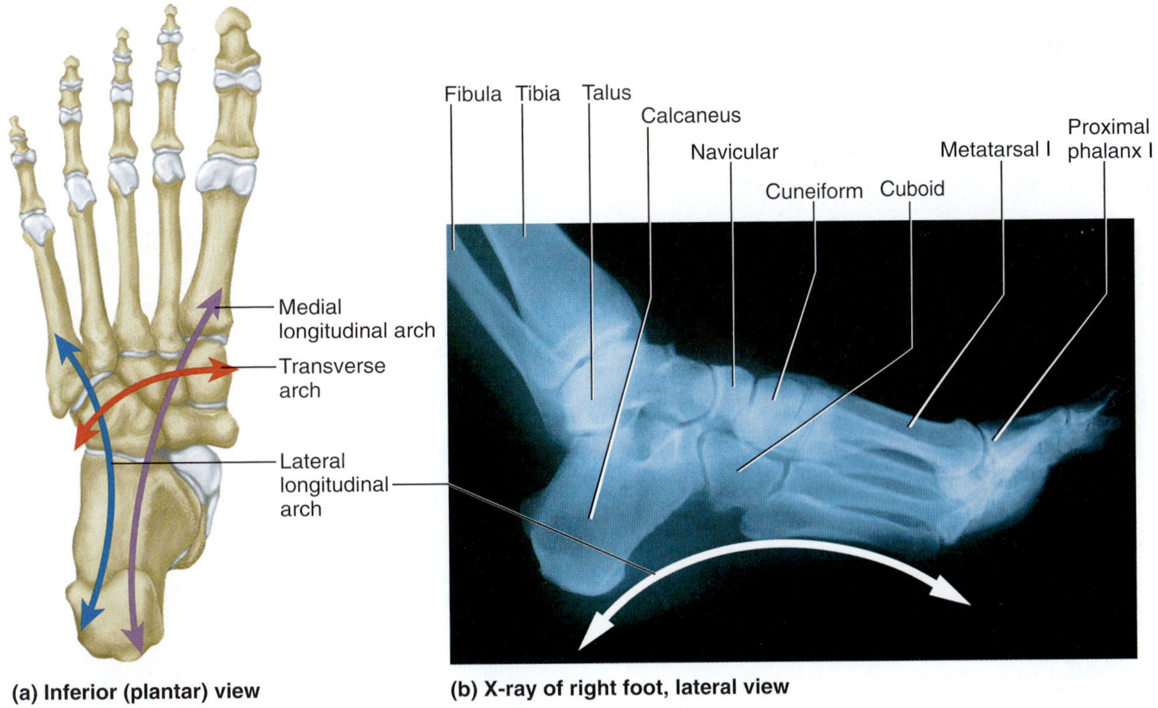

FIGURE 19.6 Arches of the foot

lateral longitudinal arch is located on the lateral side of the foot and extends from the calcaneus to the cuboid and distal ends of the 4th and 5th metatarsals. Individual long arches can be high, medium, or low, but a low arch is not necessarily a weak arch.

The **transverse arch** (figure 19.6) extends across the foot from one metatarsal bone to the other.

Movements

FLEXIBILITY & STRENGTH

Movements of the Foot and Ankle

Dorsiflexion (flexion)

Dorsal flexion; movement of the top of the ankle and foot toward the anterior tibia bone.

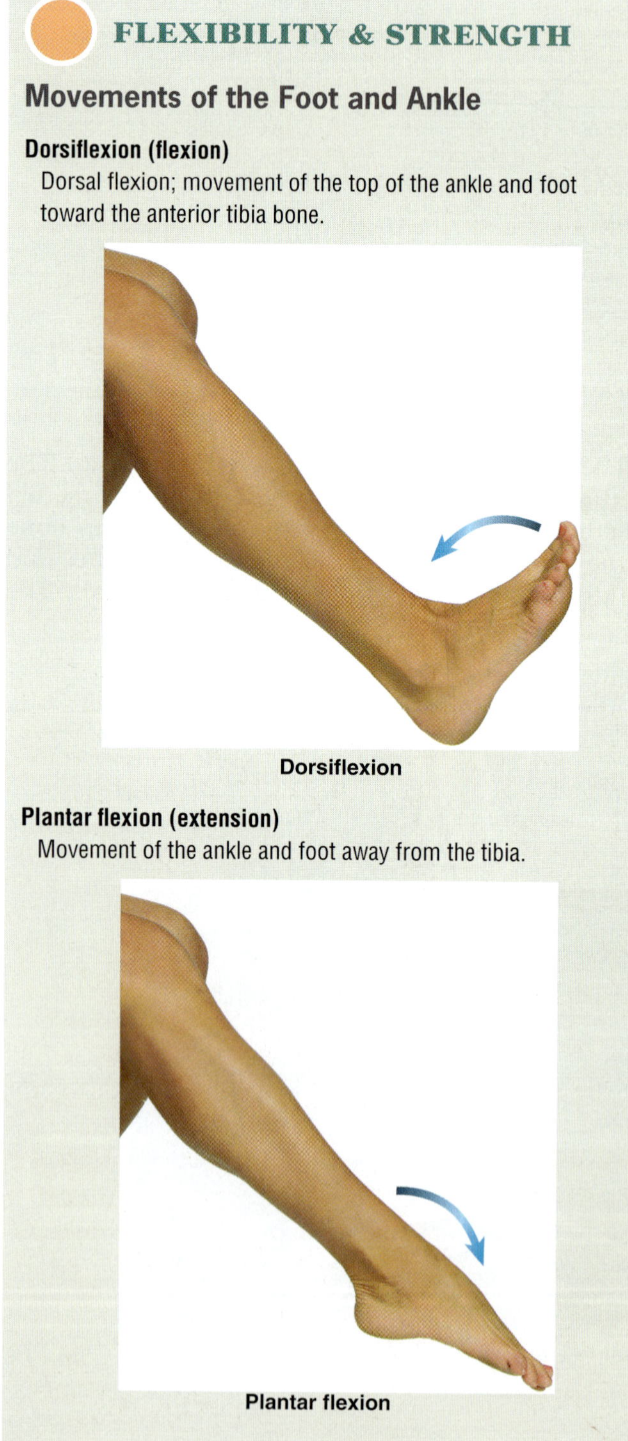

Dorsiflexion

Plantar flexion (extension)

Movement of the ankle and foot away from the tibia.

Plantar flexion

Eversion

Turning the ankle and foot outward; abduction, away from the midline. Weight is on the medial edge of the foot.

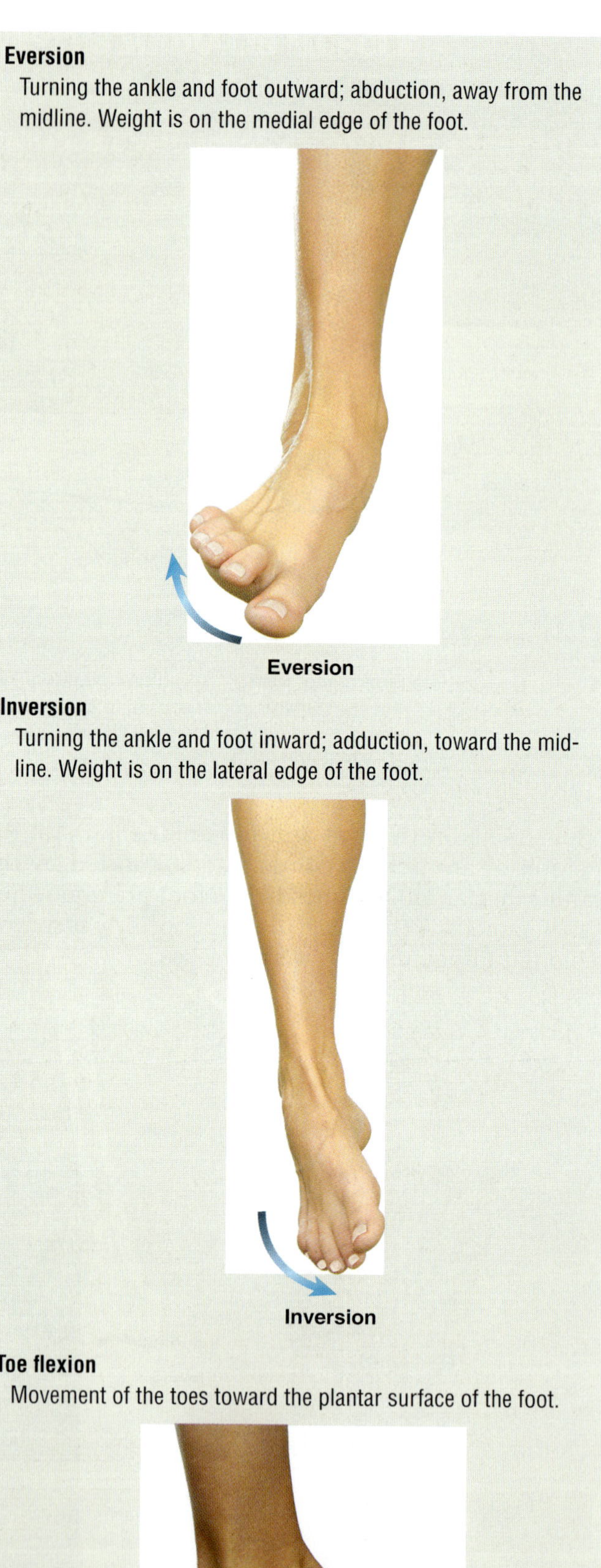

Eversion

Inversion

Turning the ankle and foot inward; adduction, toward the midline. Weight is on the lateral edge of the foot.

Inversion

Toe flexion

Movement of the toes toward the plantar surface of the foot.

Toe flexion

Toe extension
Movement of the toes away from the plantar surface of the foot.

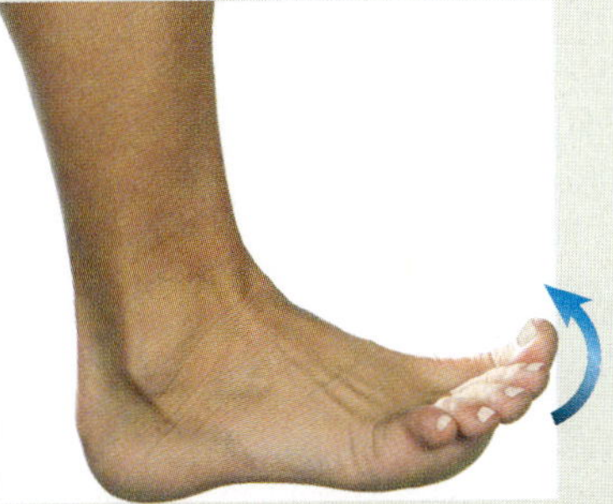

Toe extension

Pronation
A combination of ankle dorsiflexion, subtalar eversion, and forefoot abduction (toe-out).

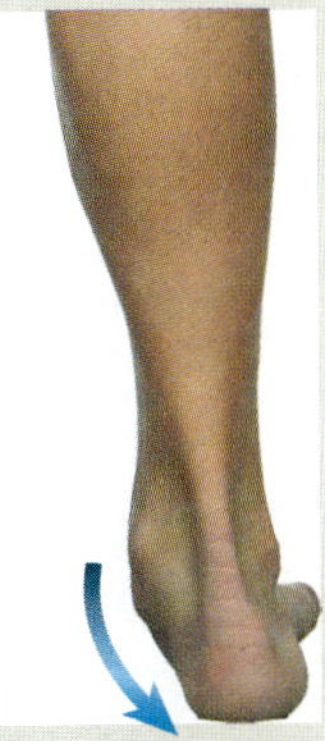

Pronation

Supination
A combination of ankle plantar flexion, subtalar inversion, and forefoot adduction (toe-in).

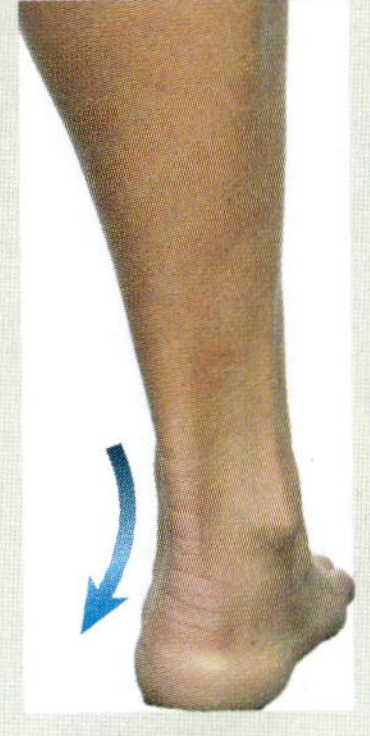

Supination

Ankle and Foot Muscles

The large number of muscles in the ankle and foot (figure 19.7) are easier to learn when grouped according to location and function. In general, the muscles located on the anterior aspect of the ankle and foot are the dorsal flexors. Those on the posterior aspect are plantar flexors. Specifically, the **gastrocnemius** and the **soleus** collectively are known as the **triceps surae,** due to their three heads, which join together to the **Achilles tendon.** Muscles that are evertors are located more to the lateral side, whereas the invertors are located medially.

The lower leg is divided into four compartments, each containing specific muscles. Tightly surrounding and binding each compartment is a dense fascia, which facilitates venous return and prevents excessive swelling of the muscles during exercise. The **anterior compartment** contains the dorsiflexor group, consisting of the **tibialis anterior, peroneus tertius, extensor digitorum longus,** and **extensor hallucis longus.** The **lateral compartment** contains the **peroneus longus** and **peroneus brevis**—the two most powerful evertors. Since *peroneus* is Greek for "fibula," anatomists have recently interchanged the terms *peroneus* and *fibularis;* hence the peroneus muscles also may be called *fibularis longus, fibularis brevis,* and *fibularis tertius.* The **posterior compartment** is divided into deep and superficial compartments. The gastrocnemius, soleus, and **plantaris** are located in the superficial posterior compartment, while the deep posterior compartment is composed of the **flexor digitorum longus, flexor hallucis longus,** popliteus, and **tibialis posterior.** The muscles of the superficial posterior compartment are primarily plantar flexors. The plantaris, absent in some humans, is a vestigial biarticular muscle that contributes minimally to ankle plantar flexion. The deep posterior compartment muscles, except for the popliteus, are plantar flexors, but they also function as invertors. (See figures 19.8, 19.9, and 19.10.)

Note: A number of the ankle and foot muscles are capable of helping produce more than one movement.

MUSCLE SPECIFIC

Muscles that move the ankle and foot—by function

Plantar flexors
- Gastrocnemius
- Flexor digitorum longus
- Flexor hallucis longus
- Peroneus (fibularis) longus
- Peroneus (fibularis) brevis
- Plantaris
- Soleus
- Tibialis posterior

(Continued)

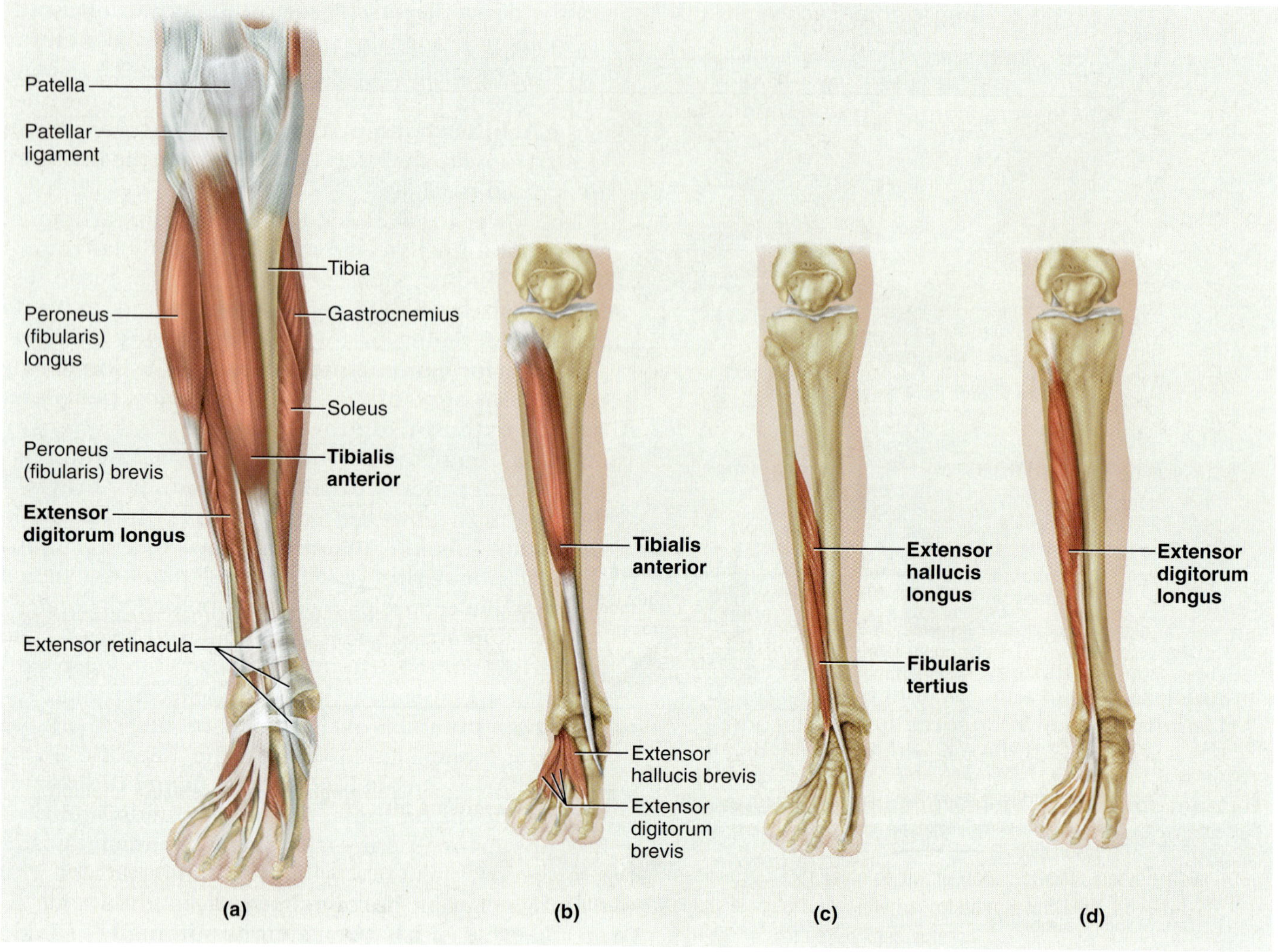

FIGURE 19.7 Muscles of the leg anterior compartment

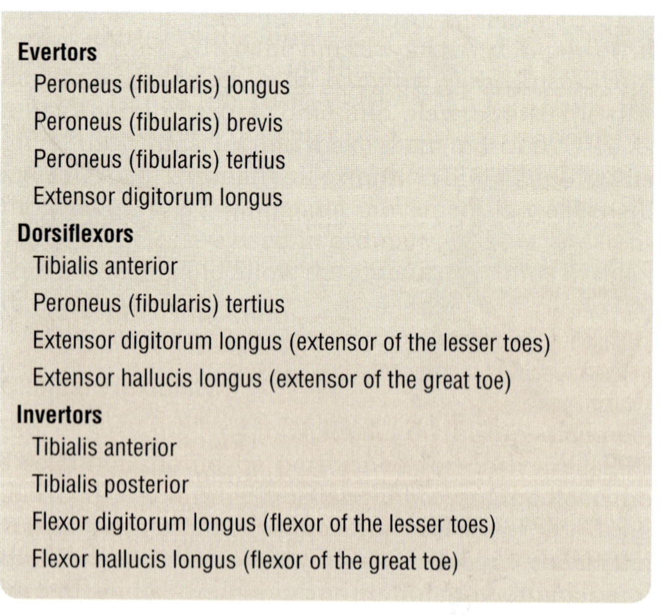

Evertors

- Peroneus (fibularis) longus
- Peroneus (fibularis) brevis
- Peroneus (fibularis) tertius
- Extensor digitorum longus

Dorsiflexors

- Tibialis anterior
- Peroneus (fibularis) tertius
- Extensor digitorum longus (extensor of the lesser toes)
- Extensor hallucis longus (extensor of the great toe)

Invertors

- Tibialis anterior
- Tibialis posterior
- Flexor digitorum longus (flexor of the lesser toes)
- Flexor hallucis longus (flexor of the great toe)

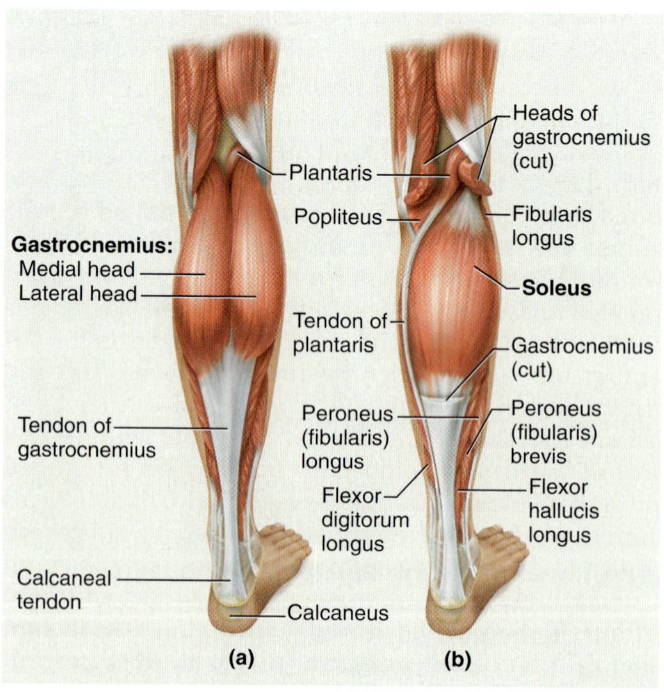

FIGURE 19.8 Superficial muscles of the leg posterior compartment

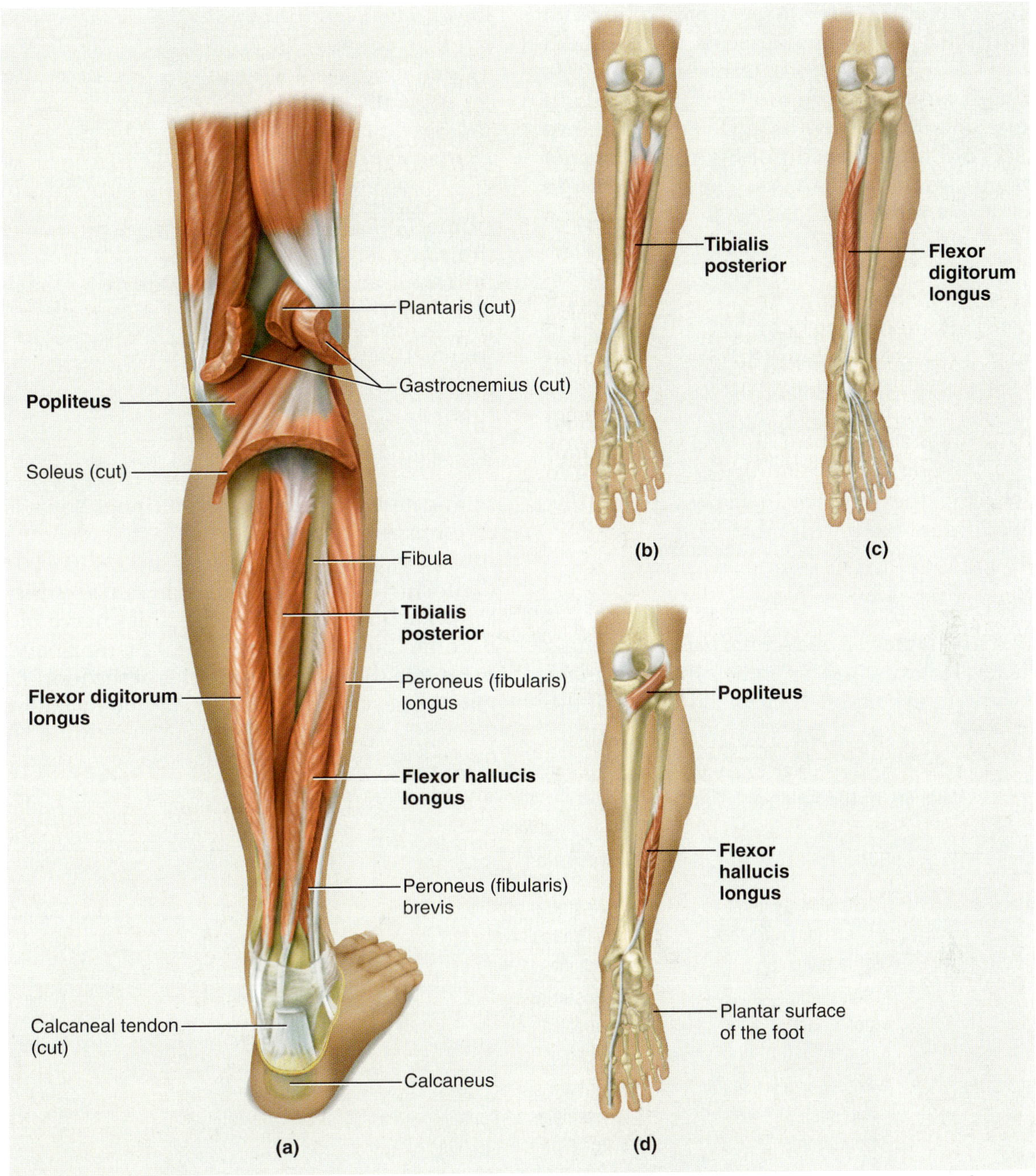

Plantaris (cut)
Gastrocnemius (cut)
Popliteus
Soleus (cut)
Fibula
Tibialis posterior
Peroneus (fibularis) longus
Flexor digitorum longus
Flexor hallucis longus
Peroneus (fibularis) brevis
Calcaneal tendon (cut)
Calcaneus
(a)

Tibialis posterior
(b)

Flexor digitorum longus
(c)

Popliteus
Flexor hallucis longus
Plantar surface of the foot
(d)

FIGURE 19.9 Deep muscles of the leg posterior and lateral compartments

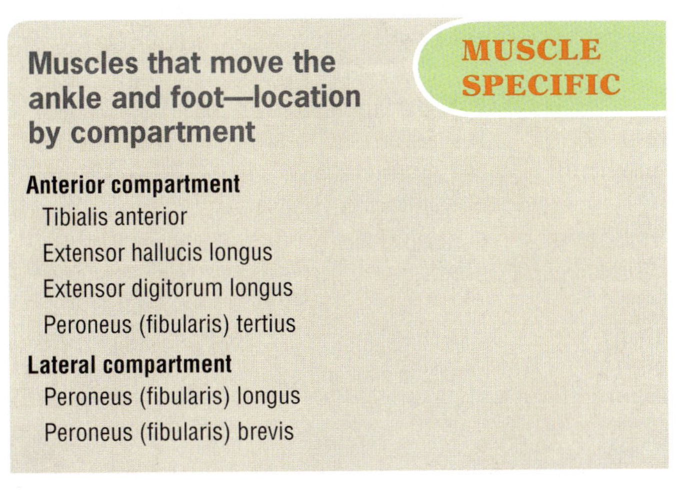

Muscles that move the ankle and foot—location by compartment

MUSCLE SPECIFIC

Anterior compartment
- Tibialis anterior
- Extensor hallucis longus
- Extensor digitorum longus
- Peroneus (fibularis) tertius

Lateral compartment
- Peroneus (fibularis) longus
- Peroneus (fibularis) brevis

Deep posterior compartment
- Flexor digitorum longus
- Flexor hallucis longus
- Tibialis posterior

Superficial posterior compartment
- Gastrocnemius (medial head)
- Gastrocnemius (lateral head)
- Soleus

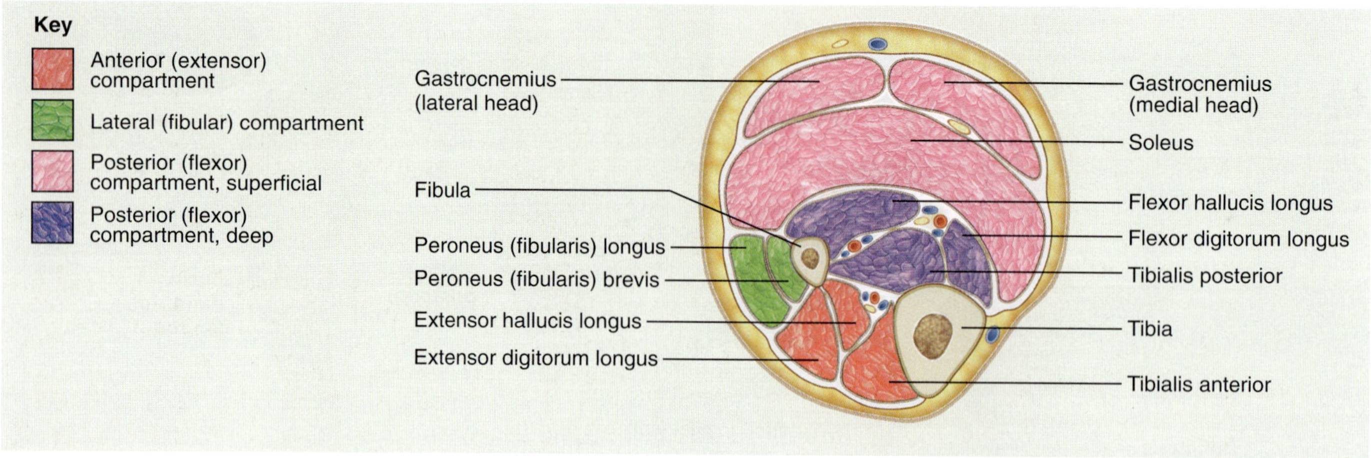

FIGURE 19.10 Cross section through the lower limb

While viewing the muscles in figures 19.8, 19.9, and 19.10, correlate them with table 19.1.

Nerves

As described in Chapter 15, the *sciatic nerve* originates from the sacral plexus and branches into the *tibial nerve* and the *peroneal nerve*. The tibial division of the sciatic nerve (figure 19.11) continues down to the posterior aspect of the lower leg to innervate the gastrocnemius (medial head), soleus, tibialis posterior, flexor digitorum longus, and flexor hallucis longus. Just before reaching the ankle, the tibial nerve branches to become the medial and lateral plantar nerves, which innervate the intrinsic muscles of the foot. The medial plantar nerve innervates the abductor hallucis, flexor

TABLE 19.1 Muscles of the Ankle and Foot Joints

Name of Muscle	Origins	Insertion	Actions	Innervations
Gastrocnemius	Medial and lateral posterior condyles of femur	Posterior surface of calcaneus via Achilles tendon	Plantar flexion of ankle, flexion of knee	Tibial nerve (S1, S2)
Soleus	Soleal line of tibia, posterior head and upper shaft of fibula	Posterior surface of calcaneus via Achilles tendon	Plantar flexion of ankle	Tibial nerve (S1, S2)
Tibialis posterior	Posterior tibia, fibula, and interosseous membrane	Plantar surface of navicular and cuneiform bones and base of 2nd, 3rd, 4th, and 5th metatarsal bones	Inversion and plantar flexion	Tibial nerve (L5, S1)
Flexor digitorum longus	Middle third of posterior tibia	Base of distal phalanx of each of four outer toes	Plantar flexion of ankle, flexion of four lateral toes at DIP joints, inversion of foot	Tibial nerve (L5, S1)
Flexor hallucis longus	Middle two-thirds of posterior surface of fibula	Plantar surface of base of distal phalanx of great toe	Plantar flexion of ankle and inversion of foot, plantar flexion of big toe	Tibial nerve (L5, S1–S2)
Peroneus longus	Head and lateral shaft of upper two-thirds of fibula	Base of 1st metatarsal and 1st medial cuneiform plantar surface	Eversion of foot, assists plantar flexion	Superficial peroneal nerve (L4–L5, S1)
Peroneus brevis	Lateral shaft of lower two-thirds of fibula	Tuberosity of lateral aspect of 5th metatarsal	Eversion of foot, assists in plantar flexion of ankle	Superficial peroneal nerve (L4–L5, S1)

TABLE 19.1 (Continued)

Name of Muscle	Origins	Insertion	Actions	Innervations
Peroneus tertius	With extensor digitorum longus, anterior distal third of fibula	Base of 5th metatarsal	Eversion of foot, assists dorsiflexion	Deep peroneal nerve (L4–L5, S1)
Tibialis anterior	Upper two-thirds of lateral surface of tibia	Base of 1st metatarsal and inner surface of medial cuneiform	Dorsiflexion and inversion of foot	Deep peroneal nerve (L4–L5, S1)
Extensor digitorum longus	Lateral condyle of tibia, head of fibula—proximal two-thirds of anterior shaft of fibula	Middle and distal phalanges of four lateral toes	Dorsiflexion of ankle, eversion of foot, extension of two to five outer toes	Deep peroneal nerve (L4–L5, S1)
Extensor hallucis longus	Middle two-thirds of medial surface of anterior fibula, interosseous membrane	Base of distal phalanx of great toe	Dorsiflexion of ankle, toe extension and inversion	Deep peroneal nerve (L4–L5, S1)

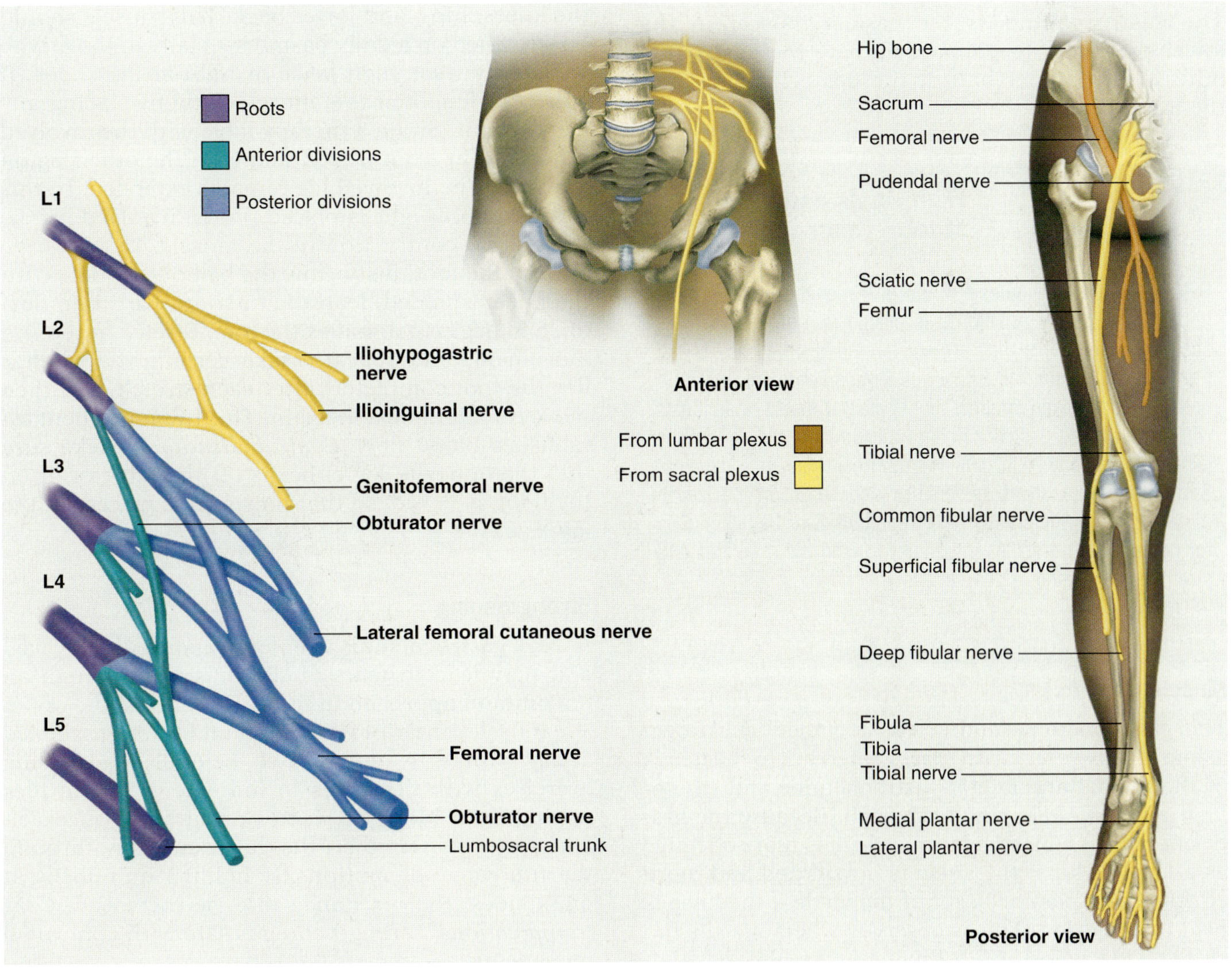

FIGURE 19.11 Lumbar plexus and nerves of the leg and foot

hallucis brevis, first lumbricale, and flexor digitorum brevis. The lateral plantar nerve supplies the adductor hallucis, quadratus plantae, lumbricales (2, 3 and 4), dorsal interossei, plantar interossei, abductor digiti minimi, and flexor digiti minimi.

The *peroneal,* or *fibular, nerve* (figure 19.11) divides just below the head of the fibula to become the superficial and deep peroneal nerves. The superficial branch innervates the peroneus longus and peroneus brevis, while the deep branch innervates the tibialis anterior, extensor digitorum longus, extensor hallucis longus, peroneus tertius, and extensor digitorum brevis.

Individual Muscles of the Leg, Ankle, and Foot—Posterior Compartment

GASTROCNEMIUS MUSCLE

Palpation

The gastrocnemius is the easiest muscle in the lower extremity to palpate. Palpate the gastrocnemius on the upper half of the posterior aspect of the lower leg.

CLINICAL NOTES **High Heels and Leg Muscle Contractures**

High heels are the nemesis of the posterior leg muscles. The body adapts to the position it is placed in, and the muscles shorten, especially if they are not stretched on a daily basis. Individuals with contracted gastrocnemius fibers are unable to perform dorsiflexion, and the foot is plantar-flexed. Individuals with a shortened gastrocnemius walk on their toes and have little push-off power in gait. Hammertoes also may develop. Some contractures are irreversible, depending on the length of time spent in the plantar-flexed position. See the techniques for posterior leg muscles in Chapter 20 and the exercises and stretches below and in Chapter 21.

Muscle Specifics

The gastrocnemius and soleus together are known as the *triceps surae,* with *triceps* referring to the heads of the medial and lateral gastrocnemius and the soleus and *surae* referring to the calf. Because the gastrocnemius is a biarticular muscle, it is more effective as a knee flexor if the ankle is dorsiflexed and more effective as a plantar flexor of the ankle if the knee is held in extension. This is observed when one sits too close to the wheel when driving a car; this position significantly shortens the entire muscle, reducing its effectiveness. When the knees are bent, the muscle becomes an ineffective plantar flexor, and it is more difficult to depress the brakes. Running, jumping, hopping, and skipping all depend significantly on the gastrocnemius and soleus to propel the body upward and forward.

Additionally, painful cramps caused by acute muscle spasms in the gastrocnemius and soleus are common, and they may be relieved through active stretching or deep pressure to the muscle fibers. Also, the complete rupture of the strong Achilles tendon, which connects these two plantar flexors to the calcaneus, can occur when these muscle tissues are shortened or in spasm.

Clinical Flexibility

Many people have a shortened gastrocnemius muscle. A limited gastrocnemius affects gait because push-off after the foot strikes the ground is limited; the body compensates by distributing vector forces to the knees, hips, and lower back. This muscle should be stretched on a daily basis, especially in those who frequently wear high heels or tight-fitting shoes. It is best to lengthen this muscle without placing any weight on it. Sit on a therapy table with the involved hip flexed in front of you and with the other leg on the floor. The involved leg remains extended. In this position no weight is placed on the involved leg, so there is no contraction in the muscle. Wrap a rope around the foot, just below the ball of the foot. With the knee extended, lean the torso forward into flexion and begin to dorsiflex the foot. Stretch at the end movement, and repeat. Make certain you plantar flex the foot completely after each stretch, and then move into dorsiflexion again. This full movement establishes blood flow. *Contraindications:* Make sure that the opposite leg either is off the table or, if on the floor, is flexed, so that no strain is placed on the low back.

Strengthening

A weak gastrocnemius will not support gait very well and may lead to tears of the muscle. Although an uncommon approach in fitness programs, the opposite muscle, anterior tibialis, should be strengthened along with this muscle (see below). Heel-raising exercises with the knees in full extension and toes resting on a block of wood or stairs are an excellent way to strengthen the gastrocnemius through the full range of motion. By holding dumbbells at one's sides, the resistance may be increased. *Contraindications:* Strengthening is safe with controlled movement.

OIAI MUSCLE CHART GASTROCNEMIUS (gas-trok-ne´mi-us) Greek for "belly"

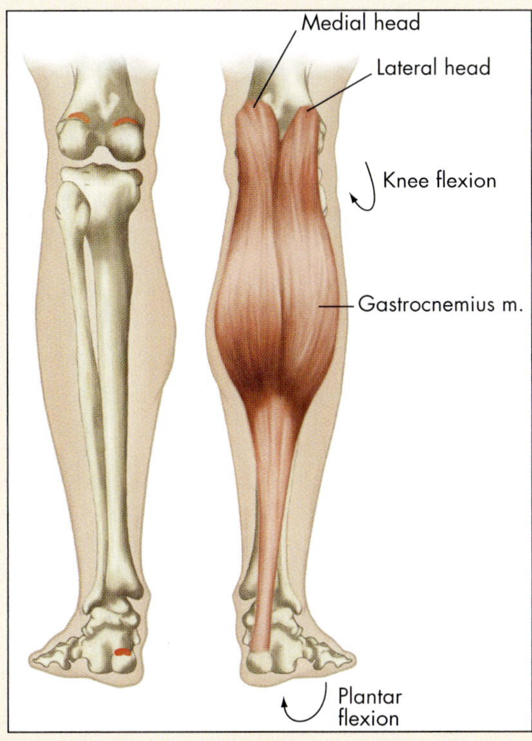

Name of Muscle	Origins	Insertion	Actions	Innervations
Gastrocnemius	Medial and lateral posterior condyles of femur	Posterior surface of calcaneus via Achilles tendon	Plantar flexion of ankle, flexion of knee	Tibial nerve (S1, S2)

SOLEUS MUSCLE

Palpation

Palpate the soleus posteriorly under the gastrocnemius muscle on the medial and lateral sides of the lower leg, particularly with the client in the prone position with the knee flexed approximately 90 degrees and during active plantar flexing of the ankle.

CLINICAL NOTES **Endangerment Zone**

Anterior to the heads of the gastrocnemius lies the soleus, a large flat muscle that covers the tibia and fibula. In the center of the muscle is the soleus canal, through which the tibial vein, artery, and nerve pass. The massage therapist should be cautious about applying pressure between the two heads of the gastrocnemius because of the proximity of the soleus canal and its vascular entities. See Chapter 20 for techniques to unwind the soleus and gastrocnemius muscles.

Muscle Specifics

The soleus muscle is one of the most important plantar flexors of the ankle, especially when the knee is flexed. When a person rises on the toes, the soleus muscle can plainly be seen on the outside of the lower leg, especially if this muscle is developed through exercise.

The soleus muscle is used whenever the ankle plantar flexes. Any movement with body weight on the foot and with the knee flexed or extended calls it into

OIAI MUSCLE CHART SOLEUS (so´le-us) Latin for "flat fish"

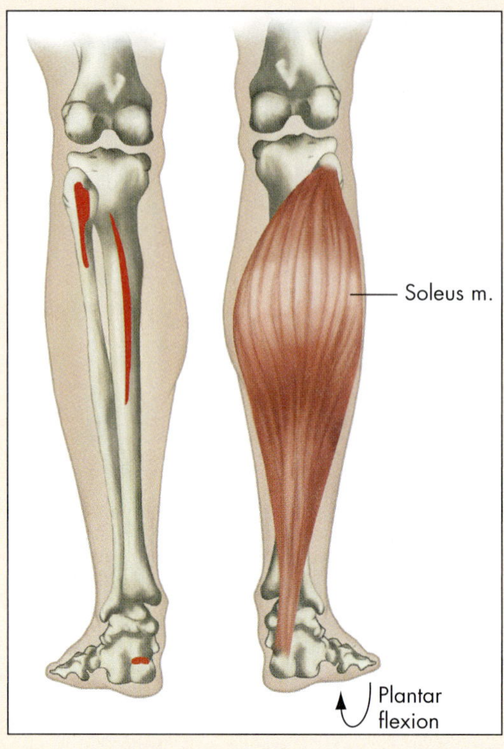

Name of Muscle	Origins	Insertion	Actions	Innervations
Soleus	Soleal line of tibia, posterior head and upper shaft of fibula	Posterior surface of calcaneus via Achilles tendon	Plantar flexion of ankle	Tibial nerve (S1, S2)

action. When the knee is flexed slightly, the effect of the gastrocnemius is reduced, thereby placing more work on the soleus. Running, jumping, hopping, skipping, and dancing on the toes are exercises that depend heavily on the soleus.

Clinical Flexibility

The soleus is stretched in the same manner as is the gastrocnemius, except that the knees must be flexed slightly. This releases the stretch on the gastrocnemius and places it more on the soleus. Flex the involved leg on the table, bringing the heel near the pelvis. Place your hands underneath the foot and dorsiflex up. The hands help stretch at the end movement. Repeat. *Contraindications:* This stretch is safe with controlled movement.

Strengthening

The soleus is strengthened the same way as gastrocnemius is, and it can be better isolated if the knee is flexed slightly to deemphasize the gastrocnemius.

TIBIALIS POSTERIOR MUSCLE

Palpation

The tendon for the tibialis posterior may be palpated both proximally and distally immediately behind the medial malleolus with inversion and plantar flexion; it is better distinguished from the flexor digitorum longus and flexor hallucis longus if the toes can be maintained in slight extension.

OIAI MUSCLE CHART TIBIALIS POSTERIOR (tib-i-a´lis pos-te´ri-or)

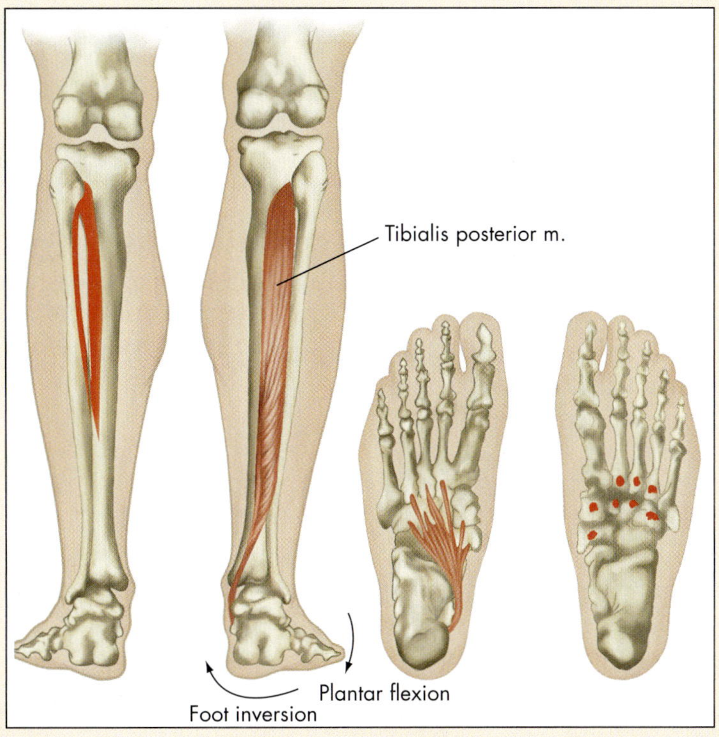

Name of Muscle	Origins	Insertion	Actions	Innervations
Tibialis posterior	Posterior tibia, fibula, and interosseous membrane	Plantar surface of navicular and cuneiform bones and base of 2nd, 3rd, 4th, and 5th metatarsal bones	Inversion and plantar flexion	Tibial nerve (L5, S1)

CLINICAL NOTES

Web of the Foot

The tibialis posterior is the deepest muscle of the posterior compartment. In fact, it is so deep that there is only the interosseous membrane separating it from the tibialis anterior. Because of its location and proximity to the anterior compartment muscles, it is easy to see why it might be involved in shin splints. (See the Clinical Notes for tibialis anterior.) Tibialis posterior is also intricately attached to seven bones at the bottom of the foot. When this muscle is chronically tight, it pulls on the arch of the foot, affecting the foot's placement in walking. Because it helps support the arch, it should be strengthened, especially in individuals with pes planus (flat feet). If any part of the tendinous insertion is torn or avulsed, it may need to be reattached surgically. The painful recovery requires no weight bearing for several months, as well as extensive physical and massage therapy and patience.

Muscle Specifics

Passing down the back of the leg, under the medial malleolus, and then forward to the navicular and medial cuneiform bones, the tibialis posterior muscle pulls down from the underside and, when contracted concentrically, inverts and plantar flexes the foot. As a result, it is in position to support the medial longitudinal arch. Use of the tibialis posterior muscle in plantar flexion and inversion gives support to the longitudinal arch of the foot.

Clinical Flexibility

The tibialis posterior may be stretched by moving the foot into extreme eversion during the gastrocnemius stretch described earlier.

Strengthening

The tibialis posterior muscle is generally strengthened by performing heel raises, as described for the gastrocnemius and soleus, as well as inversion exercises against resistance.

FLEXOR DIGITORUM LONGUS MUSCLE

Palpation

The tendon of the flexor digitorum longus may be palpated immediately posterior to the medial malleolus and tibialis posterior and immediately anterior to the flexor hallucis longus, with flexion of the lesser toes while maintaining great-toe extension, ankle dorsiflexion, and foot eversion.

CLINICAL NOTES **Cramps in the Bottom of the Foot**

The next time you are on a beach, try to pick some sand up with your toes. Flexor digitorum longus is at work with flexor hallucis longus curling the toes. If this position is held too long, it can lead to some serious cramping in the bottom of the foot, especially if the foot muscles are weak. This muscle must be included in any treatment for plantar fasciitis, as tightness in these flexor tendons will add to pain and dysfunction of the fascia. Dorsiflexion of the foot in combination with toe extension will stretch the toe flexors. See Clinical Flexibility on the next page for appropriate stretching.

OIAI MUSCLE CHART FLEXOR DIGITORUM LONGUS (fleks´or dij-i-to´rum long´gus) "Dick"

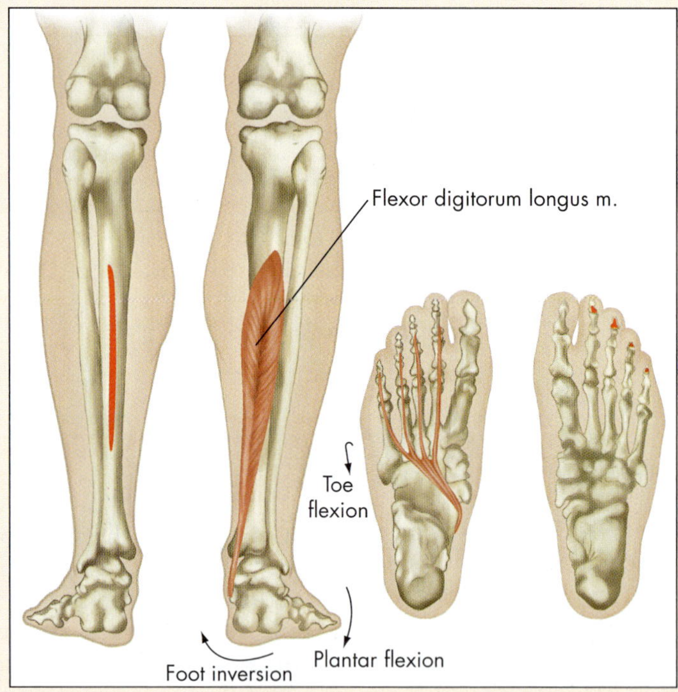

Name of Muscle	Origins	Insertion	Actions	Innervations
Flexor digitorum longus	Middle third of posterior tibia	Base of distal phalanx of each of four outer toes	Plantar flexion of ankle, flexion of four lateral toes at DIP joints; inversion of foot	Tibial nerve (L5, S1)

Muscle Specifics

Passing down the back of the lower leg under the medial malleolus and then forward, the flexor digitorum longus muscle draws the four lesser toes down into flexion toward the heel as it plantar flexes the ankle. It is very important in helping other foot muscles maintain the longitudinal arch. Walking, running, and jumping do not necessarily call the flexor digitorum longus muscle into action. Some weak foot and ankle conditions result from ineffective use of the flexor digitorum longus. Walking barefoot with the toes curled downward toward the heels and with the foot inverted will exercise this muscle.

Clinical Flexibility

The main belly of the flexor digitorum longus may be stretched by using the gastrocnemius stretch. To isolate its tendons on the four toes, actively take the four lesser toes into extreme extension while the foot is everted and dorsiflexed. You can assist with the hands and stretch each flexor tendon individually. This stretch is active because the extensors of the four toes are contracted to pull them up. Stretching the metatarsal tendons is helpful for foot dysfunctions such as plantar fasciitis.

Strengthening

Strengthen the flexor digitorum longus by performing towel grabs against resistance wherein the heel rests on the floor while the toes extend to grab a flat towel and then flex to pull the towel under the foot. This may be repeated numerous times, with a small weight placed on the opposite end of the towel for added resistance. This exercise is of great help for plantar fascia issues and pes planus. *Contraindications:* This exercise is safe with controlled movement. Cramping might occur in weak feet.

FLEXOR HALLUCIS LONGUS MUSCLE

Palpation

Palpate the flexor hallucis longus immediately behind the medial malleolus, between the medial soleus and the tibia, with active great-toe flexion while maintaining extension of the four lesser toes, ankle dorsiflexion, and foot eversion. Of the three tendons—flexor hallucis longus, tibialis posterior, and flexor digitorum longus—flexor hallucis longus is the most posterior.

CLINICAL NOTES **Follow the Big Toe**

The flexor hallucis longus (FHL) has an unpopular history associated with foot dysfunction. Gait is abnormal when the FHL is not working properly. This muscle's action is imperative to a smooth toe-off during gait. The FHL is injured frequently in ballet dancers, soccer players, and runners, as prolonged plantar flexion leads to tenosynovitis or tendinopathy. If this thick tendon becomes nodular, triggering of the great toe (hallux saltans) may develop; this often snowballs into hallux rigidus (immobile toe joint). Maintenance for this muscle includes stretching the flexor tendons and gastrocnemius, as well as using the towel exercise described for the flexor digitorum longus.

Muscle Specifics

Pulling from the underside of the great toe, the flexor hallucis longus muscle may work independently of the flexor digitorum longus muscle or in conjunction with it. If these two muscles are poorly developed, they cramp easily when they are called on to perform activities to which they are unaccustomed. These muscles are used effectively in walking if the toes are used (as they should be) in maintaining balance as each step is taken.

When the gastrocnemius, soleus, tibialis posterior, peroneus longus, peroneus brevis, flexor digitorum longus, flexor digitorum brevis, and flexor hallucis longus muscles are all used effectively in walking, ankle strength is evident. If an ankle and a foot are weak, in most cases the weakness is due to a lack of use of the muscles just mentioned. Running, walking, jumping, hopping, and skipping provide exercise for this muscle group.

Clinical Flexibility

The flexor hallucis longus may be stretched by actively taking the great toe into extreme extension. This is accomplished by using the hands to pull back the big toe and stretch the tendon at the end movement. With the other hand, push down on the four lateral toes into flexion so that the big toe is isolated during the movement. Stretching of the gastrocnemius is also helpful. *Contraindications:* These stretches are safe with controlled movement. Discomfort might be felt if tendinopathies are present.

Strengthening

The flexor hallucis longus muscle may be specifically strengthened by performing the towel grab-stretches described for the flexor digitorum longus.

OIAI MUSCLE CHART FLEXOR HALLUCIS LONGUS (fleks´or hal-u´sis long´gus) Big-toe flexor—"Harry"

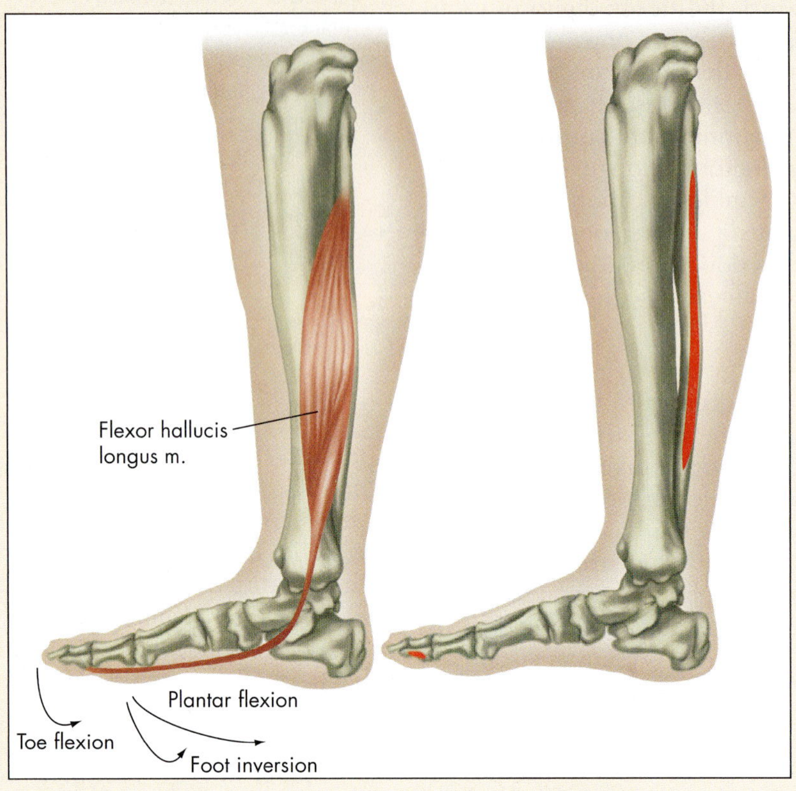

Name of Muscle	Origins	Insertion	Actions	Innervations
Flexor hallucis longus	Middle two-thirds of posterior surface of fibula	Plantar surface of base of distal phalanx of great toe	Plantar flexion of ankle and inversion of foot, plantar flexion of big toe	Tibial nerve (L5, S1–S2)

Individual Muscles of the Leg, Ankle, and Foot—Lateral Compartment

PERONEUS LONGUS MUSCLE

Palpation

Palpate the peroneus longus on the upper lateral side of the tibia, just distal to the fibular head and down to immediately posterior to the lateral malleolus and just posterolateral from the tibialis anterior and extensor digitorum longus, with active eversion.

CLINICAL NOTES **Binds the Arch**

When the peroneus longus muscle is used effectively with the other ankle flexors, it helps bind the transverse arch as it flexes. It also naturally opposes the tibialis anterior, as the two meet on the same insertion bones. This relationship requires balance in opposing tension, as imbalance will affect the position of the foot as it lands. A tight tibialis anterior pulls on the inside of the foot, lengthens the peroneus longus, and causes weight to shift to the lateral side of the foot. Frequent inversion sprains can weaken and stretch the peroneals, creating imbalance between the tibialis anterior and the peroneals. See Chapter 20 for techniques, and see Clinical Flexibility and Strengthening below and in Chapter 21.

Muscle Specifics

The peroneus longus muscle passes posteroinferiorly to the lateral malleolus and under the foot from the outside to under the inner surface. Because of its line of pull, it is a strong evertor and assists in plantar flexion.

Developed without the other plantar flexors, it would produce a weak, everted foot. In running, jumping, hopping, and skipping, the foot should be

OIAI MUSCLE CHART PERONEUS LONGUS (per-o-ne´us long´gus) Greek for "fibula"

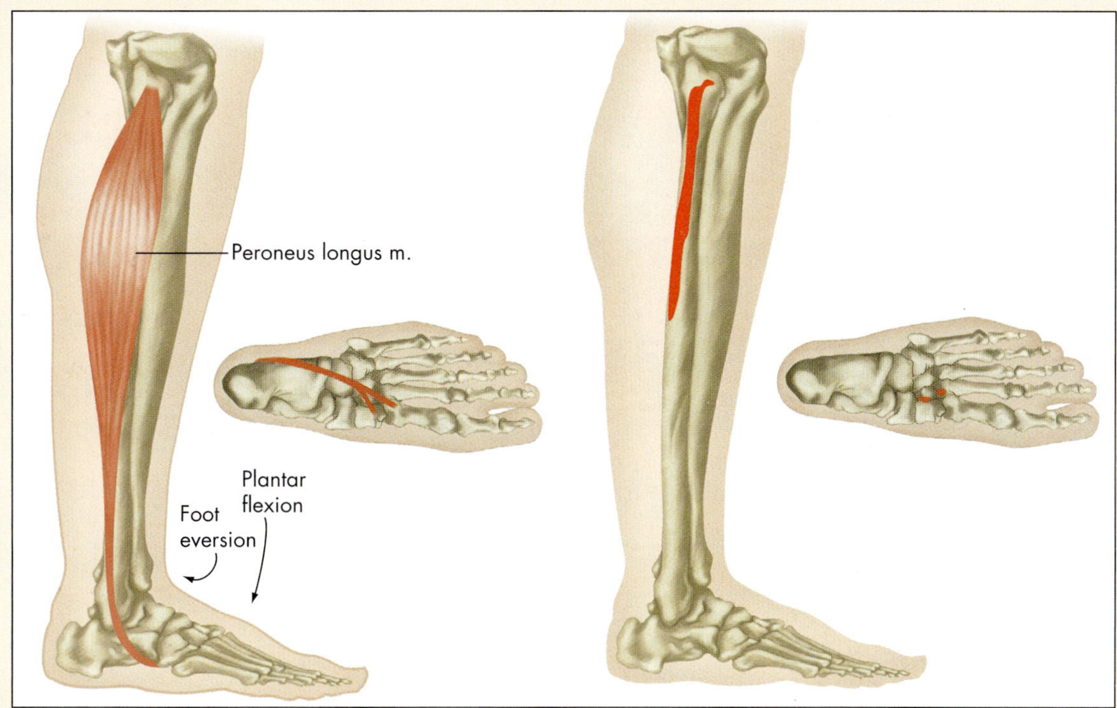

Name of Muscle	Origins	Insertion	Actions	Innervations
Peroneus longus	Head and lateral shaft of upper two-thirds of fibula	Base of 1st metatarsal and 1st medial cuneiform plantar surface	Eversion of foot, assists plantar flexion	Superficial peroneal nerve (L4–L5, S1)

placed so that it is pointing forward to ensure proper development of the group.

Clinical Flexibility

The peroneus longus may be stretched by moving the foot into extreme inversion and dorsiflexion while the knee is extended. While peroneus longus is hard to isolate, the gastrocnemius stretch will lengthen it with the foot in inversion. Use a rope to help hold the foot in inversion, and then dorsiflex the foot. This helps isolate the lateral side of the leg.

Strengthening

Eversion exercises to strengthen the peroneus longus may be performed by turning the sole of the foot outward while resistance is applied in the opposite direction. This is accomplished using a large sock filled with a weight. Tie the sock around the dorsal part of the foot, and sit at the end of a table with the feet hanging off the edge. Start with the foot in plantar flexion, with the toe pointed in. Lift the weight up into dorsiflexion, and try to evert the foot. Repeat, and return to the start position each time. *Contraindications:* This exercise is safe with controlled movement.

PERONEUS BREVIS MUSCLE

Palpation

Palpate the tendon of peroneus brevis at the proximal end of the 5th metatarsal, just proximal and posterior to the lateral malleolus and immediately deep anteriorly and posteriorly to the peroneus longus, with active eversion.

CLINICAL NOTES **Inversion Sprain**

An inversion sprain involves many structures of the foot in its severity, but it almost certainly will stretch, and possibly tear, fibers of the peroneus brevis. Edema reduces oxygen to

OIAI MUSCLE CHART PERONEUS BREVIS (per-o-ne´us bre´vis) Shorter evertor

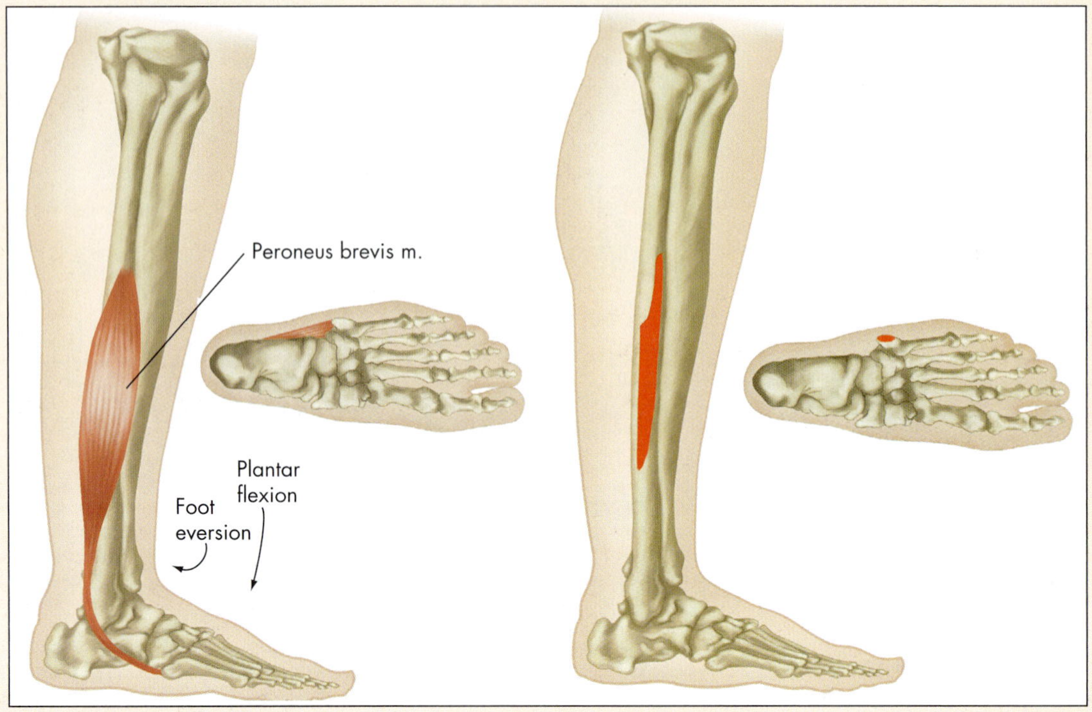

Name of Muscle	Origins	Insertion	Actions	Innervations
Peroneus brevis	Lateral shaft of lower two-thirds of fibula	Tuberosity of lateral aspect of 5th metatarsal	Eversion of foot, assists in plantar flexion of ankle	Superficial peroneal nerve (L4–L5, S1)

surrounding tissues and causes secondary trauma to muscles of the region. Inversion sprains can take a prolonged amount of time to heal because of the ligaments that may be involved and the trapped edema in the foot. See Chapter 20 for more on the inversion sprain and how to help resolve this trauma. Chapter 21 contains additional stretches and strengthening for the leg and foot muscles.

Muscle Specifics

The peroneus brevis muscle passes posteroinferiorly to the lateral malleolus to pull on the base of the 5th metatarsal. It is a primary evertor of the foot and assists in plantar flexion. In addition, it aids in maintaining the lateral longitudinal arch as it depresses the foot. The peroneus brevis muscle is exercised with other plantar flexors during running, jumping, hopping, and skipping.

Clinical Flexibility

The peroneus brevis is stretched in the manner described for the peroneus longus.

Strengthening

Strengthen the peroneus brevis in a fashion similar to that for the peroneus longus by performing eversion exercises, such as turning the sole of the foot outward against resistance.

PERONEUS TERTIUS MUSCLE

Palpation

Palpate peroneus tertius just medial to the distal fibula and lateral to the extensor digitorum longus tendon on the anterolateral aspect of the foot, down to the medial side of the base of the 5th metatarsal, with dorsiflexion and eversion.

OIAI MUSCLE CHART PERONEUS TERTIUS (per-o-ne´us ter´shi-us) Secret dorsiflexor

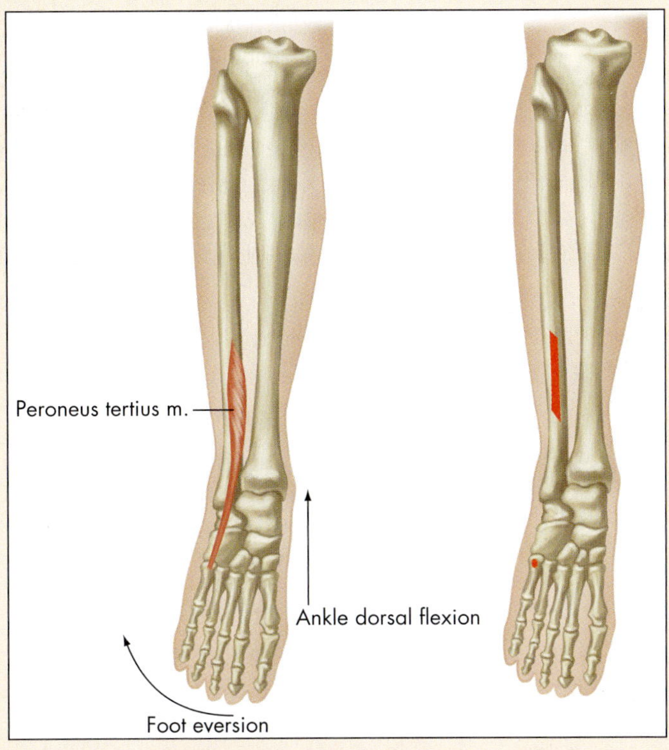

Name of Muscle	Origins	Insertion	Actions	Innervations
Peroneus tertius	With extensor digitorum longus, anterior distal third of fibula	Base of 5th metatarsal	Eversion of foot, assists dorsiflexion	Deep peroneal nerve (L4–L5, S1)

CLINICAL NOTES **The Small Helper**

This muscle, though small, is an important helper in eversion and dorsiflexion along with the larger muscles. Between 5 and 17 percent of the population does not have this muscle, and research has shown that these individuals are at risk for greater ankle injuries. For those who do have it, the muscle should be strengthened as an evertor and dorsiflexor by isolating these movements against resistance.

Muscle Specifics

The peroneus tertius, absent in some humans, is a small muscle that assists in dorsal flexion and eversion. Some authorities refer to it as the fifth tendon of the extensor digitorum longus.

Clinical Flexibility

The peroneus tertius may be stretched by moving the foot into extreme inversion and plantar flexion. The gastrocnemius stretch is suitable, but with the foot inverted during the movement.

Strengthening

Strengthen the peroneus tertius by pulling the foot up into dorsiflexion against a weight or resistance. The weighted-sock exercise is useful to help strengthen this muscle. Everting the foot against resistance, such as weighted eversion towel drags, can also be used for strength development.

Individual Muscles of the Ankle and Foot—Anterior Compartment

TIBIALIS ANTERIOR MUSCLE

Palpation

The tibialis anterior, the first muscle to the lateral side of the anterior tibial border, is particularly palpable with fully active ankle dorsiflexion; palpate the most prominent tendon of tibialis anterior as it crosses the ankle anteromedially.

CLINICAL NOTES **Shin Splints**

Due to heavy demands placed on the musculature of the legs during running activities, acute and chronic injuries are common. *Shin splints* is a common term used to describe a painful condition of the leg that is often associated with running. This condition is not a specific diagnosis but, rather, is attributed to a number of specific musculotendinous injuries. Most often the tibialis posterior, medial soleus, or tibialis anterior is involved, but the extensor digitorum longus may also contribute. Tightness in the anterior capsule of the tibia is also a culprit. Shin splints may be helped by stretching the plantar flexors and achieving a balance between opposing muscle groups. The anterior tibialis should always be strengthened along with the gastrocnemius, as the more powerfully developed calf muscle can exhaust the dorsiflexors.

Muscle Specifics

By its insertion, the tibialis anterior muscle is in a fine position to hold up the inner margin of the foot. However, as it contracts concentrically, it dorsiflexes the ankle and is used as an antagonist to the plantar

OIAI MUSCLE CHART TIBIALIS ANTERIOR (tib-i-a´lis ant-te´ri-or) Primary dorsiflexor

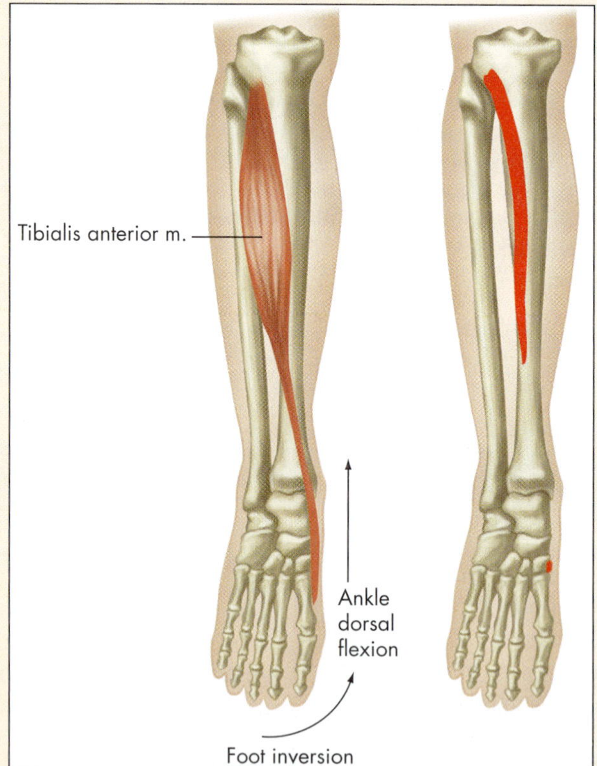

Name of Muscle	Origins	Insertion	Actions	Innervations
Tibialis anterior	Upper two-thirds of lateral surface of tibia	Base of 1st metatarsal and inner surface of medial cuneiform	Dorsiflexion and inversion of foot	Deep peroneal nerve (L4–L5, S1)

flexors of the ankle. The tibialis anterior is forced to contract strongly when a person ice skates or walks on the outside of the foot. It strongly supports the medial longitudinal arch in inversion. Walking in a hilly area will usually cause tenderness in the anterior capsule of the leg, especially if the person is not accustomed to this activity.

Clinical Flexibility

The tibialis anterior may be stretched by moving the foot into extreme plantar flexion. This is accomplished by sitting and crossing one leg over the other so that the ankle rests on the other leg. The foot is plantar-flexed as the hand assists in a gentle stretch to the anterior leg. The toes should also be flexed while performing this movement. *Contraindications:* This stretch is safe with controlled movement.

Strengthening

Use the weighted-sock exercise to strengthen this muscle. The foot should begin in an everted and plantar-flexed position. The weight is lifted into dorsiflexion and inversion.

EXTENSOR DIGITORUM LONGUS MUSCLE

Palpation

The extensor digitorum longus is the second muscle to the lateral side of the anterior tibial border; palpate the extensor digitorum longus on the upper lateral side of the tibia between the tibialis anterior medially and the fibula laterally. With active toe extension,

OIAI MUSCLE CHART EXTENSOR DIGITORUM LONGUS (eks-ten´sor dij-i-to´rum long´gus) Long toe extensors

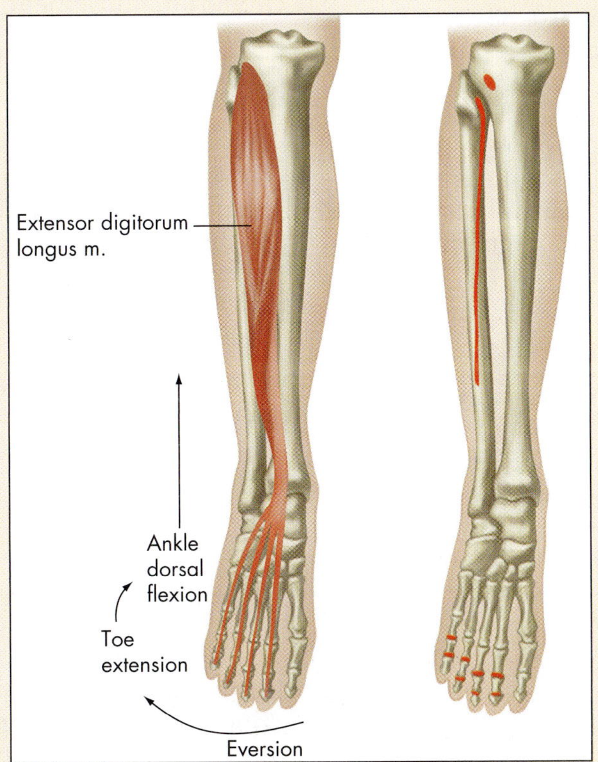

Name of Muscle	Origins	Insertion	Actions	Innervations
Extensor digitorum longus	Lateral condyle of tibia, head of fibula—proximal two-thirds of anterior shaft of fibula	Middle and distal phalanges of four lateral toes	Dorsiflexion of ankle, eversion of foot, extension of two to five outer toes	Deep peroneal nerve (L4–L5, S1)

this muscle divides into four tendons just distal to the anterior ankle.

CLINICAL NOTES **Extensor Issues**

Dorsiflexion and extension of the toes can cause cramping on the top of the foot, especially if weakness is present or the individual wears tight-fitting shoes. The peroneal nerve that supplies current to the top of the foot can be tweaked by inversion sprains. Weak muscles with damaged nerve innervation tend to cramp more often. Isolate toes 2 through 5 to better stretch the extensor tendons of this muscle. See Chapters 20 and 21 for techniques, exercises, and stretching routines.

Muscle Specifics

Strength is necessary in the extensor digitorum longus muscle to maintain balance between the plantar and the dorsal flexors. Action that involves dorsal flexion of the ankle and extension of the toes against resistance strengthens both the extensor digitorum longus and the extensor hallucis longus muscles. This may be accomplished by manually applying a downward force on the toes while attempting to extend them up.

Clinical Flexibility

The extensor digitorum longus may be stretched moving the four lesser toes into full flexion while the foot is inverted and plantar-flexed. Pressure is applied to the top of the toes as the flexion occurs, stretching the attachments of the extensor tendons. Move each toe separately into flexion while holding the other toes back. Use the thumb and fingers to apply a gentle stretch to each toe. *Contraindications:* This stretch is safe with controlled movement. Cramping might occur.

Strengthening

Use the weighted-sock exercise for the extensor digitorum longus. Move the toes into extension with the dorsiflexion during the stretch.

EXTENSOR HALLUCIS LONGUS MUSCLE

Palpation

Palpate the extensor hallucis longus from the dorsal aspect of the great toe to just lateral to the tibialis anterior and medial to the extensor digitorum longus at the anterior ankle joint.

CLINICAL NOTES **Equal Strength**

A tight extensor hallucis longus makes it almost impossible to flex the great toe. Toe flexors and extensors need to balance each other equally in strength to prevent cramping in either the top or the bottom of the foot. A subcutaneous rupture of the extensor hallucis longus tendon can occur in sports such as skiing.

Muscle Specifics

The four dorsiflexors of the foot—tibialis anterior, extensor digitorum longus, extensor hallucis longus, and peroneus tertius—are called into action when climbing stairs or while hiking. Dorsiflexion is an important movement; its strength should be balanced with the flexors.

Clinical Flexibility

The extensor hallucis longus may be stretched by moving the great toe into full flexion while the foot is everted and plantar-flexed. Apply pressure to the top of the toe as flexion occurs. *Contraindications:* This stretch is safe with controlled movement.

Strengthening

Extension of the great toe, as well as ankle dorsiflexion against resistance, will provide strengthening for the extensor hallucis longus. The weighted sock works well for this muscle. *Contraindications:* Strengthening is safe with controlled movement.

Intrinsic Muscles of the Foot

The intrinsic muscles of the foot (figure 19.12) have their origins and insertions on the bones within the foot. The extensor digitorum brevis is located on the dorsum of the foot, while the others are located in a plantar compartment in four layers on the plantar surface of the foot. The muscles located in the four layers are listed in the following box.

Four Layers **MUSCLE SPECIFIC**

First (superficial) layer

Abductor hallucis, flexor digitorum brevis, abductor digiti minimi (quinti)

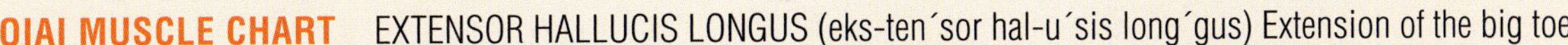

OIAI MUSCLE CHART EXTENSOR HALLUCIS LONGUS (eks-ten´sor hal-u´sis long´gus) Extension of the big toe

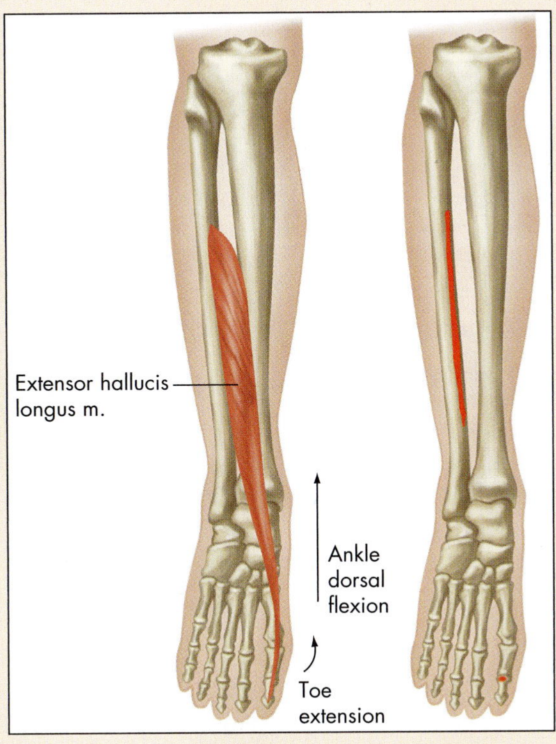

Name of Muscle	Origins	Insertion	Actions	Innervations
Extensor hallucis longus	Middle two-thirds of medial surface of anterior fibula, interosseous membrane	Base of distal phalanx of great toe	Dorsiflexion of ankle, toe extension and weak inversion	Deep peroneal nerve (L4–L5, S1)

Second layer
Quadratus plantae, lumbricales (four)

Third layer
Flexor hallucis brevis, adductor hallucis, flexor digiti minimi (quinti) brevis

Fourth (deep) layer
Dorsal interossei (four), plantar interossei (three)

The intrinsic foot muscles may be grouped by location as well as by the parts of the foot on which they act. The abductor hallucis, flexor hallucis brevis, and adductor hallucis all insert either medially or laterally on the proximal phalanx of the great toe. The abductor hallucis and flexor hallucis brevis are located somewhat medially, whereas the adductor hallucis is more centrally located beneath the metatarsals.

The quadratus plantae, four lumbricales, four dorsal interossei, three plantar interossei, flexor digitorum brevis, and extensor digitorum brevis are all somewhat centrally located. All are beneath the foot except the extensor digitorum brevis, which is the only intrinsic muscle in the foot located in the dorsal compartment. Although the entire extensor digitorum brevis has its origin on the anterior and lateral calcaneus, some anatomists refer to its first tendon as the extensor hallucis brevis in order to maintain consistency in naming according to function and location. It is often involved in severe ankle inversion sprains.

Located laterally beneath the foot are the abductor digiti minimi and the flexor digiti minimi brevis, both of which insert on the lateral aspect of the base of the proximal phalanx of the 5th phalange. Because of these two muscles' insertion and action on the 5th toe, the name *quinti* is sometimes used instead of *minimi*.

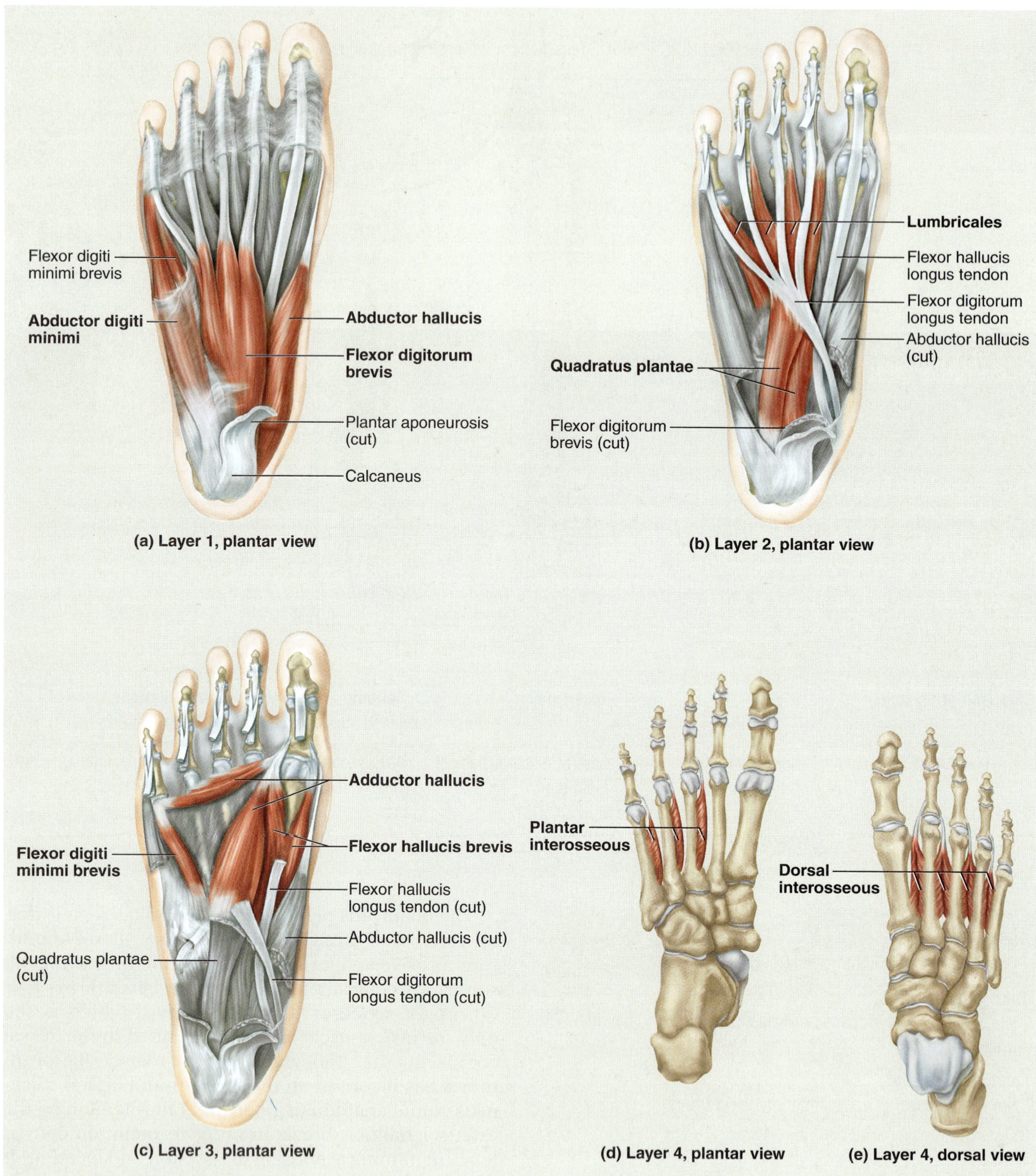

FIGURE 19.12 Intrinsic muscles of the foot

Four muscles act on the great toe. The abductor hallucis is solely responsible for abduction of the great toe, but it assists the flexor hallucis brevis in flexing the great toe at the metatarsophalangeal joint. The adductor hallucis is the sole adductor of the great toe, while the extensor digitorum brevis is the only intrinsic extensor of the great toe at the metatarsophalangeal joint.

The four lumbricales are flexors of the 2nd, 3rd, 4th, and 5th phalanges at their metatarsophalangeal joints, while the quadratus plantae are flexors of these phalanges at their distal interphalangeal joints. The three plantar interossei are adductors and flexors of the proximal phalanxes of the 3rd, 4th, and 5th phalanges, while the four dorsal interossei are abductors and flexors of the 2nd, 3rd, and 4th phalanges, also at their metatarsophalangeal joints. The flexor digitorum brevis flexes the middle phalanxes of the 2nd, 3rd, 4th, and 5th phalanges. The extensor digitorum brevis, as previously mentioned, is an extensor of the great toe but also extends the 2nd, 3rd, and 4th phalanges at their metatarsophalangeal joints.

There are two muscles that act solely on the 5th toe. The proximal phalanx of the 5th phalange is abducted by the abductor digiti minimi and is flexed by the flexor digiti minimi brevis.

Refer to table 19.2 for further details regarding the intrinsic muscles of the foot.

Many upper- and lower-extremity issues can be helped by looking at the intrinsic muscles of the foot. Muscles are developed and maintain their strength only when they are used. A lack of exercise to develop

TABLE 19.2 Intrinsic Muscles of the Foot

	Muscle	Origin	Insertion	Action	Palpation	Innervation
Superficial layer	Flexor digitorum brevis	Tuberosity of calcaneus, plantar aponeurosis	Medial and lateral aspects of 2nd, 3rd, 4th, 5th middle phalanxes	MP and PIP flexion of 2nd, 3rd, 4th, and 5th phalanges	Cannot be palpated	Medial plantar nerve (L4, L5)
	Abductor digiti minimi (quinti)	Tuberosity of calcaneus, plantar aponeurosis	Lateral aspect of 5th proximal phalanx	MP abduction of 5th phalange	Cannot be palpated	Lateral plantar nerve (S1, S2)
	Flexor hallucis brevis	Cuboid, lateral cuneiform	*Medial head:* medial aspect of 1st proximal phalanx *Lateral head:* lateral aspect of 1st proximal phalanx	MP flexion of 1st phalange	Cannot be palpated	Medial plantar nerve (L4, L5, S1)
	Abductor hallucis	Tuberosity of calcaneus, flexor retinaculum, plantar aponeurosis	Medial aspect of base of 1st proximal phalanx	MP flexion, abduction of 1st phalanx	On the plantar aspect of the foot from medial tubercle of calcaneus to medial side of great toe proximal phalanx with great toe abduction	Medial plantar nerve (L4, L5)

(Continued)

TABLE 19.2 (Continued)

	Muscle	Origin	Insertion	Action	Palpation	Innervation
Second layer	Flexor digiti minimi (quinti brevis)	Base of 5th metatarsal, sheath of peroneus longus tendon	Lateral aspect of base of 5th proximal phalanx	MP flexion of 5th phalange	Cannot be palpated	Lateral plantar nerve (S2, S3)
	Quadratus plantae	*Medial head:* medial surface of calcaneus *Lateral head:* lateral border of inferior surface of calcaneus	Lateral margin of flexor digitorum longus tendon	DIP flexion of 2nd, 3rd, 4th, and 5th phalanges	Cannot be palpated	Lateral plantar nerve (S1, S2)
	Lumbricales (4)	Tendons of flexor digitorum longus	Dorsal surface of 2nd, 3rd, 4th, and 5th proximal phalanxes	MP flexion of 2nd, 3rd, 4th, and 5th phalanges	Cannot be palpated	1st lumbricales: medial plantar nerve (L4, L5) 2nd, 3rd, 4th lumbricales: lateral plantar nerve (S1, S2)
Third layer	Adductor hallucis	*Oblique head:* 2nd, 3rd, and 4th metatarsals and sheath of peroneus longus tendon *Transverse head:* plantar metatarsophalangeal ligaments of 3rd, 4th, and 5th phalanges and transverse metatarsal ligaments	Lateral aspect of base of 1st proximal phalanx	MP adduction of 1st phalange	Cannot be palpated	Lateral plantar nerve (S1, S2)
	Plantar interossei (3)	Bases and medial shafts of 3rd, 4th, and 5th metatarsals	Medial aspects of bases of 3rd, 4th, and 5th proximal phalanxes	MP adduction and flexion of 3rd, 4th, and 5th phalanges	Cannot be palpated	Lateral plantar nerve (S1, S2)
Dorsal layer	Dorsal interossei (4)	Two heads on shafts of adjacent metatarsals	*1st interossei:* medial aspect of 2nd proximal phalanx *2nd, 3rd, and 4th interossei:* lateral aspect of 2nd, 3rd, and 4th proximal phalanxes	MP abduction and flexion of 2nd, 3rd, and 4th phalanges	Cannot be palpated	Lateral plantar nerve (S1, S2)
	Extensor digitorum brevis	Anterior and lateral calcaneus, lateral talocalcaneal ligament, inferior extensor retinaculum	Base of proximal phalanx of 1st phalange, lateral sides of extensor digitorum longus tendons of 2nd, 3rd, and 4th phalanges	Assists in MP extension of 1st phalanx and extension of middle three phalanges	As a mass anterior to and slightly below lateral malleolus on dorsum of foot	Deep peroneal nerve (L5, S1)

these muscles is one primary factor involved in the increase of weak-foot conditions. The feet are often forgotten in conditioning programs, mainly because the focus in conditioning programs remains on the larger muscle groups. Maintaining flexibility in these intrinsic muscles can help alleviate common foot ailments such as plantar fasciitis. The dorsal and plantar aspects of the foot should remain pliable as one ages, as a rigid foot does not support proper gait and places excessive force on the entire body. Walking is one of the best activities for maintaining and developing the many small muscles that help support the arch of the foot. Yet a more concentrated daily effort to stretch the foot muscles is ideal. Growing evidence suggests that walking without shoes or with newer shoes designed to enhance proper mechanics can help correct foot dysfunctions, as can applying the stretching and strengthening exercises described in this chapter.

CHAPTER *summary*

Introduction

- ✔ Appropriate shoes can support the feet and help with foot and gait mechanics.
- ✔ The gait cycle is divided into stance and swing phases.
- ✔ Designed for propulsion and support, the foot has 26 bones, 19 large muscles, many small intrinsic muscles, and more than 100 ligaments.

Bones

- ✔ There are 26 bones of the foot and ankle, not including the tibia and fibula.
- ✔ The tarsals include the calcaneus, talus, navicular, cuboid, and three cuneiforms. There are 5 metatarsals and 14 phalanges that form the toes.
- ✔ The ankle bones are the distal tibia and fibula bones, called the medial malleolus and lateral malleolus, respectively.

Joints

- ✔ The tibia and fibula form the tibiofibular joint, which is held together by ligaments.
- ✔ The ankle joint is the talocrural joint, a hinge joint.
- ✔ Inversion and eversion occur in the subtalar and transverse tarsal joints.
- ✔ Phalanges are hinge joints, and the metatarsophalangeal joints are condyloid-type joints.
- ✔ There are more than 100 ligaments in the ankle and foot. Ligaments can become injured in ankle sprains.
- ✔ There are two longitudinal arches and a transverse arch.

Movements

- ✔ Ankle and foot joint movements include dorsiflexion, plantar flexion, inversion, eversion, toe flexion, toe extension, supination, and pronation.
- ✔ Supination and pronation are combined movements.

Ankle and Foot Muscles

- ✔ The gastrocnemius, soleus, and plantaris are located in the posterior compartment and plantar flex the ankle and foot.
- ✔ The tibialis posterior, flexor digitorum, and flexor hallucis longus are located in the deep posterior compartment.
- ✔ The peroneals are located in the lateral compartment. They are the peroneus longus and brevis. The peroneals evert the foot and ankle.
- ✔ The tibialis anterior, extensor digitorum longus, extensor hallucis longus, and peroneus tertius are in the anterior compartment. The tibialis anterior is a primary dorsiflexor and inverts the foot.

Nerves

- ✔ The sciatic nerve comes from the sacral plexus and branches into the tibial and peroneal divisions.
- ✔ The tibial division innervates the posterior leg, including the gastrocnemius, soleus, tibialis posterior, flexor digitorum longus, and flexor hallucis longus.
- ✔ The peroneal nerve divides to become the superficial and deep peroneal nerves.
- ✔ The superficial peroneal nerve innervates the peroneus longus and brevis.
- ✔ The deep peroneal nerve innervates the tibialis anterior, extensor digitorum longus, extensor hallucis longus, peroneus tertius, and extensor digitorum brevis.

Individual Muscles of the Leg, Ankle, and Foot—Posterior Compartment

- ✔ *Gastrocnemius* shapes the posterior calf with two heads coming from the medial and lateral condyles of the femur and inserting in the Achilles tendon at the calcaneus. The muscle flexes the knee or plantar flexes the foot.
- ✔ *Soleus* gives a foundation to the gastrocnemius in the posterior compartment. It is a true plantar flexor, as it begins on the tibia and fibula and inserts with the gastrocnemius in the Achilles tendon at the calcaneus.
- ✔ *Tibialis posterior* is a deep posterior compartment muscle that is attached to the posterior tibia, fibula, and interosseous membrane. It inserts in the bottom of the foot like a web and plantar flexes the ankle and inverts the foot.

- ✔ *Flexor digitorum longus* is a deep posterior compartment muscle that spans from the posterior surface of the tibia and inserts at the base of the distal phalanx of the four toes. The flexor digitorum longus flexes the toes, inverts the foot, and plantar flexes the ankle.
- ✔ *Flexor hallucis longus* comes from the posterior surface of the fibula and inserts on the base of the distal phalanx of the great toe. It flexes the great toe and assists in inversion of the foot and plantar flexion of the ankle.

Individual Muscles of the Leg, Ankle, and Foot—Lateral Compartment

- ✔ *Peroneus longus* spans the length of the fibula and dives under the foot at the 5th metatarsal, runs the width of the foot, and inserts on the medial arch on the same bones as does tibialis anterior. Peroneus longus everts and plantar flexes the foot.
- ✔ *Peroneus brevis,* shorter than the longus, also begins on the fibula and inserts on the base of the 5th metatarsal. It assists the longus in eversion and plantar flexion.

Individual Muscles of the Ankle and Foot—Anterior Compartment

- ✔ *Tibialis anterior* has its origin on the anterior lateral surface of the tibia. It inserts on the medial arch at the medial cuneiform and the base of the 1st metatarsal bone. Tibialis anterior is a strong dorsiflexor of the ankle and inverts the foot.
- ✔ *Extensor digitorum longus* comes from the lateral condyle of the tibia and portions of the fibula. It inserts on the top and middle of the distal phalanges of the four toes. Its actions include extension of the toes and dorsiflexion of the ankle, and it assists with eversion of the foot.
- ✔ *Extensor hallucis longus* comes from the fibula and inserts at the base of the distal phalanx of the great toe. It extends the great toe, dorsiflexes the ankle, and assists in weak inversion of the foot.
- ✔ *Peroneus tertius* has a more anterior presentation than do the longus and brevis and thus is included as a dorsiflexor as well as an evertor. Like the peroneus brevis, it inserts on the base of the 5th metatarsal.

CHAPTER *review*

Worksheet Exercises

As an aid to learning, for in-class or out-of-class assignments, or for testing, tear-out worksheets are found at the end of the text, on pages 547–550.

True or False

Write true *or* false *after each statement.*

1. There are eight metatarsals.
2. The tibialis posterior and soleus insert in the Achilles tendon.
3. The peroneus tertius dorsiflexes the ankle.
4. The soleus is the true plantar flexor of the ankle.
5. The extensor digitorum brevis is an intrinsic muscle on the dorsum of the foot.
6. The medial and lateral condyles of the femur are the origins of the gastrocnemius muscle.
7. The tibial division of the sciatic nerve innervates the peroneals.
8. The tendon of the tibialis anterior can be seen on the top of the foot during dorsiflexion.
9. The gastrocnemius and soleus form the triceps surae.
10. The medial and lateral malleoli are formed from the talus and calcaneus.
11. The extensor hallucis longus inserts on the plantar surface of the great toe.

Short Answers

Write your answers on the lines provided.

1. Name the tarsal bones.

____

____

____

2. Name the heel of the foot.

____

____

____

3. What type of joint is the tibiofibular joint?

____

____

____

4. Which muscles are in the anterior compartment?

____

____

____

5. Name the muscles in the lateral compartment.

____

____

____

6. What nerve supplies the top of the foot?

____

____

____

7. List the muscles that dorsiflex the ankle.

____

____

____

8. List the muscles that invert the foot.

____

____

____

9. Name the nerve that innervates the gastrocnemius and soleus.

____

____

____

10. List the muscles that evert the foot.

____

____

____

Multiple Choice

Circle the correct answers.

1. How many bones are in the foot and ankle?
   a. 26
   b. 32
   c. 14
   d. none of the above
2. The two muscles that support the transverse arch are:
   a. extensor hallucis longus and flexor hallucis longus
   b. plantaris and gastrocnemius
   c. peroneus longus and tibialis anterior
   d. none of the above
3. The peroneus brevis inserts on:
   a. the talus
   b. the calcaneus
   c. the 5th metatarsal
   d. none of the above
4. The primary dorsiflexor of the ankle is:
   a. tibialis anterior
   b. gastrocnemius
   c. tibialis posterior
   d. none of the above
5. The flexor hallucis longus originates on:
   a. the posterior surface of the femur
   b. the posterior surface of the fibula
   c. the posterior surface of the tibia
   d. none of the above
6. Primary muscles that evert the foot are:
   a. tibialis anterior and peroneus longus
   b. peroneus longus, brevis, and tertius
   c. tibialis posterior and tibialis anterior
   d. none of the above
7. Inversion and eversion are performed by the:
   a. tibiofibular joint
   b. subtalar and transverse tarsal joints
   c. talocrural joint
   d. metatarsophalangeal joint
8. In order to invert, the foot muscles must cross what side of the foot?
   a. medial
   b. dorsal
   c. lateral
   d. lateral malleolus
9. The tibialis posterior inserts on:
   a. the 5th metatarsal
   b. the plantar surface of the navicular and cuneiform bones and bases of the 2nd, 3rd, 4th, and 5th metatarsal bones
   c. all the phalanges
   d. the cuboid only
10. The intrinsic muscles of the foot form ______ layers.
    a. 4
    b. 3
    c. 2
    d. none of the above

EXPLORE & practice

1. Locate the following parts of the ankle and foot on a human skeleton and on a partner:
   a. Lateral malleolus
   b. Medial malleolus
   c. Calcaneus
   d. Navicular
   e. Three cuneiform bones
   f. Metatarsal bones
   g. Phalanges
2. Palpate and locate the following muscles and their origins and insertions:
   a. Tibialis anterior
   b. Extensor digitorum longus
   c. Peroneus longus
   d. Peroneus brevis
   e. Soleus
   f. Gastrocnemius
   g. Extensor hallucis longus
   h. Flexor digitorum longus
   i. Flexor hallucis longus
3. Demonstrate and palpate the following movements, active and passive:
   a. Plantar flexion
   b. Dorsal flexion
   c. I nversion
   d. Eversion
   e. Flexion of the toes
   f. Extension of the toes
4. Why are *low arches* and *flat feet* not synonymous terms?
5. Discuss the value of proper footwear in various sports and activities.
6. What are orthotics, and how do they function?
7. Research the anatomical factors relating to the prevalence of inversion versus eversion ankle sprains. Report your findings in class.
8. Have a partner raise up on the toes (heel raise) with the knees fully extended and then repeat with the knees flexed approximately 20 degrees. Which exercise position appears to be more difficult to maintain for an extended period of time, and why? What are the implications for strengthening the involved muscles and for stretching these muscles?
9. *Muscle analysis chart:* Fill in the chart below by listing the muscles primarily involved in each joint movement.

Ankle	
Dorsiflexion	Plantar flexion
Transverse tarsal and subtalar joints	
Eversion	Inversion
Toes	
Flexion	Extension

10. *Antagonistic muscle action chart:* Fill in the chart below by listing the muscle(s) or parts of muscles that are antagonistic in their actions to the muscles in the left column.

Agonist	Antagonist
Gastrocnemius	
Soleus	
Tibialis posterior	
Flexor digitorum longus	
Flexor hallucis longus	
Peroneus longus/Peroneus brevis	
Peroneus tertius	
Extensor digitorum longus	
Extensor hallucis longus	

chapter 20

Dimensional Massage Techniques for the Muscles of the Leg, Ankle, and Foot

LEARNING OUTCOMES

After completing this chapter, you should be able to:

20-1 Define key terms.

20-2 Locate on a human skeleton bony structures of the ankle and foot.

20-3 Palpate bony landmarks of the ankle and foot on a partner.

20-4 Explore the origins and insertions of the muscles of the ankle and foot on a partner.

20-5 Review general pathologies and conditions of the muscles of the ankle and foot.

20-6 Discuss a treatment protocol for conditions of plantar fasciitis, Morton's toe, sprained ankle, and posterior leg cramps.

20-7 Demonstrate safe body mechanics.

20-8 Practice specific techniques on the leg, ankle, and foot muscles.

20-9 Incorporate dimensional massage therapy techniques in a regular routine or use them when needed.

20-10 Determine safe treatment protocols and refer clients to other health professionals when necessary.

KEY TERMS

Anterior talofibular ligament
Calcaneofibular ligament
Compartment syndrome
Extensor digitorum brevis
Foot drop
Inferior peroneal retinaculum
Inversion sprain
Morton's foot structure
Plantar fasciitis
Posterior leg cramp
Superior peroneal retinaculum

Introduction

In the same way that the hand and wrist are located at the end of the upper extremity, the foot and ankle are distally located at the end of the lower extremity. The feet are designed for propulsion and support. The weight of the entire body rests on top of the talus and calcaneus, just 2 of the 26 bones in the foot. The ankle moves in flexion, extension, inversion, and eversion. If any of the leg muscles are in a state of contraction, it will be apparent in the foot. Tight posterior leg muscles draw the foot in plantar flexion. The leg muscles pull on the attachments on the feet and add or subtract from normal foot patterns and gait. It is no wonder that the feet hurt on occasion even without any abnormalities or conditions.

Few things compare to a good foot massage. The body's weight transfers through the pelvic girdle to the tibia and finally to the feet. As an individual takes a step, the body weight concusses through the foot. Fully functioning leg muscles are important to the health and support capabilities of the feet. Massage therapy can help balance the soft tissue in the legs and feet and should be included as part of a conservative approach to rid the feet of soreness, assist in recovery from injuries, and encourage better walking patterns.

Structural Perspectives of the Foot and Ankle

Normal gait is disrupted when a person cannot roll off the toes or when dorsiflexion is not possible. The body compensates by using a different part of the foot on which to balance and walk. If the hips are in external rotation, for example, the feet tend to be pointed in that direction. The feet might roll medial to lateral to compensate for not being able to heel-strike and toe-off. In fact, there are a few separate issues at hand. The first is the structure of the foot; the second is a control of the gait pattern by structural compensation of the body either from the muscles in the leg, curvature of the spine, hip position, deformities and abnormalities, and/or rotation of the hips; the third is inappropriate footwear.

Foot structure is important. It is hard to toe-off in a gait pattern if one of the lesser toes is longer than the great toe. Even when the toes are crammed into shoes, discomfort will shift the pattern to accommodate the structure. **Morton's foot structure** is usually described as a short great toe and a second toe that is measurably an entire knuckle longer than the great toe. This sometimes results in a medial-lateral shifting in walking as well as a domino effect up the kinetic chain. The peroneals on the lateral leg shorten when walking on the medial side of the foot is more prevalent. Problems with knee position, patellar tracking, the Q angle, hip position, and compensating back muscles are not unheard of with this foot structure. Fortunately, appropriate orthotics can help balance weight distribution and this foot structure. Massage therapy can assist with unwinding the compensating muscular domino challenge.

There are two muscles in the leg that oppose each other in action, but both insert on the same two bones. The peroneus longus and tibialis anterior balance the transverse arch by their opposing actions and physical attachments. If either muscle were to shorten, this could change how the foot walks in the gait pattern. A tight tibialis anterior will pull on the medial side of the foot and place strain on the evertors. The opposite can happen with a shortened peroneus longus. Balancing the muscles that control the transverse arch will assist the foot to have a normal gait pattern. Massage therapy, exercise, and stretching work well for balancing the muscles of the transverse arch.

All the leg muscles balance and stabilize the foot. If any are overly contracted, they pull in the direction of the contraction. High heels have long been blamed for contracted gastrocnemius and soleus muscles and perpetual plantar flexion. Therapists who have not worked with clients who walk only on the toes may find it hard to visualize shortened muscles that will not lengthen. The leg muscles are like any other postural muscles in the body. They adapt to a repetitive position and, without the aid of stretching, will seek to permanently shorten their fibers into a contracted state. High-heel shoes should come with a warning: "Caution: Extended wear could result in shortened posterior leg muscles."

Other structural problems might include bone spurs in the heel, bunions, great-toe deformities, and flat feet. A good pathology text will review these common problems among clients. People have surgery, wear orthotics, use bad footwear, and sometimes try to ignore the pain. Getting a good diagnosis and understanding the problem is half the battle. Massage therapy is a useful part of a conservative approach and can relieve the stress of being in constant pain.

Injuries and Overuse Syndromes

Fractures, compartment syndromes, shin splints, cramps, sprains, and strains are only a few of the possible leg, ankle, and foot problems. Fractures and stress fractures to the leg bones can cause bleeding into the compartments. There is little structural room in the compartments because they are confined spaces. A **compartment syndrome** occurs when swelling or bleeding presses against the structures in the compartment; it is painful and can prevent blood flow to the foot. This condition needs emergency care and resolution of the compressive issues.

Fractures usually require casts, although some stress fractures may not require a cast and can even go unnoticed. Stress fractures may be caused not by a blow to the leg but by overindulgence in a sport. Runners have been known to get stress fractures. Any unidentified leg pain should be diagnosed to rule out serious emergency issues.

As discussed in Chapter 19, *shin splints* and *medial tibial stress syndrome* are terms used to describe a painful overuse syndrome in the anterior and deep posterior compartments, usually after running. In one serious scenario, the tibialis anterior and other muscles could pull the periosteum off the tibia and bleed into one or more of the compartments. Unfortunately, if the condition is not addressed immediately or if it is left untreated, it could lead to a compartment syndrome or possible stress fracture and create an emergency situation. Most shin splints, while unpleasant, do not lead to more complex problems. Involved muscles usually include the tibialis anterior, tibialis posterior, and extensor digitorum. Massage therapy, stretching, strengthening, and appropriate training reduce instances of shin splints. See Chapter 19 for more on shin splints.

Many people have experienced leg cramps in the middle of the night. Jumping out of bed at night to stand on the feet is a natural way to stretch the foot and posterior leg muscles. A **posterior leg cramp** is usually just a painful muscle spasm. Gastrocnemius and soleus cramps are common and can be a reaction to standing on cement all day, wearing high heels, or being pregnant; they can also arise from a circulatory issue (such as varicose veins) or a reaction to or deficiency of certain vitamins or minerals. Cramping in other body regions as well as in the posterior leg muscles may be related to dehydration and the depletion of electrolytes, a problem usually seen at post-marathon events. Gastrocnemius cramps are often associated with overuse; they are the most common complaint about the posterior leg muscles. Should a client develop a gastrocnemius cramp while on the massage table, therapists can simply dorsiflex the foot to relieve the cramp. Massage therapy, stretching, strengthening, and training go a long way to help prevent posterior leg cramps. For night cramps, an individual can place a prop at the bottom of the bed to help keep the foot in dorsiflexion; this should reduce gastrocnemius cramps and may promote uninterrupted sleep.

The opposite of jumping out of bed to stretch is not wanting to do so. For the individual who suffers from plantar fasciitis, the first step in the morning hurts the most, until the plantar fascia is stretched out. Later in the day, walking again becomes painful. **Plantar fasciitis** is an inflammation of the plantar fascia with possible microtears. Mostly an overuse syndrome, it can also be caused by tight fascia resulting from high arches and improper footwear. This condition is not limited to athletes; it also seems to target menopausal women who are prone to soft-tissue injuries. Although there are medical interventions for plantar fasciitis, a conservative approach, including massage therapy, clinical flexibility, stretching, strengthening, hydrotherapy, appropriate footwear, and/or orthotics, works for many.

Inversion sprains are one of the more common injuries of the ankle and foot. The foot has limited mobility, and if pushed to its limit from stepping in a hole or falling down steps, for example, the result could be an inversion sprain injury to the ligaments and soft tissue. The direction of the foot's movement gives meaning to the term **inversion sprain.** The outside of the foot lies laterally as the sole rolls into view.

Although the foot has a great deal more inversion than eversion, the weight of the body as a fall becomes imminent forces the foot into an unnatural, inverted position that puts too much strain on the ligaments of the ankle. Fluids rush into the painful area and often cause a secondary trauma to the area. The peroneal muscles become stretched in the action, and specific ligaments fall prey to the inversion sprain. The anterior talofibular ligament and the calcaneofibular ligament are the two most common structures affected by inversion sprains. The **anterior talofibular ligament** is located at the distal end of the anterior fibula, attaching distally to the talus. The **calcaneofibular ligament** is located at the very distal end of the fibula at an angle to the calcaneus. On either side of the calcaneofibular ligament, tacking down the peroneal tendons, are two tissue bridges called the **superior peroneal retinaculum** and **inferior peroneal retinaculum.** If the sprain mechanism is significant, these tissue bridges could be torn and the peroneal tendons might ride up over the lateral malleolus as a result. If the body weight comes down on the lateral side of the foot, the sprain could involve the only large intrinsic dorsal foot muscle, the **extensor digitorum brevis.** When the sprain involves the ligaments, retinacula, and possibly the extensor digitorum brevis, there will be a great deal of swelling. Ice will help reduce the inflammatory response and possible secondary trauma due to the swelling, but it has to be applied immediately for best results. It is never too late to work on the small structures of the foot. Years after being injured, old sprained ankles can harbor puffiness around the lateral malleolus. Massage therapists should treat old injuries with respect and use appropriate treatment options. Although most first-degree sprains are ignored, the leg muscles and other soft-tissue structures could be strengthened and stretched for healthy maintenance of ankle movement. Therapists should refer to the appropriate health care professional for safe exercise and strengthening guidance. See the techniques later in the chapter for treatment suggestions.

Massage therapy should be included as part of the conservative therapies in treating muscle strains. As discussed before, the compartments are fairly confining. There is no room for swelling or injuries to the muscles themselves. Muscle strains come in first-, second-, and third-degree injuries, with the worst being third degree, which includes torn tissue. Achilles tendons are often strained or ruptured. It is more likely for the Achilles tendon to rupture as a result of a stop-and-start sport, such as basketball or soccer. For a rupture, the Achilles will have to be reattached and casted. It is a long healing process that should include massage therapy and other conservative therapies in the rehabilitation efforts.

Nerve Complaints

PERONEAL NERVE ENTRAPMENT AND ISSUES

The peroneal nerve feeds the dorsum of the foot. It can be part of the injured structures in a severe inversion sprain. An individual can feel tenderness and tingling by touching the top of the foot. The deep peroneal nerve is sometimes a suspect in **foot drop,** a condition that usually involves a weak tibialis anterior. In foot drop, the toes might drag; the tibialis anterior cannot seem to contract well enough to dorsiflex the ankle properly. Whether it is muscular instability or a nerve issue, foot drop can affect gait dramatically. The peroneal nerve can be entrapped by crossing one knee over the other and pressing against the lateral side of the leg. Numbness and tingling are usually enough to move the legs into another position. Massage will not help damaged nerves, but soft-tissue bodywork can release hypertonic muscles that entrap nerves.

Arthritis and Osteoarthritis

Ankle fractures are an invitation for arthritis later in life. Like any other joint capsule, the foot and ankle have cartilage and structures of the common synovial joint. For individuals whose response to injury is arthritis, therapists may see enlarged calcified bony structures that will impede range of motion.

One example of posttraumatic arthritis occurred with Tom, a 50-year-old male who was snowmobiling and caught his foot and ankle in the sled tracks during an accident. He sustained a spiral fracture to the tibia into the ankle joint. The injury was treated and casted. The fracture healed, but Tom always experienced pain when walking, which was initially attributed to the healing process. A year later, Tom consulted with a different physician and brought his original x-rays. Broken chips of his tibia were lodged in his ankle joint and were wearing down the cartilage between the two bones. Tom had an arthroscopy, and the surgeon cleared out the bone chips and the damaged cartilage. The surgeon reported that Tom had only 40 percent of his cartilage left after the operation and that he would probably need a fusion of the ankle within a limited amount of time. The doctor indicated that the fusion would help resolve the pain but would severely limit dorsiflexion. Tom never got the fusion. Now, 10 years later, his ankle looks like burl on a tree; it has bony growths on both sides that have partially fused the ankle and limited dorsiflexion. When Tom walks, he must externally rotate his hip in order to roll medially off his foot. He walks with a limp.

It is clear, in this case, that arthritis is a reaction to the trauma of the injury. Unfortunately for Tom, his gait affects his back and contributes to his lower-back problems. Posttraumatic arthritis cannot really be helped medically. There is no medication to slow down or stop the insidious bony growth. Massage therapy can help with soft-tissue compensations and assist other conservative efforts to maintain function. For Tom, full-body massage is a necessity, not just an option.

Unwinding the Muscles of the Leg, Ankle, and Foot

The tibia, or shin, is pointed and bony and presents little, if any, soft tissue. Stay to either side of the tibia, and do not work on it. The leg is a compact structure; the compartments define the leg according to depth and location. Review the muscle locations in their compartments. Locate all the origins and insertions of the muscles. Do not be shy about pinpointing the attachments. Ask clients for appropriate feedback to help you locate specific sore areas. The attachments of the peroneus longus and tibialis anterior are almost always sore; structurally, they are taxed with their job of balancing the transverse arch.

As with all conditions, the massage therapist must determine the goal of treatment. In this instance, evaluate how the leg muscles affect balance, stability, and gait of the foot. Have the client take a little walk for you, and record your observations. Is there hip and lower-extremity external rotation? Is the condition bilateral, or is it a problem of one foot? What do the client's shoes look like? Is there a worn side to the shoe that tells a story? Which muscles are shortened, and which are lengthened? Have you evaluated active and passive motion? Always look at the agonist and antagonist relationship. If the person walks medial to lateral, for example, there is a relationship between the peroneus longus and the tibialis anterior. Which one is shortened? Strengthening and stretching may have to be a part of the conservative treatment. Therapists who have not had a class in gait and postural assessment should consider adding one to their continuing education list.

Determine if there is edema in the ankle area and why. Make sure there are no serious reasons for edema, such as congestive heart failure, and rule out any other contraindications. A lot of people carry

TREATMENT PROTOCOL

How do you unwind the foot and ankle muscles in a sequence?

- Take a careful medical history appropriate for the client, look for contraindications, assess edema, and refer the client to an appropriate professional when necessary.
- Always use treatment protocols to determine the sequence of a therapeutic session; assess active and passive ranges of motion of the leg, ankle, and foot.
- Palpate tissues.
- Follow a dimensional approach, and critically think about the involved joints and muscles.
- Determine appropriate pressure; ask for feedback from the client.
- Work superficial to deep.
- Visit all the muscles possibly involved in the problem.
- Visit all the attachments of the involved muscles.
- Passively shorten muscles whenever possible with your techniques to decrease tension.
- Do not overwork sore areas.
- Begin supine, and try the techniques below for a dimensional approach.

around swelling in the foot and ankle region. To help reduce simple swelling in the ankles, start on the thigh first and use an appropriate amount of effleurage. If the edema is the result of a sprained ankle, determine the stage of the sprain. An acute sprain may need definitive care and is a local contraindication. For a chronic sprain, reducing edema is part of the treatment. Working proximal to the area will help encourage the lymphatic system to function naturally. For more problematic edemic situations, lymphatic drainage is a modality that specializes in reducing edema and jump-starting the lymphatic system. Refer the client to a certified lymphatic drainage therapist when necessary.

For chronic sprained-ankle or foot structures, determine which ligaments and muscles are damaged. Treat the ligaments and muscles very specifically. The anterior talofibular and calcaneofibular ligaments may be very sore, but that should not deter you from treating them at the right time. See the techniques below for treatment suggestions for the muscles of the leg and the muscles and ligaments of the ankle and foot.

Sequence for the Leg, Foot, and Ankle

In the series of techniques that follows, you'll begin with the client in a supine position, treating the anterior compartment muscles first. The peroneals come next, ending with specific strokes for muscles and tendons in the foot and ankle. Next, in the prone position, the gastrocnemius, soleus, and posterior leg muscles are addressed. Notice that nonlubrication techniques are presented first. Among the posterior leg muscles, the Achilles tendon receives specific attention. The next treatments require a prone flexed knee. With the client in this position, treat the ankle and foot and even give some very specific stripping to the peroneals. The prone foot allows easy access to specific ligaments and the plantar surface of the foot. Do not be afraid to utilize movement of the knee joint, ankle, and foot in the course of the treatment. It is an added feature that contributes to the success of the techniques and can help you sink into deeper structures. At the end of your treatments, do not forget to connect the entire extremity or to utilize effleurage to advantage.

Dimensional Massage Therapy for the Muscles of the Leg, Ankle, and Foot

The following techniques can be used as a complete sequence for the leg, foot, and ankle muscles or be incorporated into a full-body routine.

SUPINE BODY POSITION—ANTERIOR LEG

Broadening Away from the Tibia

This technique separates the fibers away from the tibia. Start just below the client's knee. Straddle the tibia, and with the palms of your hands broaden away from the bone. Move distally toward the ankle. (See figure 20.1.)

Russian Effleurage

This is very brisk effleurage. Cup and shape both hands, one on top of another, over the client's anterior leg near the ankle. Briskly stroke toward the knee with one hand. As the hand reaches the knee, the other hand follows

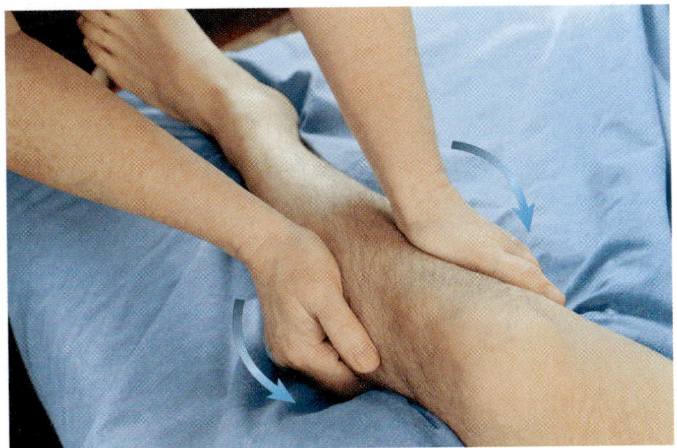

FIGURE 20.1 Broadening away from the tibia

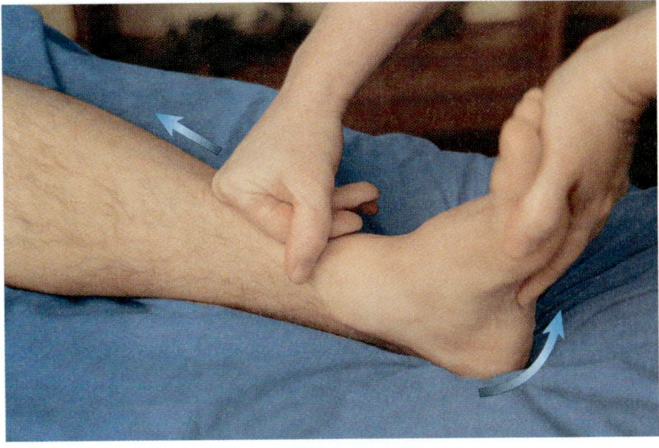

FIGURE 20.3 Stripping the tibialis anterior with passive shortening

and the whole technique is repeated. The effect must be as deep as possible and must be executed as quickly as possible. Use some lubrication. (See figure 20.2.)

Stripping the Tibialis Anterior with Passive Shortening

Dorsiflex the client's foot, and apply collapsed fingers to the base of the distal muscle. While holding the foot in passive dorsiflexion, strip proximal toward the knee. (See figure 20.3.)

Stripping the Tibialis Anterior Tendon

Place the client's foot in a slight dorsiflexion to passively shorten the tibialis anterior. Place your thumb on the tendon, and strip in a superior direction toward the belly of the muscle. (See figure 20.4.)

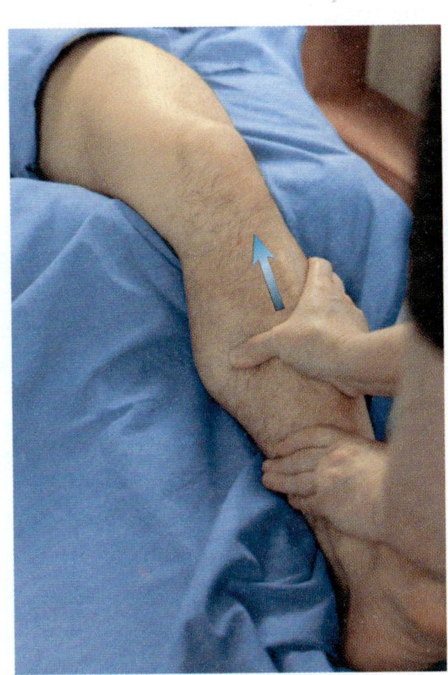

FIGURE 20.2 Russian effleurage

SUPINE BODY POSITION—LATERAL COMPARTMENT MUSCLES

Compression of the Peroneals with Lateral Rotation

Place your superior hand on the client's knee. Roll the knee inward. Compress the peroneals, starting just below the fibula and traveling down the lateral leg. Use caution around the peroneal nerve. (See figure 20.5.)

Parallel Thumbs on the Peroneals

With the client's leg in the above position, roll your thumbs over each other and on the peroneals, starting from the peroneus longus origin and working toward the ankle. (See figure 20.6.)

Compress the Superior Leg Muscles

Compress the client's anterior tibialis and extensor digitorum longus. (See figure 20.7.)

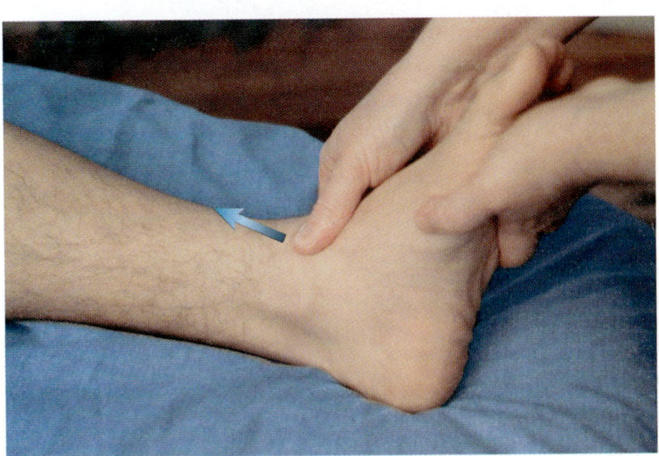

FIGURE 20.4 Stripping the tibialis anterior tendon

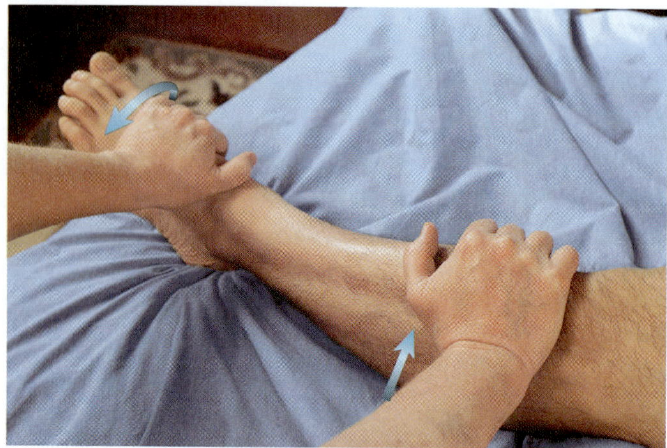

FIGURE 20.5 Compression of the peroneals with lateral rotation

Strip the Peroneals

Strip the peroneals on the client's lateral leg with any combination of fingers, with the thumb, or with collapsed fingers. Always move from the ankle toward the knee. (See figure 20.8.)

Deep Transverse Friction for the Peroneals

Using your thumbs in a seesaw motion, move up the peroneals from the client's ankle. Use double thumbs or use a single thumb. (See figures 20.9 and 20.10.)

Deep Transverse Friction on the Peroneus Longus with Passive Shortening with Fingers

Face the lower extremities, and work on the leg farthest from you, on the opposite side of the client's body.

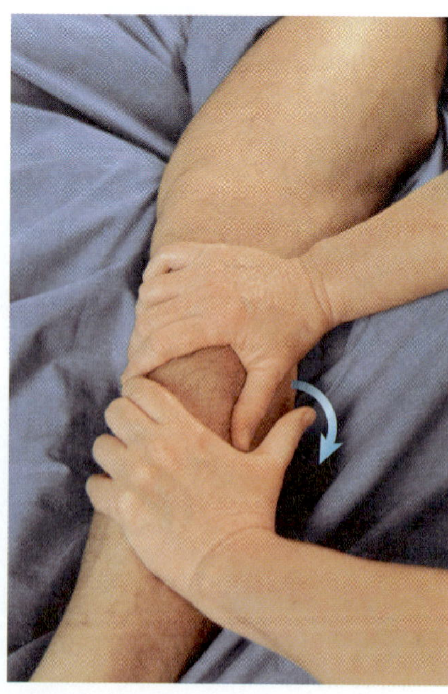

FIGURE 20.6 Parallel thumbs on the peroneals

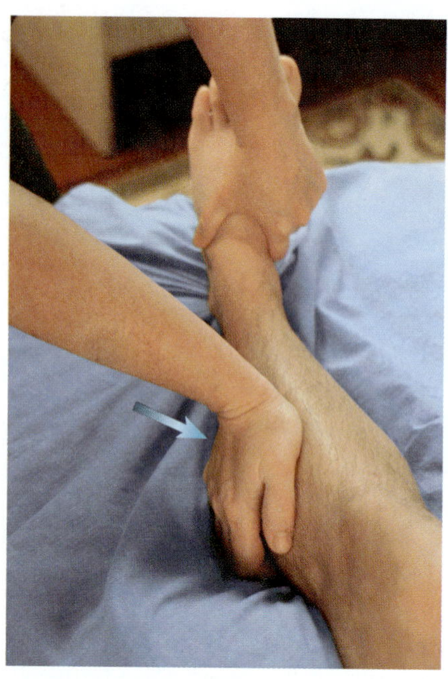

FIGURE 20.7 Compression of the superior leg muscles

Using your inferior hand, passively shorten the peroneal muscles with the foot in eversion. Brace the fingers of your superior hand, and apply deep transverse friction to the origin of the peroneus longus while you maintain the position of the foot. (See figure 20.11.)

ANKLE SUPINE

Effleurage of the Plantar Fascia

Place your thumbs on the client's dorsal foot, and place the fingers of both your hands on the plantar surface of the foot. Starting just below the toes, apply pressure on the entire sole of the foot toward the heel from the toes. The whole foot should move as you slide down the arch with appropriate pressure. Repeat. (See figure 20.12.)

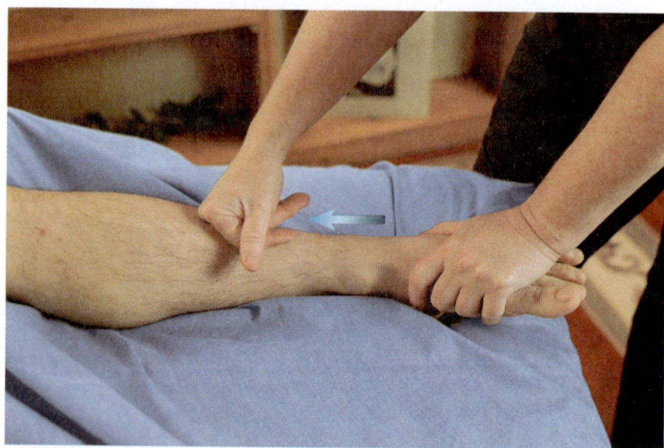

FIGURE 20.8 Deep stripping the peroneals with collapsed fingers

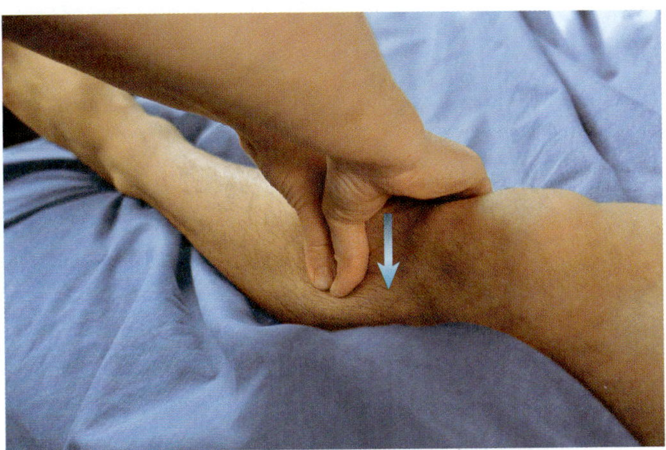

FIGURE 20.9 Deep transverse friction with double thumbs

Elliptical Movement of the Foot

Grasp the dorsal side of the client's foot with your thumbs, and place your fingers on the arch of the foot on both sides. Create clockwise and counterclockwise movements of the foot. Place your hands in different positions so that you elliptically move the areas between the tarsals and metatarsals and between the metatarsals and phalanges. (See figure 20.13 for elliptical movement of the tarsals and figure 20.14 for elliptical movement of the metatarsals.)

Circular Friction on the Extensor Digitorum Brevis

Use circular friction on specific muscles of the client's foot. Use your thumbs or fingers. (See figure 20.15.)

Windshield Wipe around the Malleolus

Use your thumbs in opposing directions around the lateral malleolus of the client's foot. (See figure 20.16.)

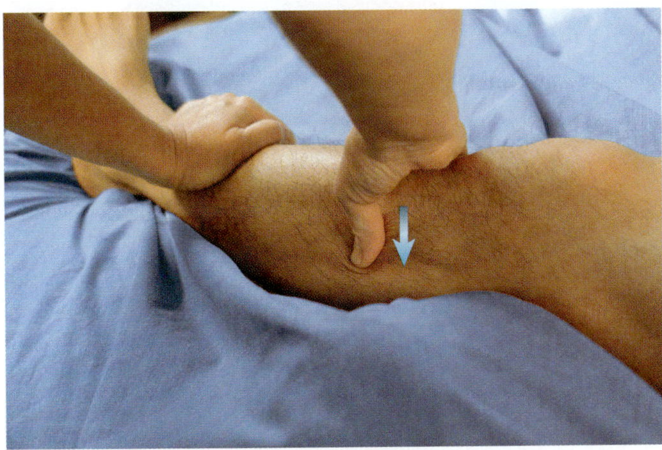

FIGURE 20.10 Deep transverse friction with a single thumb

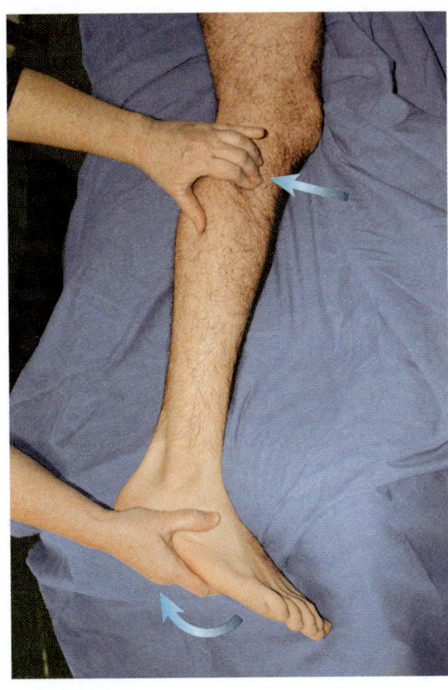

FIGURE 20.11 Deep transverse friction on the peroneus longus with passive shortening

Deep Transverse Friction to the Peroneus Longus and Tibialis Anterior Attachments

Locate the tendon of the peroneus longus starting at the 5th metatarsal on your client's foot. Apply deep transverse friction to the tendon across the bottom of the foot with the straight fingers of one hand or your thumb. (See figure 20.17.) Locate the tibialis anterior tendon on the foot, and apply deep transverse friction toward its insertion. (See figure 20.18.)

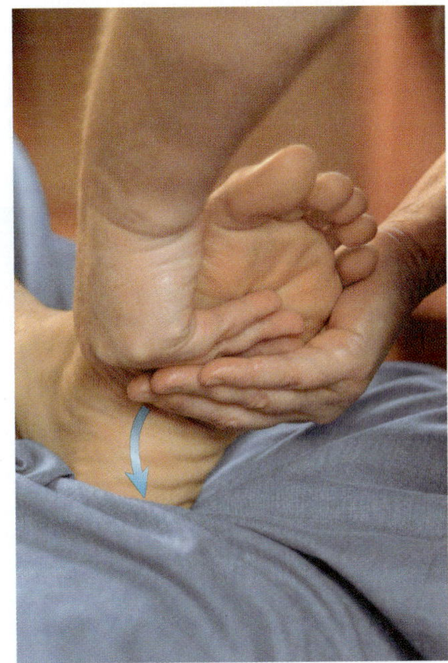

FIGURE 20.12 Effleurage of the plantar fascia

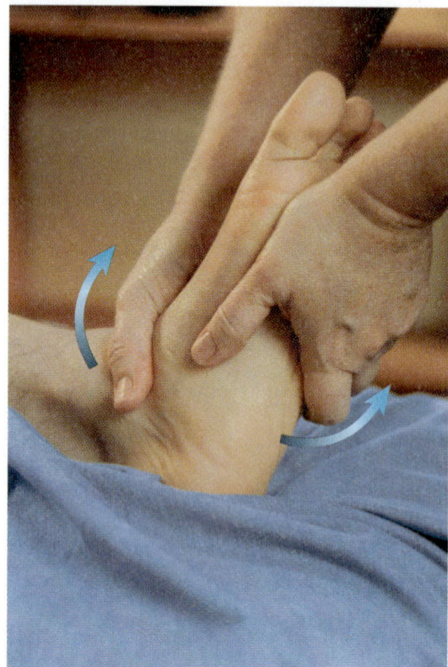

FIGURE 20.13 Elliptical movement of the foot for tarsals

Pressure with Distraction

Locate trigger points around the ankle bones on the client's foot. Apply ischemic pressure while rotating the ankle. (See figure 20.19.)

Trigger Points

Locate trigger points in a variety of muscles, and apply ischemic pressure. Passively shorten the muscles first, if possible.

Range of Motion

Dorsiflex the client's ankle by cradling the calcaneus with your palm and using your forearm to dorsiflex the foot toward the ankle. (See figure 20.20.) Plantar flex and circumduct the ankle. Shake the ankle side to side by placing the heels of both hands on either side of the ankle at the malleoli. (See figure 20.21.)

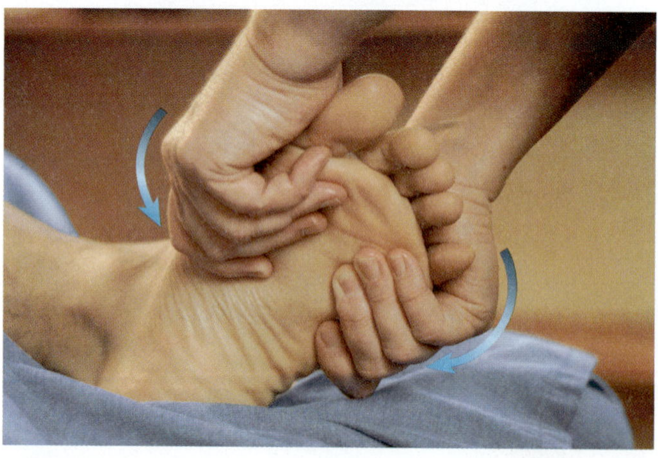

FIGURE 20.14 Elliptical movement of the foot for metatarsals

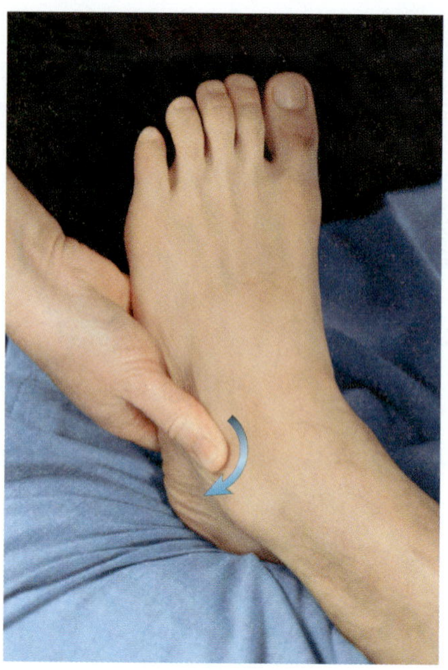

FIGURE 20.15 Circular friction on the extensor digitorum brevis

PRONE

Elliptical Movement of the Gastrocnemius and Soleus

Place both hands on either head of the gastrocnemius on the client's posterior leg. Move the muscles in a clockwise and counterclockwise manner. (See figure 20.22.)

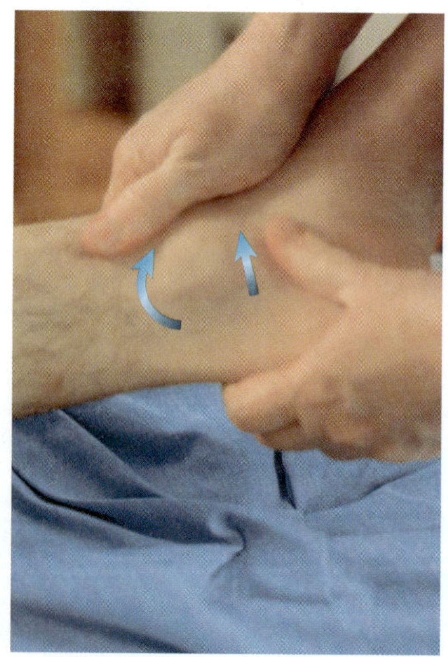

FIGURE 20.16 Windshield wiping around the malleolus

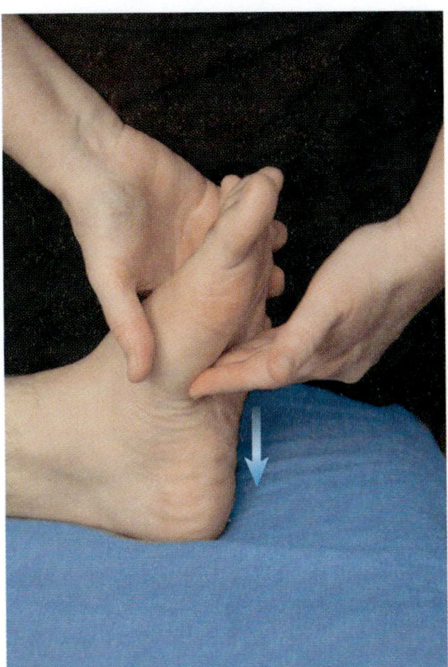

FIGURE 20.17 Deep transverse friction to the peroneus longus

Jostle the Gastrocnemius and Soleus

Grasp each head of the gastrocnemius, and shake the muscles from behind the client's knee, origin to insertion. (See figure 20.23.)

Myofascial Technique for the Gastrocnemius

Separate the heads of the muscle by drawing the center of the client's gastrocnemius toward and over your thumbs. (See figure 20.24)

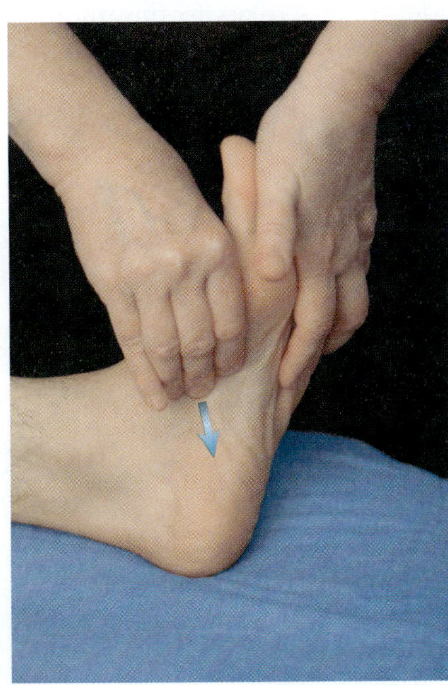

FIGURE 20.18 Deep transverse friction to the tibialis anterior

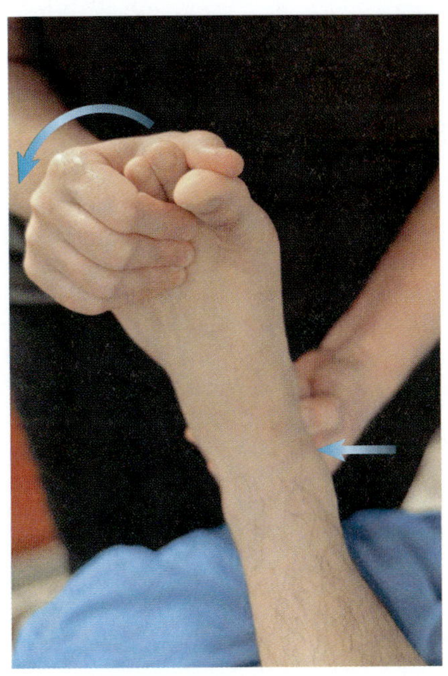

FIGURE 20.19 Pressure with distraction

Compress the Gastrocnemius and Soleus

Compress each head of the muscle, angling the client's leg and your hand to best fit the area. The leg can lie on the table, or, as pictured, you can flex the leg into your hand. (See figure 20.25.)

Flex the Knee and Stretch the Femoral Heads of the Gastrocnemius

Flex the client's knee, and let the leg rest on your inside forearm. Insert your fingers behind the knee at

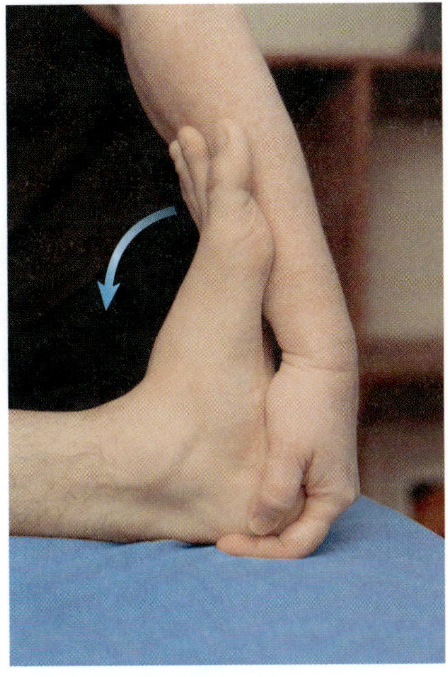

FIGURE 20.20 Dorsiflexing the ankle

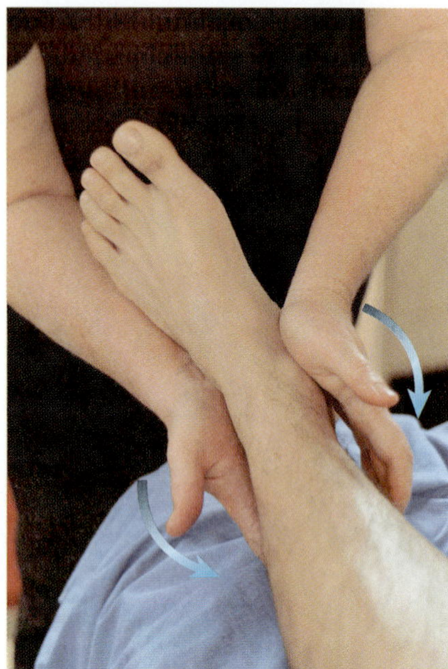

FIGURE 20.21 Ankle shaking

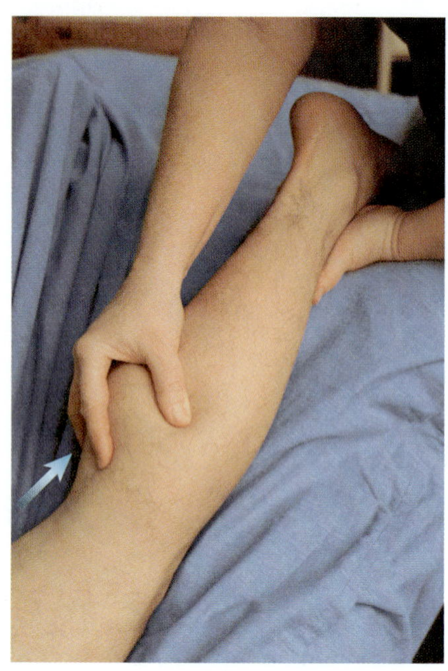

FIGURE 20.23 Jostling the gastrocnemius and soleus

the heads of the gastrocnemius. Flex the knee a tad more, and as you extend the leg, stretch the fibers that you have anchored. Repeat. (See figure 20.26.)

Russian Effleurage of the Gastrocnemius

Repeat the technique used for the client's anterior leg, but address both heads of the gastrocnemius. (See figure 20.27.)

Classic Kneading of the Gastrocnemius

This is another Russian technique. With one hand performing classic kneading, use a clockwise movement with the whole muscle. Grasp part of the client's gastrocnemius as close to the insertion as possible. Always stroke toward the heart. With a clockwise movement, rotate the hand and the muscle toward your little finger. Move along the muscle in a superior fashion. The Russians apply this technique on the gastrocnemius in groups of three—three strokes to the inside, three strokes to the middle, and three strokes laterally. (See figure 20.28.)

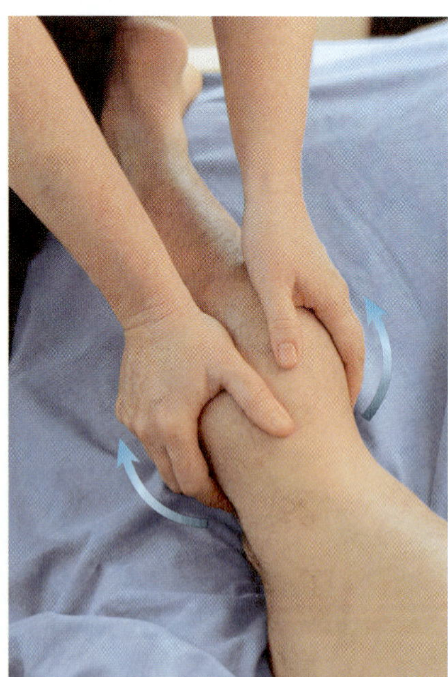

FIGURE 20.22 Elliptical movement for the gastrocnemius and soleus

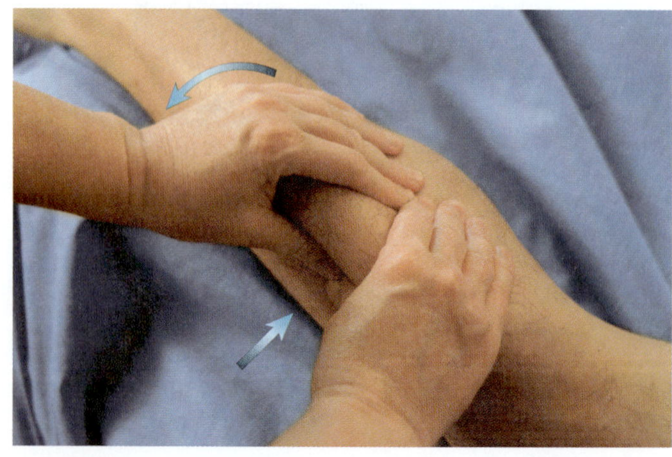

FIGURE 20.24 Myofascial technique for the gastrocnemius

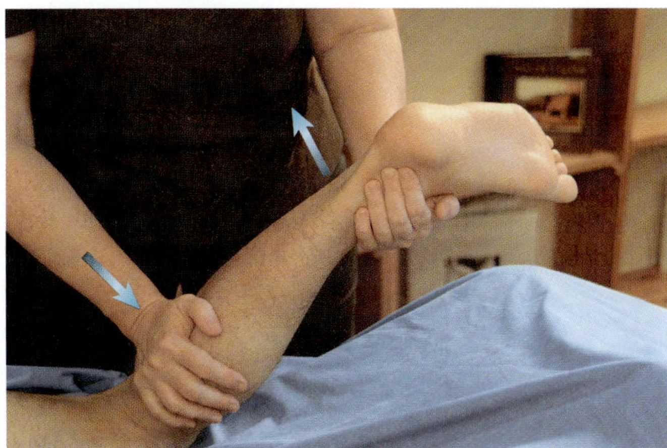

FIGURE 20.25 Compression of the gastrocnemius and soleus

Broadening the Gastrocnemius

Separate fibers by broadening each head of the client's gastrocnemius. (See figure 20.29.)

Petrissage and Circular Friction of the Gastrocnemius

Use alternating petrissage and circular friction on each head of the client's gastrocnemius.

Forearm Effleurage to the Gastrocnemius

Flatten and stroke the client's gastrocnemius with your forearm from ankle to knee. Repeat. (See figure 20.30.)

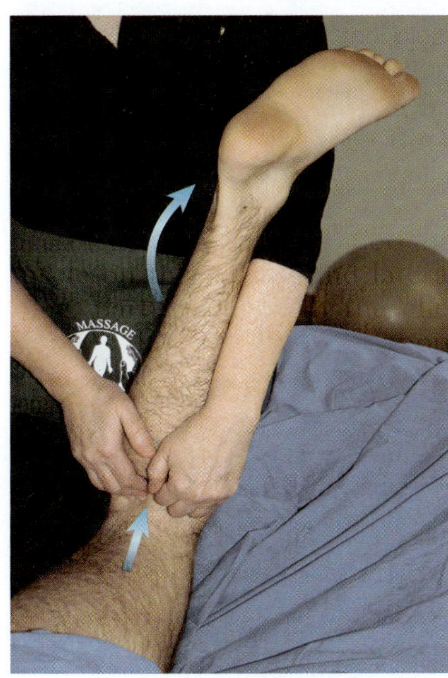

FIGURE 20.26 Stretching the femoral heads of the gastrocnemius

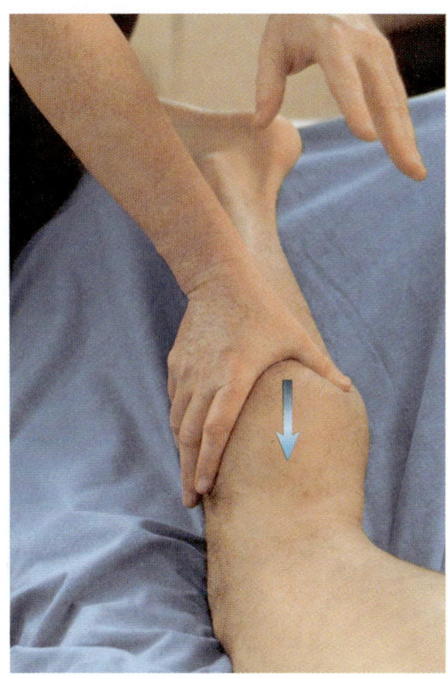

FIGURE 20.27 Russian effleurage of the gastrocnemius

This is a great time to add active engagement techniques for the posterior leg muscles.

Achilles Tendon Glide

While holding the client's plantar foot with one hand, grasp the Achilles tendon with the thumb and forefinger of the other hand. Stroke the tendon in a superior direction toward the muscle while dorsiflexing the foot. (See figure 20.31.)

Deep Transverse Friction for the Achilles Tendon

Use your thumbs in a seesaw motion over the client's Achilles tendon. (See figure 20.32.)

Flex and Strip the Achilles Tendon

Flex and extend the client's ankle while stripping the tendon. *Achilles stretch:* Dorsiflex the foot and use your fingers and thumb to stretch the tendon at the calcaneus. (See figure 20.33.)

PRONE FLEXED KNEE

Distracting the Ankle and Knee Joints

Flex the client's knee joint. Surround the calcaneus and dorsal part of the foot, and lift the whole leg off the table. Shake the leg. (See figure 20.34.)

Foot Flip-Flop

Stand to the side of the end of the table by your client's feet. Pick up the ankle closest to you, and bend the client's knee. Hold the foot so that the ankle is

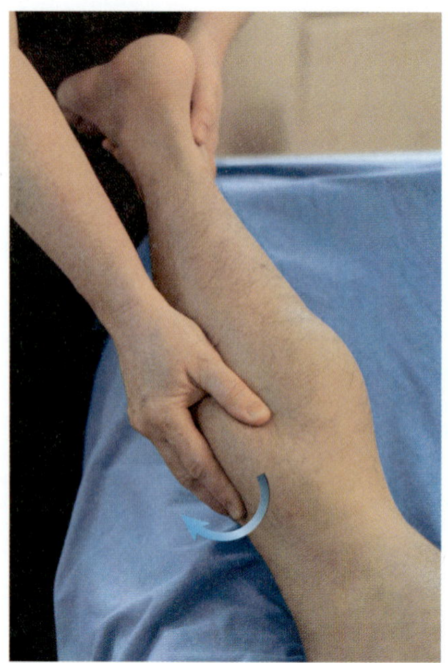

FIGURE 20.28 Classic kneading of the gastrocnemius

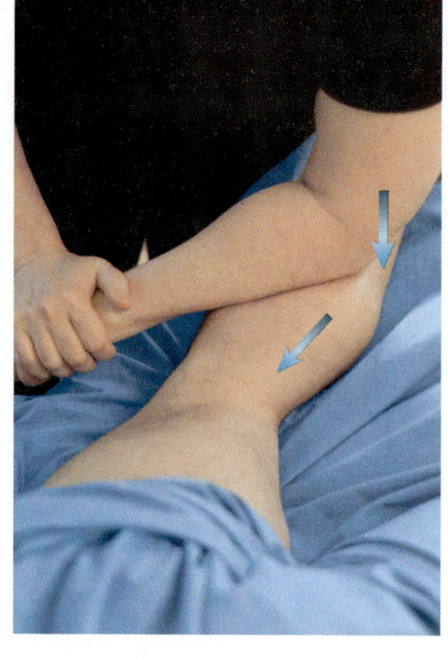

FIGURE 20.30 Forearm effleurage to the gastrocnemius

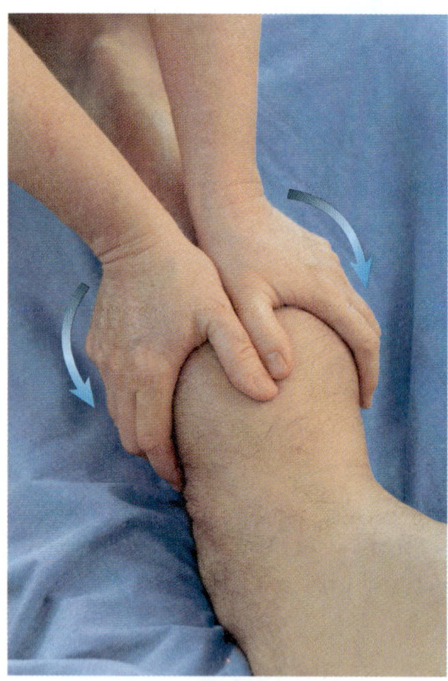

FIGURE 20.29 Broadening the gastrocnemius

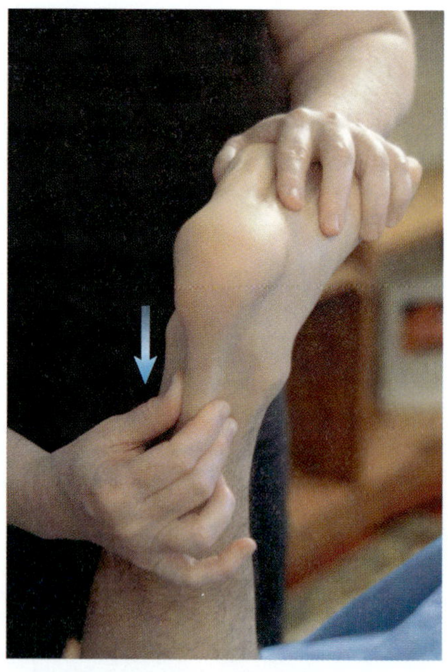

FIGURE 20.31 Achilles tendon glide

between your thumb and forefinger of each hand. Surround the Achilles tendon with one hand and the anterior ankle with the other. Alternately dorsiflex and plantar flex the ankle as you shape your hand to the structure of the ankle. Glide superiorly and inferiorly as the ankle flexes. Repeat a few times. Lift the foot by the ankle, and shake the knee joint slightly to distract the ankle joint. (See figure 20.35.)

Deep Stripping the Peroneals with Collapsed Fingers

Flex the client's knee joint. Hold the ankle with the inside hand. Position your collapsed fingers just

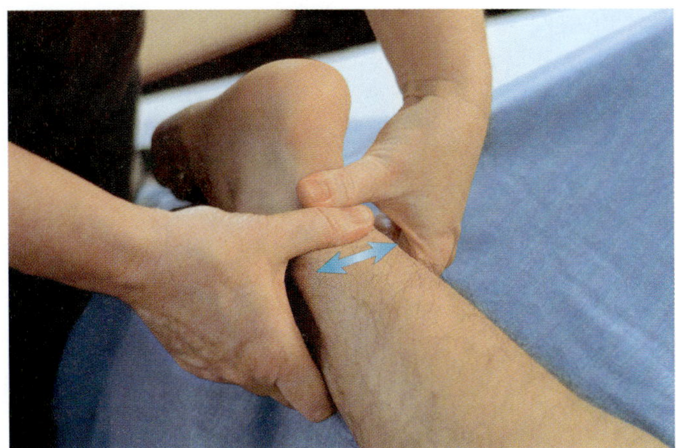

FIGURE 20.32 Deep transverse friction for the Achilles tendon

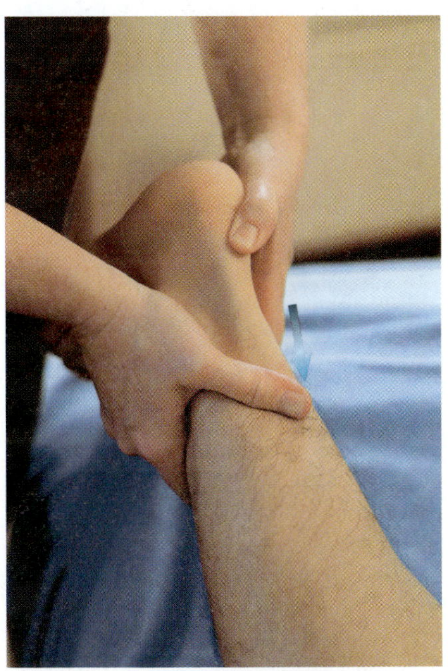

FIGURE 20.33 Flexing and stripping the Achilles tendon

superior to the lateral malleolus. As you draw the leg toward you, strip in a superior direction toward the head of the peroneus longus. (See figure 20.36.)

FOOT PRONE

Wringing the Bottom of the Foot

Flex the client's knee joint. Grasp the bottom of the foot so that one hand comes across the arch and the other hand opposes it in position. Move your hands in a wringing motion. (See figure 20.37.)

Deep Transverse Friction to the Anterior Talofibular Ligament

Flex the client's knee joint. Locate the lateral malleolus and the anterior talofibular ligament. Apply your thumb at a right angle to the ligament, and draw across it. (See figure 20.38.)

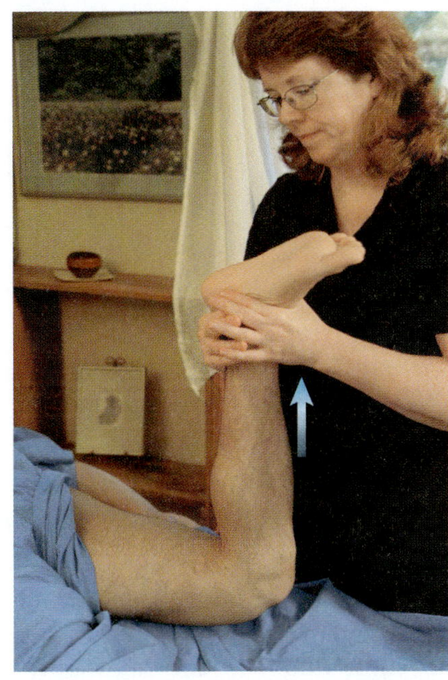

FIGURE 20.34 Distracting the ankle and knee joints

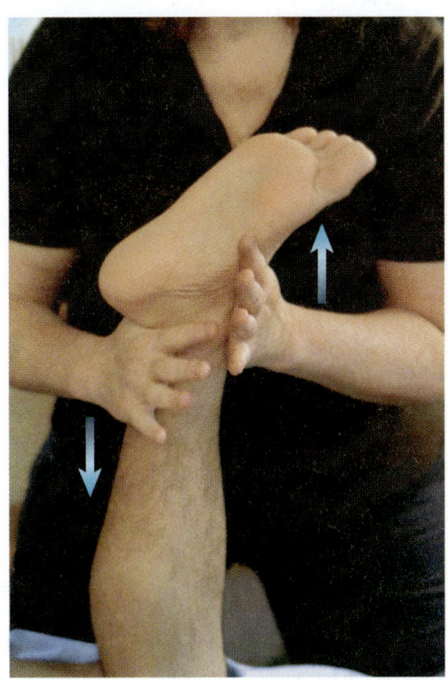

FIGURE 20.35 Foot flip-flop

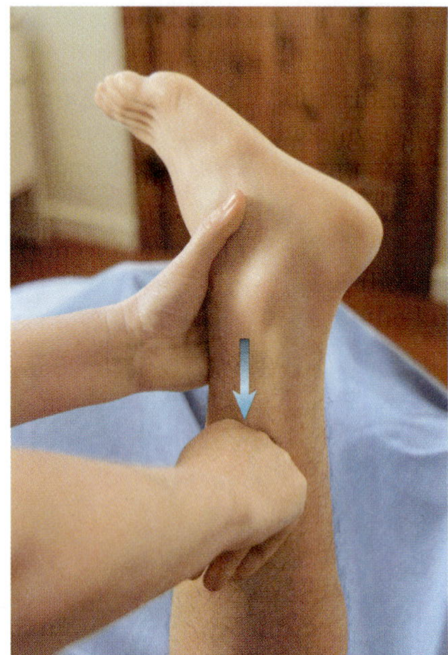

FIGURE 20.36 Deep stripping the peroneals with collapsed fingers

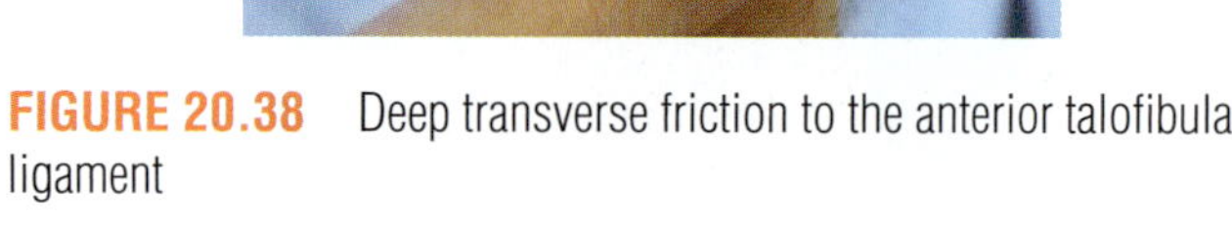

FIGURE 20.38 Deep transverse friction to the anterior talofibular ligament

Deep Transverse Friction to the Calcaneofibular Ligament

Flex the client's knee joint. Locate the lateral malleolus and the calcaneofibular ligament. Apply your thumb at a right angle to the ligament, and draw across it. (See figure 20.39.) On either side of the calcaneofibular ligament are the superior and inferior peroneal retinacula. Apply deep transverse friction to the retinacula.

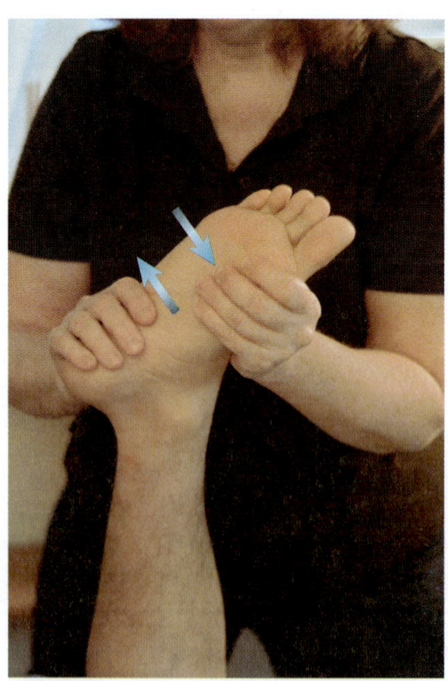

FIGURE 20.37 Wringing the bottom of the foot

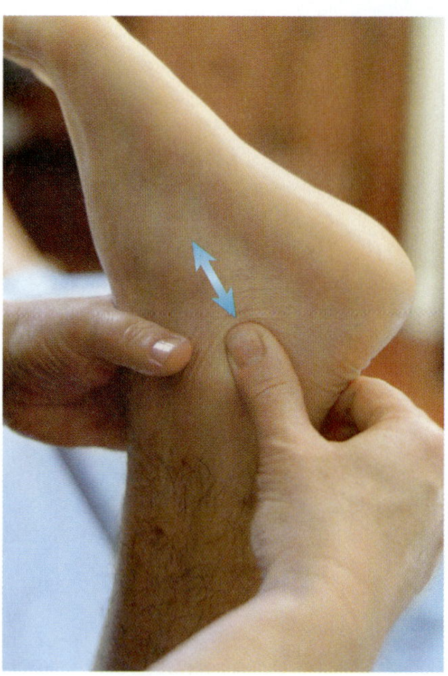

FIGURE 20.39 Deep transverse friction to the calcaneofibular ligament

Hack the Bottom of the Foot

Lightly hack the bottom of the client's foot with one hand. (See figure 20.40.)

Place the leg on the table, and apply effleurage to the client's leg and perhaps to the entire lower extremity. Finish with nerve strokes.

See Chapters 19 and 21 for stretching and strengthening of specific muscles of the leg, ankle, and foot.

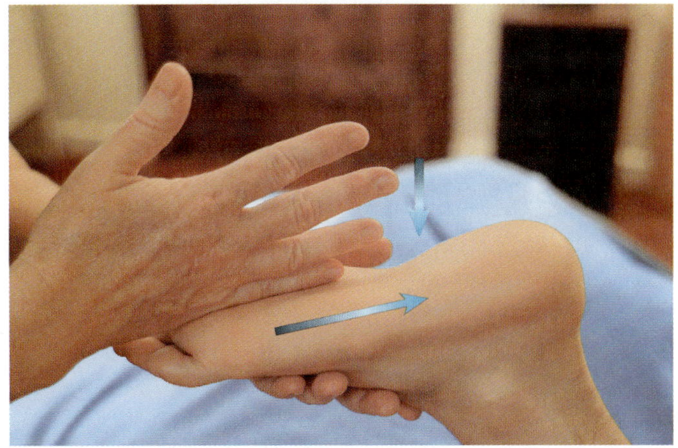

FIGURE 20.40 Hacking the bottom of the foot

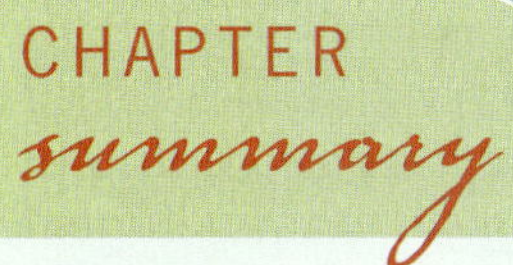

CHAPTER *summary*

Introduction

- ✔ The foot and ankle are located distally at the end of the lower extremity.
- ✔ The weight of the entire body rests on the talus and calcaneus, which are 2 of the 26 bones of the foot.
- ✔ Massage therapy can provide a great deal of relief for soft-tissue dysfunction of the leg, ankle, and foot.

Structural Perspectives of the Foot and Ankle

- ✔ Normal gait patterns include a heel-strike and a roll off the toes.
- ✔ Abnormal foot structures, curvatures of the spine and hip positions, deformities and abnormalities, and inappropriate footwear contribute to problematic gait patterns.
- ✔ Abnormal gait patterns contribute to structural problems that reverberate up the kinetic chain.

Injuries and Overuse Syndromes

- ✔ Fractures, compartment syndromes, shin splints, cramps, sprains, and strains are a few of the possible problems for the leg, ankle, and foot.
- ✔ Fractures and compartment syndromes are emergency injuries.
- ✔ Shin splints are an overuse syndrome and do not usually lead to an emergency situation.
- ✔ Posterior leg cramping can be caused by a variety of problems from poor circulation and fatigue to poor shoes, vitamin deficiency, or dehydration.
- ✔ Plantar fasciitis is an inflammation of the plantar fascia that causes pain during walking.
- ✔ Inversion sprains can involve ligament tears, swelling, and nerve damage.
- ✔ Although many problems of the foot and ankle are of an emergency nature, massage therapy can help resolve soft-tissue complaints with other conservative therapies.

Nerve Complaints

- ✔ The peroneal nerve can be damaged in inversion sprains.
- ✔ The deep peroneal nerve has been implicated in foot drop, a condition that involves a weak tibialis anterior.
- ✔ Crossing the legs at the knee can entrap the peroneal nerve.

Arthritis and Osteoarthritis

- ✔ Posttraumatic arthritis may affect gait patterns.

Unwinding the Muscles of the Leg, Ankle, and Foot

- ✔ The tibia, or shin, is pointed and superficial on the anterior leg. It should be avoided during treatment.
- ✔ Review the muscles of the compartments. Locate the origins and insertions of the muscles.
- ✔ Always use treatment protocols to determine the sequence of a therapeutic session.
- ✔ Refer clients to appropriate health care professionals when necessary.

Sequence for the Leg, Foot, and Ankle

- ✔ The suggested sequence begins with the client supine for treatment of the anterior and lateral compartment muscles.
- ✔ With the client in a prone position, treatment includes techniques for the posterior compartment muscles,

strokes for the Achilles tendon, a flexed-knee position with strokes for lateral compartment muscles, ankle and foot techniques, and prone foot strokes.

Dimensional Massage Therapy for the Muscles of the Leg, Ankle, and Foot

- ✔ Begin using specific strokes for the muscles of the anterior foot and ankle.
- ✔ Approach techniques methodically, unwinding soft tissue superficially to deep.
- ✔ Apply techniques to the lateral compartment muscles.
- ✔ The prone position allows the use of range of motion with the foot while applying techniques to the posterior compartment muscles.
- ✔ Treat trigger points toward the end of treatment and do range of motion of joints last.

CHAPTER *review*

True or False

Write true *or* false *after each statement.*

1. Massage is appropriate for an acute anterior compartment syndrome.
2. A client who has worn high heels for 10 years and cannot bring the foot out of plantar flexion has complete flexibility after just one massage treatment.
3. Plantar fasciitis is a problem only for athletes.
4. Individuals who have had an inversion sprain can have puffiness around the lateral malleolus years later.
5. Morton's foot structure can contribute to an abnormal gait pattern.
6. The calcaneofibular ligament is insignificant and never injured.
7. Shin splints could lead to a compartment syndrome.
8. Arthritis is so rare that the massage therapist will never see it in practice.
9. Plantar fasciitis usually hurts when you first step on your feet in the morning.
10. Problems in the feet such as gait and structure can contribute to back pain.

Short Answers

Write your answers on the lines provided.

1. What is the difference between an inversion sprain and an eversion sprain?

____

____

____

2. What two ligaments in the ankle get injured the most in inversion sprains?

____

____

____

3. Name three things that can contribute to posterior leg cramping.

____

____

____

4. Is a compartment syndrome a dangerous problem?

____

____

____

5. Define *plantar fasciitis.*

____

____

____

6. Name an intrinsic muscle that is on the top of the foot on the lateral side.

____

____

____

7. Name two muscles that balance the transverse arch.

____

____

____

8. What problem can result from a weak tibialis anterior muscle?

____

____

____

9. Name two things that might affect a gait pattern.

____

____

____

10. Name the actions of the ankle and foot.

____

____

____

Multiple Choice

Circle the correct answers.

1. If you had a client on your table who had a gastrocnemius cramp, you would:
   a. plantar flex the foot
   b. dorsiflex the foot
   c. ask the client to stop whining
   d. none of the above
2. The major muscles that might be involved in posterior leg cramping are:
   a. gastrocnemius and soleus
   b. tibialis anterior and extensor digitorum longus
   c. peroneus longus and brevis
   d. all of the above
3. The muscles most likely to be involved in shin splints are:
   a. peroneals
   b. gastrocnemius and soleus
   c. tibialis anterior, tibialis posterior, and extensor digitorum longus
   d. none of the above
4. Morton's foot structure appears to have:
   a. a short great toe and a second toe that is a whole knuckle longer than the great toe
   b. all the toes equal in size and length
   c. a bunion at the first metatarsal
   d. none of the above
5. Which of the following might prevent you from working on a sprained ankle?
   a. extreme swelling
   b. extensive bruising
   c. 10 on the pain scale
   d. all of the above
6. Muscles that might be involved in inversion sprains include:
   a. gastrocnemius
   b. peroneals
   c. soleus
   d. none of the above
7. If a client was cramping all over, you would:
   a. start prone and work only on the back muscles
   b. start in a supine position and work superficial to deep
   c. work on the lower extremity first
   d. refer the client to an appropriate health care professional
8. Two of the muscles that dorsiflex the ankle are:
   a. gastrocnemius and soleus
   b. tibialis anterior and extensor digitorum longus
   c. flexor hallucis longus and tibialis posterior
   d. none of the above
9. Foot drop may be a weakness in:
   a. tibialis anterior
   b. peroneus longus
   c. tibialis posterior
   d. none of the above
10. If a client came in with an undiagnosed pain in the leg from a direct-blow trauma, you would:
    a. massage the client and make repeated appointments
    b. make an appropriate referral
    c. examine the leg by applying pressure to the hematoma
    d. do nothing

EXPLORE & *practice*

1. Locate bony landmarks of the ankle and foot on a partner.
2. Locate on a partner the origins and insertions of the muscles discussed in this chapter and in Chapter 19.
3. Demonstrate how to passively shorten the dorsiflexors, plantar flexors, invertors, and evertors of the ankle and foot.
4. Demonstrate passive range of motion of the ankle and foot with a partner.
5. Demonstrate active range of motion of the ankle and foot with a partner.
6. List which muscles are agonists and synergists for dorsiflexion of the ankle and foot.
7. List which muscles are agonists and synergists for plantar flexion of the ankle and foot.
8. List which muscles are agonists and synergists for inversion and eversion of the ankle and foot.
9. Describe how you might work on a client who had a sprained ankle in a chronic stage.
10. Practice dimensional techniques individually and in a sequence on a partner.

chapter 21

Muscular Analysis of the Trunk and Lower-Extremity Exercises

LEARNING OUTCOMES

After completing this chapter, you should be able to:

21-1 Analyze movements to determine the joint actions and the types of contractions occurring in the specific muscles involved in those movements.

21-2 Categorize groups of individual muscles that produce certain joint movements.

21-3 Demonstrate specific clinical flexibility and strengthening exercises for the lower extremity.

21-4 Explain how certain muscle groups might have an effect on lower-extremity dysfunctions.

21-5 Apply the concept of the open kinetic chain to the lower extremity.

21-6 Identify the contraindications in performing the exercises in this chapter.

21-7 Recognize the concepts of analyzing and prescribing exercises to strengthen major muscle groups.

KEY TERMS

Contraction

Core

Sarcopenia

Traditional kinesiology

Introduction

The lower extremities allow the body to propel itself against gravity, participate in sports requiring skill and precision, and participate in myriad other activities. The body's system of levers and muscles works synergistically to produce smooth, powerful *movement*. When movement is compromised by shortened and weak muscle tissue, pain usually results, thereby setting off a snowball of mechanical disadvantages. The lower extremities have a vital connection to the upper extremities, discussed in Chapter 12. Dysfunctional gait, for example, directly affects upper-body movement. An individual might hold her head in an awkward position that places torque on the cervical disks, or lower-extremity limitations might change a person's sports ability and skill. Specific stretching and resistance exercises that condition this area and isolate the muscle groups can help individuals maintain natural movement, abate injury, and enjoy a better quality of life. This chapter includes some of these simple exercises, and it will be helpful for the student to review the principles of clinical flexibility and therapeutic exercise in Chapter 12.

The exercises and activities in this chapter focus on the muscles in the trunk and lower extremity. Strength, endurance, and flexibility of these muscles are important for skillful physical performance and body maintenance. Prescribed exercises for the lower extremity should focus on ignored and/or underworked muscles, which are also mentioned in this chapter.

Muscle Contraction

The type of **contraction** of a muscle is determined by whether the muscle is lengthening or shortening during the movement. However, muscles may shorten or lengthen in the absence of a contraction through passive movement caused by other contracting muscles, momentum, gravity, or external forces, such as manual assistance and exercise machines.

A *concentric* contraction is a shortening contraction of the muscles against gravity or resistance, whereas an *eccentric* contraction is a contraction in which the muscle lengthens under tension to control the joints moving with gravity or resistance. This lengthening movement is an important component in challenging muscle hypertrophy.

Contraction against gravity is evident in the lower extremities when the body moves into a vertical position, such as when rising from sleeping. Gravity acts on joints and muscles, and contractions must occur against the force of gravity for movement to occur.

The quadriceps muscle group contracts eccentrically when the body slowly lowers in a weight-bearing movement through lower-extremity action. The quadriceps functions as a decelerator to knee joint flexion in weight-bearing movements by contracting eccentrically to prevent too rapid downward movement. One can easily demonstrate this by palpating this muscle group when slowly moving from a standing position to a half-squat. Almost as much work is done in this type of contraction as in concentric contractions.

In this example involving the quadriceps, the slow descent is *eccentric,* or lengthening, and the ascent from the squatted position is concentric. If the descent were under no muscular control, it would be at the same speed as gravity and the muscle lengthening would be passive. That is, the movement and change in length of the muscle would be both caused and controlled by gravity and not by active muscular contractions.

In recent years, an increasing number of medical and allied health professionals have emphasized the development of muscle groups through resistance-training and circuit-training activities. Athletes and nonathletes, both male and female, require overall muscular development. Even individuals who do not necessarily desire significant muscle mass are advised to develop and maintain muscle mass through resistance training; moreover, simple exercises designed to maintain strength and flexibility can be performed without joining a health club. Resistance exercises have multiple benefits. As the body ages, muscle mass decreases, a condition called **sarcopenia;** as a result, the body is more susceptible to injuries as well as decreased metabolism. This factor, combined with improper eating habits, results in unhealthy fat accumulation and excessive weight gain. The United States is currently seeing an increase in adolescent obesity, a percentage that could be decreased through education about proper diet and exercise. Through increasing muscle mass, the body burns more calories and is less likely to gain excessive fat.

Despite common myths, sports participation does not ensure sufficient development of muscle groups. Additionally, more emphasis is being placed on **traditional kinesiology** in physical education and athletic skill teaching. Traditional kinesiology is the study of the science of muscle movement, which involves biomechanics, prescribed exercise, and anatomy. Traditional kinesiology can help bring about more skillful performance; however, one must remember that mechanical principles will be of little or no value to performers without adequate strength and endurance of the muscular system, which are developed through specific exercises and activities. In recent years, greater emphasis has been placed on exercises and activities that improve one's physical fitness, strength, endurance, and flexibility. Some of the exercises presented in this chapter consist of *Active Isolated Stretching (AIS),* described in Chapter 12, and strengthening of the same muscles that were lengthened (antagonists), which makes understanding the functional actions of the agonist and antagonist easier. Refer to table 12.1 on page 244, which shows the protocol for performing AIS. An 8-foot rope is used in some of the stretches; rope is recommended over an elastic band or towel.

This chapter continues analyzing muscles through specific exercises. When these techniques are mastered, individuals will have a better understanding of analyzing and prescribing exercises and activities for the muscular strength and endurance needed in sports activities and for healthy living. *A word of caution:* Therapists must stay within their scope of practice when recommending exercises to patients. This chapter is only a guide to fully understanding the principles of prescribed exercises.

Analysis of Clinical Flexibility and Therapeutic Exercise of the Trunk and Lower Extremity

The next several pages present Active Isolated Stretching movements that can be used in a clinical setting to increase range of motion in specific muscles. After each section on stretches, a section on strengthening techniques is presented for the same muscle group that was lengthened (antagonists) so that the student can better understand functional anatomy. See the table after each resistance exercise to better understand agonist, joint, and muscle action. For all movements, the individual should exhale deeply on the work phase and inhale on the relaxation phase. Generally, these exercises consist of 10 repetitions and 2 to 3 sets. All exercises are performed in slow and controlled movements and never in a "swinging" motion.

Since the core is an important element in conditioning, the exercises below begin with stretching and strengthening of the abdominals and low back.

FLEXIBILITY ANALYSIS—TRUNK HYPEREXTENSION

Stretching the Rectus Abdominis and Internal and External Obliques

Stretching the rectus abdominis and obliques, or the **core** of the body, has many benefits. The abdominals often become shortened from overuse as core muscles. They also have the enormous responsibility of supporting the body internally as well as externally. Hyperextension of the spine should be performed on a daily basis to help "open" the anterior core of the body. Start prone on a table or floor, with the palms down, as shown in figure 21.1. Individuals with low-back issues may benefit from a pad under the pelvis. Begin the movement by retracting the scapula as the torso lifts up from the table. Exhale on the lift, following the eyes upward, for a gentle 2-second stretch (figure 21.2). Return and repeat. The arms help hyperextend the spine much like a yoga movement. Performing this exercise with arms at sides has the added benefit of strengthening the antigravity muscles of the upper back. The antigravity muscles of the upper back perform the lifting movement. *Contraindications:* This stretch is safe with controlled movement.

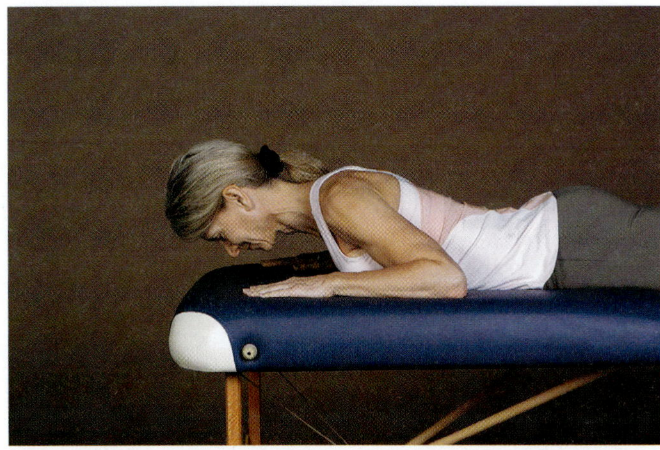

FIGURE 21.1 Trunk hyperextension, start

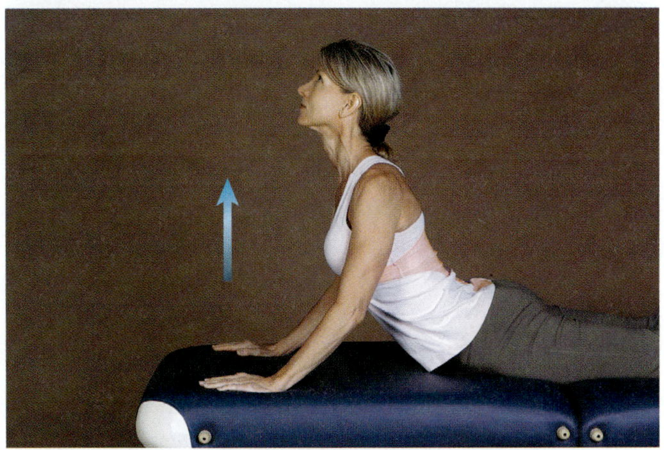

FIGURE 21.2 Trunk hyperextension, end

STRENGTHENING ANALYSIS—REVERSE-CRUNCH FLEXION

Strengthening the Rectus Abdominis and External and Internal Obliques

This exercise targets the lower abdominals and the internal and external obliques. While regular crunches (sit-ups) work the rectus abdominis, this reverse crunch is a way to isolate more fibers of the rectus abdominis and get the obliques involved. Because the trunk is flexed lifting the knees and not the torso, the abdominals are forced to work dynamically, especially on the eccentric (down) phase of this movement. Start in a supine position on a bench or table, with the knees bent (figure 21.3). Clasp the end of the table with the hands. Tilt the pelvis posteriorly, flattening the low back against the table. Maintain a 90-degree angle in the knees and between

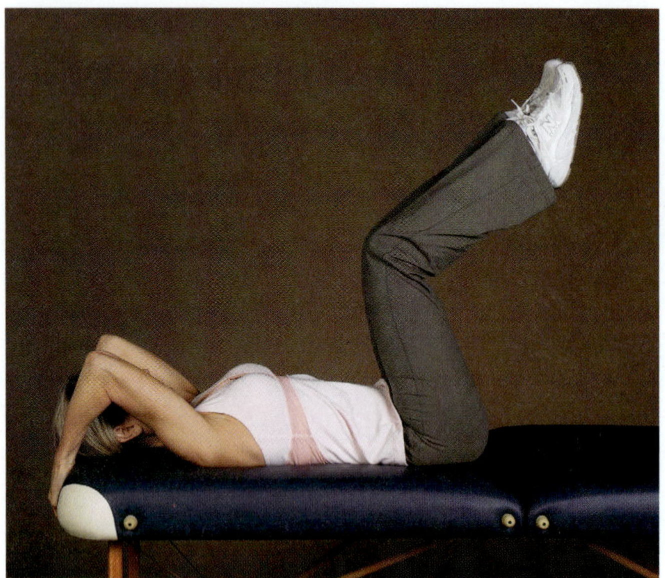

FIGURE 21.3 Reverse trunk flexion, start

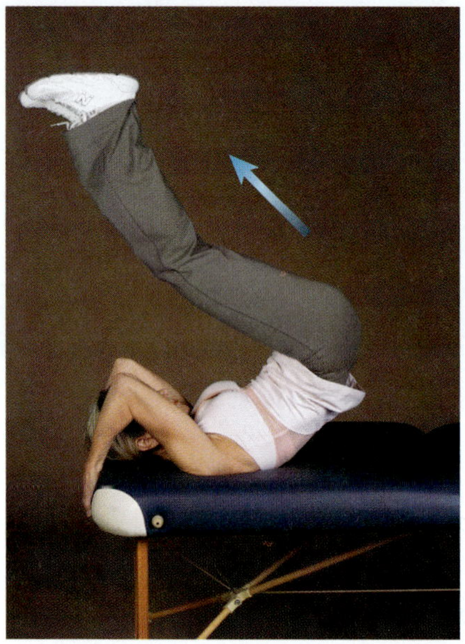

FIGURE 21.4 Reverse trunk flexion, end

the trunk and the thigh throughout this movement. While contracting the lower abdominals and exhaling, lift the pelvis and lower back off the table one vertebra at a time. Continue the movement until the shoulder blades touch the table level. For the return movement, inhale and slowly return to the start position, letting each vertebra slowly touch the table (figure 21.4). This eccentric part of the exercise is the most important and the most difficult; the movement should always be slow and controlled, maintaining the 90-degree angle. *Contraindications:* This exercise is safe with controlled movement; abdominals may become sore in persons who are not accustomed to this exercise. Individuals with herniated disks in the lumbar spine should use caution when performing this exercise.

This movement may take practice. The arms should stabilize the upper body and not assist in the movement. See table 21.1 for the muscle actions.

FLEXIBILITY ANALYSIS—BENT-KNEE TRUNK FLEXION

Stretching the Erector Spinae and Sacrospinalis

Flexing the legs during this exercise helps better isolate the low-back musculature; moreover, less pressure is applied to the lumbar disks from the hamstrings. Care should be taken in less flexible individuals or those with a history of disk problems. While these individuals can certainly perform this movement, there may need to be adjustments to the level of stretch applied. This movement can be performed while seated in a chair, which is safer for individuals who are inflexible or have pain. Begin seated upright on a table (figure 21.5) or seated in a chair. With the knees flexed about 10 degrees, tuck the chin on the exhale, contract the abdominals, and curl the body into flexion. Use the arms to assist at the end movement (figure 21.6). Return to the start

TABLE 21.1 Reverse-Crunch Flexion Muscle Actions

	Lifting Phase		Lowering Phase	
Joint	Action (concentric)	Agonists	Action (eccentric)	Agonists
Hip	Flexion	Iliopsoas, rectus femoris, pectineus	Extension	Iliopsoas, rectus femoris, pectineus
Trunk	Flexion	Rectus abdominis (pelvic tilt), internal and external obliques	Extension	Rectus abdominis (pelvic tilt), internal and external obliques

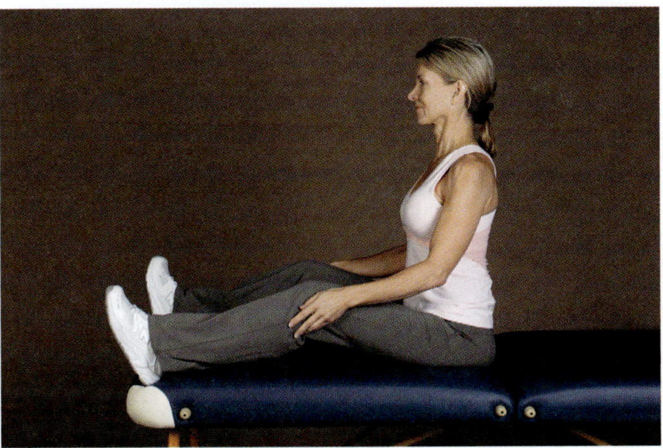

FIGURE 21.5 Bent-knee trunk flexion, start

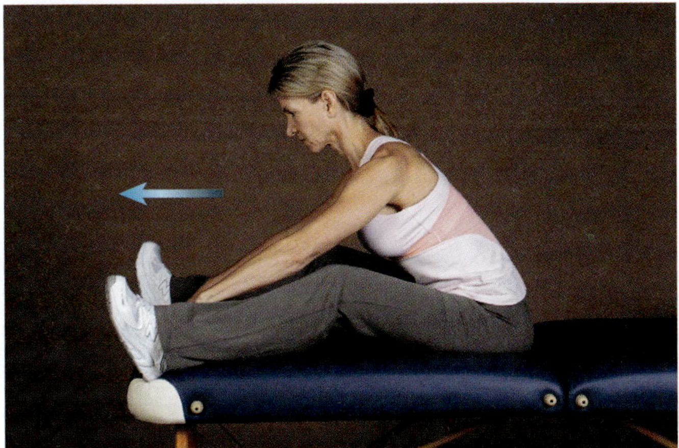

FIGURE 21.6 Bent-knee trunk flexion, end

position, and repeat. Take care not to bounce or move too quickly during the movement. There are many variations of this movement to achieve different goals. One variation, for example, is to keep the shoulders back while leaning forward, leading with the chest. *Contraindications:* This exercise is safe with controlled movement. It should never be performed with extended legs.

STRENGTHENING ANALYSIS—TRUNK STABILIZATION

Strengthening the Erector Spinae, Multifidus, Quadratus Lumborum, Gluteus Maximus, Proximal Biceps Femoris, Semimembranosus, and Semitendinosus

This exercise is a good way to bilaterally develop the upper shoulder muscles and the lower spinal and hip musculature. Because the movement occurs on opposite sides of the spinal column, stability of the trunk is encouraged through the resistance. Start in the prone

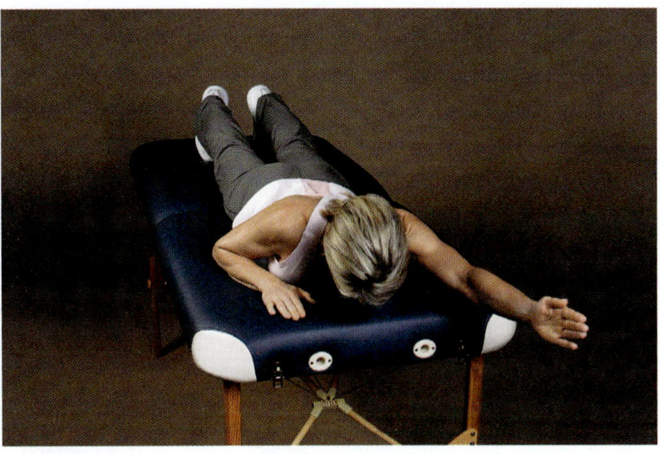

FIGURE 21.7 Trunk stabilization, start

position, face-down, with one arm extended out in front, thumbs up (figure 21.7). Extend the opposite-side leg, with the foot dorsiflexed throughout the movement. Begin lifting the extended arm up while also lifting the opposite extended leg into extension (figure 21.8). Perform 8 to 10 repetitions, and return to the start position each time. Weight can be added to this movement as strength improves: Hold a dumbbell in the hand, and attach a weight to the ankle. *Contraindications:* This exercise is safe with controlled movement.

See table 21.2 for the muscle actions.

FLEXIBILITY ANALYSIS—STRAIGHT-LEG HAMSTRING STRETCH

Stretching the Proximal Biceps Femoris, Semitendinosus, and Semimembranosus

The importance of hamstring flexibility in sports and daily movement cannot be overstated. While the opposite muscle group, the quadriceps, is often shortened, a limited-flexibility hamstring group,

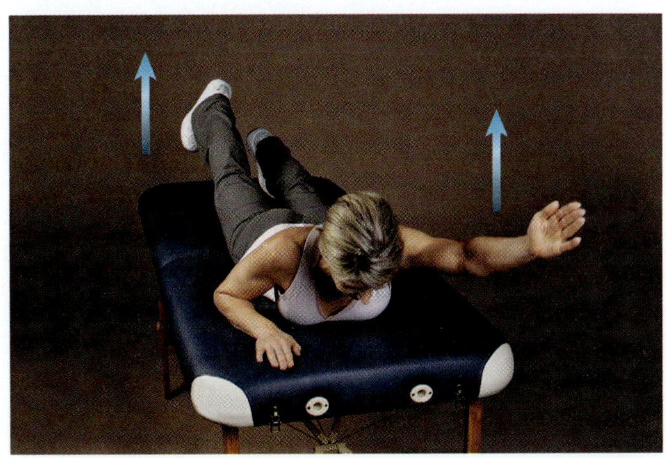

FIGURE 21.8 Trunk stabilization, end

TABLE 21.2 Trunk Stabilization Muscle Actions

	Lifting Phase		Lowering Phase	
Joint	**Action (concentric)**	**Agonists**	**Action (eccentric)**	**Agonists**
Hip	Extension	Biceps femoris, semimembranosus, semitendinosus, gluteus maximus	Extension (return to neutral position)	Biceps femoris, semimembranosus, semitendinosus gluteus maximus
Trunk	Extension	Quadratus lumborum, erector spinae, splenius	Extension (return to neutral position)	Quadratus lumborum, erector spinae, splenius
Shoulder	Flexion	Anterior deltoid, biceps brachii, pectoralis major (clavicular head), coracobrachialis	Extension	Anterior deltoid, biceps brachii, pectoralis major (clavicular head), coracobrachialis
Shoulder girdle	Adduction	Trapezius, rhomboids	Abduction	Trapezius, rhomboids

especially the biceps femoris, places extreme force on the lower back and hips. A solid treatment always includes treating both anterior and posterior muscle groups (see the quadriceps stretch on page 462). Individuals with chronic disk problems can perform this movement as long as caution is used with the range of motion. Individuals with disk problems are advised to start with small movements and then slowly increase the range of motion and amount of stretch. From a supine position, wrap an 8-foot-long rope around the foot of the involved leg. Flex the opposite leg (figure 21.9), and lock the involved leg throughout the movement. Contracting the quadriceps, lift the leg into flexion and apply a gentle 2-second stretch at the end movement using the rope (figure 21.10). The rope does not do the work; the proximal quadriceps and psoas contract to lift the thigh into flexion. Extend the knee into the stretch; the end point should be measured by the feel of the stretch on the proximal hamstring. *Contraindications:* This stretch is safe with controlled movement.

The uninvolved leg should remain relaxed throughout the movement to protect the lower back.

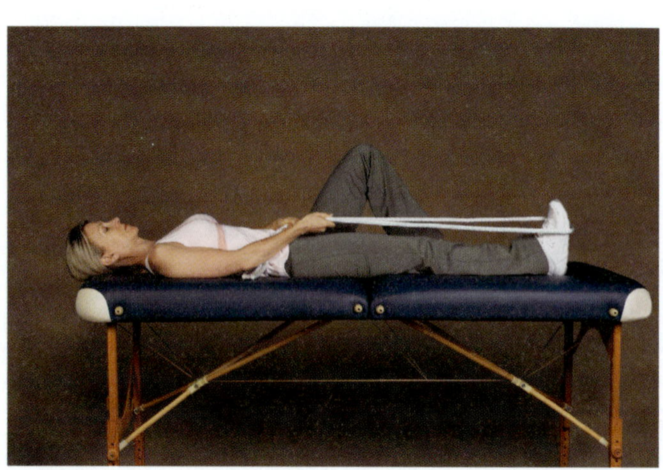

FIGURE 21.9 Straight-leg hamstring stretch, start

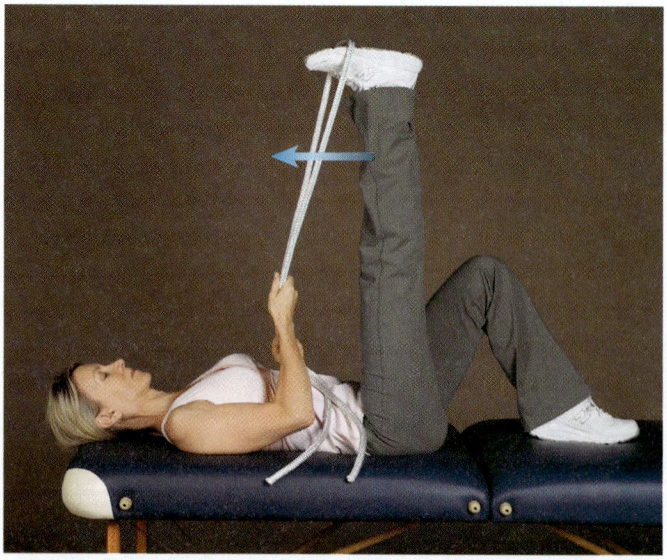

FIGURE 21.10 Straight-leg hamstring stretch, end

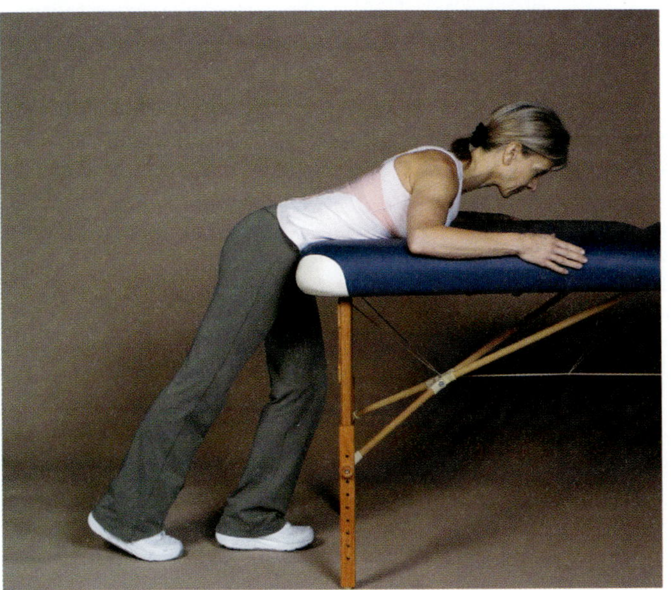

FIGURE 21.11 Straight-leg hip hyperextension, start

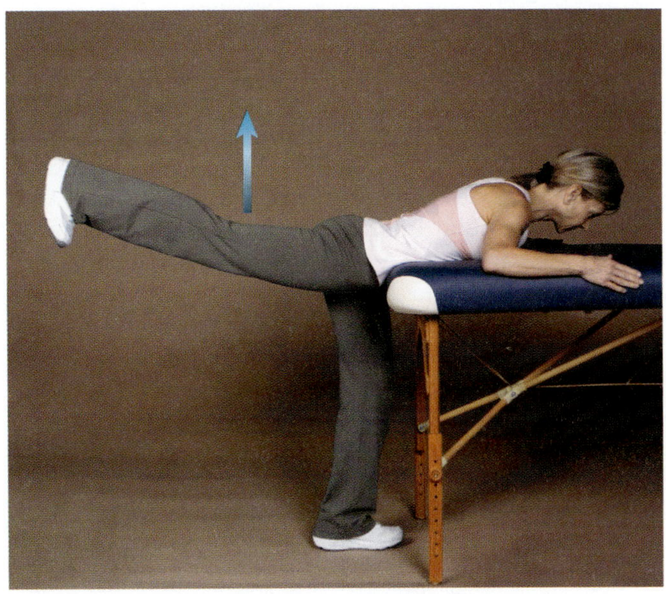

FIGURE 21.12 Straight-leg hip hyperextension, end

STRENGTHENING ANALYSIS—STRAIGHT-LEG HIP HYPEREXTENSION

Strengthening the Proximal Hamstrings and Gluteus Maximus

This exercise strengthens the proximal hamstring group and the gluteus maximus. While it is common to strengthen the belly of the hamstring group, the proximal part is often ignored, especially in individuals with low-back and hip dysfunctions. This area should be strong to support the lower back and to help improve gait. Strengthening this area is also helpful for sciatic issues. It is best to perform this exercise over a therapy table (pictured) or bench. Using ankle weights of 5 to 10 pounds (less if pain and weakness are present), bend over the edge of the table and reach forward with the arms to clasp the front of the table (figure 21.11). The pelvis and upper body remain relaxed and supported on the table, with no movement in the upper torso. Extend the involved leg out with the knee locked while slightly flexing the other leg for support. Contracting the hamstrings and gluteus maximus, lift the leg up into extension just level with the body; then return to the start position. The involved-side pelvis stays on the table as much as possible, and no weight is placed on the support leg (figure 21.12). *Contraindications:* This exercise is safe with controlled movement. The return position is always slow and controlled.

See table 21.3 for the muscle actions.

TABLE 21.3 Straight-Leg Hip Hyperextension Muscle Actions

	Lifting Phase		Lowering Phase	
Joint	**Action (concentric)**	**Agonists**	**Action (eccentric)**	**Agonists**
Hip	Hyperextension	Biceps femoris, semimembranosus, semitendinosus, gluteus maximus	Flexion	Biceps femoris, semimembranosus, semitendinosus, gluteus maximus
Trunk	Extension	Quadratus lumborum, erector spinae, splenius	Extension (return to neutral position)	Quadratus lumborum, splenius

FLEXIBILITY ANALYSIS—QUADRICEPS STRETCH

Stretching the Rectus Femoris, Vastus Lateralis, Vastus Medialis, and Vastus Intermedius

The rectus femoris is a powerful thigh muscle that has a direct relationship to the knee and patella. When it is shortened, extreme vector forces produce torque on the patella and can cause dysfunctions such as chondromalacia or patellar tendonitis. Because it also contributes to hip flexion, the rectus femoris can help skew the pelvis and make gait dysfunctional. This stretch helps lengthen the belly of this muscle and can help correct Osgood-Schlatter disease (inflammation of the growth plate at the tibial tuberosity) and patellar tendonitis in young athletes. This stretch is performed in the side-lying position instead of standing; thus the muscle is better stretched and isolated because it is relaxed. Bring the uninvolved leg into flexion by "hugging" the thigh to the chest (figure 21.13). This helps isolate the involved hip. Contract the abdominals throughout this movement to prevent hip rotation, with the involved leg in adduction (hip lined up with the shoulders). Contracting the gluteus maximus, extend the leg back while using the hand to stretch at the end movement (figure 21.14). Return the hip into flexion each time. Individuals who have difficulty reaching the ankle can try using a rope wrapped around the foot. For arthritis and disk issues, the abdominals must stay contracted to protect and stabilize the spine. *Contraindications:* This stretch is safe with controlled movement. It is safe for individuals with arthritis, but the movements must be adjusted to the condition. The "pumping" motion of this stretch—that is, flexion and extension of the knee—is most beneficial for getting blood and oxygen to the knee capsule.

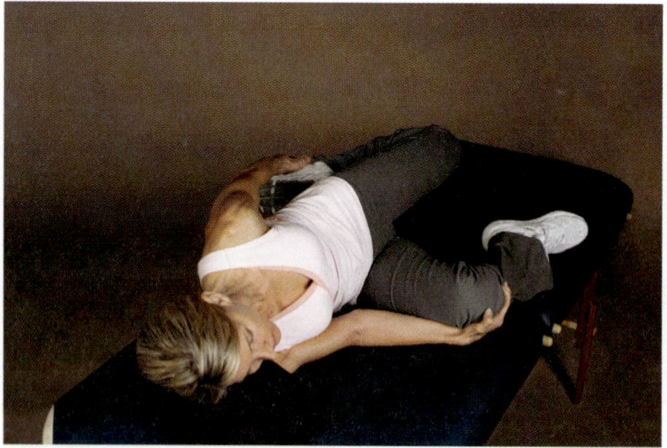

FIGURE 21.13 Stretching of the quadriceps, start

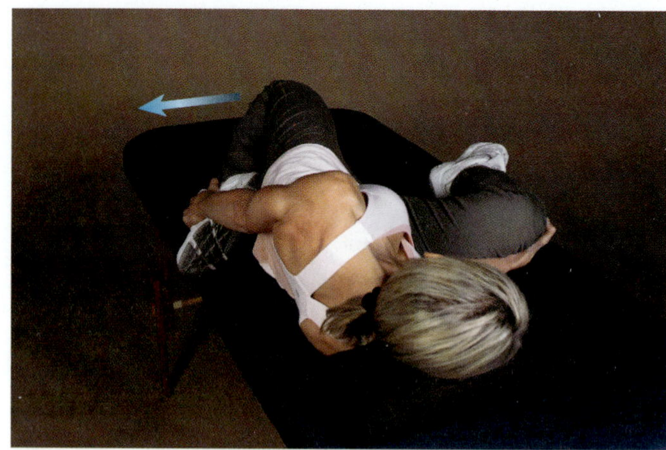

FIGURE 21.14 Stretching of the quadriceps, end

STRENGTHENING ANALYSIS—PHYSIO-BALL WALL SQUATS

Strengthening the Quadriceps, Gluteus Maximus, Tensor Fasciae Latae, Hamstrings, and Sartorius

This exercise targets many of the hip and knee muscles. It is safe because it utilizes a physio ball for support. Standing with the back to the wall, place a midsize physio ball between the lumbar spine and the wall (figure 21.15). The body should be at a slight angle from the wall. Keeping pressure against the ball, slowly lower the hips, letting the ball roll

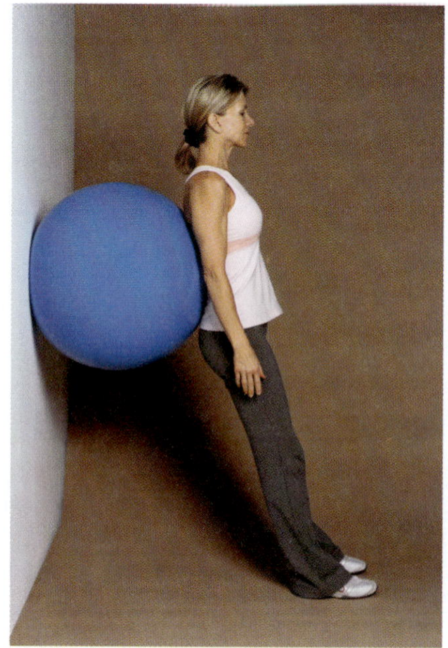

FIGURE 21.15 Physio-ball squats, start

TABLE 21.4 Physio-Ball Wall Squat Muscle Actions

	Lowering Phase (squat)		Raising Phase	
Joint	**Action (eccentric)**	**Agonists**	**Action (concentric)**	**Agonists**
Hip	Flexion	Psoas, quadriceps, adductors, sartorius	Extension	Quadriceps, gluteals, tensor fasciae latae, sartorius, biceps femoris, semimembranosus, semitendinosus
Knee	Flexion	Quadriceps, adductors	Extension	Quadriceps

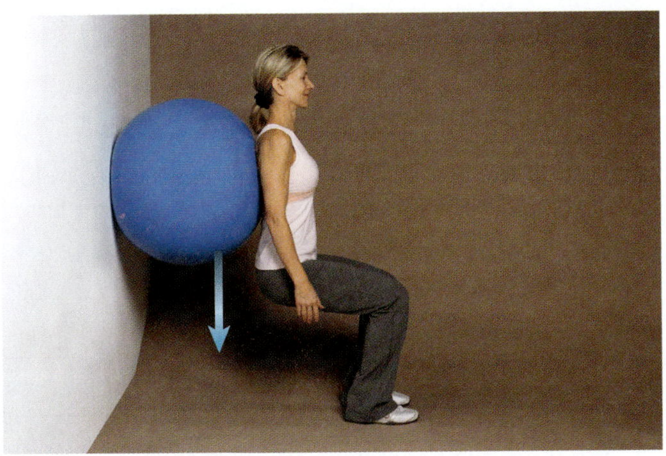

FIGURE 21.16 Physio-ball squats, end

up the back. After about 50 to 60 degrees of squat, return to the start position, letting the ball roll down the back and sacrum (figure 21.16). Before beginning the exercise, contract the abdominals. The head and spine remain in the neutral position throughout the movement. During the movement, contract the adductors to help support the knees and hips. *Contraindications:* This exercise is safe with controlled movement.

See table 21.4 for the muscle actions.

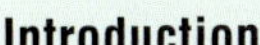

CHAPTER *summary*

Introduction

- ✔ The lower extremities allow the body to propel itself against gravity, participate in sports requiring skill and precision, and participate in myriad other activities. The body's system of levers and muscles works synergistically to produce smooth, powerful *movement*. When this movement is compromised by shortened and weak muscle tissue, pain usually results, thereby setting off a snowball of mechanical disadvantages. The lower extremities have a vital connection to the upper extremities.

Muscle Contraction

- ✔ The type of contraction of a muscle is determined by whether the muscle is lengthening or shortening during the movement. However, muscles may shorten or lengthen in the absence of a contraction through passive movement caused by other contracting muscles, momentum, gravity, or external forces such as manual assistance and exercise machines.

Analysis of Clinical Flexibility and Therapeutic Exercise of the Trunk and Lower Extremity

- ✔ Active Isolated Stretching movements can be used in a clinical setting to increase range of motion in specific muscles.
- ✔ Stretching the rectus abdominis and obliques, or the *core* of the body, has many benefits. The abdominals often become shortened from overuse as core muscles.
- ✔ Trunk stabilization is a good way to bilaterally develop the upper shoulder muscles and the lower spinal and hip musculature.

CHAPTER *review*

True or False

Write true *or* false *after each statement.*

1. The eccentric contraction in resistance exercises challenges muscle fibers to grow.
2. The lower extremities have a vital connection to the upper extremities.
3. The rectus femoris has no involvement in chondromalacia.
4. Traditional kinesiology has become popular in athletic training and physical therapy programs.
5. The rectus abdominis has no role in the backhand tennis swing.
6. The weakest part of the biceps femoris in many athletes is the proximal end.
7. One benefit of performing trunk hyperextension is that it stretches the abdominals.
8. Strength, endurance, and lower-extremity muscle flexibility will not help improve movement.
9. A concentric contraction is a shortening contraction of the muscles against gravity or resistance.
10. An individual with sciatic pain will benefit from daily stretching.

Short Answers

Write your answers on the lines provided.

1. What is considered the *core* of the body?
2. What is Osgood-Schlatter disease?
3. What is the benefit of stretching the quadriceps in a side-lying position?
4. What other part of the abdominals does the reverse crunch work?
5. What is sarcopenia?
6. In a clinical setting, is it considered safe to hold a muscle longer than 2 seconds if the client has lumbar disk herniations?
7. What are the agonists in the straight-leg hamstring stretch?
8. If an athlete has a hamstring injury that makes him limp, over time will this affect his neck or shoulders?
9. What kind of muscle contraction occurs in the rectus femoris during the lowering phase of a wall squat?

10. What is one benefit of specific flexibility for someone with gait issues?

____

____

____

Multiple Choice

Circle the correct answers.

1. Reverse sit-ups challenge:
   a. erector spinae
   b. quadratus lumborum
   c. lower abdominals and obliques
   d. none of the above
2. When movement in the lower extremity is compromised, this will affect:
   a. toe-off on one leg only
   b. the anterior cruciate ligament
   c. patellar tracking
   d. the upper extremities
3. In a fitness program, one of the most ignored muscular areas to strengthen is:
   a. quadriceps
   b. proximal hamstring
   c. abdominals
   d. erector spinae
4. A professional tennis player who does not perform specific flexibility and resistance work during the season:
   a. has a high chance of injury
   b. has developed enough through constant tennis movements
   c. has weak lateral movements
   d. has weak external rotation of the hips
5. Active Isolated Stretching utilizes:
   a. breathing
   b. 2-second holds
   c. both a and b
   d. passive movements
6. A teen basketball player has pain below her patella. An assessment shows limited ROM in flexion. Most likely she has:
   a. chondromalacia
   b. a torn ACL
   c. patellar tendonitis
   d. Baker's cyst
7. Lengthening the hamstring group through specific stretching can:
   a. relieve low-back dysfunction
   b. help knee tracking
   c. improve tensor fasciae latae contraction
   d. help genu varum
8. An individual undergoing physical therapy for a lumbar herniation should:
   a. never stretch
   b. gauge the level of stretch carefully
   c. perform gentle 2-second stretches with the opposite leg bent
   d. both b and c
9. The core of the body has what function?
   a. provides balance and support
   b. makes one feel dizzy during a workout
   c. prevents the body from becoming injured
   d. stores energy
10. Loss of skeletal muscle tissue is called:
    a. atrophic osmosis
    b. sarcopenia
    c. wastings disease
    d. hypertrophy

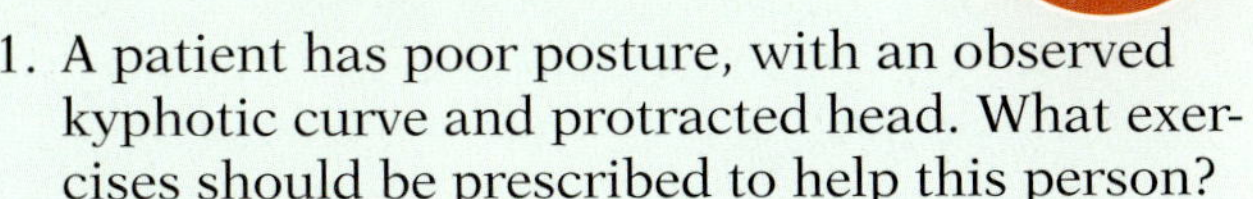

1. A patient has poor posture, with an observed kyphotic curve and protracted head. What exercises should be prescribed to help this person?
2. A patient complains of low-back pain but has no active herniations. What exercises will help this person?
3. During trunk hyperextension, which agonists act on the shoulder girdle?
4. Perform the straight-leg hamstring stretch with a rope. Then try it while first tilting the pelvis posteriorly, flattening the low back

against the floor. Describe how this changes the stretch to the hamstrings.

5. If an individual strengthens his abdominals at the gym, what other exercise should he do to ensure that balance to the core is maintained?

6. After observing a person's gait, describe how this observation could help in exercise prescription.

7. Explain why it is beneficial to stretch muscles before resistance training.

8. Describe how stretching the rectus femoris will help an individual with Osgood-Schlatter disease.

9. What are two functions of the psoas muscle?

10. Define traditional kinesiology.

Appendix A

References and Resources

chapter 1

Anthony C, Thibodeau G: *Textbook of anatomy and physiology,* ed 10, St. Louis, 1979, Mosby.

Booher JM, Thibodeau GA: *Athletic injury assessment,* ed 4, New York, 2000, McGraw-Hill.

Goss CM: *Gray's anatomy of the human body,* ed 29, Philadelphia, 1973, Lea & Febiger.

Hamilton N, Luttgens K: *Kinesiology: scientific basis of human motion,* ed 10, New York, 2002, McGraw-Hill.

Lindsay DT: *Functional human anatomy,* St. Louis, 1996, Mosby.

Logan GA, McKinney WC: *Anatomic kinesiology,* ed 3, Dubuque, IA, 1982, Brown.

National Strength and Conditioning Association; Baechle TR, Earle RW, eds.: *Essentials of strength training and conditioning,* ed 2, Champaign, IL, 2000, Human Kinetics.

Neumann DA: *Kinesiology of the musculoskeletal system: foundations for physical rehabilitation,* St. Louis, 2002, Mosby.

Northrip JW, Logan GA, McKinney WC: *Analysis of sport motion: anatomic and biomechanic perspectives,* ed 3, Dubuque, IA, 1983, Brown.

Prentice WE: *Arnheim's principles of athletic training,* ed 11, New York, 2003, McGraw-Hill.

Prentice WE: *Rehabilitation techniques in sports medicine,* ed 4, New York, 2004, McGraw-Hill.

Seeley RR, Stephens TD, Tate P: *Anatomy & physiology,* ed 7, New York, 2006, McGraw-Hill.

Shier D, Butler J, Lewis R: *Hole's essentials of human anatomy and physiology,* ed 9, New York, 2006, McGraw-Hill.

Stedman TL: *Stedman's medical dictionary,* ed 27, Baltimore, 2000, Lippincott Williams & Wilkins.

Steindler A: *Kinesiology of the human body,* Springfield, IL, 1970, Thomas.

Van De Graaff KM: *Human anatomy,* ed 6, New York, 2002, McGraw-Hill.

Van De Graaff KM, Fox SI, LaFleur KM: *Synopsis of human anatomy & physiology,* Dubuque, IA, 1997, Brown.

chapter 2

Bernier MR: Perturbation and agility training in the rehabilitation for soccer athletes, *Athletic Therapy Today* 8(3):20–22, 2003.

Blackburn T, Guskiewicz KM, Petschauer MA, Prentice WE: Balance and joint stability: the relative contributions of proprioception and muscular strength, *Journal of Sport Rehabilitation* 9(4):315–328, 2000.

Carter AM, Kinzey SJ, Chitwood LF, Cole JL: Proprioceptive neuromuscular facilitation decreases muscle activity during the stretch reflex in selected posterior thigh muscles, *Journal of Sport Rehabilitation* 9(4):269–278, 2000.

Dover G, Powers ME: Reliability of joint position sense and force-reproduction measures during internal and external rotation of the shoulder, *Journal of Athletic Training* 38(4):304–310, 2003.

Hall SJ: *Basic biomechanics,* ed 4, New York, 2003, McGraw-Hill.

Hamill J, Knutzen KM: *Biomechanical basis of human movement,* ed 2, Baltimore, 2003, Lippincott Williams & Wilkins.

Hamilton N, Luttgens K: *Kinesiology: scientific basis of human motion,* ed 10, Boston, 2002, McGraw-Hill.

Knight KL, Ingersoll CD, Bartholomew J: Isotonic contractions might be more effective than isokinetic contractions in developing muscle strength, *Journal of Sport Rehabilitation* 10(2):124–131, 2001.

Kreighbaum E, Barthels KM: *Biomechanics: a qualitative approach for studying human movement,* ed 4, Boston, 1996, Allyn & Bacon.

Lindsay DT: *Functional human anatomy,* St. Louis, 1996, Mosby.

Logan GA, McKinney WC: *Anatomic kinesiology,* ed 3, Dubuque, IA, 1982, Brown.

Mattes AL: *Active Isolated Stretching,* Sarasota, FL, 1995.

McArdle WD, Katch FI, Katch VI: *Exercise physiology: energy, nutrition, and human performance,* ed 5, Baltimore, 2001, Lippincott Williams & Wilkins.

McCrady BJ, Amato HK: Functional strength and proprioception testing of the lower extremity, *Athletic Therapy Today* 9(5):60–61, 2005.

Myers JB, Guskiewicz KM, Schneider, RA, Prentice WE: Proprioception and neuromuscular control of the shoulder after muscle fatigue, *Journal of Athletic Training* 34(4):362–367, 1999.

National Strength and Conditioning Association; Baechle TR, Earle RW, eds.: *Essentials of strength training and conditioning,* ed 2, Champaign, IL, 2000, Human Kinetics.

Neumann DA: *Kinesiology of the musculoskeletal system: foundations for physical rehabilitation,* St. Louis, 2002, Mosby.

Norkin CC, Levangie PK: *Joint structure and function: a comprehensive analysis,* Philadelphia, 1983, Davis.

Northrip JW, Logan GA, McKinney WC: *Analysis of sport motion,* ed 3, Dubuque, IA, 1983, Brown.

Olmsted-Kramer LC, Hertel J: Preventing recurrent lateral ankle sprains: an evidence-based approach, *Athletic Therapy Today* 9(2):19–22, 2004.

Powers ME, Buckley BD, Kaminski TW, Hubbard TJ, Ortiz C: Six weeks of strength and proprioception training does not affect muscle fatigue and static balance in functional ankle stability, *Journal of Sport Rehabilitation* 13(3):201–227, 2004.

Powers SK, Howley ET: *Exercise physiology: theory and application of fitness and performance,* ed 5, New York, 2004, McGraw-Hill.

Rasch PJ: *Kinesiology and applied anatomy,* ed 7, Philadelphia, 1989, Lea & Febiger.

Riemann BL, Lephart SM: The sensorimotor system, part I: the physiological basis of functional joint stability, *Journal of Athletic Training* 37(1):71–79, 2002.

Riemann BL, Lephart SM: The sensorimotor system, part II: the role of proprioception in motor control and functional joint stability, *Journal of Athletic Training* 37(1):80–84, 2002.

Riemann BL, Myers JB, Lephart SM: Sensorimotor system measurement techniques, *Journal of Athletic Training* 37(1):85–98, 2002.

Riemann BL, Tray NC, Lephart SM: Unilateral multiaxial coordination training and ankle kinesthesia, muscle strength, and postural control, *Journal of Sport Rehabilitation* 12(1):13–30, 2003.

Ross S, Guskiewicz K, Prentice W, Schneider R, Yu B: Comparison of biomechanical factors between the kicking and stance limbs, *Journal of Sport Rehabilitation* 13(2):135–150, 2004.

Saladin SK: *Anatomy and physiology: the unity of form and function,* ed 4, New York, 2007, McGraw-Hill.

Sandrey MA: Using eccentric exercise in the treatment of lower extremity tendinopathies, *Athletic Therapy Today* 9(1):58–59, 2004.

Seeley RR, Stephens TD, Tate P: *Anatomy & physiology,* ed 7, New York, 2006, McGraw-Hill.

Shier D, Butler J, Lewis R: *Hole's essentials of human anatomy and physiology,* ed 9, New York, 2006, McGraw-Hill.

Shier D, Butler J, Lewis R: *Hole's human anatomy and physiology,* ed 9, New York, 2002, McGraw-Hill.

Van De Graaff KM: *Human anatomy,* ed 6, New York, 2002, McGraw-Hill.

Van De Graaf KM, Fox SI, LaFleur KM: *Synopsis of human anatomy & physiology,* Dubuque, IA, 1997, Brown.

Yaggie J, Armstrong WJ: Effects on lower extremity fatigue on indices of balance, *Journal of Sport Rehabilitation* 10(2):124–131, 2004.

chapter 3

Adrian MJ, Cooper JM: *The biomechanics of human movement,* Indianapolis, IN, 1989, Benchmark.

American Academy of Orthopaedic Surgeons; Schenck RC, ed.: *Athletic training and sports medicine,* ed 3, Rosemont, IL, 1999, American Academy of Orthopaedic Surgeons.

Barham JN: *Mechanical kinesiology,* St. Louis, 1978, Mosby.

Broer MR: *An introduction to kinesiology,* Englewood Cliffs, NJ, 1968, Prentice-Hall.

Broer MR, Zernicke RF: *Efficiency of human movement,* ed 3, Philadelphia, 1979, Saunders.

Bunn JW: *Scientific principles of coaching,* ed 2, Englewood Cliffs, NJ, 1972, Prentice-Hall.

Cooper JM, Adrian M, Glassow RB: *Kinesiology,* ed 5, St. Louis, 1982, Mosby.

Donatelli R, Wolf SL: *The biomechanics of the foot and ankle,* Philadelphia, 1990, Davis.

Hall SJ: *Basic biomechanics,* ed 4, New York, 2000, McGraw-Hill.

Hamill J, Knutzen KM: *Biomechanical basis of human movement,* ed 2, Baltimore, 2003, Lippincott Williams & Wilkins.

Hinson M: *Kinesiology,* ed 4, New York, 1981, McGraw-Hill.

Kegerreis S, Jenkins WL, Malone TR: Throwing injuries, *Sports Injury Management* 2:4, 1989.

Kelley DL: *Kinesiology: fundamentals of motion description,* Englewood Cliffs, NJ, 1971, Prentice-Hall.

Kreighbaum E, Barthels KM: *Biomechanics: a qualitative approach for studying human movement,* ed 3, New York, 1990, Macmillan.

Logan GA, McKinney WC: *Anatomic kinesiology,* ed 3, New York, 1982, McGraw-Hill.

Luttgens K, Hamilton N: *Kinesiology: scientific basis of human motion,* ed 10, New York, 2002, McGraw-Hill.

McCreary EK, Kendall FP, Rodgers MM, Provance PG, Romani WA: *Muscles: testing and function with posture and pain,* ed 5, Philadelphia, 2005, Lippincott Williams & Wilkins.

McGinnis PM: *Biomechanics of sport and exercise,* ed 2, Champaign, IL, 2005, Human Kinetics.

Neumann DA: *Kinesiology of the musculoskeletal system: foundations for physical rehabilitation,* St. Louis, 2002, Mosby.

Nordin M, Frankel VH: *Basic biomechanics of the musculoskeletal system,* ed 2, Philadelphia, 1989, Lea & Febiger.

Norkin CC, Levangie PK: *Joint structure and function: a comprehensive analysis,* Philadelphia, 1983, Davis.

Northrip JW, Logan GA, McKinney WC: *Analysis of sport motion: anatomic and biomechanic perspectives,* ed 3, New York, 1983, McGraw-Hill.

Oatis CA: *Kinesiology: the mechanics and pathomechanics of human movement,* Philadelphia, 2004, Lippincott Williams & Wilkins

Piscopo J, Baley J: *Kinesiology: the science of movement,* New York, 1981, Wiley.

Prentice WE: *Arheim's principles of athletic training,* ed 11, New York, 2003, McGraw-Hill.

Rasch PJ: *Kinesiology and applied anatomy,* ed 7, Philadelphia, 1989, Lea & Febiger.

Scott MG: *Analysis of human motion,* ed 2, New York, 1963, Appleton-Century-Crofts.

Segedy A: Braces' joint effects spur research surge, *Biomechanics,* February 2005.

Weineck J: *Functional anatomy in sports,* ed 2, St. Louis, 1990, Mosby.

Whiting WC: *Biomechanics of musculoskeletal injury,* Champaign, IL, 1998, Human Kinetics.

Wirhed R: *Athletic ability and the anatomy of motion,* London, 1984, Wolfe.

chapter 4

Andrews JR, Wilk KE: *The athlete's shoulder,* New York, 1994, Churchill Livingstone.

Andrews JR, Zarins B, Wilk KE: *Injuries in baseball,* Philadelphia, 1998, Lippincott-Raven.

Dail N: *Kinesiology manual,* Waldoboro, ME, 2006, Lincoln County Publishing.

DePalma MJ, Johnson EW: Detecting and treating shoulder impingement syndrome: the role of scapulothoracic dyskinesis, *The Physician and Sportsmedicine* 31(7), 2003.

Field D: *Anatomy: palpation and surface markings,* ed 3, Oxford, 2001, Butterworth-Heinemann.

Hislop HJ, Montgomery J: *Daniels and Worthingham's muscle testing: techniques of manual examination,* ed 7, Philadelphia, 2002, Saunders.

Johnson RJ: Acromioclavicular joint injuries: identifying and treating "separated shoulder" and other conditions, *The Physician and Sportsmedicine* 29(11), 2001.

Mattes AL: *Active Isolated Stretching,* Sarasota, FL, 1995.

McMurtrie H, Rikel JK: *The coloring review guide to human anatomy,* New York, 1991, McGraw-Hill.

Muscolino JE: *The muscular system manual: the skeletal muscles of the human body,* ed 2, St. Louis, 2003, Elsevier Mosby.

Neumann DA: *Kinesiology of the musculoskeletal system: foundations for physical rehabilitation,* St. Louis, 2002, Mosby.

Norkin CC, Levangie PK: *Joint structure and function: a comprehensive analysis,* Philadelphia, 1983, Davis.

Rasch PJ: *Kinesiology and applied anatomy,* ed 7, Philadelphia, 1989, Lea & Febiger.

Seeley RR, Stephens TD, Tate P: *Anatomy & physiology,* ed 7, Dubuque, IA, 2006, McGraw-Hill.

Smith LK, Weiss EL, Lehmkuhl LD: *Brunnstrom's clinical kinesiology,* ed 5, Philadelphia, 1996, Davis.

Sobush DC, et al.: The Lennie test for measuring scapula position in healthy young adult females: a reliability and validity study, *Journal of Orthopaedic and Sports Physical Therapy* 23:39, January 1996.

Soderburg GL: *Kinesiology—application to pathological motion,* Baltimore, 1986, Williams & Wilkins.

Travell J, Simons D, Simons L: *Myofascial pain and dysfunction: the trigger point manual, vol. 1: upper half of body,* ed 2, Baltimore, 1999, Williams & Wilkins.

Van De Graaff KM: *Human anatomy,* ed 6, Dubuque, IA, 2002, McGraw-Hill.

Werner R: *A massage therapist's guide to pathology,* ed 3, Baltimore, 2005, Lippincott Williams & Wilkins.

Williams CC: Posterior sternoclavicular joint dislocation emergencies series, Howe WB, ed., *The Physician and Sportsmedicine* 27(2), 1999.

chapter 5

Barnes J: Myofascial release in treatment of thoracic outlet syndrome, *Journal of Bodywork and Movement Therapies* 1(1):53–57, 1996.

Cyriax J: *Textbook of orthopaedic medicine, vol. 2: treatment by manipulation, massage, and injection,* London, 1984, Bailliere Tindall.

Dail N: *Kinesiology manual,* Waldoboro, ME, 2006, Lincoln County Publishing.

Dail N: *Manual for a gift of touch,* Waldoboro, ME, 2008, Lincoln County Publishing.

Dail N: *Massage manual,* Waldoboro, ME, 2008, Lincoln County Publishing.

Field T: *Touch therapy,* Edinburgh, 2000, Churchill Livingstone.

Hall SJ: *Basic biomechanics,* ed 4, New York, 2003, McGraw-Hill.

Hamill J, Knutzen KM: *Biomechanical basis of human movement,* ed 2, Baltimore, 2003, Lippincott Williams & Wilkins.

Hamilton N, Luttgens K: *Kinesiology: scientific basis of human motion,* ed 10, Boston, 2002, McGraw-Hill.

Hoppenfeld S: *Physical examination of the spine & extremities,* Norwalk, CT, 1976, Appleton & Lange.

King R: *Myofascial techniques for the shoulder girdle and shoulder joint* (Manual), Chicago, 2003, Robert King Seminars.

Lowe W: *Orthopedic massage,* Edinburgh, 2003, Mosby.

Meagher J: *Sportsmassage,* New York, 1980, Station Hill Press.

Moore T: *Care of the soul,* New York, 1992, HarperCollins.

Saladin K: *Anatomy & physiology,* ed 4, New York, 2007, McGraw-Hill.

Tappan FM, Benjamin P: *Tappan's handbook of healing massage techniques,* ed 3, Stamford, 1998, Appleton & Lange.

Travell J, Rinzler SH: The myofascial genesis of pain, *Postgraduate Medical Journal* 11:425–431, 1952.

Travell J, Simons D, Simons L: *Myofascial pain and dysfunction: the trigger point manual, vol 1: upper half of body,* ed 2, Baltimore, 1999, Williams & Wilkins.

Van De Graaff KM: *Human anatomy,* ed 6, Dubuque, IA, 2002, McGraw-Hill.

chapter 6

Andrews JR, Wilk KE: *The athlete's shoulder,* New York, 1994, Churchill Livingstone.

Andrews JR, Zarins B, Wilk KE: *Injuries in baseball,* Philadelphia, 1988, Lippincott-Raven.

Dail N: *Kinesiology manual,* Waldoboro, ME, 2006, Lincoln County Publishing.

Field D: *Anatomy: palpation and surface markings,* ed 3, Oxford, 2001, Butterworth-Heinemann.

Garth WP, et al.: Occult anterior subluxations of the shoulder in noncontact sports, *American Journal of Sports Medicine* 15:579, November–December 1987.

Hislop HJ, Montgomery J: *Daniels and Worthingham's muscle testing: techniques of manual examination,* ed 7, Philadelphia, 2002, Saunders.

Khan KM, Cook JL, Taunton JE, Bonar F: Overuse tendinosis, not tendonitis, part 1: a new paradigm for a difficult clinical problem, *The Physician and Sportsmedicine* 28(5):38 ff, 2000.

Lowe W: *Orthopedic massage,* Edinburgh, 2003, Mosby.

Muscolino JE: *The muscular system manual: the skeletal muscles of the human body,* ed 2, St. Louis, 2003, Elsevier Mosby.

Oatis CA: *Kinesiology: the mechanics and pathomechanics of human movement,* Philadelphia, 2004, Lippincott Williams & Wilkins.

Perry JF, Rohe DA, Garcia AO: *The kinesiology workbook,* Philadelphia, 1992, Davis.

Poppen NK, Walker PS: Normal and abnormal motion of the shoulder, *Journal of Bone and Joint Surgery* [American] 58:195–201, 1976.

Rasch PJ: *Kinesiology and applied anatomy,* ed 7, Philadelphia, 1989, Lea & Febiger.

Seeley RR, Stephens TD, Tate P: *Anatomy & physiology,* ed 7, New York, 2006, McGraw-Hill.

Sieg KW, Adams SP: *Illustrated essentials of musculoskeletal anatomy,* ed 2, Gainesville, FL, 1985, Megabooks.

Smith LK, Weiss EL, Lehmkuhl LD: *Brunnstrom's clinical kinesiology,* ed 5, Philadelphia, 1996, Davis.

Stacey E: Pitching injuries to the shoulder, *Athletic Journal* 65:44, January 1984.

Travell J, Simons D, Simons L: *Myofascial pain and dysfunction: the trigger point manual, vol 1: upper half of body,* ed 2, Baltimore, 1999, Williams & Wilkins.

Werner R: *A massage therapist's guide to pathology,* ed 3, Baltimore, 2005, Lippincott Williams & Wilkins.

chapter 7

Caillet R: *Shoulder pain,* ed 3, Philadelphia, 1991, Davis.

Chaitow L: *Muscle energy techniques,* London, 1998, Churchill Livingstone.

Cyriax J: *Textbook of orthopaedic medicine, vol. 2: treatment by manipulation, massage, and injection,* London, 1984, Bailliere Tindall.

Dail N: *Kinesiology manual,* Waldoboro, ME, 2006, Lincoln County Publishing.

Dail N: *Massage manual,* Waldoboro, ME, 2008, Lincoln County Publishing.

Dail N: *Manual for a gift of touch,* Waldoboro, ME, 2008, Lincoln County Publishing

Field T: *Touch therapy,* Edinburgh, 2000, Churchill Livingstone.

Fritz S: *Mosby's fundamentals of therapeutic massage,* ed 3, St. Louis, 2004, Mosby.

Goold GB: *First aid in the workplace,* ed 2, Upper Saddle River, NJ, 1998, Prentice-Hall.

Hoppenfeld S: *Physical examination of the spine & extremities,* Norwalk, CT, 1976, Appleton & Lange.

King R: *Myofascial techniques for the shoulder girdle and shoulder joint* (Manual), Chicago, 2003, Robert King Seminars.

Lowe W: *Orthopedic massage,* Edinburgh, 2003, Mosby.

Magee DJ: *Orthopedic physical assessment,* ed 4, Philadelphia, 2002, Saunders.

Meagher J: *Sportsmassage,* New York, 1980, Station Hill Press.

Oatis CA: *Kinesiology: the mechanics and pathomechanics of human movement,* Philadelphia, 2004, Lippincott Williams & Wilkins.

Saladin K: *Anatomy & physiology,* ed 4, New York, 2007, McGraw-Hill.

Stedman TL: *Stedman's medical dictionary,* ed 27, Baltimore, 2000, Lippincott Williams & Wilkins.

Travell J, Simons D, Simons L: *Myofascial pain and dysfunction: the trigger point manual, vol. 1: upper half of body,* ed 2, Baltimore, 1999, Williams & Wilkins.

Van De Graaff KM: *Human anatomy,* ed 6, Dubuque, IA, 2002, McGraw-Hill.

Werner R: *A massage therapist's guide to pathology,* ed 3, Baltimore, 2005, Lippincott Williams & Wilkins.

chapter 8

Andrews JR, Wilk KE: *The athlete's shoulder,* New York, 1994, Churchill Livingstone.

Andrews JR, Zarins B, Wilk KE: *Injuries in baseball,* Philadelphia, 1998, Lippincott-Raven.

Back BR Jr, et al.: Triceps rupture: a case report and literature review, *American Journal of Sports Medicine* 15:285, May–June 1987.

Dail N: *Kinesiology manual,* Waldoboro, ME, 2006, Lincoln County Publishing.

Gabbard CP, et al.: Effects of grip and forearm position on flexed-arm hang performance, *Research Quarterly for Exercise and Sport,* July 1983.

Guarantors of *Brain: Aids to the examination of the peripheral nervous system,* ed 4, London, 2000, Saunders.

Herrick RT, Herrick S: Ruptured triceps in powerlifter presenting as cubital tunnel syndrome—a case report, *American Journal of Sports Medicine* 15:514, September–October 1987.

Hislop HJ, Montgomery J: *Daniels and Worthingham's muscle testing: techniques of manual examination,* ed 7, Philadelphia, 2002, Saunders.

Magee DJ: *Orthopedic physical assessment,* ed 4, Philadelphia, 2002, Saunders.

Mattes AL: *Active Isolated Stretching,* Sarasota, FL, 1995.

Muscolino JE: *The muscular system manual: the skeletal muscles of the human body,* ed 2, St. Louis, 2003, Elsevier Mosby.

Oatis CA: *Kinesiology: the mechanics and pathomechanics of human movement,* Philadelphia, 2004, Lippincott Williams & Wilkins.

Rasch PJ: *Kinesiology and applied anatomy,* ed 7, Philadelphia, 1989, Lea & Febiger.

Shier D, Butler J, Lewis R: *Hole's human anatomy and physiology,* ed 9, New York, 2002, McGraw-Hill.

Sieg KW, Adams SP: *Illustrated essentials of musculoskeletal anatomy,* ed 2, Gainesville, FL, 1985, Megabooks.

Sisto DJ, et al.: An electromyographic analysis of the elbow in pitching, *American Journal of Sports Medicine* 15:260, May–June 1987.

Smith LK, Weiss EL, Lehmkuhl LD: *Brunnstrom's clinical kinesiology,* ed 5, Philadelphia, 1996, Davis.

Springer SI: Racquetball and elbow injuries, *National Racquetball* 16:7, March 1987.

Travell J, Simons D, Simons L: *Myofascial pain and dysfunction: the trigger point manual, vol. 1: upper half of body,* ed 2, Baltimore, 1999, Williams & Wilkins.

Van De Graaff KM: *Human anatomy,* ed 6, Dubuque, IA, 2002, McGraw-Hill.

Werner R: *A massage therapist's guide to pathology,* ed 3, Baltimore, 2005, Lippincott Williams & Wilkins.

chapter 9

Chaitow L: *Muscle energy techniques,* London, 1998, Churchill Livingstone.

Cyriax J: *Textbook of orthopaedic medicine, vol. 1: diagnosis of soft tissue lesions,* London, 1982, Bailliere Tindall.

Cyriax J: *Textbook of orthopaedic medicine, vol. 2: treatment by manipulation, massage, and injection,* London, 1984, Bailliere Tindall.

Dail N: *Kinesiology manual,* Waldoboro, ME, 2006, Lincoln County Publishing.

Dail N: *Manual for a gift of touch,* Waldoboro, ME, 2008, Lincoln County Publishing.

Dail N: *Massage manual,* Waldoboro, ME, 2008, Lincoln County Publishing.

Field T: *Touch therapy,* Edinburgh, ME, 2000, Churchill Livingstone.

Fritz S: *Mosby's fundamentals of therapeutic massage,* ed 3, St. Louis, 2004, Mosby.

Hoppenfeld S: *Physical examination of the spine & extremities,* Norwalk, CT, 1976, Appleton & Lange.

King R: *Myofascial techniques for the upper extremity* (Manual), Chicago, 2002, Robert King Seminars.

Knight K: *Cryotherapy: theory, technique and physiology,* Chattanooga, TN, 1985, Chattanooga Corporation.

Lowe W: *Orthopedic massage,* Edinburgh, 2003, Mosby.

Magee D: *Orthopedic physical assessment,* ed 3, Philadelphia, 1997, Saunders.

Meagher J: *Sportsmassage,* New York, 1980, Station Hill Press.

Saladin K: *Anatomy & physiology,* ed 4, New York, 2007, McGraw-Hill.

Stedman TL: *Stedman's medical dictionary,* ed 27, Baltimore, 2000, Lippincott Williams & Wilkins.

Travell J, Simons D, Simons L: *Myofascial pain and dysfunction: the trigger point manual, vol. 1: upper half of body,* ed 2, Baltimore, 1999, Williams & Wilkins.

Upton AR, McComas AJ: The double crush in nerve entrapment syndromes, *Lancet* 2(7825):359–362, 1973.

Van De Graaff KM: *Human anatomy,* ed 6, Dubuque, IA, 2002, McGraw-Hill.

Werner R: *A massage therapist's guide to pathology,* ed 3, Baltimore, 2005, Lippincott Williams & Wilkins.

chapter 10

Dail N: *Kinesiology manual,* Waldoboro, ME, 2006, Lincoln County Publishing.

Gabbard CP, et al.: Effects of grip and forearm position on flexed-arm hang performance, *Research Quarterly for Exercise and Sport,* July 1983.

Gench BE, Hinson MM, Harvey PT: *Anatomical kinesiology,* Dubuque, IA, 1995, Bowers.

Guarantors of *Brain: Aids to the examination of the peripheral nervous system,* ed 4, London, 2000, Saunders.

Hislop HJ, Montgomery J: *Daniels and Worthingham's muscle testing: techniques of manual examination,* ed 7, Philadelphia, 2002, Saunders.

Hoppenfeld S: *Physical examination of the spine & extremities,* Norwalk, CT, 1976, Appleton & Lange.

Lindsay DT: *Functional human anatomy,* St. Louis, 1996, Mosby.

Luttgens K, Hamilton N: *Kinesiology: scientific basis of human motion,* ed 10, New York, 2002, McGraw-Hill.

Magee DJ: *Orthopedic physical assessment,* ed 4, Philadelphia, 2002, Saunders.

Mattes AL: *Active Isolated Stretching,* Sarasota, FL, 1995.

Muscolino JE: *The muscular system manual: the skeletal muscles of the human body,* ed 2, St. Louis, 2003, Elsevier Mosby.

Norkin CC, Levangie PK: *Joint structure and function: a comprehensive analysis,* Philadelphia, 1983, Davis.

Norkin CC, White DJ: *Measurement of joint motion: a guide to goniometry,* Philadelphia, 1985, Davis.

Oatis CA: *Kinesiology: the mechanics and pathomechanics of human movement,* Philadelphia, 2004, Lippincott Williams & Wilkins.

Rasch PJ: *Kinesiology and applied anatomy,* ed 7, Philadelphia, 1989, Lea & Febiger.

Seeley RR, Stephens TD, Tate P: *Anatomy & physiology,* ed 7, New York, 2006, McGraw-Hill.

Sieg KW, Adams SP: *Illustrated essentials of musculoskeletal anatomy,* ed 2, Gainesville, FL, 1985, Megabooks.

Sisto DJ, et al.: An electromyographic analysis of the elbow in pitching, *American Journal of Sports Medicine* 15:260, May–June 1987.

Smith LK, Weiss EL, Lehmkuhl LD: *Brunnstrom's clinical kinesiology,* ed 5, Philadelphia, 1996, Davis.

Springer SI: Racquetball and elbow injuries, *National Racquetball* 16:7, March 1987.

Stone RJ, Stone JA: *Atlas of the skeletal muscles,* New York, 1990, McGraw-Hill.

Travell J, Simons D: *Myofascial pain and dysfunction: the trigger point manual, vol. 1: upper half of body,* Baltimore, 1983, Williams & Wilkins.

Van De Graaff KM: *Human anatomy,* ed 6, Dubuque, IA, 2002, McGraw-Hill.

Werner R: *A massage therapist's guide to pathology,* ed 3, Baltimore, 2005, Lippincott Williams & Wilkins.

chapter 11

Chaitow L: *Muscle energy techniques,* London, 1998, Churchill Livingstone.

Cyriax J: *Textbook of orthopaedic medicine, vol. 1: diagnosis of soft tissue lesions,* London, 1982, Bailliere Tindall.

Cyriax J: *Textbook of orthopaedic medicine, vol. 2: treatment by manipulation, massage, and injection,* London, 1984, Bailliere Tindall.

Dail N: *Kinesiology manual,* Waldoboro, ME, 2006, Lincoln County Publishing.

Dail N: *Manual for a gift of touch,* Waldoboro, ME, 2008, Lincoln County Publishing.

Dail N: *Massage manual,* Waldoboro, ME, 2008, Lincoln County Publishing.

Field T: *Touch therapy,* Edinburgh, 2000, Churchill Livingstone.

Hoppenfeld S: *Physical examination of the spine & extremities,* Norwalk, CT, 1976, Appleton & Lange.

King R: *Myofascial techniques for the upper extremity* (Manual), Chicago, 2002, Robert King Seminars.

Lowe W: *Orthopedic massage,* Edinburgh, 2003, Mosby.

Magee DJ: *Orthopedic physical assessment,* ed 4, Philadelphia, 2002, Saunders.

Meagher J: *Sportsmassage,* New York, 1980, Station Hill Press.

Oatis CA: *Kinesiology: the mechanics and pathomechanics of human movement,* Philadelphia, 2004, Lippincott Williams & Wilkins.

Travell J, Simons D, Simons L: *Myofascial pain and dysfunction: the trigger point manual, vol. 1: upper half of body,* ed 2, Baltimore, 1999, Williams & Wilkins.

Van De Graaff KM: *Human anatomy,* ed 6, Dubuque, IA, 2002, McGraw-Hill.

Werner R: *A massage therapist's guide to pathology,* ed 3, Baltimore, 2005, Lippincott Williams & Wilkins.

chapter 12

Adrian M: Isokinetic exercise, *Training and Conditioning* 1:1, June 1991.

Agnew TA: *Dynamic flexibility: a safe and effective self-stretching manual,* Sarasota, FL, 1993, Intent.

Andrews JR, Wilk KE: *The athlete's shoulder,* New York, 1994, Churchill Livingstone.

Andrews JR, Zarins B, Wilk KE: *Injuries in baseball,* Philadelphia, 1998, Lippincott-Raven.

Booher JM, Thibodeau GA: *Athletic injury assessment,* ed 4, Dubuque, IA, 2000, McGraw-Hill.

Ellenbecker TS, Davies GJ: *Closed kinetic chain exercise: a comprehensive guide to multiple-joint exercise,* Champaign, IL, 2001, Human Kinetics.

Fleck SJ: Periodized strength training: a critical review, *Journal of Strength and Conditioning Research,* 13(1):82–89, 1999.

Geisler P: Kinesiology of the full golf swing—implications for intervention and rehabilitation, *Sports Medicine Update* 11(9):2, 1996.

Hamilton N, Luttgens K: *Kinesiology: scientific basis of human motion,* ed 10, Boston, 2002, McGraw-Hill.

Matheson O, et al.: Stress fractures in athletes, *American Journal of Sports Medicine* 15:46, January–February 1987.

Mattes AL: *Active Isolated Stretching,* Sarasota, FL, 1995.

National Strength and Conditioning Association; Baechle TR, Earle RW, eds.: *Essentials of strength training and conditioning,* ed 2, Champaign, IL, 2000, Human Kinetics.

Northrip JW, Logan GA, McKinney WC: *Analysis of sport motion: anatomic and biomechanic perspectives,* ed 3, New York, 1983, McGraw-Hill.

Powers SK, Howley ET: *Exercise physiology: theory and application to fitness and performance,* ed 5, New York, 2004, McGraw-Hill.

Smith LK, Weiss EL, Lehmkuhl LD: *Brunnstrom's clinical kinesiology,* ed 5, Philadelphia, 1996, Davis.

Steindler A: *Kinesiology of the human body,* Springfield, IL, 1970, Thomas.

chapter 13

Clarkson HM, Gilewich GB: *Musculoskeletal assessment: joint range of motion and manual muscle strength,* Baltimore, 1989, Williams & Wilkins.

Dail N: *Kinesiology manual,* Waldoboro, ME, 2006, Lincoln County Publishing.

Day AL: Observation on the treatment of lumbar disk disease in college football players, *American Journal of Sports Medicine* 15:275, January–February 1987.

Field D: *Anatomy: palpation and surface markings,* ed 3, Oxford, 2001, Butterworth-Heinemann.

Gench BE, Hinson MM, Harvey PT: *Anatomical kinesiology,* Dubuque, IA, 1995, Bowers.

Hamilton N, Luttgens K: *Kinesiology: scientific basis of human motion,* ed 10, Boston, 2002, McGraw-Hill.

Hislop HJ, Montgomery J: *Daniels and Worthingham's muscle testing: techniques of manual examination,* ed 7, Philadelphia, 2002, Saunders.

Holden DL, Jackson DW: Stress fractures of ribs in female rowers, *American Journal of Sports Medicine* 13:277, July–August 1987.

Lindsay DT: *Functional human anatomy,* St. Louis, 1996, Mosby.

Magee DJ: *Orthopedic physical assessment,* ed 4, Philadelphia, 2002, Saunders.

Martens MA, et al.: Adductor tendonitis and muscular abdominis tendonopathy, *American Journal of Sports Medicine* 15:353, July–August 1987.

Marymont JV: Exercise-related stress reaction of the sacroiliac joint, an unusual cause of low back pain in athletes, *American Journal of Sports Medicine* 14:320, July–August 1986.

Muscolino JE: *The muscular system manual: the skeletal muscles of the human body,* ed 2, St. Louis, 2003, Elsevier Mosby.

National Strength and Conditioning Association; Baechle TR, Earle RW, eds.: *Essentials of strength training and conditioning,* ed 2, Champaign, IL, 2000, Human Kinetics.

Oatis CA: *Kinesiology: the mechanics and pathomechanics of human movement,* Philadelphia, 2004, Lippincott Williams & Wilkins.

Perry JF, Rohe DA, Garcia AO: *The kinesiology workbook,* Philadelphia, 1992, Davis.

Prentice WE: *Arnheim's principles of athletic training,* ed 12, New York, 2006, McGraw-Hill.

Rasch PJ: *Kinesiology and applied anatomy,* ed 7, Philadelphia, 1989, Lea & Febiger.

Seeley RR, Stephens TD, Tate P: *Anatomy & physiology,* ed 7, New York, 2006, McGraw-Hill.

Sieg KW, Adams SP: *Illustrated essentials of musculoskeletal anatomy,* ed 2, Gainesville, FL, 1985, Megabooks.

Stone RJ, Stone JA: *Atlas of the skeletal muscles,* New York, 1990, McGraw-Hill.

Thibodeau GA, Patton KT: *Anatomy & physiology,* ed 9, St. Louis, 1993, Mosby.

Travell J, Simons D, Simons L: *Myofascial pain and dysfunction: the trigger point manual, vol. 1: upper half of body,* ed 2, Baltimore, 1999, Williams & Wilkins.

Van De Graaff KM: *Human anatomy,* ed 6, Dubuque, IA, 2002, McGraw-Hill.

Werner R: *A massage therapist's guide to pathology,* ed 3, Baltimore, 2005, Lippincott Williams & Wilkins.

chapter 14

Ad Hoc Committee on Classifications of Headache, National Institute of Neurological Diseases and Blindness: Classifications of headache, *Journal of the American Medical Association* 179:717–718, 1962.

Berkow R, Fletcher A: *Merck manual, vol 1* (Headache, pp. 1228–1233). Rahway, NJ, 1992, Merck Research Labs.

Chaitow L: *Muscle energy techniques,* London, 1998, Churchill Livingstone.

Constantine L, Scott S: *Migraine: the complete guide* (American Council for Headache Education), New York, 1994, Dell.

Cyriax J: *Textbook of orthopaedic medicine, vol. 1: diagnosis of soft tissue lesions,* London, 1982, Bailliere Tindall.

Cyriax J: *Textbook of orthopaedic medicine, vol. 2: treatment by manipulation, massage, and injection,* London, 1984, Bailliere Tindall.

Dail N: *Headache handbook,* Waldoboro, ME, 2007, Lincoln County Publishing.

Dail N: *Kinesiology manual,* Waldoboro, ME, 2006, Lincoln County Publishing.

Dail N: *Manual for a gift of touch,* Waldoboro, ME, 2008, Lincoln County Publishing.

Dail N: *Massage manual,* Waldoboro, ME, 2008, Lincoln County Publishing.

DeGood D: *The headache and neck pain workbook,* Oakland, CA, 1997, New Harbingers.

Field T: *Touch therapy,* Edinburgh, 2000, Churchill Livingstone.

Fritz S: *Mosby's fundamentals of therapeutic massage,* ed 3, St. Louis, 2004, Mosby.

Headache Classification Committee of the International Headache Society: Classification and diagnostic criteria for headache disorders, cranial neuralgias and facial pain, *Cephalalgia* 8(7), 1988.

Hoppenfeld S: *Physical examination of the spine & extremities,* Norwalk, CT, 1976, Appleton & Lange.

King R: *Clinical massage for head, neck and upper back pain* (Manual), Chicago, 2008, Robert King Seminars.

Kunkel R, Tollison CD: *Headache diagnosis and treatment,* Baltimore, 1993, Williams & Wilkins.

Lowe W: *Orthopedic massage,* Edinburgh, 2003, Mosby.

Meagher J: *Sportsmassage,* New York, 1980, Station Hill Press.

Robinson W: Tense neck muscles may cause headaches, Associated Press in *Portland Press Herald* (Baltimore), February 16, 1995, 8A.

Rohen J, Yokochi C: *Color atlas of anatomy,* ed 3, New York, 1993, Igaku-Shoin.

Stedman TL: *Stedman's medical dictionary,* ed 27, Baltimore, 2000, Lippincott Williams & Wilkins.

Travell J, Simons D, Simons L: *Myofascial pain and dysfunction: the trigger point manual, vol. 1: upper half of body,* ed 2, Baltimore, 1999, Williams & Wilkins.

Van De Graaff KM: *Human anatomy,* ed 6, Dubuque, IA, 2002, McGraw-Hill.

Werner R: *A massage therapist's guide to pathology,* ed 3, Baltimore, 2005, Lippincott Williams & Wilkins.

chapter 15

Dail N: *Kinesiology manual,* Waldoboro, ME, 2006, Lincoln County Publishing.

Field D: *Anatomy: palpation and surface markings,* ed 3, Oxford, 2001, Butterworth-Heinemann.

Grey H: *Grey's anatomy,* Philadelphia: Lea & Febiger, 1918, New York: Bartleby.com, 2000.

Hamilton N, Luttgens K: *Kinesiology: scientific basis of human motion,* ed 10, Boston, 2002, McGraw-Hill.

Hislop HJ, Montgomery J: *Daniels and Worthingham's muscle testing: techniques of manual examination,* ed 7, Philadelphia, 2002, Saunders.

Kendall FP, McCreary EK, Provance, PG: *Muscles: testing and function,* ed 4, Baltimore, 1993, Lippincott Williams & Wilkins.

Lindsay DT: *Functional human anatomy,* St. Louis, 1996, Mosby.

Lysholm J, Wikland J: Injuries in runners, *American Journal of Sports Medicine* 15:168, September–October 1986.

Magee DJ: *Orthopedic physical assessment,* ed 4, Philadelphia, 2002, Saunders.

Mattes AL: *Active Isolated Strengthening,* Sarasota, FL, 2006.

Mattes AL: *Active Isolated Stretching,* Sarasota, FL, 1995.

Muscolino JE: *The muscular system manual: the skeletal muscles of the human body,* ed 2, St. Louis, 2003, Elsevier Mosby.

Noakes TD, et al.: Pelvic stress fractures in long distance runners, *American Journal of Sports Medicine* 13:120, March–April 1985.

Oatis CA: *Kinesiology: the mechanics and pathomechanics of human movement,* Philadelphia, 2004, Lippincott Williams & Wilkins.

Prentice WE: *Arnheim's principles of athletic training,* ed 12, New York, 2006, McGraw-Hill.

Seeley RR, Stephens TD, Tate P: *Anatomy & physiology,* ed 7, New York, 2006, McGraw-Hill.

Sieg KW, Adams SP: *Illustrated essentials of musculoskeletal anatomy,* ed 2, Gainesville, FL, 1985, Megabooks.

Stone RJ, Stone JA: *Atlas of the skeletal muscles,* New York, 1990, McGraw-Hill.

Tank PW: *Grant's dissector,* ed 13, Hagerstown, MD, 2005, Lippincott Williams & Wilkins.

Thibodeau GA, Patton KT: *Anatomy & physiology,* ed 9, St. Louis, 1993, Mosby.

Van De Graaff KM: *Human anatomy,* ed 6, Dubuque, IA, 2002, McGraw-Hill.

Werner R: *A massage therapist's guide to pathology,* ed 3, Baltimore, 2005, Lippincott Williams & Wilkins.

Wheeless CR III: *Wheeless' textbook of orthopaedics,* www.wheelessonline.com.

chapter 16

Chaitow L: *Muscle energy techniques,* London, 1998, Churchill Livingstone.

Cyriax J: *Textbook of orthopaedic medicine, vol. 1: diagnosis of soft tissue lesions,* London, 1982, Bailliere Tindall.

Cyriax J: *Textbook of orthopaedic medicine, vol. 2: treatment by manipulation, massage, and injection,* London, 1984, Bailliere Tindall.

Dail N: *Kinesiology manual,* Waldoboro, ME, 2006, Lincoln County Publishing.

Dail N: *Manual for a gift of touch,* Waldoboro, ME, 2008, Lincoln County Publishing.

Dail N: *Massage manual,* Waldoboro, ME, 2008, Lincoln County Publishing.

Hoppenfeld S: *Physical examination of the spine & extremities,* Norwalk, CT, 1976, Appleton & Lange.

King R: *Myofascial techniques for the low back and pelvic girdle* (Manual), Chicago, 2006, Robert King Seminars.

Lowe W: *Orthopedic massage,* Edinburgh, 2003, Mosby.

Magee DJ: *Orthopedic physical assessment,* ed 4, Philadelphia, 2002, Saunders.

Meagher J: *Sportsmassage,* New York, 1980, Station Hill Press.

Oatis CA: *Kinesiology: the mechanics and pathomechanics of human movement,* Philadelphia, 2004, Lippincott Williams & Wilkins.

Travell J, Simons D, Simons L: *Myofascial pain and dysfunction: the trigger point manual, vol. 1: upper half of body,* ed 2, Baltimore, 1999, Williams & Wilkins.

Travell J, Simons D, Simons L: *Myofascial pain and dysfunction: the trigger point manual, vol. 2: lower half of body,* ed 2, Baltimore, 1999, Williams & Wilkins.

Ullrich P: Common causes of back pain and neck pain, *Spine-health.com,* February 28, 2001.

Van De Graaff KM: *Human anatomy,* ed 6, Dubuque, IA, 2002, McGraw-Hill.

Werner R: *A massage therapist's guide to pathology,* ed 3, Baltimore, 2005, Lippincott Williams & Wilkins.

chapter 17

Baker BE, et al.: Review of meniscal injury and associated sports, *American Journal of Sports Medicine* 13:1, January–February 1985.

Dail N: *Kinesiology manual,* Waldoboro, ME, 2006, Lincoln County Publishing.

Field D: *Anatomy: palpation and surface markings,* ed 3, Oxford, 2001, Butterworth-Heinemann.

Garrick JG, Regna RK: Prophylactic knee bracing, *American Journal of Sports Medicine* 15:471, September–October 1987.

Hamilton N, Luttgens K: *Kinesiology: scientific basis of human motion,* ed 10, Boston, 2002, McGraw-Hill.

Hislop HJ, Montgomery J: *Daniels and Worthingham's muscle testing: techniques of manual examination,* ed 7, Philadelphia, 2002, Saunders.

Kelly DW, et al.: Patellar and quadriceps tendon ruptures—jumping knee, *American Journal of Sports Medicine* 12:375, September–October 1984.

Lysholm J, Wikland J: Injuries in runners, *American Journal of Sports Medicine* 15:168, September–October 1986.

Magee DJ: *Orthopedic physical assessment,* ed 4, Philadelphia, 2002, Saunders.

Mattes AL: *Active Isolated Strengthening,* Sarasota, FL, 2006.

Mattes AL: *Active Isolated Stretching,* Sarasota, FL, 1995.

Muscolino JE: *The muscular system manual: the skeletal muscles of the human body,* ed 2, St. Louis, 2003, Elsevier Mosby.

Oatis CA: *Kinesiology: the mechanics and pathomechanics of human movement,* Philadelphia, 2004, Lippincott Williams & Wilkins.

Prentice WE: *Arnheim's principles of athletic training,* ed 12, New York, 2006, McGraw-Hill.

Seeley RR, Stephens TD, Tate P: *Anatomy & physiology,* ed 7, New York, 2006, McGraw-Hill.

Sieg KW, Adams SP: *Illustrated essentials of musculoskeletal anatomy,* ed 2, Gainesville, FL, 1985, Megabooks.

Stone RJ, Stone JA: *Atlas of the skeletal muscles,* New York, 1990, McGraw-Hill.

Travell J, Simons D, Simons L: *Myofascial pain and dysfunction: the trigger point manual, vol. 2: lower half of body,* ed 2, Baltimore, 1999, Williams & Wilkins.

Van De Graaff KM: *Human anatomy,* ed 6, Dubuque, IA, 2002, McGraw-Hill.

Werner R: *A massage therapist's guide to pathology,* ed 3, Baltimore, 2005, Lippincott Williams & Wilkins.

Wroble RR, et al.: Pattern of knee injuries in wrestling: a six-year study, *American Journal of Sports Medicine* 14:55, January–February 1986.

chapter 18

Chaitow L: *Muscle energy techniques,* London, 1998, Churchill Livingstone.

Cyriax J: *Textbook of orthopaedic medicine, vol. 1: diagnosis of soft tissue lesions,* London, 1982, Bailliere Tindall.

Cyriax J: *Textbook of orthopaedic medicine, vol. 2: treatment by manipulation, massage, and injection,* London, 1984, Bailliere Tindall.

Dail N: *Kinesiology manual,* Waldoboro, ME, 2006, Lincoln County Publishing.

Dail N: *Manual for a gift of touch,* Waldoboro, ME, 2008, Lincoln County Publishing.

Dail N: *Massage manual,* Waldoboro, ME, 2008, Lincoln County Publishing.

Hoppenfeld S: *Physical examination of the spine & extremities,* Norwalk, CT, 1976, Appleton & Lange.

King R: *Myofascial techniques for the thigh and knee joint* (Manual), Chicago, 2005, Robert King Seminars.

Lowe W: *Orthopedic massage,* Edinburgh, 2003, Mosby.

Magee DJ: *Orthopedic physical assessment,* ed 4, Philadelphia, 2002, Saunders.

Meagher J: *Sportsmassage,* New York, 1980, Station Hill Press.

Oatis CA: *Kinesiology: the mechanics and pathomechanics of human movement,* Philadelphia, 2004, Lippincott Williams & Wilkins.

Travell J, Simons D, Simons L: *Myofascial pain and dysfunction: the trigger point manual, vol. 2: lower half of body,* ed 2, Baltimore, 1999, Williams & Wilkins.

Van De Graaff KM: *Human anatomy,* ed 6, Dubuque, IA, 2002, McGraw-Hill.

Werner R: *A massage therapist's guide to pathology,* ed 3, Baltimore, 2005, Lippincott Williams & Wilkins.

chapter 19

Agnew TA: *Dynamic flexibility: a safe and effective self-stretching manual,* Sarasota, FL, 1993, Intent.

Astrom M, Arvidson T: Alignment and joint motion in the normal foot, *Journal of Orthopaedic and Sports Physical Therapy* 22:5, November 1995.

Booher JM, Thibodeau GA: *Athletic injury assessment,* ed 4, New York, 2000, McGraw-Hill.

Dail N: *Kinesiology manual,* Waldoboro, ME, 2006, Lincoln County Publishing.

Field D: *Anatomy: palpation and surface markings,* ed 3, Oxford, 2001, Butterworth-Heinemann.

Franco AH: Pes cavus and pes planus—analysis and treatment, *Physical Therapy* 67:688, May 1987.

Gench BE, Hinson MM, Harvey PT: *Anatomical kinesiology,* Dubuque, IA, 1995, Bowers.

Hamilton N, Luttgens K: *Kinesiology: scientific basis of human motion,* ed 10, Boston, 2002, McGraw-Hill.

Henderson J: Baring the soles, *Runner's World* 22:14, November 1987.

Hislop HJ, Montgomery J: *Daniels and Worthingham's muscle testing: techniques of manual examination,* ed. 7, Philadelphia, 2002, Saunders.

Hoppenfeld S: *Physical examination of the spine & extremities,* Norwalk, CT, 1976, Appleton & Lange.

Lindsay DT: *Functional human anatomy,* St. Louis, 1996, Mosby.

Magee DJ: *Orthopedic physical assessment,* ed 4, Philadelphia, 2002, Saunders.

Mattes AL: *Active Isolated Stretching,* Sarasota, FL, 1995.

Muscolino JE: *The muscular system manual: the skeletal muscles of the human body,* ed 2, St. Louis, 2003, Elsevier Mosby.

Oatis CA: *Kinesiology: the mechanics and pathomechanics of human movement,* Philadelphia, 2004, Lippincott Williams & Wilkins.

Prentice WE: *Arnheim's principles of athletic training,* ed 12, New York, 2006, McGraw-Hill.

Robinson M: Feet first, *Coach and Athlete* 44:30, August–September 1981.

Rockar PA: The subtalar joint: anatomy and joint motion, *Journal of Orthopaedic and Sports Physical Therapy* 21:6, June 1995.

Sammarco GJ: Foot and ankle injuries in sports, *American Journal of Sports Medicine* 14:6, November–December 1986.

Seeley RR, Stephens TD, Tate P: *Anatomy & physiology,* ed 7, New York, 2006, McGraw-Hill.

Sieg KW, Adams SP: *Illustrated essentials of musculoskeletal anatomy,* ed 2, Gainesville, FL, 1985, Megabooks.

Stone RJ, Stone JA: *Atlas of the skeletal muscles,* New York, 1990, McGraw-Hill.

Thibodeau GA, Patton KT: *Anatomy & physiology,* ed 9, St. Louis, 1993, Mosby.

Travell J, Simons D, Simons L: *Myofascial pain and dysfunction: the trigger point manual, vol. 2: lower half of body,* ed 2, Baltimore, 1999, Williams & Wilkins.

Van De Graaff KM: *Human anatomy,* ed 6, Dubuque, IA, 2002, McGraw-Hill.

Werner R: *A massage therapist's guide to pathology,* ed 3, Baltimore, 2005, Lippincott Williams & Wilkins.

chapter 20

Chaitow L: *Muscle energy techniques,* London, 1998, Churchill Livingstone.

Cyriax J: *Textbook of orthopaedic medicine, vol. 1: diagnosis of soft tissue lesions,* London, 1982, Bailliere Tindall.

Cyriax J: *Textbook of orthopaedic medicine, vol. 2: treatment by manipulation, massage, and injection,* London, 1984, Bailliere Tindall.

Dail N: *Kinesiology manual,* Waldoboro, ME, 2006, Lincoln County Publishing.

Dail N: *Manual for a gift of touch,* Waldoboro, ME, 2008, Lincoln County Publishing.

Dail N: *Massage manual,* Waldoboro, ME, 2008, Lincoln County Publishing.

Hoppenfeld S: *Physical examination of the spine & extremities,* Norwalk, CT, 1976, Appleton & Lange.

King R: *Myofascial techniques for the ankle and foot* (Manual), Chicago, 2004, Robert King Seminars.

Lowe W: *Orthopedic massage,* Edinburgh, 2003,Mosby.

Magee DJ: *Orthopedic physical assessment,* ed 4, Philadelphia, 2002, Saunders.

Meagher J: *Sportsmassage,* New York, 1980, Station Hill Press.

Oatis CA: *Kinesiology: the mechanics and pathomechanics of human movement,* Philadelphia, 2004, Lippincott Williams & Wilkins.

Savchenko V: *Russian massage,* Moscow, 1997, University of Belgorod.

Snow RE, Williams KR: High heel shoes: their effect on center of mass position, posture, three-dimensional kinematics, rearfoot motion, and ground reaction forces, *Archives of Physical Medicine and Rehabilitation* 75(5):568–576, 1994.

Travell J, Simons D, Simons L: *Myofascial pain and dysfunction: the trigger point manual, vol. 2: lower half of body,* ed 2, Baltimore, 1999, Williams & Wilkins.

Van De Graaff KM: *Human anatomy,* ed 6, Dubuque, IA, 2002, McGraw-Hill.

Werner R: *A massage therapist's guide to pathology,* ed 3, Baltimore, 2005, Lippincott Williams & Wilkins.

chapter 21

Adrian M: Isokinetic exercise, *Training and Conditioning* 1:1, June 1991.

Agnew TA: *Dynamic flexibility: a safe and effective self-stretching manual,* Sarasota, FL, 1993, Intent.

Altug Z, Hoffman JL, Martin JL: *Manual of clinical exercise testing, prescription and rehabilitation,* Norwalk, CT, 1993, Appleton & Lange.

Andrews JR, Harrelson GL: *Physical rehabilitation of the injured athlete,* Philadelphia, 1991, Saunders.

Ellenbecker TS, Davies GJ: *Closed kinetic chain exercise: a comprehensive guide to multiple-joint exercise,* Champaign, IL, 2001, Human Kinetics.

Fahey TD: *Athletic training: principles and practices,* Mountain View, CA, 1986, Mayfield.

Logan GA, McKinney WC: *Anatomic kinesiology,* ed 3, New York, 1982, McGraw-Hill.

Matheson O, et al.: Stress fractures in athletes, *American Journal of Sports Medicine* 15:46, January–February 1987.

Mattes AL: *Active Isolated Strengthening,* Sarasota, FL, 2006.

Mattes AL: *Active Isolated Stretching,* Sarasota, FL, 1995.

National Strength and Conditioning Association; Baechle TR, Earle RW, eds.: *Essentials of strength training and conditioning,* ed 2, Champaign, IL, 2000, Human Kinetics.

Northrip JW, Logan GA, McKinney WC: *Analysis of sport motion: anatomic and biomechanic perspectives,* ed 3, New York, 1983, McGraw-Hill.

Powers SK, Howley ET: *Exercise physiology: theory and application to fitness and performance,* ed 5, New York, 2004, McGraw-Hill.

Prentice WE: *Rehabilitation techniques in sports medicine,* ed 3, New York, 1999, McGraw-Hill.

Steindler A: *Kinesiology of the human body,* Springfield, IL, 1970, Thomas.

Torg JS, Vegso JJ, Torg E: *Rehabilitation of athletic injuries: an atlas of therapeutic exercise,* Chicago, 1987, Year Book.

Wirhed R: *Athletic ability and the anatomy of motion,* London, 1984, Wolfe.

Appendix B

Downeast School of Massage

Head, Neck, Shoulder Pain History Questionnaire

Name ____

Address ____

Date ____________ DOB ____________

Occupation ____

Repetitive Actions ____

____

____

1. Chief Complaint(s) (circle all that apply)
   Headache   Neck Pain   Shoulder/Arm Pain
   Other (describe)
2. Circle where you have the worst pain
   Head   Neck   Shoulder/Arm
3. Rate your overall problem
   Getting Better   Getting Worse   Staying the Same
4. How did your pain begin? Describe in detail the event.

   Auto Accident ____

   Other Trauma ____

   Unknown ____

   Other cause (describe) (environmental, hormonal, menstrual, menopausal, genetic, atmospheric, stress, etc.) ____

   ____
5. When did your pain begin?

   Date ____

6. **Where do you have pain? Mark the chart with appropriate symbols.**

Throbbing TTTT **Burning BBB** **Stabbing SSS** **Ache AAA**

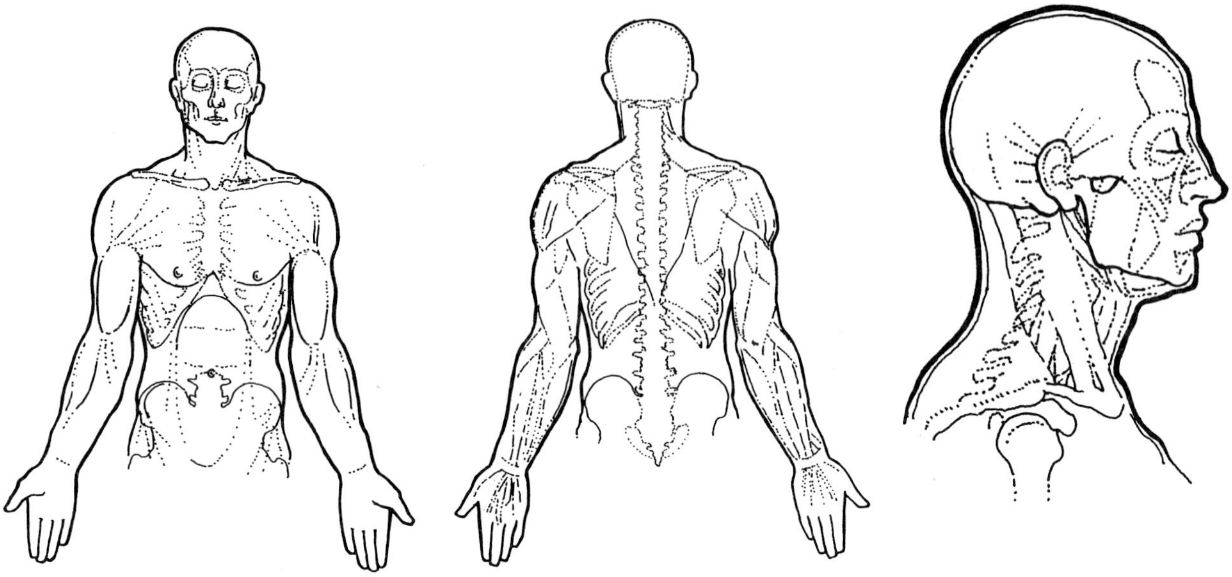

Does your pain stay in one place or refer or radiate to someplace else? Explain.

____

____

7. **Have you been to a physician, chiropractor, osteopath, health care provider? What was your diagnosis if any? (Cervical strain, herniated disk, shoulder problem, hormones, other)**

Diagnosis: ____

____

No Diagnosis: ____

____

8. **What makes your pain better?** ____

____

9. **What makes your pain worse?** ____

____

10. **Is your pain worse on the left?** **Right?** **Both?**

11. On a scale of one to ten, how severe is your pain?

0 ____ 1 ____ 2 ____ 3 ____ 4 ____ 5 ____ 6 ____ 7 ____ 8 ____ 9 ____ 10

No pain **Worst possible pain**

12. Does your head throb or pound? **Yes** **No**

13. Do you feel a headache "coming on" or experience an "aura" (warning signs)?

Yes **No**

14. Do you have any other symptoms accompanying your headache? (Numbness, tingling, dizziness, visual or hearing problems, nausea, vomiting, diarrhea, seizures, etc.) List all that apply.

____

15. How often do you have a headache? **Daily,** **A week,** **A month**

16. How long does it last? Hours, days? Does it reoccur in a pattern?

____

17. Does it coincide with special circumstances or at any special time? (in sunlight, fluorescent lights, at end of day, at night, before or after food, etc.?

____

____

18. Do you have more than one type of headaches? ______________________

19. Are you incapacitated during your headache? ______________________

20. Do you have a family history of headaches? Please list all.

____

____

21. How much water do you drink in a day? ______________________

22. Do you keep a headache log or diary? ______________________

22. List all medications, vitamins, homeopathic remedies, etc. used for neck pain/ headaches:

Over-the-counter: ______________________________

Prescribed: ______________________________

List all previous treatment you have received. Include Physician, Physical Therapy, Chiropractic, Massage Therapy, Acupuncture, Osteopathic, Biofeedback, Surgeries, etc. List length of treatment, where you received it, and if it helped or not.

____

____

____

____

____

____

____

____

____

____

List all medical diagnostic tests: X-rays, CT Scan, MRI Scan, Myelogram, Nerve Conduction Test, other. Include Date and Where taken.

____

____

____

____

____

____

____

____

____

____

This questionnaire should accompany a complete medical history. It is not meant to replace the medical history.

Glossary

A

Abduction A lateral movement away from the midline of the trunk in the frontal plane. An example is raising the arms or legs to the side horizontally.

Abductor pollicis longus A muscle in the forearm that abducts the thumb.

Acceleration The rate of change in velocity. To attain speed in moving the body, a strong muscular force is generally necessary.

Acetabular femoral joint The multiaxial enarthrodial-type (ball-and-socket) hip joint.

Acetabulum The cup-shaped socket of the pelvic girdle that houses the head of the femur.

Achilles tendon The tendon that inserts at the calcaneus or heel and is the attachment for both the gastrocnemius and the soleus.

Acromioclavicular (AC) joint The joint located where the clavicle and acromion of the scapula meet and attach.

Action The specific movement of a joint that results from a concentric contraction of a muscle that crosses the joint.

Active Isolated Stretching (AIS) A method of stretching that involves the use of the body's natural movements (flexion, extension, rotation, etc.) and physiology to achieve greater range of motion.

Active movement Movement that shortens muscles as it contracts and pulls on the engaged bone.

Acute The inflammatory stage of inflammation. It has all the signs and symptoms of inflammation: redness, heat, pain, swelling, and loss of function.

Adduction Movement medially toward the midline of the trunk in the frontal plane. Examples are lowering the arm to the side or moving the thigh back to the anatomical position.

Adductor brevis A small hip adductor connecting from the pubic bone to the femur.

Adductor longus A hip adductor connecting from the pubic bone to the femur.

Adductor magnus The largest muscle of the hip adductors; fills in most of the medial thigh from the pelvis to the knee.

Adhesion A scar that is often painful.

Adhesive capsulitis A progressive, painful condition that starts with limited motion of the shoulder joint and progresses to a frozen stage. Small adhesions form in the joint capsule, creating an extremely debilitating condition.

Aggregate muscle action The ability of muscles working in groups, rather than independently, to achieve a given joint motion.

Agonists Muscles that, when contracting concentrically, cause joint motion through a specified plane of motion. Also known as *primary* or *prime movers* and *muscles most involved*.

All-or-none principle The principle of motion which states that the individual muscle fibers within a given motor unit will fire and contract either maximally or not at all.

Amphiarthrodial (cartilaginous) joints Slightly movable joints.

Amplitude The range of muscle-fiber length between maximal and minimal lengthening.

Anatomical position A reference position used as a basis to describe joint movement. The individual stands in an upright posture, facing straight ahead, with feet parallel and close and palms facing forward.

Anconeus A small muscle on the posterior distal humerus and proximal ulna that assists the triceps with extension of the forearm.

Angle of pull The angle between the line of pull of the muscle and the bone on which it inserts.

Angular motion Motion that involves rotation around an axis. Also known as *rotary motion*.

Antagonists Muscles that are usually located on the opposite side of the joint from the agonist and have the opposite concentric action. They work in cooperation with agonist muscles by relaxing and allowing movement, but when contracting concentrically, they perform the joint motion opposite that of the agonist. Also known as *contralateral muscles*.

Anterior compartment The anterior compartment of the lower leg contains the dorsiflexor group, consisting of the tibialis anterior, peroneus tertius, extensor digitorum longus, and extensor hallucis longus.

Anterior cruciate ligament (ACL) A ligament located inside the knee joint. It crosses with the posterior cruciate ligament between the tibia and the femur and maintains stability in the knee joint.

Anterior talofibular ligament A ligament located at the distal end of the anterior fibula, attaching distally to the talus.

Aponeurosis A plastic wrap–like flat tissue that serves as a tendinous attachment for muscle. The latissimus dorsi has a large aponeurosis in its lower-back attachments.

Arc of pain A pain response during a portion of active or passive movement.

Arthritis An inflammation of a joint. It is common in the aging process.

Arthrodial joint A type of diarthrodial joint that is characterized by two flat, or plane, bony surfaces that butt against each other. This type of joint permits limited gliding movement.

Arthrosis Another term for *joint.*

Articulation A joint comprised of two or more bones that allows for various types of movement.

Atlantoaxial joint The pivot joint formed by the atlas and the axis.

Atlantooccipital joint The first joint of the axial skeleton. It is formed by the occipital condyles of the skull sitting on the articular fossa of the first vertebra, which allows flexion and extension.

Atlas The first cervical vertebra.

Axial pain A type of pain that can be sharp or dull, constant or intermittent, and mild or severe and can be confined to the low back.

Axis (1) The second cervical vertebra. (2) The point of rotation about which a lever moves.

Axis of rotation The movement occurring in a given plane. The joint moves or turns around an axis that has a 90-degree relationship to the plane.

B

Back-pocket sciatica A painful condition due to keeping a wallet in the back pocket of pants that, over time, applies compression to the sciatic nerve as the individual sits on it.

Balance The ability to control equilibrium, either static or dynamic.

Biarticular A type of muscle that crosses and acts directly on two different joints.

Biceps brachii A two-headed muscle that is located on the anterior arm, performs weak flexion for the shoulder joint, and flexes the forearm in a supinated position.

Biceps femoris A hamstring muscle that is located on the posterior thigh and inserts on the lateral tibia and fibula. It is a two-headed muscle that extends the hip and flexes the knee.

Biomechanics The study of mechanics as it relates to the functional and anatomical analysis of biological systems.

Body mechanics Ergonomically safe methods and practices of executing techniques that can prevent injury, support self-care, provide balanced energy, and promote a long career in manual therapies.

Brachial plexus A group of nerves consisting of the 5th cervical to 1st thoracic that provide a base for the nerves that innervate the upper extremity.

Brachialis An anterior arm muscle that inserts on the ulna and performs only flexion of the forearm.

Brachioradialis The "neutral-position" muscle that spans from the supracondyloid ridge of the humerus to the styloid process of the radius. It is used in all neutral-position actions.

Breathing The act of respiration in which air is forced into and out of the lungs.

Bursa A synovial sac of fluid needed to lubricate joints.

Bursitis A pathologic condition that is an inflammation of a bursa.

C

Calcaneofibular ligament A ligament located at the very distal end at an angle to the calcaneus.

Calcaneus A tarsal bone that is the heel of the foot.

Capitate A carpal bone.

Cardinal planes The specific planes that divide the body exactly into two halves.

Carpal tunnel syndrome A median nerve disorder that may be caused by soft-tissue entrapment, repetitive action, incorrect mechanics, or bony compression of the median nerve.

Carpals Bones that include the capitate, lunate, hamate, trapezium, trapezoid, pisiform, scaphoid, and triquetrum.

Carpometacarpal (CMC) The joint between the carpals and the metacarpals.

Cartilaginous (amphiarthrodial) joints Slightly movable joints.

Cervical plexus A group of nerves consisting of the first four cervical nerves.

Cervical vertebrae Seven bony structures that surround the spinal cord in the neck and are attached to the thoracic vertebrae after C7.

Chondromalacia Wear and tear of the cartilage on the underside of the patella.

Chronic The stage of the inflammatory process that has leveled-off signs and symptoms. The chronic stage can last for months or years.

Circumduction A circular movement of a limb that delineates an arc or describes a cone. It is a combination of flexion, extension, abduction, and adduction. An example occurs when the shoulder joint and the hip joint move in a circular fashion around a fixed point, either clockwise or counterclockwise. Also known as *circumflexion.*

Clavicle One of the two bones of the shoulder girdle. It attaches to the trunk via the sternum and to the scapula via the acromioclavicular joint. Also known as *collarbone.*

Clinical flexibility Flexibility used in a clinical setting and usually assisted by a therapist.

Clinical Flexibility and Therapeutic Exercise (CFTE) A modality that consists of stretching and strengthening the muscles of the body. It is designed to improve human movement and prevent current or past dysfunctions from worsening.

Closed kinetic chain A closed system in which movement of one joint in an extremity cannot occur without causing predictable movements of the other joints in the extremity; occurs when the distal end of the extremity is fixed, as in a push-up, dip, squat, or dead lift.

Collagen The white fibers of connective tissue; consists mostly of protein.

Compartment syndromes Conditions that occur when swelling or bleeding presses against the structures in a compartment and could prevent blood flow to the foot.

Compression A deep-tissue technique designed to flatten the soft tissue repeatedly with the heel of the palm.

Concentric contractions Contractions in which the muscle develops tension as it shortens.

Condyloid joint A type of diarthrodial joint in which the bones permit movement in two planes without rotation.

Contracted iliotibial band A condition in which the tract or band becomes taut from overuse as the muscles that lead into it shorten.

Contractibility The ability of a muscle to contract and develop tension or an internal force against resistance when stimulated.

Contraction The action of a muscle being lengthened or shortened. In skeletal muscle, this is one of three types: eccentric, concentric, or isometric.

Contralateral The movement, position, or landmark locations on the opposite side.

Coracobrachialis A muscle named for its attachments on the coracoid process of the scapula and the humerus. It flexes and horizontally adducts the humerus.

Core The center of the body where muscles are located anterior and posterior to the spine, including the rectus abdominis, the external and internal obliques, transversus abdominis, psoas major, and quadratus lumborum.

Crepitus Any grinding, grating, or popping elicited during the movement of a joint.

Cross-fiber friction See **Deep transverse friction.**

Cryotherapy The safe use of ice to reduce inflammation and acute responses.

Cuboid A tarsal bone in the foot.

Cuneiforms Three tarsal bones in the foot.

D

Deep-tissue therapy A series of specific techniques designed to unwind the soft tissue in a particular pattern or sequence with the end result of specific goals.

Deep transverse friction A deep-tissue technique executed deliberately at a right angle to the fibers of the soft tissue. Also called *cross-fiber friction*.

Degenerative disk disease The literal depletion of the disk space between the vertebrae.

Deltoid A multiple superficial lateral muscle that is divided into three sections: anterior, middle, and posterior. The deltoid originates on the clavicle and scapula and inserts on the humerus. It is a major abductor of the humerus and is its own agonist and antagonist, as the anterior and posterior deltoid reflect opposite actions. The anterior deltoid performs flexion, medial rotation, and horizontal adduction, whereas the posterior deltoid performs extension, lateral rotation, and horizontal abduction. The middle deltoid has very strong abduction to 90 degrees.

Depression Shoulder girdle inferior movement in the frontal plane. An example is returning to the normal position from a shoulder shrug.

Dermatome A defined area of skin supplied by a specific spinal nerve.

Diagonal plane A combination of more than one plane. Also known as *oblique plane*.

Diarthrodial joints Freely movable joints. Also known as *synovial joints*.

Dimensional massage therapy A philosophical approach to using a variety of techniques for the benefit of the client; based on science, structure, and functions of the soft tissue.

Displacement A change in the position or location of an object from its original point of reference.

Distal interphalangeal (DIP) A hinge joint for the distal phalanx.

Distance The actual sum length of measurement traveled. Also known as *path of movement*.

Dorsiflexion (dorsal flexion) (1) Of the ankle: The flexion movement of the ankle that results in the top of the foot moving toward the anterior tibia bone in the sagittal plane. (2) Of the wrist: An extension movement in the sagittal plane with the dorsal or posterior side of the hand moving toward the posterior side of the lateral forearm.

Double-crush syndrome A condition that includes the soft-tissue entrapment of the median nerve by the pectoralis minor and by the pronator teres.

Dupuytren's contracture Named after a French surgeon, a problem that involves the palmar aponeurosis or fascia and nodules that develop in the fibrous tissue, causing a permanent flexion of mostly the 4th or 5th finger in one or both hands.

E

Eccentric contractions Contractions in which the muscle lengthens under tension.

Eccentric force A force that is applied in a direction not in line with the center of rotation of an object with a fixed axis.

Elasticity The ability of muscle to return to its original resting length following stretching.

Elbow joint A hinge joint formed by the ulna and humerus.

Elevation The superior movement of the shoulder girdle in the frontal plane. An example is shrugging the shoulders.

Elliptical movement An alternating clockwise and counterclockwise distraction movement sometimes done on joints such as the shoulder girdle and most often done while engaged with muscles.

Enarthrodial joint A type of diarthrodial joint that permits movement in all planes.

Erector spinae A group of muscles that extends on each side of the spinal column from the sacrum to the occiput. It is divided into three muscles: the spinalis, the longissimus, and the iliocostalis.

Eversion An ankle and foot movement that turns the sole of the foot outward or laterally in the frontal plane (abduction). An example is standing with the weight on the inner edge of the foot.

Extensibility The ability of muscle to be passively stretched beyond its normal resting length.

Extension A straightening movement that results in an increase of the angle in a joint by moving bones apart, usually in the sagittal plane. An example is the movement in the elbow joint when the hand moves away from the shoulder.

Extension of the spine The return of the spinal column in the frontal plane to the anatomical position from lateral flexion; adduction of the spine.

Extensor carpi radialis brevis A hand and wrist muscle that extends the wrist.

Extensor carpi radialis longus A hand and wrist muscle that extends the wrist.

Extensor carpi ulnaris A hand and wrist muscle that extends the wrist and performs ulnar flexion.

Extensor digiti minimi A hand and wrist muscle that extends the wrist and performs extension of the little finger.

Extensor digitorum A hand and wrist muscle that performs extension of the fingers and wrist.

Extensor digitorum brevis A large intrinsic muscle on the dorsal lateral side of the foot that is often involved in inversion sprains.

Extensor digitorum longus An anterior leg muscle that extends the toes of the foot.

Extensor digitorum minimi A hand and wrist muscle that performs extension of the little finger.

Extensor hallucis longus An anterior leg muscle that extends the big toe.

Extensor indicis A hand and wrist muscle that extends the index finger.

Extensor pollicis brevis A hand and wrist muscle that extends the thumb.

Extensor pollicis longus A hand and wrist muscle that extends the thumb.

External oblique A large superficial abdominal muscle that surrounds the side of the body and is involved in lumbar movement and organ compression and is an accessory respiratory muscle.

External rotation A rotary movement around the longitudinal axis of a bone away from the midline of the body; occurs in the transverse plane. Also known as *rotation laterally, outward rotation,* and *lateral rotation.*

Extrinsic A term that usually pertains to muscles that arise or originate outside (proximal to) the body part on which they act.

F

Femoral nerve A large nerve in the anterior thigh that innervates anterior thigh muscles and knee extensors.

Fibula The lateral bone of the leg.

Fibular (lateral) collateral ligament (LCL) A ligament located on the lateral side of the knee that connects the femur with the fibula. It helps to maintain lateral knee stability.

Flexibility The end motion of a segment. It can occur by active contraction of the agonist (active range of motion) or by motion of an external force (passive range of motion).

Flexion A bending movement that results in a decrease of the angle in a joint by bringing bones together, usually in the sagittal plane. An example is the movement in the elbow joint when the hand is drawn to the shoulder.

Flexor carpi radialis A hand and wrist muscle that flexes the wrist and helps perform radial flexion.

Flexor carpi ulnaris A hand and wrist muscle that flexes the wrist and helps perform ulnar flexion.

Flexor digitorum longus A deep posterior leg muscle that flexes the toes.

Flexor digitorum profundus A hand and wrist muscle that flexes the wrist and fingers and helps with a strong grip.

Flexor digitorum superficialis A hand and wrist muscle that flexes the wrist and fingers and supports a strong grip.

Flexor hallucis longus A deep posterior leg muscle that flexes the big toe.

Flexor pollicis longus A hand and wrist muscle that flexes the thumb.

Follow-through phase In the movement cycle, the phase in which the velocity of the body segment progressively decreases, usually over a wide range of motion. Also known as *deceleration phase.*

Foot drop A condition that usually involves a weak tibialis anterior. The toes might drag as the tibialis anterior cannot seem to contract well enough to dorsiflex the foot properly.

Foraminal stenosis The narrowing of the hole through which the spinal nerve exits; due to bone spurs or arthritis.

Force The product of mass times acceleration.

Force arm The shortest distance from the axis of rotation to the line of action of the force.

Friction The force that results from the resistance between the surfaces of two objects moving against one another.

Frontal plane The plane that divides the body into front and back halves. Also known as *lateral* or *coronal plane.*

Frozen shoulder A condition in which the scapula is unable to move in its regular patterns without pain. The term *frozen shoulder* is often used interchangeably with *adhesive capsulitis,* but frozen shoulder can be caused by other conditions besides adhesive capsulitis.

Functional anatomy The functional actions of muscles.

Functional unit Muscles cooperating to work in groups and in paired opposition.

G

Ganglion A cyst that often protrudes on the dorsal side of the wrist.

Gaster The central, fleshy portion (belly or body) of a muscle that generally increases in diameter as the muscle contracts. It is the contractile portion of the muscle.

Gastrocnemius A superficial posterior leg muscle. It is a two-joint muscle that flexes the knee or plantar flexes the foot.

Gemellus inferior A lateral hip rotator that is located on the posterior pelvis.

Gemellus superior A lateral hip rotator that is located on the posterior pelvis.

Genu valgum A walking pattern marked by a lateral angulation of the leg in relation to the thigh. The thigh responds by being medially rotated, thus putting strain on the hip muscles and torque on the medial knee and resulting in probable patellar tracking issues and an apparent corrective foot pattern. Also known as *knock-knees.*

Genu varum A walking pattern marked by a medial angulation of the leg in relation to the thigh. This puts strain on the lateral side of the knee and often presents with walking on the lateral side of the foot. Also known as *bowlegs.*

Gerdy's tubercle A landmark attachment site for the iliotibial tract.

Ginglymus joint A type of diarthrodial joint that permits a wide range of movement in only one plane. Elbow and knee joints are examples. Also known as *hinge joint.*

Glenohumeral A multiaxial ball-and-socket joint classified as enarthrodial.

Glenoid labrum A cartilaginous ring that surrounds the glenoid fossa just inside its periphery.

Gluteus maximus The largest posterior buttock muscle; performs forceful hip extension.

Gluteus medius A small posterior buttock muscle that abducts the hip.

Gluteus minimus The smallest posterior buttock muscle; works with and is located beneath the gluteus medius.

Golfer's elbow Tendonitis of the medial epicondyle area. Also known as *medial epicondylitis.*

Golgi tendon organs (GTOs) Proprioceptors that are serially located in the tendon close to the muscle-tendon junction and are continuously sensitive to both muscle tension and active contraction.

Gomphosis A type of synarthrodial joint in which a conical peg fits into a socket, as found in teeth sockets.

Goniometer An instrument used to compare the change in joint angles.

Gracilis A long muscle that spans from the pubic bone to the medial tibia and is a hip adductor.

Greater trochanter A large process that provides attachments for muscles on the femur.

H

Hamate A carpal bone.

Hamstrings Posterior thigh muscles that extend the hip and flex the knee. They are the biceps femoris, semitendinosus, and semimembranosus.

Headache A diffuse pain in various areas of the head that is not confined to the distribution of a nerve.

Heel-strike A component of the stance phase of running or walking that is characterized by landing on the heel with the foot in supination and the leg in external rotation.

Hematoma A bruise.

Herniated disk A condition in which the gelatinous nucleus pulposus protrudes into or through the annulus fibrosus. This herniation produces a bulging of the disk tissue posteriorly into the vertebral canal and pinches the spinal cord and/or nerves of the spinal cord.

Horizontal abduction Shoulder movement of the humerus in the horizontal plane away from the midline of the body. Also known as *horizontal extension* and *transverse abduction.*

Horizontal adduction Shoulder joint movement of the humerus in the horizontal plane toward the midline of the body. Also known as *horizontal flexion* and *transverse adduction.*

Humerus An arm bone superior to the radius and ulna. It is a part of the shoulder joint, with the clavicle and scapula.

Hypertonic A condition of muscles in which they exhibit symptoms of pain and discomfort after continuous activity and may fatigue or have diminished function.

I

Iliacus A part of the iliopsoas that is located on the inner surface of the ilium and performs primary hip flexion.

Iliopsoas A deep core muscle that provides primary hip flexion. It consists of three muscles: the iliacus, psoas minor, and psoas major.

Iliotibial tract A structure that runs from the hip to the lateral tibia and provides muscular attachment to the tensor fasciae latae and the gluteus maximus.

Ilium The upper two-fifths of the pelvic bones.

Inertia Resistance to action or change.

Inferior peroneal retinaculum A tissue bridge that tacks down the peroneal tendons inferior to the calcaneofibular ligament.

Infraspinatus A rotator cuff muscle that originates on the infraspinous fossa and inserts on the middle facet of the greater tubercle. It performs extension, lateral rotation, and horizontal abduction.

Innervation The aspect of the nervous system that is responsible for providing a stimulus to muscle fibers within a specific muscle or portion of a muscle.

Insertion Structurally, the distal attachment or the part that attaches farthest from the midline or center of the body. Functionally and historically, the most movable part.

Internal oblique The abdominal muscle that is layered below the external oblique and is involved in lumbar movement and organ compression and is an accessory respiratory muscle.

Internal rotation A rotary movement around the longitudinal axis of a bone toward the midline of the body; occurs in the transverse plane. Also known as *rotation medially, inward rotation,* and *medial rotation.*

Interspinales Extensor muscles that connect from the spinous process of one vertebra to the spinous process of the adjacent vertebra.

Intertransversarii Muscles that flex the vertebral column laterally by connecting to the transverse processes of adjacent vertebrae.

Intervertebral disks The structures between the vertebrae that provide cushioning and shock absorption.

Intrinsic Pertaining to muscles within or belonging solely to the body part on which they act. The small intrinsic muscles found entirely within the hand are examples.

Inversion An ankle and foot movement that turns the sole of the foot inward or medially in the frontal plane; adduction. An example is standing with the weight on the outer edge of the foot.

Inversion sprain A sprain that forces the foot into an unnatural inverted position, putting too much strain on the ligaments of the foot. Injury includes torn ligament(s), swelling, torn tissue, and bleeding into the surrounding area.

Ipsilateral Pertaining to a movement, position, or landmark location that is on the same side as a reference point.

Ischemic compression Technique for relieving a trigger point by either digital pressure or pincer palpation by placing the tissue between the thumb and the forefinger. The purpose of the digital pressure is to try to interrupt the pain pattern by robbing the tissue of oxygen for a short period of time. Also known as *trigger point release*.

Ischial tuberosity A bony prominence that serves as an attachment for the hamstrings. It is located posteroinferiorly on the ischium.

Ischium The posterior and lower two-fifths of the pelvic bones.

Isokinetics A type of dynamic exercise, usually using concentric and/or eccentric muscle contractions, in which the speed (or velocity) of movement is constant and muscular contraction (ideally, maximum contraction) occurs throughout the movement.

Isometric contraction A contraction that occurs when tension is developed within the muscle but the joint angle remains constant; may be thought of as a static contraction, because a significant amount of tension may be developed in the muscle to maintain the joint angle in a relatively static or stable position, without an actual shortening of muscle fibers.

Isotonic contraction A contraction in which the muscle develops tension to either cause or control joint movement; may be thought of as a dynamic contraction, because the varying degrees of tension in the muscle are causing the joint angle to change.

J

Joint capsule A sleevelike covering of ligamentous tissue that surrounds the bony ends forming the joints.

Jostling A deep-tissue technique that is a form of vibration and is designed to shake tissues back and forth.

K

Kinematics A component of biomechanics that is concerned with the description of motion and includes consideration of time, displacement, velocity, acceleration, and space factors of a system's motion.

Kinesiology The science of muscle movement.

Kinesthesis The conscious awareness of the body's position and movement in space.

Kinetic chain The bony segments and their linkage system of joints in the body.

Kinetics A component of biomechanics that is concerned with the forces associated with the motion of a body.

Knee replacement The replacement of an injured or worn-out hinge joint with a prosthesis.

Kyphosis An anterior concavity of the normal thoracic curve.

L

Laminectomy A surgery in which the posterior arch and spinous processes of the midline of the vertebrae are removed, giving the spinal cord room.

Lateral collateral ligament See **Fibular collateral ligament.**

Lateral compartment A lateral part of the leg where evertors of the foot and ankle are found containing the peroneus longus and the peroneus brevis.

Lateral epicondylitis Tendonitis of the lateral epicondyle area. Commonly known as *tennis elbow.*

Lateral femoral condyle See **Medial and lateral femoral condyles.**

Lateral flexion The movement of the head and/or trunk in the frontal plane laterally away from the midline; abduction of the spine. Also known as *side bending.*

Lateral longitudinal arch The arch located on the lateral side of the foot and extending from the calcaneus to the cuboid and distal ends of the 4th and 5th metatarsals.

Lateral meniscus The lateral semilunar cartilage that acts as a cushion inside the knee, preventing friction and providing shock absorption.

Latissimus dorsi A shoulder joint muscle that spans superficially over most of the posterior trunk and inserts on the bicipital groove of the humerus. Its functions are adduction and extension, medial rotation, and horizontal abduction of the humerus.

Law of acceleration (Newton's law) The principle which states that (1) a change in the acceleration of a body occurs in the same direction as the force that caused it and (2) the change in acceleration is directly proportional to the force causing it and inversely proportional to the mass of the body.

Law of inertia One of Newton's laws, which states that (1) a body in motion tends to remain in motion at the same speed in a straight line unless acted on by a force and (2) a body at rest tends to remain at rest unless acted on by a force.

Law of reaction One of Newton's laws, which states that for every action there is an opposite and equal reaction.

Lesser trochanter A smaller process that serves as a bony landmark for the iliopsoas.

Levator scapulae A shoulder girdle muscle that lifts the scapula. It lies underneath the trapezius and spans from the cervical vertebrae to the superior angle of the scapula.

Line of pull The line of action for a contracting muscle.

Linea alba A structure that runs vertically from the xiphoid process through the umbilicus to the pubis. It divides each rectus abdominis and serves as its medial border.

Linea aspera The line on the posterior femur that provides attachment sites for many muscles, including the adductors, quadriceps, and short head of the biceps femoris.

Linea semilunaris A crescent, or moon-shaped, line that runs vertically and lateral to each rectus abdominis. This line represents the aponeurosis connecting the lateral border of the rectus abdominis and the medial border of the external and internal abdominal obliques.

Linear motion Motion along a line. Also known as *translatory motion.*

Lordosis An increased posterior concavity of the lumbar and cervical curves.

Lumbar kyphosis A reduction of the lumbar spine's normal lordotic curve, resulting in a flat-back appearance.

Lumbar vertebrae The five bony structures that surround the spinal cord in the lower back and are attached superiorly to the thoracic vertebrae and inferiorly to the sacrum.

Lumbosacral plexus A group of nerves from the lumbar and sacral plexuses. The femoral nerve is a major nerve stemming from the lumbar plexus.

Lunate A carpal bone.

M

Malleoli Bony protrusions at the distal end of the fibula and tibia.

Manubrium The body of the sternum.

Mass The amount of matter in a body; affects the speed and acceleration in physical movements.

Mechanical advantage A principle which states that machines enable us to apply a relatively small force, or effort, to move a much greater resistance. It is determined by dividing the load by the effort.

Medial collateral ligament (MCL) A ligament located on the medial side of the knee joint; maintains medial stability by resisting valgus forces or by preventing the knee joint from being abducted.

Medial epicondylitis Tendonitis, or "golfer's elbow," of the medial epicondyle area.

Medial and lateral femoral condyles Bony prominences on the distal end of the femur that articulate with the tibia and provide attachment sites for muscles.

Medial longitudinal arch The arch located on the medial side of the foot and extending from the calcaneus bone to the talus, the navicular, the three cuneiforms, and the distal ends of the three medial metatarsals.

Medial meniscus The medial semilunar cartilage that acts as a cushion inside the knee, preventing friction and providing shock absorption.

Medial tibial condyle The bony process that provides an area of attachment for the semimembranosus.

Median nerve The nerve that spans from the brachial plexus and can be compromised in the carpal tunnel and by other soft tissue; provides sensation to the hand and the first three fingers.

Median nerve disorders The pathologic conditions of carpal tunnel syndrome, pronator teres syndrome, and double-crush syndrome; may be caused by soft-tissue entrapment of the median nerve as well as repetitive action.

Meralgia paresthetica Pain in the anterior thigh; can be attributed to branches of the femoral nerve being compromised at some location, often from soft tissue.

Metacarpophalangeal (MCP) The condyloid joint between the metacarpal and the phalange; allows action in flexion, extension, abduction, and adduction. Commonly known as *knuckle*.

Metatarsals The five bones connected to the phalanges of the toes and to the tarsals of the foot.

Metatarsophalangeal (MP) joint The joint between the metatarsal and the phalange.

Midstance The stance phase of running or walking that occurs during pronation and internal rotation of the foot and leg, respectively.

Morton's foot structure The structure in which the second toe is an entire knuckle longer than the great toe.

Movement phase In the movement cycle, the phase that is the action part of the skill. Also known as *acceleration, action, motion,* or *contact phase.*

Multiarticular Pertaining to muscles that act on three or more joints because the line of pull between their origin and insertion crosses multiple joints.

Muscle spindles Proprioceptors that are concentrated primarily in the muscle belly between the fibers and are sensitive to stretch and rate of stretch.

Musculocutaneous nerve The nerve that spans from the brachial plexus and innervates the biceps brachii and brachialis muscles.

Myofascial pain Pain that is associated with soft tissue, may or may not hurt at the location of the trigger point, and is not linked with the distribution of a nerve.

Myofascial stretches A series of techniques designed to stretch and warm up the tissues.

Myotatic reflex arc See **Stretch reflex.**

Myotome A muscle or group of muscles supplied by a specific spinal nerve.

N

Navicular A tarsal bone in the foot.

Nerve compression A nerve impingement caused by abnormal bony growth.

Nerve entrapment A nerve impingement caused by pressure from soft-tissue structures.

Nerve impingement The compression or entrapment of a nerve, caused by hard tissue (bone) or soft tissue. Commonly known as *pinched nerve.*

Neurons Nerve cells that are the basic functional units of the nervous system, responsible for generating and transmitting impulses.

Neutralizers Muscles that counteract or neutralize the action of other muscles to prevent undesirable movements such as inappropriate muscle substitutions. They contract to resist specific actions of other muscles. Also known as *neutralizing muscles*.

O

Ober's test An orthopedic test for a contracted iliotibial tract.

Obturator externus A lateral hip rotator that is located on the posterior pelvis.

Obturator internus A lateral hip rotator that is located on the posterior pelvis.

Obturator nerve A major nerve stemming from the lumbar plexus.

Occipital nerve entrapment A condition in which the soft tissue of the trapezius and semispinalis capitis entraps the occipital nerve, causing numbness, pain, and tingling in the back of the head.

Occipitofrontalis A scalp muscle that is a combination of the occipitalis and frontalis muscles.

Open kinetic chain An open system in which one joint in an extremity can move or function separately without necessitating movement of other joints in the extremity; occurs when the distal end of the extremity is not fixed to any surface.

Opposition of the thumb A diagonal movement of the thumb across the palmar surface of the hand to make contact with the fingers.

Origin (1) From a structural perspective, the proximal attachment of a muscle or the part that attaches closest to the midline or center of the body. (2) From a functional and historical perspective, the least movable part or attachment of the muscle.

Osgood-Schlatter disease A dysfunction with the growth plate of the tibia that causes pain in the superior anterior tibial region, probable tracking issues, and tendonitis of the patella.

Osteoarthritis A pathologic condition causing abnormal bony growth.

Overload principle A basic physiologic principle of exercise which states that within appropriate parameters, a muscle or muscle group increases in strength in direct proportion to the overload placed on it.

P

Palmar flexion A wrist flexion movement in the sagittal plane with the volar or anterior side of the hand moving toward the anterior side of the forearm.

Palmaris longus A superficial muscle of the forearm that assists in flexing the wrist.

Parallel thumbs A deep-tissue technique executed by alternately applying pressure with the thumbs in a rolling-over motion. The thumbs face and are parallel to each other, and they should be at a right angle to the muscle fibers.

Passive movement Action that does not shorten the soft tissues.

Patella A sesamoid, or floating, bone that is embedded in the tendon on the anterior of the knee joint.

Patellar tracking A condition that is often the result of unusual gait problems that prevent the patella from normally riding over the knee in a superior and inferior direction during flexion and extension. Should the knee be torqued in a more medial or lateral position, it does not help the patella to track over the knee properly in movement, thus causing pain in and around the knee.

Pectineus A deep small hip adductor and hip flexor located between the pubic bone and the femur.

Pectoralis major A shoulder joint muscle that has attachments on the clavicle, sternum, and costal ribs of the anterior trunk. Because of its fanlike structure coming from different directions on the trunk, it performs all shoulder joint movements with the exception of lateral rotation and horizontal abduction.

Pectoralis minor A shoulder girdle muscle that is an anterior muscle originating on the ribs and inserting on the coracoid process of the scapula. It abducts and depresses the scapula and is an accessory respiratory muscle.

Pelvic bones The ilium, the ischium, and the pubis.

Periodization The intentional variance in a training program in which the training is set at regular intervals.

Peroneal nerves Nerves that come from the sciatic nerve and provide sensation to the anterolateral lower leg and dorsum of the foot.

Peroneus brevis A lateral leg muscle that everts the foot.

Peroneus longus A lateral leg muscle that everts and plantar flexes the foot.

Peroneus tertius An anterior leg muscle that assists in dorsiflexion and eversion.

Pes anserinus A location on the medial proximal tibia that provides an area of attachment for the sartorius, gracilis and semitendinosus muscles.

Phalanges The bones that make up the toes of the feet and fingers of the hand. There are 14 phalanges in the fingers and 14 in the toes.

Piriformis A lateral hip rotator located on the posterior pelvis that can entrap the sciatic nerve.

Piriformis syndrome The entrapment of the sciatic nerve by the piriformis in a prolonged state of external rotation or by different structural scenarios of the nerve actually passing around or through the piriformis itself.

Pisiform A carpal bone.

Pivot joint See **Trochoid joint.**

Plane of motion An imaginary two-dimensional surface through which a limb or body segment is moved.

Plantar fasciitis An inflammation of the plantar fascia with possible microtears.

Plantar flexion The extension movement of the ankle that results in the foot and/or toes moving away from the body in the sagittal plane.

Plantaris The biarticulate muscle that is located posterior to the knee. It flexes the knee and minimally contributes to plantar flexion. It is absent in some humans.

Plica A synovial fold of tissue.

PNF stretching See **Proprioceptive neuromuscular facilitation stretching.**

Popliteus A muscle located on the posterior knee that flexes and internally rotates the knee joint.

Posterior compartment The posterior leg is divided into deep and superficial spaces. The gastrocnemius, soleus, and plantaris are located superficially and the tibialis posterior, flexor hallucis longus, flexor digitorum longus, and popliteus are located in the deep compartment.

Posterior cruciate ligament (PCL) A ligament located inside the knee joint. It crosses with the anterior cruciate ligament between the tibia and the femur and maintains stability in the knee joint.

Posterior leg cramp A painful muscle spasm in the gastrocnemius and/or soleus.

Preparatory phase In the movement cycle, the phase in which appropriate muscles are lengthened so that they will be in position to generate more force and momentum as they concentrically contract in the next phase. Also known as *wind-up phase*.

Pronation (1) Of the foot: a combination of ankle dorsiflexion, subtalar eversion, and forefoot abduction (toe-out). (2) Of the radioulnar joint: the internal rotation of the radius in the transverse plane so that it lies diagonally across the ulna, resulting in the palm-down position of the forearm.

Pronator quadratus A small forearm muscle that is located distally on the radius and ulna and performs pronation.

Pronator teres The forearm muscle that is located on the medial side of the ulna and radius and performs pronation.

Pronator teres syndrome A median nerve disorder that may include repetitive pronation.

Proprioceptive neuromuscular facilitation (PNF) stretching Stretching that utilizes the components of muscle physiology to obtain a great range of motion in muscles.

Proprioceptors Internal receptors located in the skin, joints, muscles, and tendons that provide us feedback relative to the tension, length, and contraction state of muscle, the position of the body and limbs, and movements of the joints.

Prosthesis A substitute that replaces a worn or injured joint.

Protraction A shoulder girdle forward movement in the horizontal plane away from the spine; abduction of the scapula.

Proximal interphalangeal (PIP) A hinge joint between the distal interphalangeal joint (DIP) and the metacarpophalangeal (MCP) joints.

Psoas major The muscle of the iliopsoas group that primarily provides hip flexion. It is a deep core muscle that also provides stability for the lumbar spine.

Psoas minor A small muscle of the iliopsoas group that does not provide hip flexion as it does not insert on the femur.

Pubis The anterior and lower one-fifth of the pelvic bones.

Q

Q angle The quadriceps angle formed by the intersection of the central line of pull of the quadriceps and the line of pull of the patella.

Quadratus femoris A lateral hip rotator that is located on the posterior pelvis.

Quadratus lumborum A muscle that is located in the deep posterior lumbar region and is involved in lumbar movements and spinal stabilization.

R

Radial flexion (radial deviation) A wrist abduction movement in the frontal plane of the thumb side of the hand toward the lateral forearm.

Radial nerve A nerve spanning from the brachial plexus that innervates muscles and provides sensation for the arm, forearm, and hand.

Radial nerve entrapment Compromise of the radial nerve by soft tissue.

Radicular pain A type of pain that is unilateral, deep, steady, and reproducible with certain activities (walking or sitting) and that follows the involved dermatome.

Radioulnar joint A pivot joint consisting of the articulation of the radius and ulna.

Radius A bone next to the ulna in the forearm.

Range of motion (ROM) The area through which a joint may normally be freely and painlessly moved.

Reciprocal innervation An effect that occurs through reciprocal inhibition of antagonists. Activation of the motor units of the agonists causes a reciprocal neural inhibition of the motor units of the antagonists. This reduction in the neural activity of the antagonists allows them to subsequently lengthen under less tension.

Recovery phase In the movement cycle, the phase after follow-through in which balance and positioning are regained to be ready for the next sports demand.

Rectus abdominis A large superficial abdominal muscle that projects from ribs 5, 6, and 7 and the xiphoid process to the pubic bone. It flexes the trunk and helps compress organs.

Rectus femoris A quadriceps muscle that provides hip flexion and knee extension.

Reduction The return movement from lateral flexion to neutral in the frontal plane.

Referred pain Pain that can be achy, dull, migratory, and intermittent with varied intensity. It can radiate from the low back to the groin, buttock, and upper thigh.

Reposition of the thumb A diagonal movement of the thumb as it returns to the anatomical position from opposition with the hand and/or fingers.

Resistance arm The distance between the axis and the point of resistance application.

Retraction A shoulder girdle backward movement in the horizontal plane toward the spine; adduction of the scapula.

Rhomboids Shoulder girdle muscles that insert on the vertebral border of the scapula. The rhomboid major and minor are deep to the trapezius. Shaped like a bilateral Christmas tree, they connect the spinous processes of the thoracic spine to the vertebral edge of the scapula. Their major functions are adduction and downward rotation.

RICE An acronym for "rest, ice, compression, and elevation." It is a first aid recipe for immediate response to acute injuries such as an acute sprain.

Rotation Spinal movement in the transverse plane. The spine can rotate 90 degrees.

Rotation downward A shoulder girdle rotary movement of the scapula in the frontal plane with the inferior angle of the scapula moving medially and downward; occurs primarily in the return from upward rotation. The inferior angle may actually move upward slightly as the scapula continues in extreme downward rotation.

Rotation upward A shoulder girdle rotary movement of the scapula in the frontal plane with the inferior angle of the scapula moving laterally and upward.

Rotator cuff group A group of muscles whose tendons line up on the head of the humerus for stabilization. It comprises the supraspinatus, infraspinatus, teres minor, and subscapularis. See entries for the individual muscles for descriptions.

S

Sacroiliac joint The joint between the sacrum and the ilium.

Sacrum An extension of the spinal column that has five fused vertebrae. Extending inferior to the sacrum is the coccyx.

Saddle-type joint See **Sellar joint.**

Sagittal plane The anteroposterior, or AP, plane that divides the body into right and left symmetrical halves.

SAID See Specific adaptations to imposed demands.

Sarcopenia A condition that causes a gradual loss of skeletal muscle.

Sartorius A strap muscle that provides hip flexion, external rotation, and knee flexion. It is a superficial muscle running from the iliac crest to the medial tibia.

Scaphoid A carpal bone.

Scapula A flat bone that is one of the bones of the shoulder girdle. It attaches to the clavicle and provides a place for the upper extremity to attach.

Scapulothoracic Pertaining to the actions of the shoulder girdle as it moves in various directions over the rib cage. It is not a true joint.

Sciatic nerve A nerve composed of the tibial and common peroneal nerves, which are wrapped in connective tissue until reaching midway down the posterior thigh.

Sciatica The inflammation of the sciatic nerve.

Scoliosis A lateral curvature of the spine.

Sellar joint A type of diarthrodial joint of reciprocal reception that is found only in the thumb at the carpometacarpal joint and permits ball-and-socket movement, with the exception of slight rotation. Also known as *saddle joint.*

Semimembranosus A hamstring muscle that is located on the posterior thigh and inserts on the medial tibia. It extends the hip and flexes and internally rotates the knee.

Semitendinosus A hamstring muscle that is located on the posterior thigh and inserts on the medial tibia. It extends the hip and flexes and internally rotates the knee.

Sequence A specific series of techniques chosen to accomplish a particular goal in a massage session.

Serratus anterior A shoulder girdle muscle that spans from the upper nine ribs and inserts into the anterior medial scapula. It abducts and upwardly rotates the scapula and is an accessory muscle of respiration.

Sesamoid A bone that is not attached to another bone but "floats" in soft tissue.

Sherrington's law The law of reciprocal innervation, which states that for every neural activation of a muscle, there is a corresponding inhibition of the opposing muscle.

Shoulder girdle The bony arch made up of the clavicle and scapula. It surrounds the trunk and attaches to the sternum.

Skeletal system All the bones of the body; consists of two regions, the appendicular skeleton and the axial skeleton.

Sliding-filament theory A researched model of how a muscle contracts. Hugh Huxley and Jean Hanson proposed in 1954 that the myofilaments in muscle do not shorten during a contraction but that the thin filaments slide over the thick ones and pull the Z disks behind them, causing each sarcomere as a unit to shorten.

Soleus A deep posterior leg muscle under the gastrocnemius. It plantar flexes the foot.

Somatic pain Pain from muscle, skin, or joints.

Specific adaptations to imposed demands (SAID) A principle which states that the body will gradually, over time, adapt very specifically to the various stresses and overloads to which it is subjected. It is applicable in every form of muscle training, as well as to all the systems of the body.

Specificity The concentrated approach to a specific area of focus.

Speed A measure of how fast an object is moving, or the distance an object travels in a specific amount of time.

Spinal extension The return from flexion; posterior movement of the spine in the sagittal plane.

Spinal rotation The rotary movement of the spine in a transverse plane.

Splenius capitis A posterior cervical muscle that inserts into the occiput. Bilaterally, it extends the head; unilaterally, it laterally flexes and rotates the head.

Splenius cervicis A posterior cervical muscle that inserts on the transverse processes of C1–C3. Bilaterally, it extends the head; unilaterally, it laterally flexes and rotates the head.

Splinting A supportive action that a muscle or muscles may perform so that another joint and group of muscles can function appropriately.

Sprains Injuries with various levels of severity that often tear ligaments, bruise nerves, and tear soft tissue. All the signs and symptoms of inflammation are present.

Spurs Bony growths on the side of the vertebrae.

Stabilizers Muscles that surround a joint or body part and contract to fixate or stabilize the area to enable another limb or body segment to exert force and move. They are essential in establishing a relatively firm base for the more distal joints to work from when carrying out movements. Also known as *fixators*.

Stance phase (1) A phase of the gait (running or walking) cycle. (2) In the movement cycle, the phase in which the athlete assumes a comfortable and appropriately balanced body position from which to initiate the sports skill.

Sternoclavicular (SC) The gliding joint made up of the sternum and clavicle.

Sternocleidomastoid (SCM) An anterior and lateral neck muscle named for its attachments. It flexes, rotates, and laterally flexes the head.

Stiff neck A catchall term for limitations in neck movements.

Strains Injuries to the soft tissue, with various levels of severity.

Stretch reflex A muscle contraction in response to the lengthening, or stretching, of a muscle. This reflex acts as a defense mechanism to prevent the overstretching of a muscle. Also known as *myotatic reflex arc*.

Stretching Taking a muscle in its resting length and expanding it.

Stripping A deep-tissue technique designed to push fluids from distal to proximal.

Structural kinesiology The study of muscles, bones, and joints as they are involved in the science of movement.

Subacute The stage of inflammation that carries the same signs and symptoms as those of the acute stage but without escalation.

Subacute flare-up A response to a chronic injury that is not allowed to rest. The site exhibits the signs and symptoms of the acute stage.

Subclavius A shoulder girdle muscle that is a stabilizer and protects the sternoclavicular joint.

Subluxation A joint that is slightly ajar. It is not dislocated, but it has articular surfaces that are somewhat out of alignment.

Suboccipitals Deep posterior neck muscles known for rocking and tilting the head. They are the rectus capitis posterior minor, rectus capitis posterior major, and obliquus capitis superior and inferior.

Subscapularis A muscle that originates on the subscapular fossa and inserts on the lesser tubercle. It adducts, extends, and medially rotates the humerus.

Subtalar and transverse tarsal joints Gliding joints that allow the ankle to complete inversion and eversion.

Superior peroneal retinaculum A tissue bridge that tacks down the peroneal tendons superior to the calcaneofibular ligament.

Supination (1) Of the foot: a combination of ankle plantar flexion, subtalar inversion, and forefoot adduction (toe-in). (2) Of the radioulnar joint: the external rotation of the radius in the transverse plane so that it lies parallel to the ulna, resulting in the palm-up position of the forearm.

Supinator A muscle in the forearm that performs supination.

Supraspinatus A rotator cuff muscle that originates on the supraspinous fossa and whose insertion lines up next to the infraspinatus and teres minor on the greater tubercle of the humerus. It performs weak abduction.

Suture A type of synarthrodial joint found in the skull.

Swing A phase of the gait (running or walking) cycle that occurs when the foot leaves the ground and the leg moves forward to another point of contact.

Symphysis An amphiarthrodial joint separated by a fibrocartilage pad that allows very slight movement between the bones.

Symphysis pubis An amphiarthrodial joint that joins the pelvic bones anteriorly.

Synarthrodial joints Immovable joints.

Synchondrosis An amphiarthrodial joint separated by hyaline cartilage that allows very slight movement between the bones.

Syndesmosis A type of synarthrodial joint that is held together by strong ligaments.

Synergists Muscles that assist in the action of agonists but are not necessarily prime movers for the action. They assist in refined movement and rule out undesired motions. Also known as *guiding muscles.*

T

Talocrural joint A hinge joint that allows the foot to dorsiflex and plantar flex. It is made up of the talus, distal tibia, and distal fibula.

Talus A tarsal bone in the foot.

Tarsals Bones consisting of the talus, calcaneus, navicular, three cuneiforms, and cuboid in the foot.

Technique goals The outcomes expected from choosing techniques for a particular purpose.

Temporalis A scalp muscle that is located above the ear on each side of the head. It attaches to five different bones of the face and skull.

Temporomandibular joint (TMJ) syndrome A condition that causes pain in the jaw, headaches, and problems opening and closing the jaw. It is caused by trauma, grinding teeth, braces, dental procedures, the jaw being open too long, cervical traction, and other factors.

Tendinous inscriptions Horizontal indentations that transect the rectus abdominis at three or more locations, giving the muscle its segmented appearance.

Tendon A fibrous connective tissue, often cordlike in appearance, that connects muscles to bones and other structures.

Tendon sheath A plastic wrap–like connective tissue, surrounding individual groups of tendons, that can become inflamed from the repetitive action and continual torque received in the region.

Tendonitis A pathologic condition of the soft tissue that is characterized by inflammation of a tendon.

Tendonosis A pathologic condition of the soft tissue that is characterized by a breakdown in collagen fibers.

Tennis elbow See **Lateral epicondylitis.**

Tensor fasciae latae An anterior hip muscle that provides hip flexion and abduction.

Teres major A posterior muscle that originates on the inferior angle of the scapula and inserts on the bicipital groove of the humerus. With latissimus dorsi, it forms the back aspect of the axilla region. It is a strong extensor and adductor and medially rotates the humerus.

Teres minor A rotator cuff muscle that originates on the upper axillary border of the scapula and inserts on the inferior facet of the greater tubercle of the humerus. It performs extension, lateral rotation, and horizontal abduction.

Thoracic vertebrae The 12 bony structures that surround the spinal cord in the chest and are attached superiorly to the cervical vertebrae and inferiorly to the lumbar vertebrae.

Tibia The medial bone of the leg.

Tibial medial condyle A bony process that provides an area of attachment for the semimembranosus.

Tibial nerve The nerve that comes from the sciatic nerve and provides sensation to the posterolateral lower leg and the plantar aspect of the foot.

Tibial plateau The smooth bony surface of the medial and lateral epicondyles of the tibia that articulates with the condylar surface of the femur.

Tibial tuberosity A bony landmark where the quadriceps inserts into the tibia.

Tibialis anterior An anterior leg muscle that dorsiflexes and inverts the foot.

Tibialis posterior A posterior leg muscle deep to the soleus. It is a strong invertor of the foot.

Tibiofemoral joint A hinge joint of the knee that provides flexion and extension.

Tibiofibular joint A syndesmotic amphiarthrodial joint held together by ligaments and supported by the interosseus membrane; located at the proximal and distal tibia and fibula.

TMJ syndrome See **Temporomandibular joint syndrome.**

Toe extension Movement of the toes away from the plantar surface of the foot.

Toe flexion Movement of the toes toward the plantar surface of the foot.

Toe-off The third component of the stance phase of running or walking that occurs after the foot returns to supination and the leg returns to external rotation.

Torque The turning effect of an eccentric force. Also known as *moment of force.*

Torticollis A spasmodic contraction of the neck muscles, mostly the trapezius and sternocleidomastoid, since they are supplied by the spinal accessory nerve. Also known as *wry neck.*

Traditional kinesiology The study of the science of muscle movement.

Transverse arch The arch that extends across the foot from one metatarsal bone to the other.

Transverse plane The plane that divides the body horizontally into superior and inferior halves.

Transverse tarsal joints See **Subtalar and transverse tarsal joints.**

Transversus abdominis A deep abdominal muscle that connects to the other abdominal muscles by aponeurosis. It attaches to the diaphragm, helps in forced expiration, and compresses abdominal organs.

Trapezium A carpal bone.

Trapezius A four-sided superficial posterior muscle that is divided into three sections: upper, middle, and lower. It lifts and depresses the clavicle and scapula and adducts and upwardly rotates the scapula. Bilaterally, it extends the head; unilaterally, it can flex the head to the ipsilateral side.

Trapezoid A carpal bone.

Treatment protocol A synopsis of an overall approach to a massage session.

Trendelenburg test An orthopedic test used to assess gluteus medius weakness.

Treppe A phenomenon of muscle contraction that occurs when multiple maximal stimuli are provided at a low enough frequency to allow complete relaxation between contractions to rested muscle.

Triceps brachii A three-headed muscle located on the posterior surface of the arm. All three heads extend the forearm.

Triceps surae A term used collectively for the gastrocnemius and soleus.

Trigger point release See **Ischemic compression.**

Trigger points Irritated or hyperactive areas, often located in hypertonic tissue, that are either *active* (refer pain to a specific area) or *latent* (have a positive reaction to pain in the area of the trigger point).

Triquetrum A carpal bone.

Trochoid joint A type of diarthrodial joint with a rotational movement around a long axis; depicts its movement of rotation as supination and pronation. Also known as *pivot joint* and *screw joint*.

U

Ulna The bone next to the radius in the forearm. It articulates with the humerus and with the radius.

Ulnar flexion (ulnar deviation) A wrist adduction movement in the frontal plane of the little-finger side of the hand toward the medial forearm.

Ulnar nerve The nerve branching from C8 and T1 that supplies the flexor digitorum profundus for the 4th and 5th fingers and the flexor carpi ulnaris. Additionally, it innervates the remaining intrinsic muscles of the hand (the deep head of the flexor pollicis brevis, adductor pollicis, palmar interossei, dorsal interossei, 3rd and 4th lumbricals, opponens digiti minimi, abductor digiti minimi, and flexor digiti minimi brevis). Sensation to the ulnar side of the hand, the ulnar half of the ring finger, and the entire little finger is provided by the ulnar nerve.

Ulnar nerve compression A restriction of the ulnar nerve by a bony structure.

Uniarticular A type of muscle that acts directly on only the joint that it crosses.

V

Vastus intermedius A quadriceps muscle that is deep to the rectus femoris and extends the knee.

Vastus lateralis A quadriceps muscle that inserts laterally into the patellar tendon and extends the knee.

Vastus medialis A quadriceps muscle that inserts medially into the patellar tendon and extends the knee.

Velocity The direction and rate of displacement.

W

Whiplash An injury resulting from a sudden impact and causing a violent hyperextension of the head and neck, followed by hyperflexion and perhaps an additional hyperextension.

Wry neck See **Torticollis.**

X

Xiphoid process The structure at the base of the sternum.

Index

Page reference followed by f indicates figure; t, table.

A

B

C

D

E

F

G

H

I

J

K

L

M

N

T

U

V

W

X

Credits

Photo Credits

Part Openers:

1: © The McGraw-Hill Companies, Inc./Barbara Banks, photographer; 2: © The McGraw-Hill Companies, Inc./Leigh Kelly Monroe, photographer; 3: © Nancy Dail; 4: © The McGraw-Hill Companies, Inc./Barbara Banks, photographer.

Chapter 1

Figure 1.1: © The McGraw-Hill Companies, Inc./Joe DeGrandis, photographer; 1.2, 1.3: © The McGraw-Hill Companies, Inc./Joe DeGrandis, photographer; pp. 15, 16, 17, 18(male), 19, 20: © The McGraw-Hill Companies, Inc./Timothy L. Vacula, photographer; p. 18(female): © The McGraw-Hill Companies, Inc./Barbara Banks, photographer.

Chapter 2

Figures 2.5a–c, 2.16a–c: Britt Jones.

Chapter 3

Figure 3.11: © Karl Weatherly/Getty Images RF; 3.12: © Digital Vision/Getty Images RF; 3.14: © Rubberball Productions/Index Stock.

Chapter 5

Figures 5.1–5.3: © The McGraw-Hill Companies, Inc./Leigh Kelly Monroe, photographer; 5.4: © Nancy Dail; 5.5–5.7: © The McGraw-Hill Companies, Inc./Leigh Kelly Monroe, photographer; 5.8: © Nancy Dail; 5.9–5.29: © The McGraw-Hill Companies, Inc./ Leigh Kelly Monroe, photographer.

Chapter 6

Page 119, p. 120(top left): © The McGraw-Hill Companies, Inc./ Timothy L. Vacula, photographer; p. 120(bottom left), p. 120(top right), p. 120(bottom right), p. 121: © The McGraw-Hill Companies, Inc./Barbara Banks, photographer.

Chapter 7

Figures 7.1–7.28: © The McGraw-Hill Companies, Inc./Leigh Kelly Monroe, photographer.

Chapter 9

Figures 9.1–9.19: © The McGraw-Hill Companies, Inc./Leigh Kelly Monroe, photographer.

Chapter 10

Figure 10.7(all): Britt Jones.

Chapter 11

Figures 11.1–11.24: © The McGraw-Hill Companies, Inc./Leigh Kelly Monroe, photographer.

Chapter 12

Figures 12.1: © Royalty-Free/Corbis; 12.2–12.14: © The McGraw-Hill Companies, Inc./Barbara Banks, photographer.

Chapter 13

Figure 13.10(all): Britt Jones.

Chapter 14

Figures 14.1–14.9: © Nancy Dail; 14.10, 14.11: © The McGraw-Hill Companies, Inc./Leigh Kelly Monroe, photographer; 14.12, 14.13: © Nancy Dail; 14.14: © The McGraw-Hill Companies, Inc./Leigh Kelly Monroe, photographer; 14.15: © Nancy Dail; 14.16, 14.17: © The McGraw-Hill Companies, Inc./Leigh Kelly Monroe, photographer; 14.18–14.21: © Nancy Dail.

Chapter 15

Figure 15.6, 15.7: Britt Jones.

Chapter 16

Figure 16.1–16.32: © The McGraw-Hill Companies, Inc./Leigh Kelly Monroe, photographer.

Chapter 17

Figure 17.5(all): © The McGraw-Hill Companies, Inc./Barbara Banks, photographer.

Chapter 18

Figures 18.1–18.27: © The McGraw-Hill Companies, Inc./Leigh Kelly Monroe, photographer.

Chapter 19

Figure 19.6b: © Walter Reiter/Phototake; pp. 408, 409: Britt Jones.

Chapter 20

Figures 20.1–20.25: © The McGraw-Hill Companies, Inc./Leigh Kelly Monroe, photographer; 20.26: © Nancy Dail; 20.27–20.40: © The McGraw-Hill Companies, Inc./Leigh Kelly Monroe, photographer.

Chapter 21

Figure 21.1–21.16: © The McGraw-Hill Companies, Inc./Barbara Banks, photographer.

Illustration and Text Credits

Chapter 1

Saladin, KS: *Anatomy & Physiology: The Unit of Form and Function,* 5th edition, NY, copyright 2010, McGraw-Hill: Table 1.1-Directional Terms in Human Anatomy; Figures: 1.4; 1.5; 1.6; 1.7; 1.8; 1.9; 1.10; 1.11; & 1.12

Chapter 2

Floyd, RT: *Manual of Structural Kinesiology,* 17th edition, NY, copyright 2009, McGraw-Hill: Table 2.1-Muscle Contraction and Movement Matrix; Table 2.2-Spinal Nerve Root Dermatomes, Myotomes, Reflexes, and Functional Application; and Table 2.3-Sensory Receptors; Figures: 2.15; & 2.17

Adapted from: Hall SJ: *Basic Biomechanics of Human Motion,* 10th edition, NY, copyright 2003, McGraw-Hill: Figure: 2.18

Adapted from: Powers SK, Howley ET: *Exercise Physiology: Theory and Application to Fitness and Performance,* 4th edition, NY, copyright 2001, McGraw-Hill: Figures 2.12; & 2.13

Adapted from: Seeley RR, Stephens TD, Tate P: *Anatomy & Physiology,* 7th edition, NY, copyright 2006, McGraw-Hill: Figures: 2.11; & 2.14

Saladin, KS: *Anatomy & Physiology: The Unit of Form and Function,* 5th edition, NY, copyright 2010, McGraw-Hill: Figures: 2.1; 2.2; 2.3; 2.4; 2.6; 2.7; 2.8; 2.9; & 2.10

Chapter 3

Floyd, RT: *Manual of Structural Kinesiology,* 17th edition, NY, copyright 2009, McGraw-Hill: Table 3.1-Classification of Levers and Characteristics of Each; Figures: 3.3; 3.4; 3.5; 3.6; 3.7; 3.8; 3.9; 3.10; & 3.13

Adapted from: Hamilton N, Luttgems K: *Kinesiology: Scientific Basis of Human Motion,* 6th edition, NY, copyright 2002, McGraw-Hill: Figure: 3.12

Saladin, KS: *Anatomy & Physiology: The Unit of Form and Function,* 5th edition, NY, copyright 2010, McGraw-Hill: Figures: 3.1; & 3.2

Chapter 4

Floyd, RT: *Manual of Structural Kinesiology,* 17th edition, NY, copyright 2009, McGraw-Hill: Figures:

Adapted from: Ernest W. Beck: Figures: TA 4.1; TA 4.2; TA 4.3; & TA 4.5

Adapted from: Linda Kimbrough: Figures: 4.1; 4.2A; TA 4.4A&B; & TA 4.6

Adapted from: Shier D, Butler J, Lewis R: *Hole's Human Anatomy and Physiology,* 9th edition, NY, copyright 2002, McGraw-Hill: Figure: 4.2B

McKinley, M: *Human Anatomy,* 2nd edition, NY, copyright 2008, McGraw-Hill: Figures: 4.3; 4.4; 4.5; 4.6; 4.7; & 4.8

Chapter 6

Floyd, RT: *Manual of Structural Kinesiology,* 17th edition, NY, copyright 2009, McGraw-Hill: Table 6.1-Pairing of Shoulder Girdle and Shoulder Joint Movements; Figures:

Adapted from: Ernest W. Beck: Figures: TA 6.11; TA 6.17; & TA 6.19

Adapted from: Ernest W. Beck with inserts with Linda Kimbrough: Figure: TA 6.16

Adapted from: Booher JM, Thibodeau GA, *Athletic Injury Assessment,* 4th edition; Dubuque, IA; copyright 2003; McGraw-Hill: Figure: 6.4

Adapted from: Linda Kimbrough: Figures: 6.1; 6.2; 6.3; TA 6.13; TA 6.14; TA 6.15; TA 6.18; & TA 6.20

Saladin, KS: *Anatomy & Physiology: The Unit of Form and Function,* 5th edition, NY, copyright 2010, McGraw-Hill: Figures: 6.5; 6.6; & TA 6.12

Chapter 8

Saladin, KS: *Anatomy & Physiology: The Unit of Form and Function,* 5th edition, NY, copyright 2010, McGraw-Hill: Figures: 8.1; 8.3; 8.6; 8.7; 8.8; & 8.9

Floyd, RT: *Manual of Structural Kinesiology,* 17th edition, NY, copyright 2009, McGraw-Hill: Figures:

Adapted from: Booher JM, Thibodeau GA, *Athletic Injury Assessment,* 4th edition, Dubuque, IA, copyright 2003, McGraw-Hill: Figures: 8.4 & 8.5

Adapted from: Linda Kimbrough: Figures: 8.2; TA 8.1; TA 8.2; TA 8.3; TA 8.4; TA 8.5; TA 8.6; TA 8.7; & TA 8.8

Adapted from: Van De Graaff KM: *Human Anatomy,* 6th edition, Dubuque, IA, copyright 2002, McGraw-Hill: Figures: 8.10; & 8.11

Chapter 10

Floyd, RT: *Manual of Structural Kinesiology,* 17th edition, NY, copyright 2009, McGraw-Hill: Table 10.2-Intrinsic Muscles of the Hand; Figures:

Adapted from: Booher JM, Thibodeau GA, *Athletic Injury Assessment,* 4th edition, Dubuque, IA, copyright 2003, McGraw-Hill: Figures: 10.3; 10.5; & 10.6

Adapted from: Linda Kimbrough: Figures: 10.2; TA 10.1; TA 10.2; TA 10.3; TA 10.4; TA 10.5; TA 10.6; TA 10.7; TA 10.8; TA 10.9; TA 10.10; TA 10.11; TA 10.12; TA 10.13; TA 10.14; & TA 10.15

Adapted from: Van De Graaff KM: *Human Anatomy,* 6th edition, Dubuque, IA, copyright 2002, McGraw-Hill: Figures: 10.4 & 10.11

Saladin, KS: *Anatomy & Physiology: The Unit of Form and Function,* 5th edition, NY, copyright 2010, McGraw-Hill: Figures: 10.1; 10.8; 10.9; 10.10; &10.12

Chapter 12

Floyd, RT: *Manual of Structural Kinesiology,* 17th edition, NY, copyright 2009, McGraw-Hill: Table 12.1-Differences between Open- and Closed-Chain Exercises

**Adapted from Ellenbecker TS, Davies GJ: *Closed Kinetic Chain Exercise: A Comprehensive Guide to Multiple-Joint Exercise,* Champaign, IL, 2001, Human Kinetics

Chapter 13

Floyd, RT: *Manual of Structural Kinesiology,* 17th edition, NY, copyright 2009, McGraw-Hill: Table 13.2-Muscles That Move the Head; Table 13.3-Muscles of the Vertebral Column; Table 13.4-Muscles of the Thorax; Figures:

Adapted from: Booher JM, Thibodeau GA, *Athletic Injury Assessment,* 4th edition; Dubuque, IA; copyright 2003; McGraw-Hill: Figures: 13.8 & 13.9

Adapted from: Ernest W. Beck: Figure: TA 13.6

Adapted from: Linda Kimbrough: Figures: TA 13.1; TA 13.2; TA 13.3; TA 13.4; TA 13.5; TA 13.7; TA 13.8; & TA 13.9

Adapted from: Seeley RR, Stephens TD, Tate P: *Anatomy & Physiology,* 7th edition, NY, copyright 2006, McGraw-Hill: Figure: 13.14

Adapted from: Seeley RR, Stephens TD, Tate P: *Anatomy & Physiology,* 8th edition, NY, copyright 2008, McGraw-Hill: Figure: 13.1

Jurch, S: *Clinical Massage Therapy,* 1st edition, NY, copyright 2009, McGraw-Hill: Figure: 13.12

Saladin, KS: *Anatomy & Physiology: The Unit of Form and Function,* 5th edition, NY, copyright 2010, McGraw-Hill: Figures: 13.2; 13.3; 13.4; 13.5; 13.6; 13.7; 13.11; 13.13; 13.15; 13.16; & 13.17

Chapter 15

Floyd, RT: *Manual of Structural Kinesiology,* 17th edition, NY, copyright 2009, McGraw-Hill: Table 15.1-Motions Accompanying Pelvic Rotation; Figures:
Adapted from: Booher JM, Thibodeau GA, *Athletic Injury Assessment,* 4th edition, Dubuque, IA, copyright 2003, McGraw-Hill: Figure: 15.5
Adapted from: Ernest W. Beck: Figure: 15.11
Adapted from: Linda Kimbrough: Figures: TA 15.1; TA 15.2; TA 15.3; TA 15.4; TA 15.5; TA 15.6; TA 15.7; TA 15.8; TA 15.9; TA 15.10; TA 15.11; TA 15.12; & TA 15.13
Saladin, KS: *Anatomy & Physiology: The Unit of Form and Function,* 5th edition, NY, copyright 2010, McGraw-Hill: Figures: 15.1; 15.2; 15.3; 15.4; 15.8; 15.9; 15.10; 15.12; & 15.13

Chapter 17

Floyd, RT: *Manual of Structural Kinesiology,* 17th edition, NY, copyright 2009, McGraw-Hill: Figures:
Adapted from: Hamilton N, Weimar W, Luttgems K: *Kinesiology: Scientific Basis of Human Motion,* 11th edition, NY, copyright 2008, McGraw-Hill: Figure: 17.4
Adapted from: Linda Kimbrough: Figures: 17.6; TA 17.2; TA 17.3; TA 17.4; 17.7; TA 17.5; TA 17.6; TA 17.7; & TA 17.8
Saladin, KS: *Anatomy & Physiology: The Unit of Form and Function,* 5th edition, NY, copyright 2010, McGraw-Hill: Figures: 17.1; 17.2; 17.3; & TA 17.1

Chapter 19

Floyd, RT: *Manual of Structural Kinesiology,* 17th edition, NY, copyright 2009, McGraw-Hill: Table 19.2-Intrinsic Muscles of the Foot; Figures:
Adapted from: Booher JM, Thibodeau GA, *Athletic Injury Assessment,* 4th edition, Dubuque, IA, copyright 2003, McGraw-Hill: Figure: 19.5
Adapted from: Ernest W. Beck: Figures: TA 19.9; TA 19.10; TA 19.11; TA 19.12; TA 19.13; TA 19.14; TA 19.15; TA 19.17; TA 19.18; & TA 19.19
Adapted from: Linda Kimbrough: Figure: TA 19.16
Jurch, S: *Clinical Massage Therapy,* 1st edition, NY, copyright 2009, McGraw-Hill: Figure: 19.1
Saladin, KS: *Anatomy & Physiology: The Unit of Form and Function,* 5th edition, NY, copyright 2010, McGraw-Hill: Figures: 19.2; 19.3; 19.4; 19.6A; 19.7; 19.8; 19.9; 19.10; 19.11; & 19.12

Worksheet

chapter 4

For in- or out-of-class assignments, or for testing, utilize this tear-out worksheet.

Worksheet 1

Using crayons or colored markers, draw and label on the worksheet the following muscles. Indicate the origin and insertion of each muscle with an "O" and an "I," respectively, and draw in the origin and insertion on the contralateral side of the skeleton.

a. Trapezius
b. Rhomboid major and minor
c. Serratus anterior
d. Levator scapulae
e. Pectoralis minor

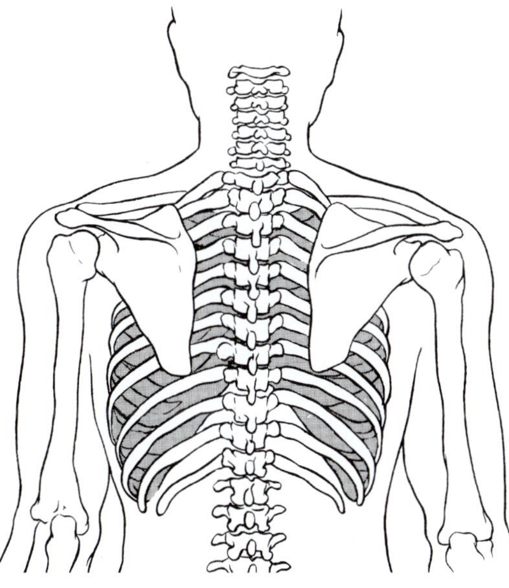

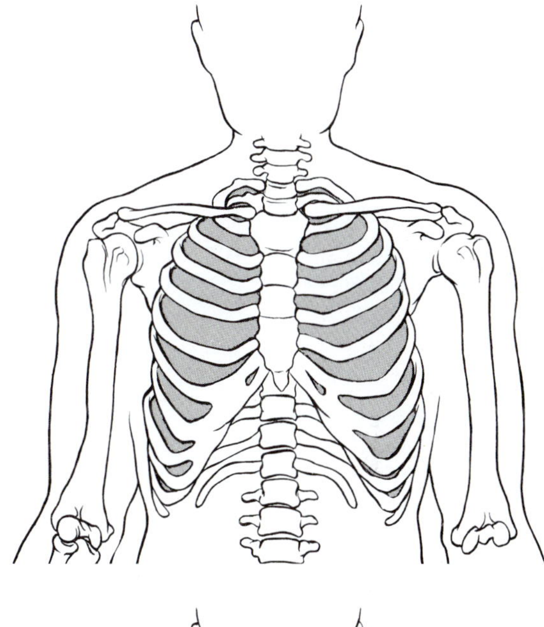

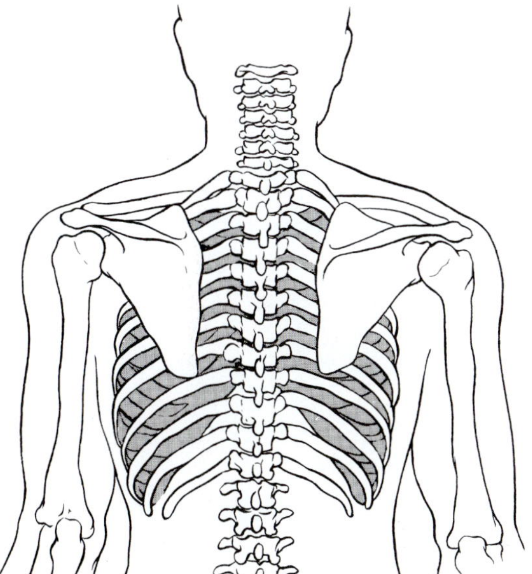

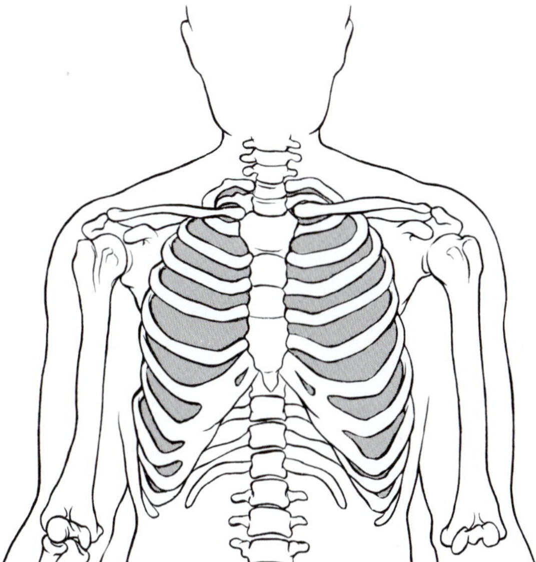

Worksheet

chapter 4

For in- or out-of-class assignments, or for testing, utilize this tear-out worksheet.

Worksheet 2

Label each of lines 1 through 6 on the drawing with the letter, from the following list, that corresponds to the movements of the shoulder girdle indicated by the arrow.

a. Adduction (retraction)
b. Abduction (protraction)
c. Rotation upward
d. Rotation downward
e. Elevation
f. Depression

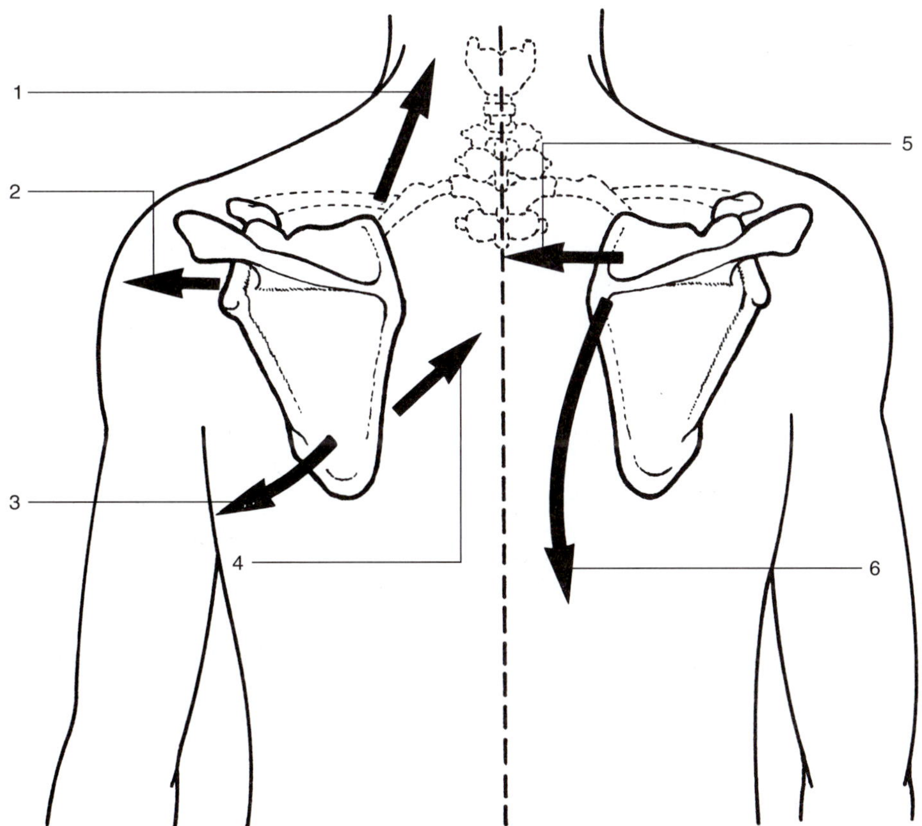

On the lines below, which correspond to the numbers of the arrows above, list the muscles or parts of muscles primarily responsible for causing the movements.

1. ______
2. ______
3. ______
4. ______
5. ______
6. ______

Worksheet

chapter 6

For in- or out-of-class assignments, or for testing, utilize this tear-out worksheet.

Worksheet 1

Using crayons or colored markers, draw and label on the worksheet the following muscles. Indicate the origin and insertion of each muscle with an "O" and an "I," respectively, and draw in the origin and insertion on the contralateral side of the skeleton.

a. Deltoid
b. Supraspinatus
c. Subscapularis
d. Teres major
e. Infraspinatus
f. Teres minor
g. Latissimus dorsi
h. Pectoralis major
i. Coracobrachialis

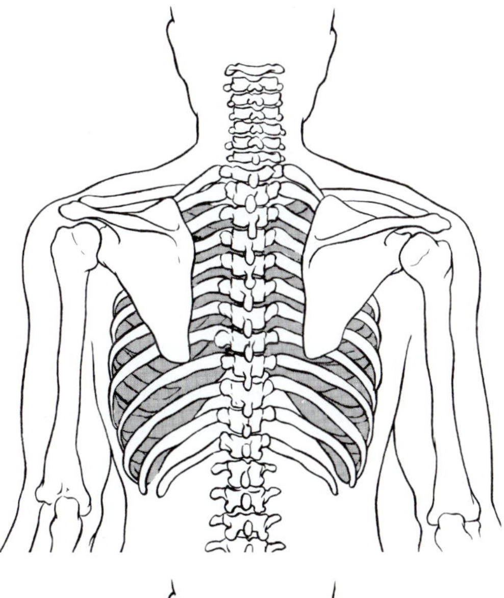

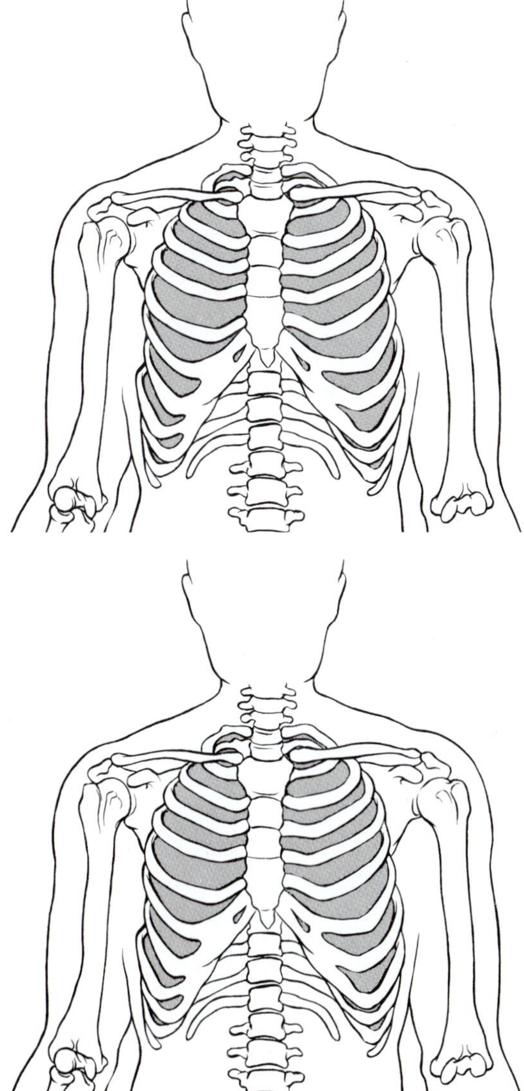

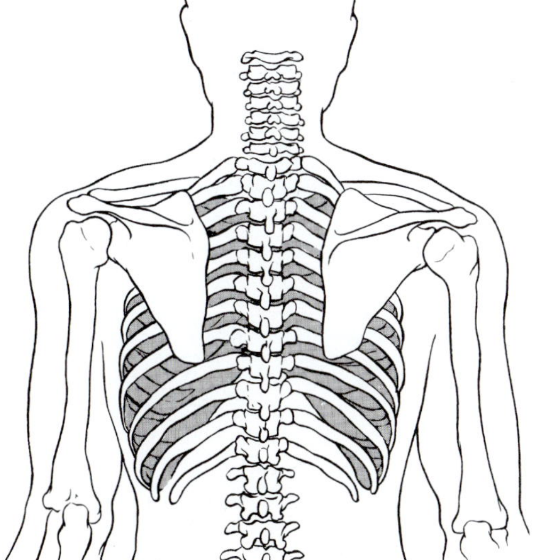

Worksheet

chapter 6

For in- or out-of-class assignments, or for testing, utilize this tear-out worksheet.

Worksheet 2

Label and indicate with arrows the following movements of the shoulder joint. For each motion, complete the sentence by supplying the plane in which it occurs and the axis of rotation.

a. Abduction occurs in the ______________ plane about the ______________ axis.
b. Adduction occurs in the ______________ plane about the ______________ axis.
c. Flexion occurs in the ______________ plane about the ______________ axis.
d. Extension occurs in the ______________ plane about the ______________ axis.
e. Horizontal adduction occurs in the ______________ plane about the ______________ axis.
f. Horizontal abduction occurs in the ______________ plane about the ______________ axis.

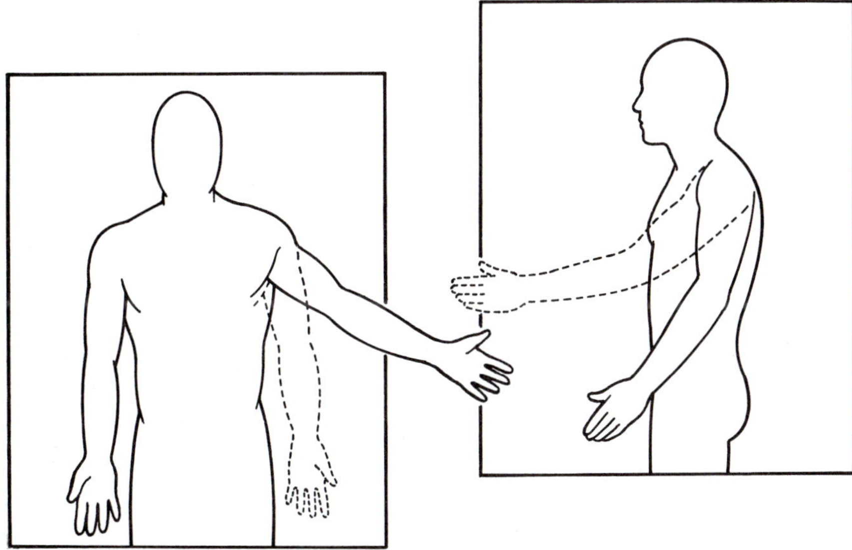

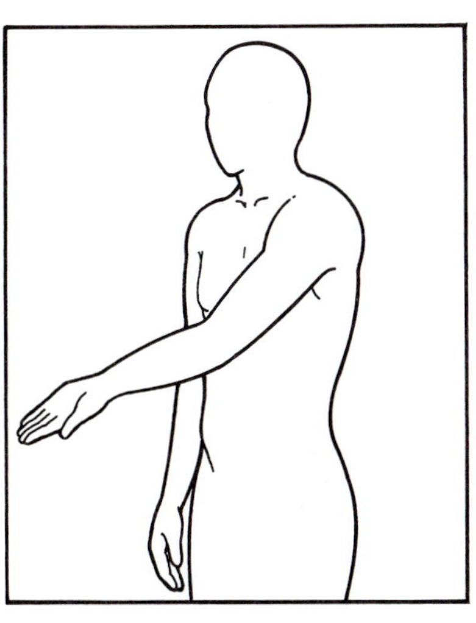

Worksheet

chapter 8

For in- or out-of-class assignments, or for testing, utilize this tear-out worksheet.

Worksheet 1

Using crayons or colored markers, draw and label on the worksheet the following muscles. Indicate the origin and insertion of each muscle with an "O" and an "I," respectively.

a. Biceps brachii
b. Brachioradialis
c. Brachialis
d. Pronator teres
e. Supinator
f. Triceps brachii
g. Pronator quadratus
h. Anconeus

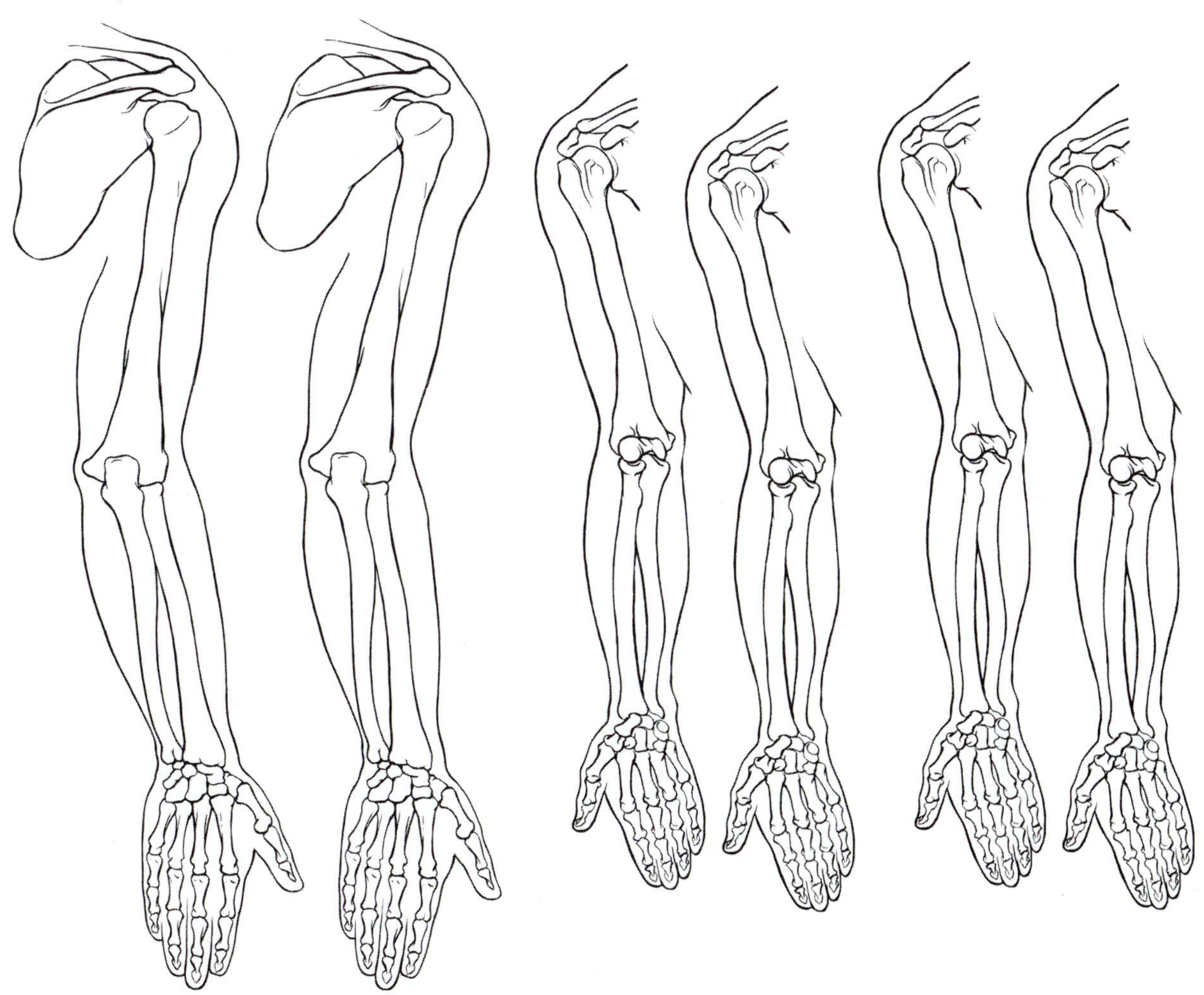

Worksheet

chapter 8

For in- or out-of-class assignments, or for testing, utilize this tear-out worksheet.

Worksheet 2

Label and indicate by arrows the following movements of the elbow and radioulnar joints. Then below, for each motion, list the agonist muscles, the plane in which the motion occurs, and its axis of rotation.

1. Elbow joints
   a. Flexion
   b. Extension
2. Radioulnar joints
   a. Pronation
   b. Supination

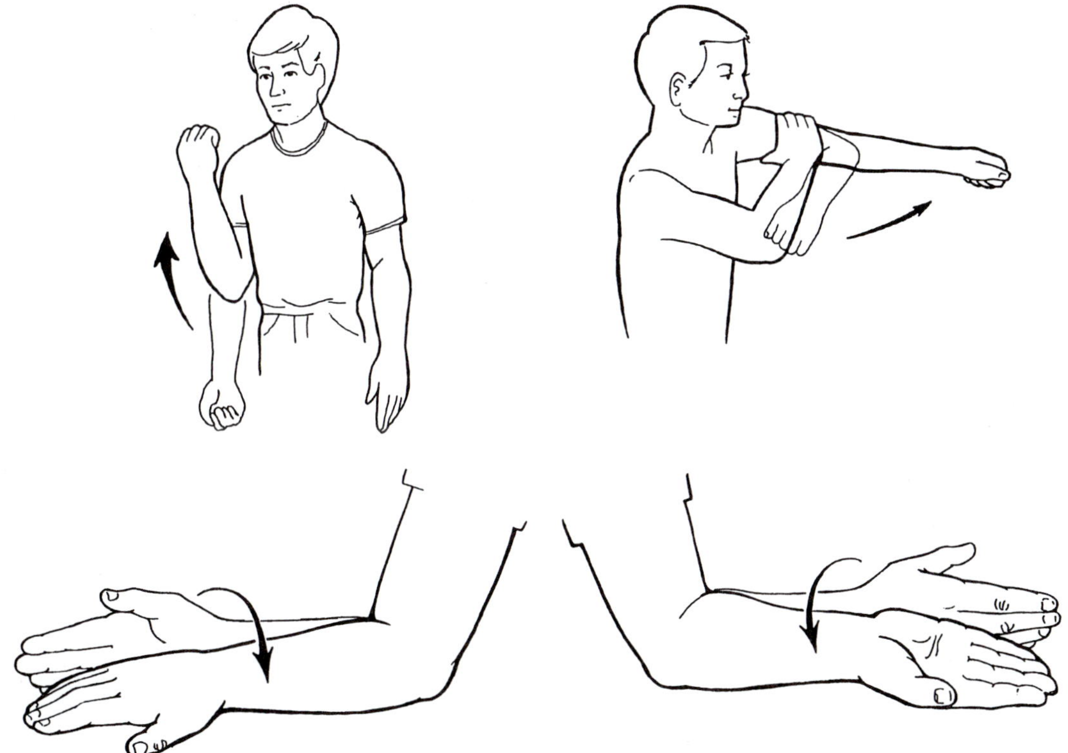

1. a. The ____________ muscle(s) cause(s) ____________ to occur in the ____________ plane about the ____________ axis.

   b. The ____________ muscle(s) cause(s) ____________ to occur in the ____________ plane about the ____________ axis.

2. a. The ____________ muscle(s) cause(s) ____________ to occur in the ____________ plane about the ____________ axis.

   b. The ____________ muscle(s) cause(s) ____________ to occur in the ____________ plane about the ____________ axis.

Worksheet

chapter 10

For in- or out-of-class assignments, or for testing, utilize this tear-out worksheet.

Worksheet 1

Using crayons or colored markers, draw and label on the worksheet the following muscles. Indicate the origin and insertion of each muscle with an "O" and an "I," respectively.

a. Flexor pollicis longus
b. Flexor carpi radialis
c. Flexor carpi ulnaris
d. Extensor digitorum
e. Extensor pollicis longus
f. Extensor carpi ulnaris
g. Extensor pollicis brevis
h. Palmaris longus
i. Extensor carpi radialis longus
j. Extensor carpi radialis brevis
k. Extensor digiti minimi
l. Extensor digitorum indicis
m. Flexor digitorum superficialis
n. Flexor digitorum profundus
o. Abductor pollicis longus

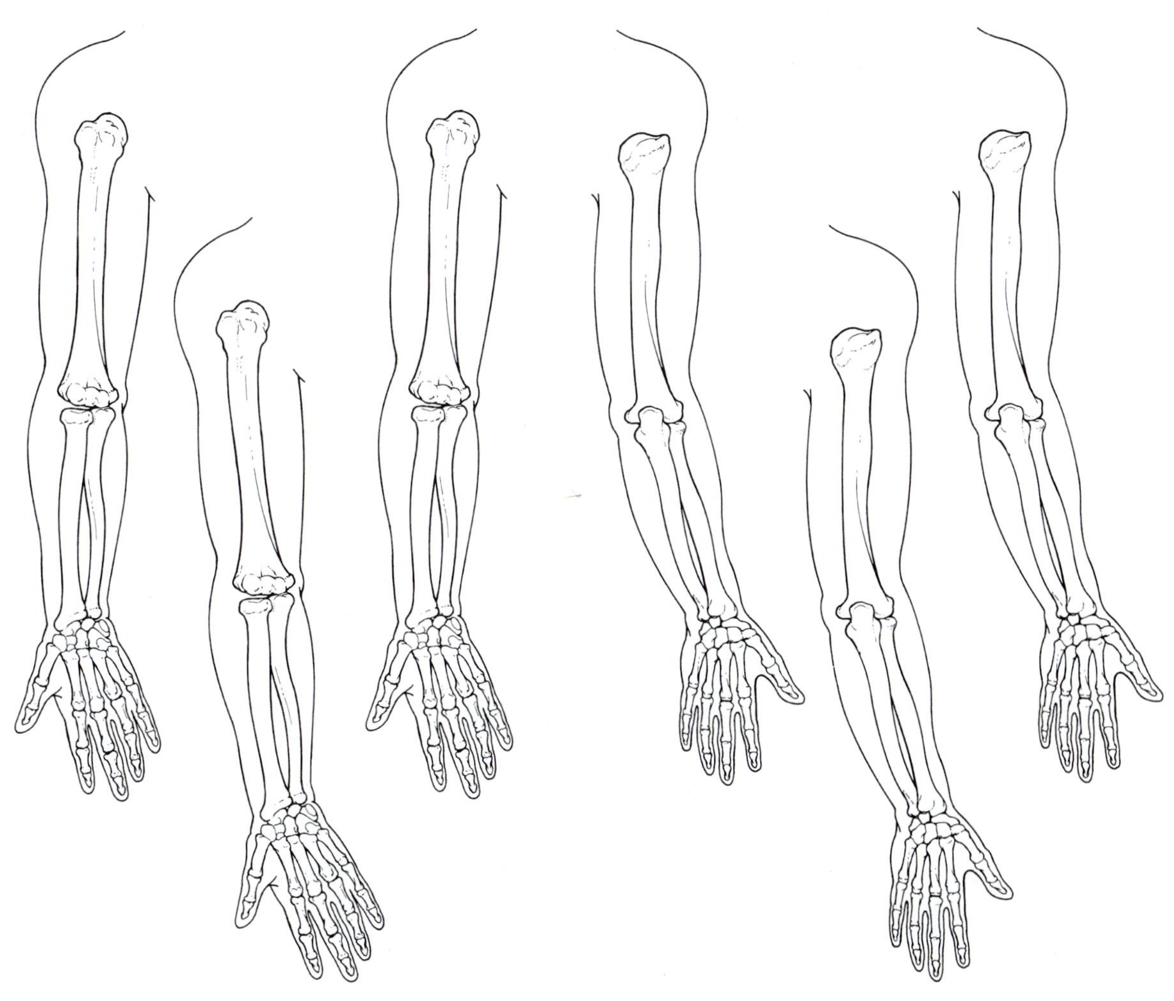

1. For each specific motion in the left column, provide the basic motion that it represents in the right column by using flexion, extension, abduction, adduction, or rotation (external or internal).

Specific Motion	Basic Motion
Eversion	**abduction**
Inversion	**adduction**
Dorsal flexion	**flexion**
Plantar flexion	**extension**
Pronation	**internal rotation**
Supination	**external rotation**
Lateral flexion	**abduction**
Radial flexion	**abduction**
Ulnar flexion	**adduction**

2. For each diarthrodial classification, give a joint example, the plane it moves in, and type of movement.

Classification	Joint	Plane Examples	Movements
Ginglymus	**Elbow, knee, ankle**	**Sagittal**	**Flexion, extension**
Trochoid	**Radioulnar atlantoaxial**	**Transverse**	**Rotation**
Condyloid	**2-5th metacarpophalangeal metarasophalangeal**	**Sagittal, frontal**	**Flexion, extension, abduction, adduction**
Arthrodial	**Transverse tarsal, C2 to S1**	**Variable, frontal, sagittal, transverse**	**Flexion, extension, adduction, abduction, rotation**
Enarthrodial	**Glenohumeral, acetabularfemoral**	**Sagittal, frontal, transverse**	**Flexion, extension, adduction, abduction, rotation**
Sellar	**1st carpometacarpal**	**Sagittal, frontal, transverse**	**Flexion, extension, adduction, abduction, rotation**

muscle name / action /

(1) The muscles that adduce the hip ae

(2) what muscles flex the hip / extend the hip

hamstrings quadriceps

(3)

Friction – Surface of two objects ~~...~~ rubbing against each other result in resistance

Running – Feet & ground have friction slippery surface will red. friction

Static friction – objects haven't began to move – resting friction

Kinetic friction – Objects that are moving – friction

Always more difficult to initiate dragging an object across a surface than continuing a motion

ance – Ability to control equilibrium (state of zero acceleration)

~~Nee~~ Static Equilibrium – Body at rest

Dynamic " = all forces in moving body are in balance

Stability resistance to a change in body's acceleration

Center of gravity – mass & wt. balanced.

R — Δ — F

F · R — Δ

R — F — Δ

Worksheet

chapter 10

For in- or out-of-class assignments, or for testing, utilize this tear-out worksheet.

Worksheet 2

Label and indicate with arrows the following movements of the wrist and hands. For each motion, list the agonist muscles, the plane in which the motion occurs, and its axis of rotation.

a. Flexion

b. Extension

c. Abduction (ulnar flexion)

d. Adduction (radial flexion)

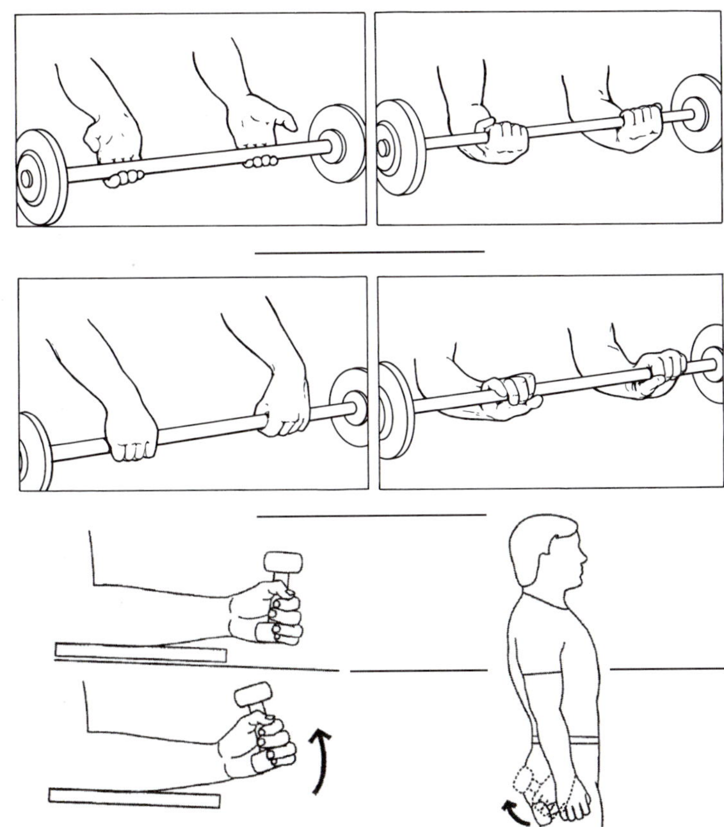

a. The ____________ muscle(s) cause(s) ____________ to occur in the ____________ plane about the ____________ axis.

b. The ____________ muscle(s) cause(s) ____________ to occur in the ____________ plane about the ____________ axis.

c. The ____________ muscle(s) cause(s) ____________ to occur in the ____________ plane about the ____________ axis.

d. The ____________ muscle(s) cause(s) ____________ to occur in the ____________ plane about the ____________ axis.

Worksheet

chapter 13

For in- or out-of-class assignments, or for testing, utilize this tear-out worksheet.

Worksheet 1

Using crayons or colored markers, draw and label on the worksheet the following muscles. Indicate the origin and insertion of each muscle with an "O" and an "I," respectively, and draw in the origin and insertion on the anterior view as applicable.

a. Rectus abdominis
b. External oblique abdominal
c. Internal oblique abdominal
d. Sternocleidomastoid

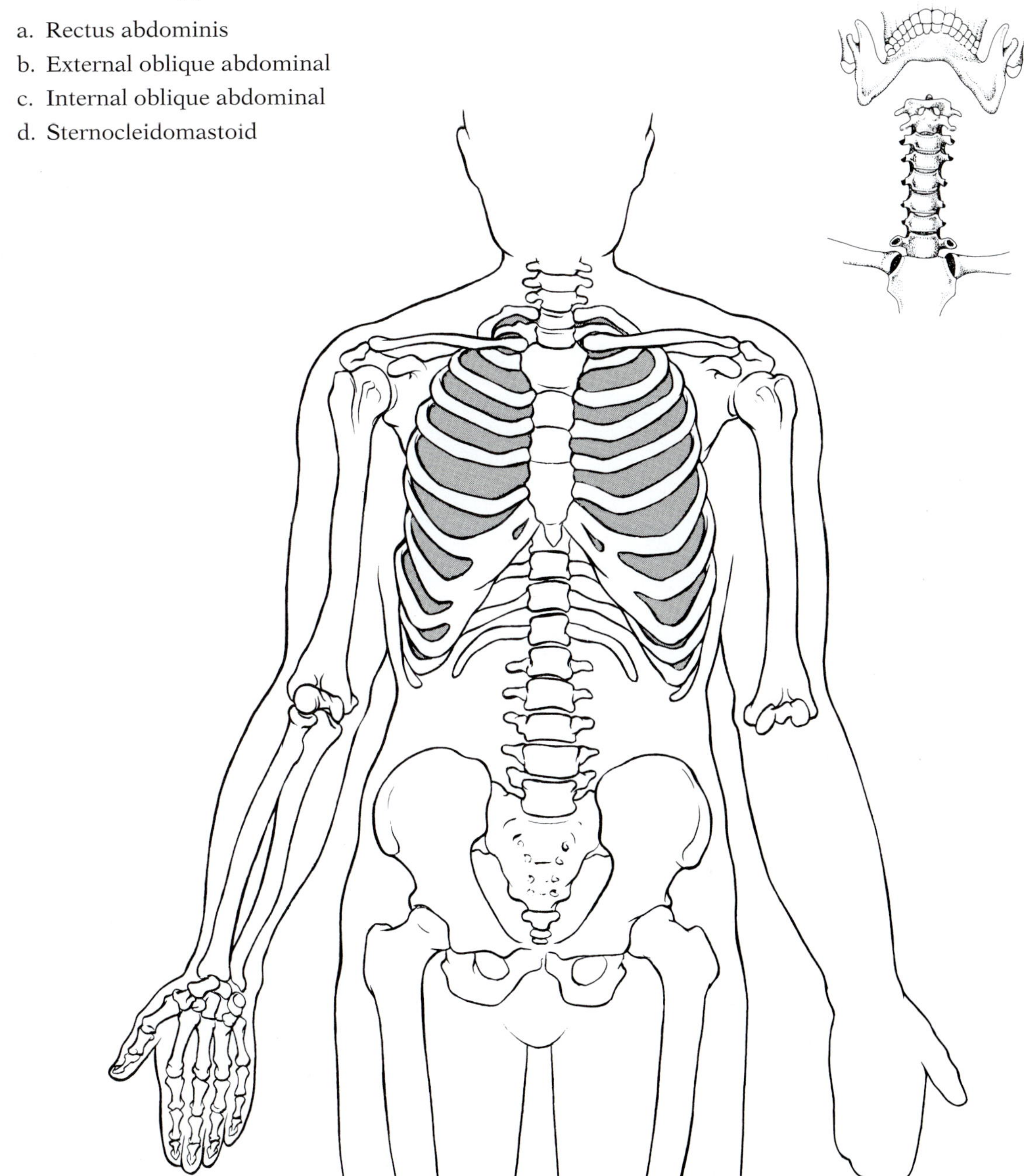

Worksheet

chapter 13

For in- or out-of-class assignments, or for testing, utilize this tear-out worksheet.

Worksheet 2

Using crayons or colored markers, draw and label on the worksheet the following muscles. Indicate the origin and insertion of each muscle with an "O" and an "I," respectively, and draw in the origin and insertion on the posterior view as applicable.

a. Erector spinae
b. Quadratus lumborum
c. Splenius—cervicis and capitis

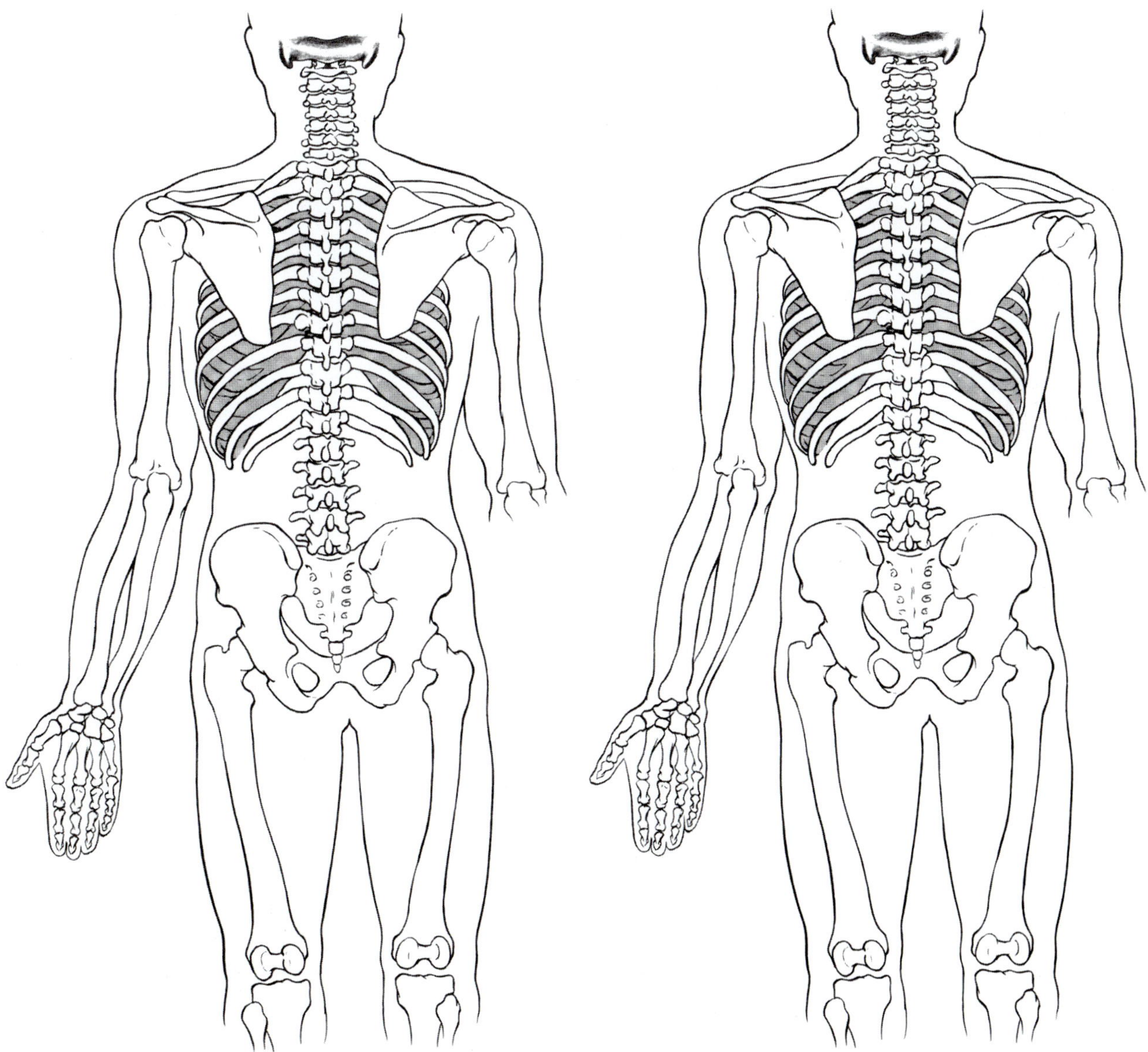

Worksheet

chapter 15

For in- or out-of-class assignments, or for testing, utilize this tear-out worksheet.

Worksheet 1

Using crayons or colored markers, draw and label on the worksheet the following muscles. Indicate the origin and insertion of each muscle with an "O" and an "I," respectively, and draw in the origin and insertion on the contralateral side of the skeleton.

a. Iliopsoas
b. Rectus femoris
c. Sartorius
d. Pectineus
e. Adductor brevis
f. Adductor longus
g. Adductor magnus
h. Gracilis

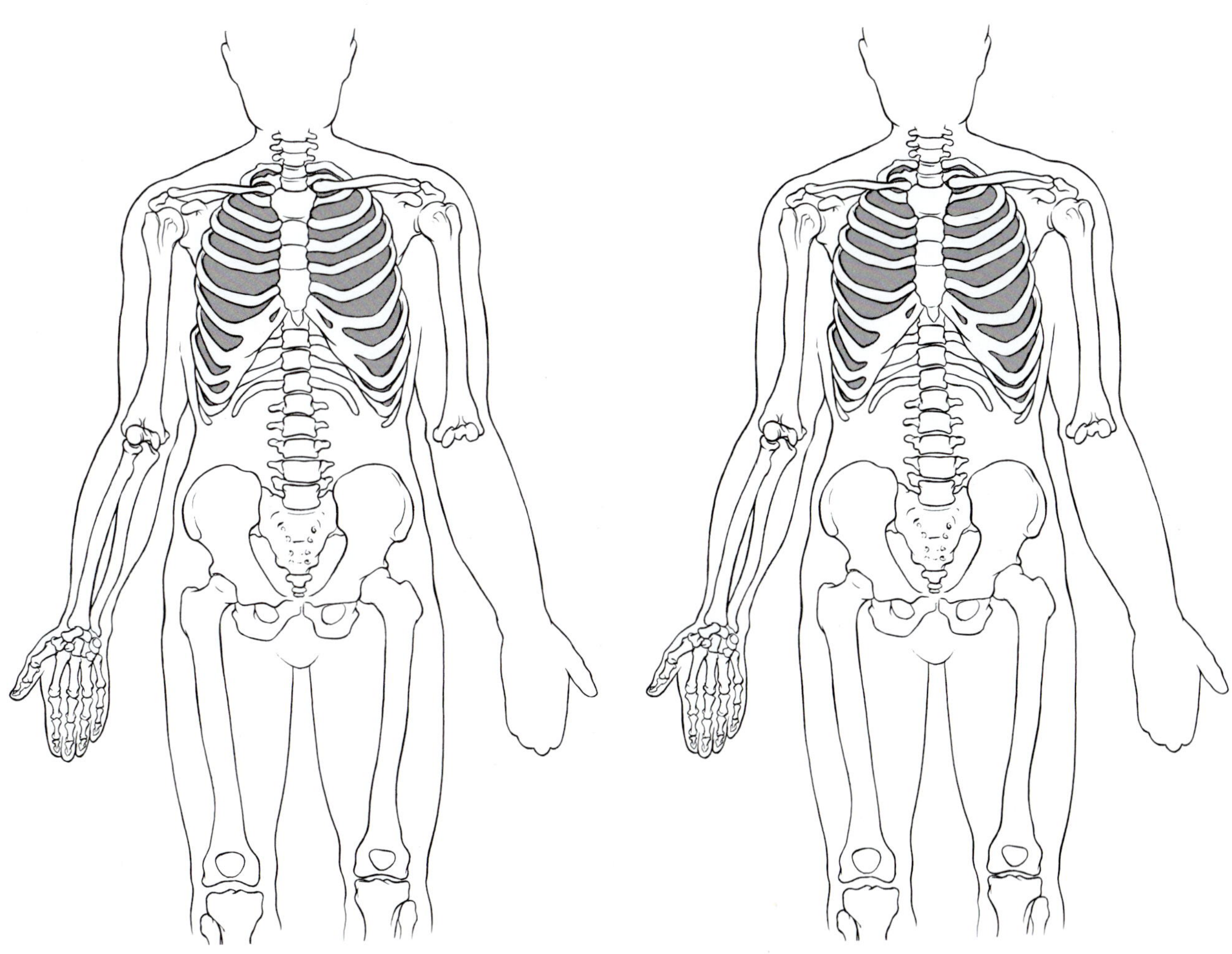

Worksheet

chapter 15

For in- or out-of-class assignments, or for testing, utilize this tear-out worksheet.

Worksheet 2

Using crayons or colored markers, draw and label on the worksheet the following muscles. Indicate the origin and insertion of each muscle with an "O" and an "I," respectively, and draw in the origin and insertion on the contralateral side of the skeleton.

a. Semitendinosus
b. Semimembranosus
c. Biceps femoris
d. Gluteus maximus
e. Gluteus medius
f. Gluteus minimus
g. Tensor fasciae latae

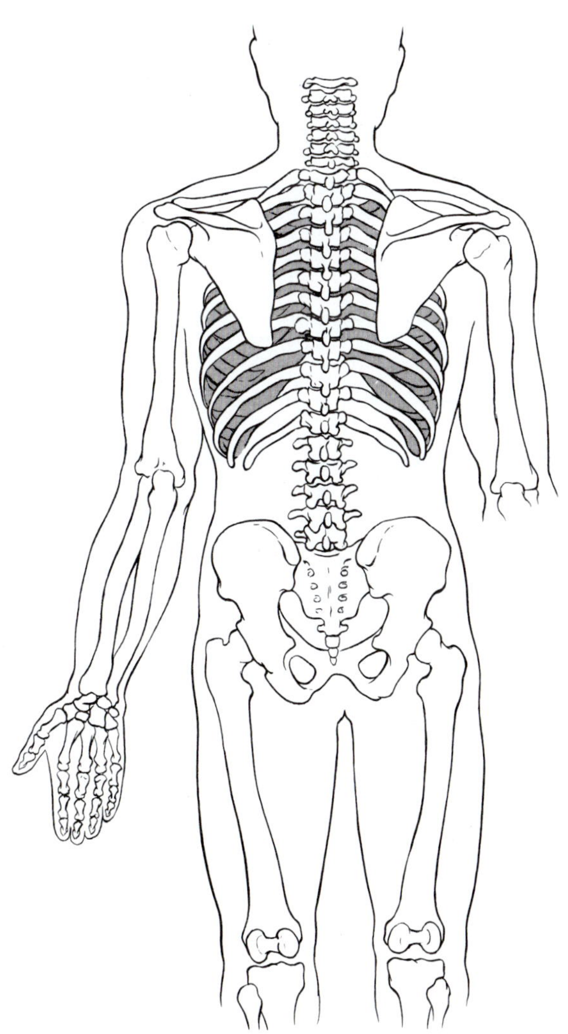

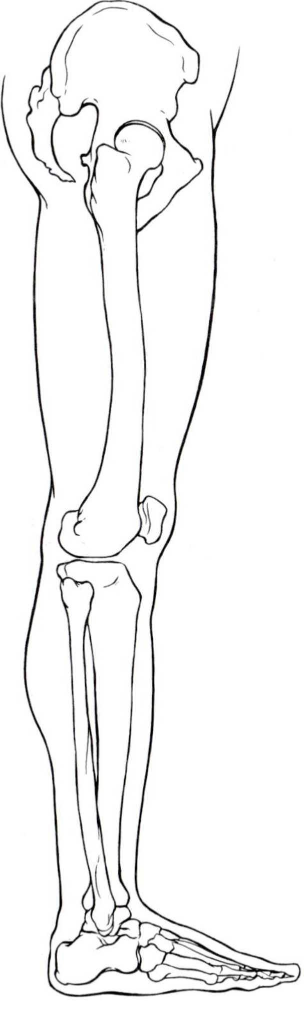

Worksheet

chapter 17

For in- or out-of-class assignments, or for testing, utilize this tear-out worksheet.

Worksheet 1

Using crayons or colored markers, draw and label on the worksheet the following muscles. Indicate the origin and insertion of each muscle with an "O" and an "I," respectively, and draw in the origin and insertion on the contralateral side of the skeleton.

a. Rectus femoris
b. Vastus lateralis
c. Vastus intermedius
d. Vastus medialis
e. Biceps femoris
f. Semitendinosus
g. Semimembranosus
h. Popliteus

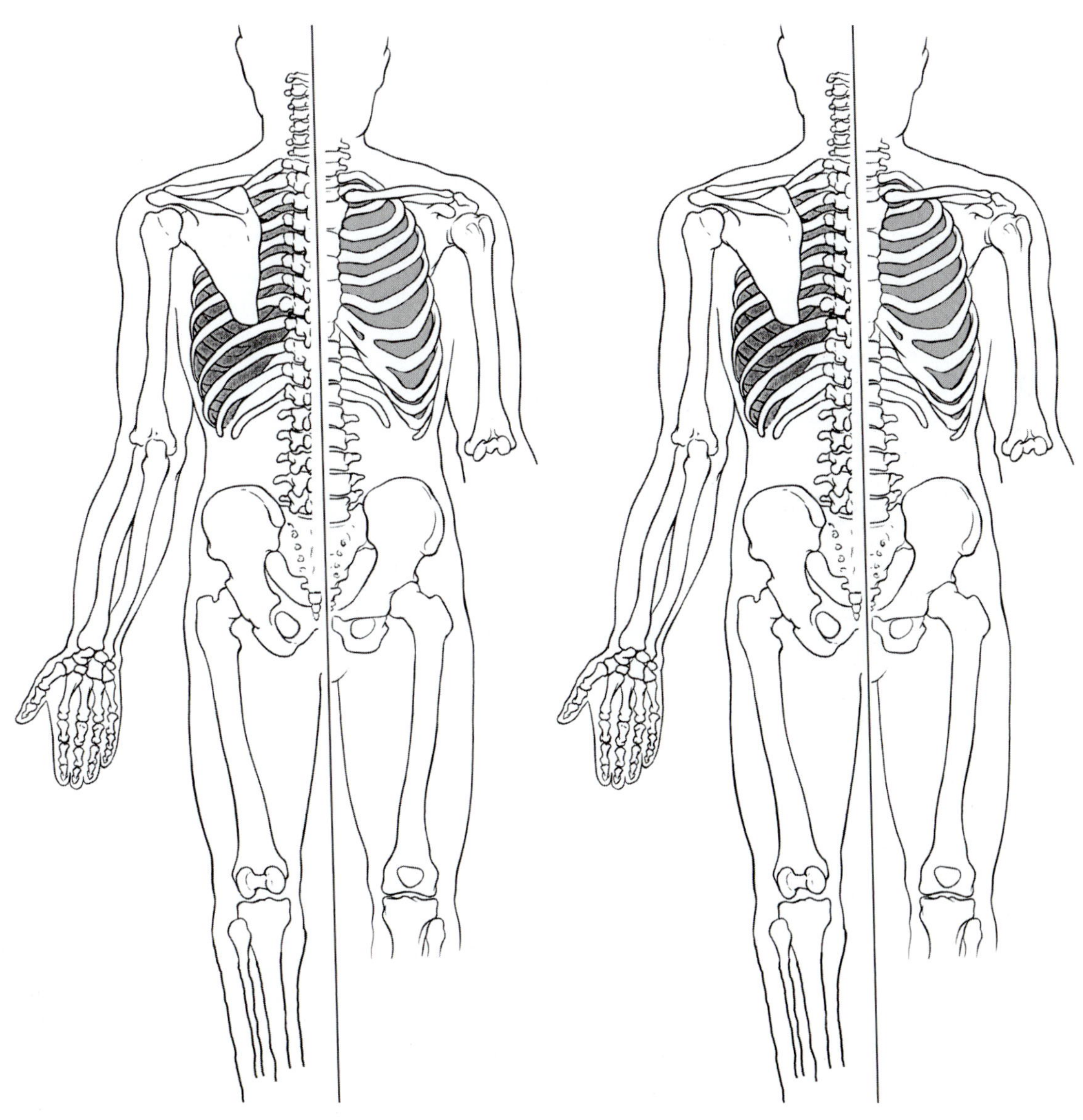

Worksheet

chapter 17

For in- or out-of-class assignments, or for testing, utilize this tear-out worksheet.

Worksheet 2

Label and indicate with arrows the following movements of the knee joint. For each motion, complete the sentence by supplying the plane in which it occurs and the axis of rotation as well as the muscles causing the motion.

a. Flexion occurs in the ______________ plane about the ______________ axis and is accomplished by concentric contractions of the ______________ ______________ muscles.

b. Extension occurs in the ______________ plane about the ______________ axis and is accomplished by concentric contractions of the ______________ ______________ muscles.

c. Internal rotation occurs in the ______________ plane about the ______________ axis and is accomplished by concentric contractions of the ______________ ______________ muscles.

d. External rotation occurs in the ______________ plane about the ______________ axis and is accomplished by concentric contractions of the ______________ ______________ muscles.

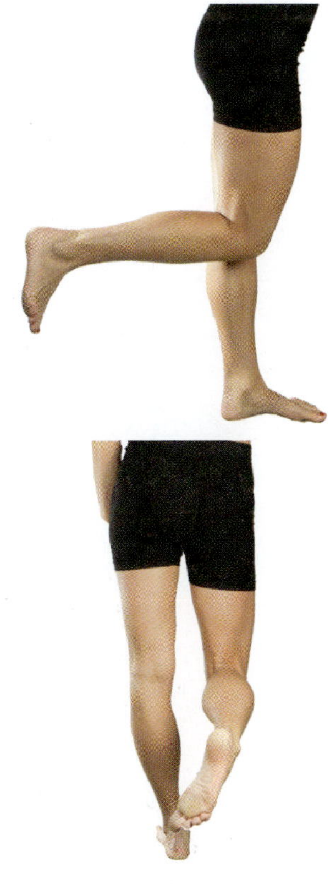

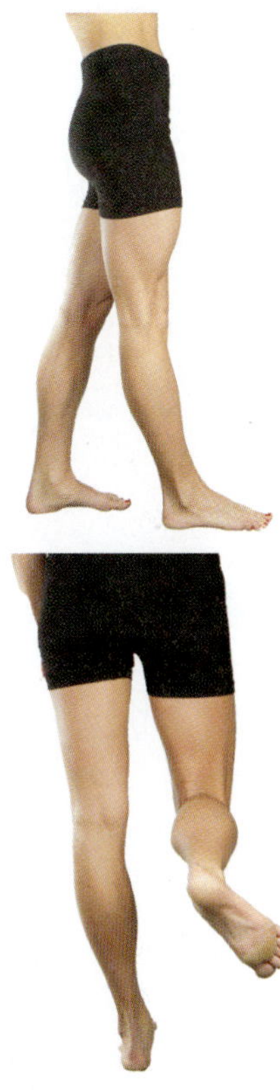

Worksheet

chapter 19

For in- or out-of-class assignments, or for testing, utilize this tear-out worksheet.

Worksheet 1

Using crayons or colored markers, draw and label on the worksheet the following muscles. Indicate the origin and insertion of each muscle with an "O" and an "I," respectively, and draw in the origin and insertion on the anterior or posterior view as applicable.

a. Tibialis anterior
b. Extensor digitorum longus
c. Peroneus longus
d. Peroneus brevis
e. Peroneus tertius
f. Soleus
g. Gastrocnemius
h. Extensor hallucis longus
i. Tibialis posterior
j. Flexor digitorum longus
k. Flexor hallucis longus

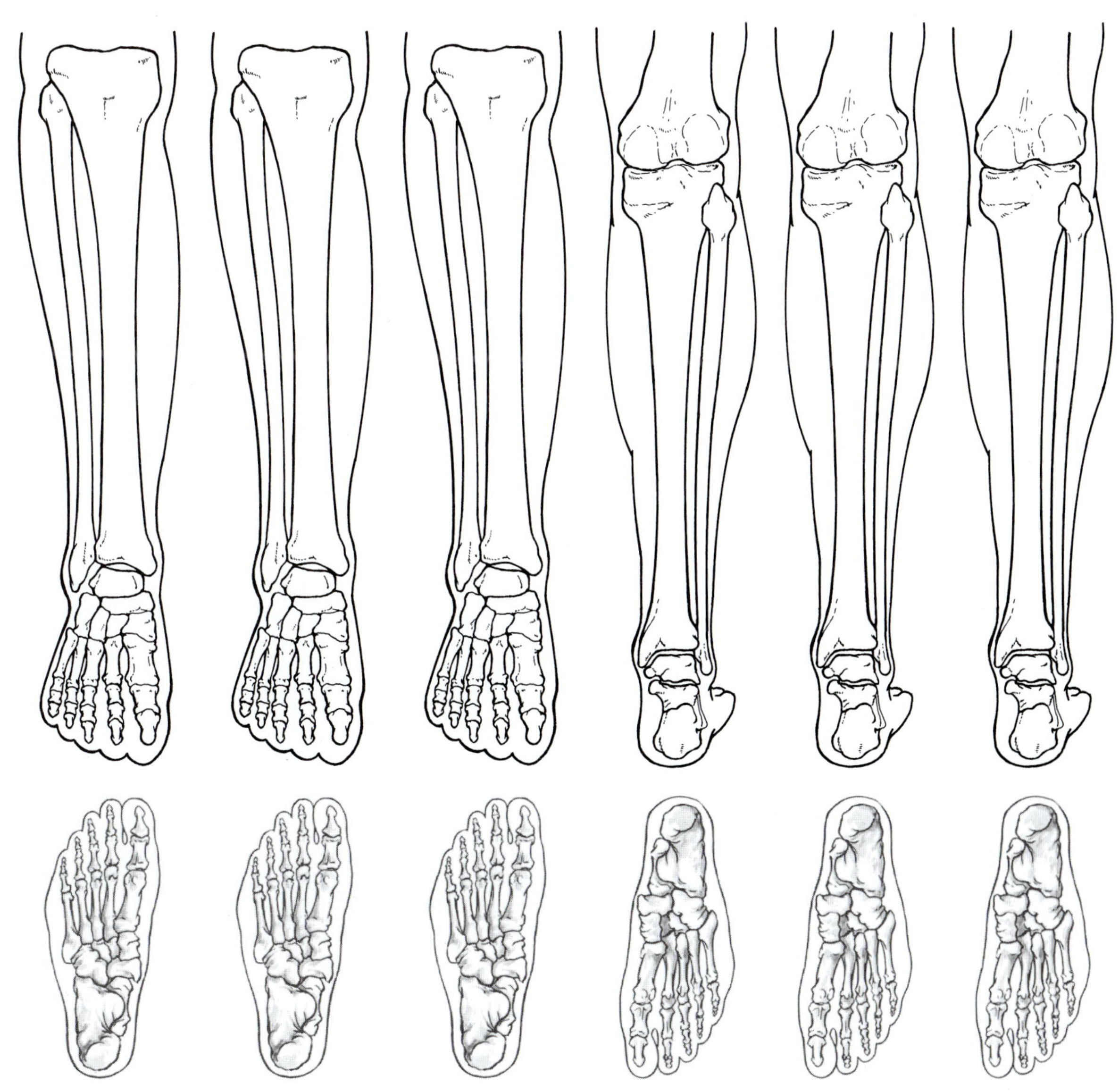

Worksheet

chapter 19

For in- or out-of-class assignments, or for testing, utilize this tear-out worksheet.

Worksheet 2

Label and indicate with arrows the following movements of the talocrural, transverse tarsal, and subtalar joints. For each motion, complete the sentence by supplying the plane in which it occurs and the axis of rotation as well as the muscles causing the motion.

a. Dorsiflexion occurs in the ________________ plane about the ________________ axis and is accomplished by concentric contractions of the ________________ ________________ muscles.

b. Plantar flexion occurs in the ________________ plane about the ________________ axis and is accomplished by concentric contractions of the ________________ ________________ muscles.

c. Eversion occurs in the ________________ plane about the ________________ axis and is accomplished by concentric contractions of the ________________ ________________ muscles.

d. Inversion occurs in the ________________ plane about the ________________ axis and is accomplished by concentric contractions of the ________________ ________________ muscles.

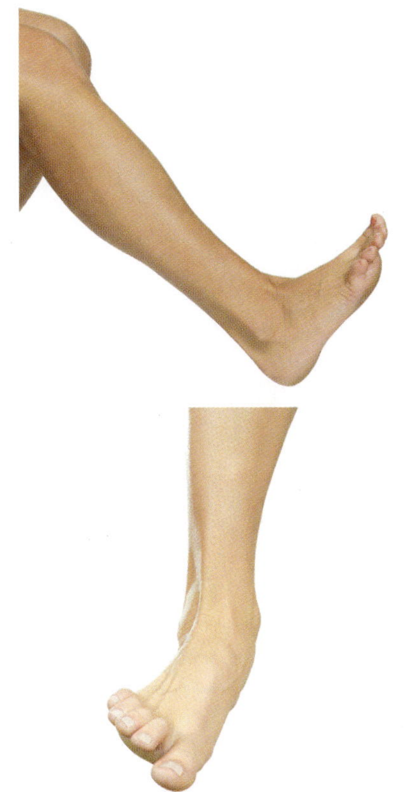

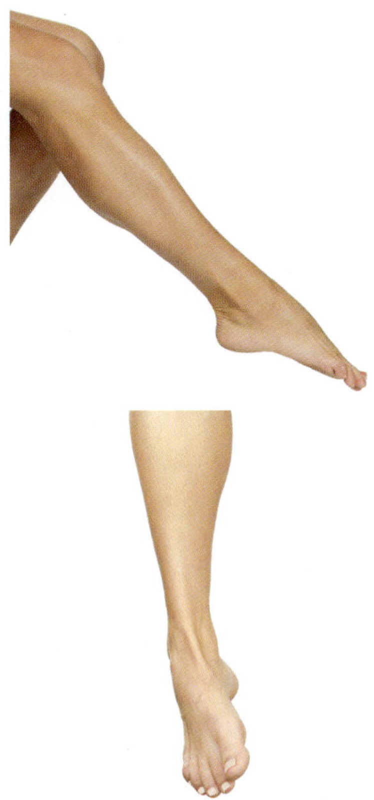